ESSENTIALS OF
Dental Assisting

SEVENTH EDITION

Debbie S. Robinson, CDA, MS

Retired/Dental Assisting
University of North Carolina
Chapel Hill, North Carolina

ELSEVIER

Elsevier
3251 Riverport Lanc
St. Louis, Missouri 63043

ESSENTIALS OF DENTAL ASSISTING, SEVENTH EDITION   ISBN: 978-0-323-764025

Previous editions copyrighted 2017, 2013, 2007, 2001, 1996, 1992.

Content Strategist: Joslyn Dumas/Kelly Skelton
Senior Content Development Manager: Luke Held
Senior Content Development Specialist: Maria Broeker
Publishing Services Manager: Deepthi Unni
Project Manager: Aparna Venkatachalam
Design Manager: Julia Dummit

Printed in India

Last digit is the print number: 9 8 7 6 5 4 3 2

About the Author

DEBBIE S. ROBINSON retired in 2020 from the University of North Carolina, where she was engaged in clinical research within the Department of Operative Dentistry and later in the Department of Nutrition at the Gilling's School of Global Public Health. Her educational background evolved from receiving an associate degree in Dental Assisting from Broward Community College to a bachelor's degree in Health Administration from Florida Atlantic University and then a master's degree in Dental Auxiliary Teachers Education from the University of North Carolina.

Her clinical experience consisted of being a clinical chairside assistant for 7 years in a pediatric/orthodontic dental practice in Florida, as well as working in the dental research center and the special patient care clinic at the University of North Carolina (UNC) School of Dentistry.

She taught dental assisting for more than 20 years within the community/technical/university settings in Florida and North Carolina. She also served as Clinical Assistant Professor and then Director of the Dental Assisting Program and Dental Assisting Specialty Program at UNC School of Dentistry. She has presented continuing education for practicing dental assistants at local, state, and international meetings. During her tenure, she served as a member of the Dental Assisting National Board (DANB) test construction committee and has authored and coauthored journal articles for *The Dental Assistant*. Additional endeavors include consulting with community colleges and proprietary schools on the development of new dental assisting programs across the country.

Preface

Welcome to the seventh edition of *Essentials of Dental Assisting*. Our goal for this edition was to design a textbook, along with ancillaries, to meet the needs of specific groups in the population of dental assisting (i.e., individuals who are gaining general background knowledge and skills, those who are in entry-level positions in a clinical setting, and those on-the-job–trained dental assistants who are preparing to take the Dental Assisting National Board certification examinations).

Many of the chapters in this edition have been revised and enhanced to include the most up-to-date knowledge and skills that are being taught in dentistry and practiced in clinical settings. The book is divided into 10 parts, beginning with historical information, legal and ethical issues, and scientific background, leading into preclinical and clinical areas, and finishing with preparation for employment and national board examinations. Each chapter provides specific objectives for the reader to achieve, terms for the reader to review to ensure comprehension of the content, specific figures and tables that are designed to assist the reader in grasping the material, and, finally, procedures that provide detail and exercises designed to test comprehension.

The role of the dental assistant in today's dental practice requires an individual who is well informed and skilled in everything from the very basic level of patient care to the performance of advanced intraoral procedures. To be an efficient and competent member of the dental team, the clinical assistant of today must have critical-thinking abilities when solving problems, as well as knowledge and understanding when making legal and ethical decisions.

A career as a dental assistant can be challenging and rewarding. Becoming a well-educated and clinically competent dental assistant will require dedication, determination, and desire. This may sound like quite the challenge, but you can do it!

The Learning Package

The seventh edition of *Essentials of Dental Assisting* is designed as a comprehensive learning package.

The student package includes:
- Textbook
- Evolve Resources
- Student Workbook (sold separately)

The faculty package includes all of the student resources plus:
- Test bank
- TEACH Instructor Resources

Textbook

Specific updated guidelines and recommendations are integrated into this edition, which provides:
- Comprehensive coverage that spans the clinical aspects of the dental assisting curriculum
- Current content in a comprehensible writing style
- Expert authorship
- Top-notch artwork
- Step-by-step procedures for basic and expanded functions
- The most recent Centers for Disease Control and Prevention (CDC) Guidelines for Infection Control in Dentistry to promote adherence to the most advanced infection control procedures for patients and dental professionals
- Intraoral, panoramic, and digital radiographic techniques used in dentistry today
- Standards that apply to performing cardiopulmonary resuscitation (CPR)
- Health Insurance Portability and Accountability Act (HIPAA) requirements that address patient confidentiality as ensured by the health care system
- Nutritional guidelines as determined by the Food and Nutrition Board of the National Academy of Sciences
- The anesthesia color-coding system designed by the American Dental Association Council on Scientific Affairs
- Excellent clinical photographs

The following tools guide the reader:
- **Key Terms** are introduced throughout the chapter. Each chapter features two different types of highlighted terms: terms that appear in bold and blue and terms that appear in bold and black. The terms appearing in blue are key terms and appear in the Key Terms list at the beginning of each chapter. The terms that appear in bold and black are important to the material being discussed in the chapter (and are therefore emphasized) but were first introduced in an earlier chapter. All terms are also included in a comprehensive Glossary at the back of the book, which provides chapter cross-references. The definitions reinforce these new terms.
- **Learning Objectives** are introduced at the beginning of each chapter so that readers will know what is expected of them at both the theoretical and performance levels.
- **Ethical Implications** help readers focus on ethical and legal behaviors that they must know to protect themselves, dental patients, and dental practices.

- **Multiple-Choice Questions** are found at the end of each chapter for readers to use to test their immediate knowledge. Answers are available to instructors in the *Instructor's Resource Manual* on the Evolve Web site.
- **Apply Your Knowledge** allows readers to analyze and initiate discussions in the classroom setting or with the dental team.
- **Procedures** are presented in a step-by-step sequence with illustrations, lists of equipment and supplies that the dental assistant will need, and the rationale behind each step. Procedural icons are included to remind the reader of the preparation and precautions that are needed. Examples of how the procedure might be entered in the patient's chart are provided at the end of many procedures.

It should be noted that there may be more than one way to perform a procedure correctly. Some dental assistants may perform a procedure one way, whereas others may choose to perform the same procedure using a slightly different technique. We have chosen to feature the methods used by most dental assisting programs.

Evolve Resources

Elsevier has created a Web site to support this learning package at http://evolve.elsevier.com/Robinson/essentials/. This Evolve site includes both student and instructor resources.

Student Resources

- Chapter quizzes in instant-feedback format
- A multiple-choice practice examination (250 questions)
- Interactive Dental Office
- Procedural videos (more information follows)

Videos

Visual presentation is vital to learning clinical skills. The student Evolve Resources provide 70 video clips of specific skills that the dental assistant may perform in the clinical setting; they are organized into the following categories:
- Oral Health and Prevention of Disease
- Infection Prevention in Dentistry
- Occupational Health and Safety
- Patient Information and Assessment
- Clinical Dentistry
- Dental Imaging
- Dental Materials
- Comprehensive Dental Care

Emphasis in these videos is placed on the expanded functions delegated to the credentialed dental assistant. Again, it should be noted that there may be more than one way to perform a technique correctly. We have chosen to feature the techniques used by most dental assisting programs.

The videos also feature:
- Interactive review questions
- Optional English and Spanish closed captioning
- Scripts in English and Spanish

Instructor Resources

- Access to all student resources
- Competency skill sheets for all procedures

- CODA Standards Mapping Guide
- Image collection
- Conversion guide
- A test bank with 1,250 questions and answers, rationales for all choices, page number references for remediation, cognitive level, Certified Dental Assistant (CDA) examination blueprint category, and chapter objectives to which the question maps, available in ExamView.
- TEACH Instructor Resources (more information follows)

TEACH Instructor Resources

TEACH for *Essentials of Dental Assisting* is an all-in-one resource designed to save educators time and take the guesswork out of classroom planning and preparation. TEACH includes detailed lesson plans that align with chapter objectives and identify national standards covered, student preparation for the lesson, learning activities and critical thinking questions, and simulations, all designed to fit inot 50-minute classroom increments to ease the work involved in classroom preparation. These lesson plans are centered on mapping textbook and ancillary content (by chapter heading) to specific chapter learning and performance outcomes. Answers to the chapter exercises and the student workbook questions and exercises are also available with TEACH. In addition, lecture outlines reference the detailed PowerPoint presentations with teaching notes or talking points as a ready-to-use classroom resource for educators.

Note: If you are unable to access TEACH on the Evolve Resources site, contact your Elsevier Education Solutions Consultant.

Student Workbook

The student workbook is a supplement to the learning process. The workbook includes review exercises for all chapters, competency skills sheets for all procedures in the textbook, and 42 flashcards as a bonus study aid.

Acknowledgments

Thank you to our publishing family at Elsevier: Joslyn Dumas and Kelly Skelton, Content Strategists; Maria Broeker, Senior Content Development Specialist; Deepthi Unni, Publishing Services Manager; Project Manager: Aparna Venkatachalam; Julia Dummitt, Design Direction; Donnalyn De Chavez, Marketing Manager. In addition, a huge thank you to the sales associates nationwide who really do the legwork to get "EDA" to instructors and programs. I truly appreciate everyone's support, advice, contributions, and collaboration in creating such a comprehensive learning package.

I sincerely appreciate and thank the reviewers who took the time to evaluate the work carefully and to provide constructive suggestions and recommendations.

Finally, a special thank you to my family, friends, and colleagues for their ongoing patience, adjustments to their schedules, and support that go hand in hand with working in the publishing world.

Debbie

How to use
Essentials of Dental Assisting

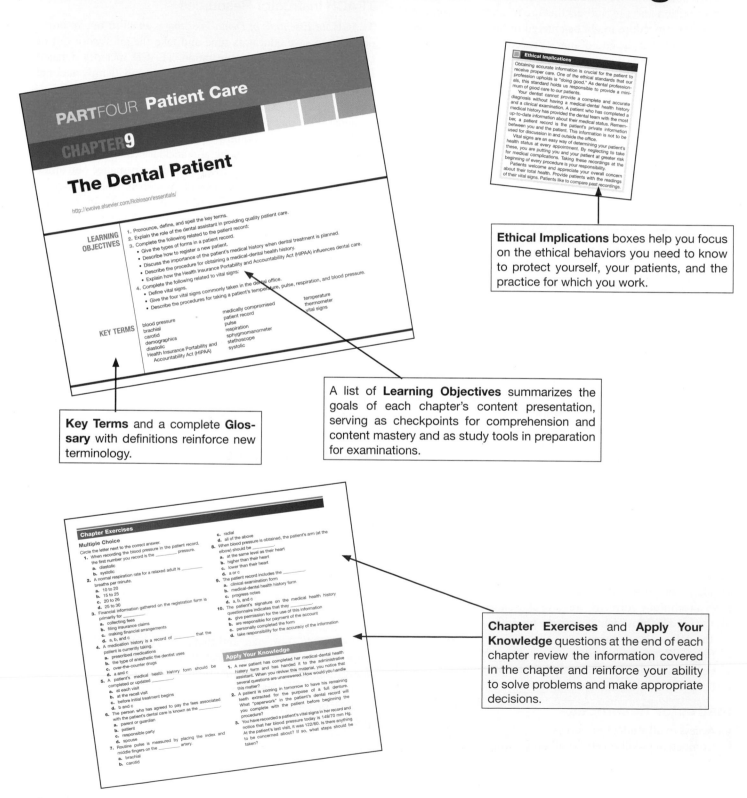

Ethical Implications boxes help you focus on the ethical behaviors you need to know to protect yourself, your patients, and the practice for which you work.

Key Terms and a complete **Glossary** with definitions reinforce new terminology.

A list of **Learning Objectives** summarizes the goals of each chapter's content presentation, serving as checkpoints for comprehension and content mastery and as study tools in preparation for examinations.

Chapter Exercises and **Apply Your Knowledge** questions at the end of each chapter review the information covered in the chapter and reinforce your ability to solve problems and make appropriate decisions.

Step-by-step procedures in the textbook include illustrations, the equipment and supplies you will need, icons, and the rationale behind certain steps. An example of how you might enter the procedure in the patient's chart is provided at the end of many procedures.

Procedural Icons are located with each procedure to remind you at a glance of those important precautions that are required during the performance of a procedure.

Expanded function procedures are identified with this icon and feature a different-colored background to differentiate them from more foundational procedures.

Icon Key

The procedure should be documented in the patient record.

In some states, the procedure is considered an expanded function if it is delegated to the dental assistant. Always review the regulations in the Dental Practice Act of your state.

The procedure involves contact with materials that are considered hazardous. Review the safety data sheet (SDS) on this procedure. Special handling, labeling, or disposal techniques may be required.

The student should be able to identify the instruments required for the stated procedure and to recognize their use.

The procedure is sensitive to moisture contamination. Special precautions, such as cotton roll placement, oral evacuation, and the use of a dental dam, must be applied to avoid moisture in the oral cavity.

The procedure involves exposure to potentially infectious materials and requires the use of appropriate personal protective equipment (PPE), such as protective clothing, mask, eyewear, and gloves.

The procedure is featured in a video on the Evolve Resources Web site.

Contents

Introduction to Dental Assisting

http://evolve.elsevier.com/Robinson/essentials/

LEARNING OBJECTIVES

1. Pronounce, define, and spell the key terms.
2. Describe the historical highlights in dentistry, including:
   - Describe the importance of Egypt, China, Mayans, Greeks, Romans, and Muslims in dentistry.
   - Name the individual considered to be the "father of dentistry."
   - Name the first dentist to employ a dental assistant.
   - Name the first dentist to use nitrous oxide for relief of dental pain.
   - Name the individual who was called the "Grand Old Man of Dentistry."
   - Name the individual who discovered x-rays.
3. Provide the members of the dental team:
   - Name each member of the dental team and describe the role of each.
   - Describe the various positions of the dental assistant.
   - List and describe the specialties of dentistry.
4. Identify and describe the areas of a dental office.

KEY TERMS

C. Edmund Kells
certified dental technician (CDT)
Commission on Dental
   Accreditation (CODA) of the
   American Dental Association
   (ADA)
dental anesthesiology
dental assistant
dental health care team
dental laboratory technician

dental public health
dental specialties
dentist
Doctor of Dental Surgery (DDS)
Doctor of Medical Dentistry
   (DMD)
endodontics
expanded-functions dental
   assistant (EFDA)
oral and maxillofacial radiology

oral and maxillofacial surgery
oral and maxillofacial pathology
oral medicine
orthodontics
pediatric dentistry
prosthodontics
radiographs
registered dental hygienist (RDH)
Wilhelm Conrad Roentgen

D ental assistants have been an instrumental member of the **dental health care team** for over a hundred years. A career in dental assisting is an exciting, challenging, and rewarding profession with many opportunities to choose from.

This chapter will guide you through the highlights of the history of dentistry, including how the **Lady in Attendance** evolved into the highly skilled dental health professional recognized today as the dental assistant. You will learn the roles and responsibilities of each member of the dental health care team, the dental specialties recognized, and an overview of the dental office.

History of Dentistry

Dentistry has a long and fascinating history. From the earliest times, humans have cleaned and cared for their teeth. They have also suffered from dental pain and have sought a variety of means to treat it. Early toothbrushes ranged from wooden sticks with frayed ends to ivory-handled brushes with animal-hair bristles for cleaning their teeth. Today, many people go to the dentist to improve the appearance of their teeth, but even back in the ninth century, skulls showed Mayans with numerous inlays of

TABLE 1.1

Highlights in the History of Dentistry

Date	Group/Individual	Event
3000–2151 BC	Egyptians	Hesi-Re is the earliest dentist known by name.
900–300 BC	Mayans	Teeth receive attention for religious reasons or self-adornment.
460–322 BC	Greeks	Hippocrates and Aristotle write about tooth decay.
166–201 AD	Romans	Decayed teeth are restored with gold crowns.
570–950	Muslims	Siwak (twigs) is used as a primitive toothbrush
1510–1590	Ambroise Paré	Writes extensively about dentistry, including extractions.
1678–1761	Pierre Fauchard	Becomes the "father of modern dentistry."
1760–1780	Isaac Greenwood	First American born dentist.
1844	Horace Wells	Uses nitrous oxide for the relief of dental pain.
1859		The American Dental Association is founded.
1885	C. Edmund Kells	Employs the first dental assistant.
1895	W.C. Roentgen	Discovers the x-ray beam.
1908	Frederick McKay	Discovers that fluoride is associated with the prevention of dental caries.
1908	G.V. Black	Becomes the "Grand Old Man of Dentistry" and perfects amalgam.
1913	Alfred C. Fones	Establishes the first dental hygiene school in Bridgeport, Connecticut.
1924		The American Dental Assistants Association is founded.
1947		The Dental Assisting National Board is founded.
1970	Congress	Creates the Occupational Safety and Health Administration (OSHA).
1978	*Journal of the American Dental Association*	Publishes a report on infection control for dental offices.
1982		The first hepatitis B vaccine becomes commercially available.
2000		*Oral Health in America: A Report of the Surgeon General* is released.
2003	Centers for Disease Control and Prevention	Releases *Guidelines for Infection Control in Dental Health-Care Settings—2003*.

decorative jade and turquoise on front teeth. Skulls of the Incas discovered in Ecuador had gold pounded into prepared holes in the teeth, which resemble modern gold inlay restorations from today. As B.W. Weinberger noted in *Dentistry: An Illustrated History,* a profession that is ignorant of its past experiences has lost an asset because "it has missed its best guide to the future." Besides the prominent individuals discussed, Table 1.1 lists major highlights in the history of dentistry.

Pierre Fauchard (1678–1761) was known as the "father of dentistry" and was a physician who developed dentistry as an independent profession. He was ahead of his time in understanding the importance of keeping teeth clean to prevent gum disease (Fig. 1.1).

Wilhelm Conrad Roentgen (rent-ken) (1845–1923) was a Bavarian physicist who discovered the x-ray beam in 1895 (Fig. 1.2). His discovery revolutionized diagnostic capabilities and forever changed the practice of medicine and dentistry. The images produced by x-ray beams on film are now referred to as **radiographs**.

C. Edmund Kells (1856–1928), a New Orleans dentist, is credited with employing the first dental assistant (Fig. 1.3). In 1885 the first "lady assistant" was actually a "lady in attendance" who made it respectable for an unaccompanied woman patient

FIGURE 1.1 Pierre Fauchard, the "father of modern dentistry." (From Fauchard P: *Le Chirurgien dentiste ou traité des dents,* Paris, 1746, Pierre-Jean Mariette.)

FIGURE 1.2 Wilhelm Conrad Roentgen discovered the early potential of the x-ray beam in 1895.

FIGURE 1.3 Dr. C. Edmund Kells and his "working unit."

to visit a dental office. By 1900, the assistant was working as a chairside dental assistant and secretarial assistant. Soon other dentists saw the value of dental assistants and began to train dental assistants in their own offices.

Today, the dental assistant is a key member of the dental health team, performing a wide variety of functions.

Members of the Dental Health Care Team

The members of the dental health care team strive to provide quality oral care for patients in a dental practice. Although each member of the dental team plays an important role, the most important person in the dental office is always the **patient.** The dental health care team consists of the following members:

1. Dentist (general dentist or specialist)
2. Dental assistant (clinical, expanded functions, business)
3. Dental hygienist
4. Dental laboratory technician

Dentist

The dentist is a licensed practitioner who is skilled in the prevention, diagnosis, and treatment of diseases and injuries and malformations of the teeth, jaws, and mouth. As a dentist, they are legally and ultimately responsible for the care of patients and for the supervision of all other members of the team. Within the United States, the dentist is a graduate from a dental school approved by the Commission on Dental Accreditation (CODA) of the American Dental Association (ADA). Dental education programs typically last 4 academic years after an undergraduate degree. When dentists graduate, they are awarded either the **Doctor of Dental Surgery (DDS)** or the **Doctor of Medical Dentistry (DMD),** depending on which dental school they attended. Before going into practice, all dentists must pass a written national board examination

and are then required to take a clinical board examination for licensure in the state in which they choose to practice. Dentists have a variety of practice options available to them. Some will choose to practice alone, some may choose to have a practice partner, and others may choose to join a large group practice. Other career options for dentists include the military, public health, community clinics, research, teaching, or returning to school for specialty training. Although a general dentist is trained and legally permitted to perform all dental functions, many dentists will refer more difficult cases to specialists who have advanced training in certain areas. Most dentists are members of their professional organization, the ADA.

Roles and Responsibilities of the Dentist

- Diagnosing diseases
- Promoting oral health and disease prevention
- Creating treatment plans to maintain or restore the oral health of their patients
- Interpreting x-rays and diagnostic tests
- Ensuring the safe administration of anesthetics
- Monitoring growth and development of the teeth and jaws
- Performing surgical procedures on teeth, bone, and soft tissues of the oral cavity

---

Dental Specialists

The licensed dentist receives an essential education from all areas of dentistry. Nevertheless, many choose to pursue advanced education and training in a specialty area. As of 2020, the ADA recognizes 11 dental specialties. Depending on the specialty, the time to complete advanced education can vary from 2 to 6 years. Most dentists who specialize will join the professional organization for their specialty, in addition to membership in the ADA.

Dental Specialties Recognized by the American Dental Association

- **Dental anesthesiology,** recognized in 2019, involves the art and science of managing the pain, anxiety, and overall health of a patient before, during, and after a procedure.
- **Dental public health** was first recognized as a dental specialty in 1950. This area is unique in that it involves developing policies at the county, state, and national levels for programs to control and prevent disease. Examples include dental public health professionals involved with fluoridation issues, community oral health education, and Head Start programs. Dental public health also includes dental screenings within a community to assess the needs of the community.
- **Endodontics** was recognized as a specialty by the American Dental Association (ADA) in 1964. This specialty involves the causes, diagnosis, prevention, and treatment of diseases and injuries of the pulp and associated structures. The common term for most of the treatment is *root canal therapy*. The specialist is referred to as an endodontist.
- **Oral and maxillofacial pathology** was first recognized as a specialty in 1946 and involves the nature, identification, and management of diseases affecting the oral cavity and adjacent structures. The specialist is an oral pathologist. One major function of an oral pathologist is to perform biopsies and work closely with oral surgeons to provide a diagnosis.
- **Oral and maxillofacial radiology** was granted recognition in 1999. The dental radiologist uses new and sophisticated imaging techniques to locate tumors and infectious diseases of the jaws, head, and neck and assists in the diagnosis of patients with trauma and temporomandibular disorders.
- **Oral and maxillofacial surgery,** recognized in 1918, involves the diagnosis and surgical treatment of diseases, injuries, and defects of the oral and maxillofacial regions. It involves both the functional and esthetic aspects of the hard and soft tissues of the mouth. The specialist is an oral and maxillofacial surgeon.
- **Oral medicine** is the newest recognized specialty in 2020. This specialty provides primary dental care to individuals with complex medical issues that require long-term management or modifications in the delivery of the care.
- **Orthodontics** became the first dental specialty in 1900. It includes the diagnosis, prevention, interception, and correction of malocclusion of the teeth and associated structures. The specialist is an orthodontist.
- **Pediatric dentistry,** recognized in 1947, provides both primary and comprehensive preventive and restorative health care for infants and children through adolescence, including those with special needs.
- **Periodontics,** recognized in 1947, involves the diagnosis and treatment of diseases of the oral tissues supporting and surrounding the teeth. The specialist is a periodontist.
- **Prosthodontics,** recognized in 1948, involves the diagnosis of missing or deficient teeth; treatment planning; rehabilitation through artificial constructs; and maintenance of the oral function, comfort, and appearance of artificial teeth.

Dental Assistant

The **dental assistant** is a valuable member of the dental team and one of the fastest growing occupations. Each dental practice will have a distinctive atmosphere but requires both interpersonal and technical skills from the practicing dental assistant and the dental team. Because of their education and training, a qualified dental assistant is quick to adapt to new situations as needs arise to take on various responsibilities throughout a dental practice to increase efficiency in the delivery of oral health.

CODA standards require a dental assisting program to be approximately 1 academic year in length and to be conducted at a post–high school educational institution. The curriculum must include didactic, laboratory, clinical, and business content. Dental assistants may also receive training at a vocational or proprietary program that is accredited through the state's board of dentistry.

Dental assistants may be members of their professional organization, the **American Dental Assistants Association (ADAA).** For additional information on dental assisting, visit the Web site at http://www.adaa.org.

The **chairside dental assistant** is directly involved in patient care and can be the most comprehensive and varied in the dental office (Fig. 1.4). Along with basic laboratory and clinical procedures, dental assistants can further their education and training to be legally certified or registered as an expanded function dental assistant (EFDA) to provide certain intraoral patient care procedures beyond the general duties traditionally performed by a dental assistant (Fig. 1.5).

Specific responsibilities assigned to the chairside dental assistant and credentialing are regulated by the Dental Practice Act of the state in which the assistant practices (see Chapter 2). Knowing which functions are legal in a state and performing only those functions are important for dental assistants.

The **circulating assistant** serves as an extra pair of hands when needed throughout the clinical areas of the practice and is referred to as **six-handed dentistry** (Fig. 1.6). In many practices, the circulating assistant is responsible for seating and dismissing patients and for preparing and caring for instruments and treatment rooms.

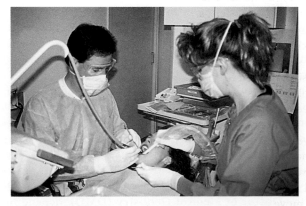

FIGURE 1.4 Dentist and chairside dental assistant working together.

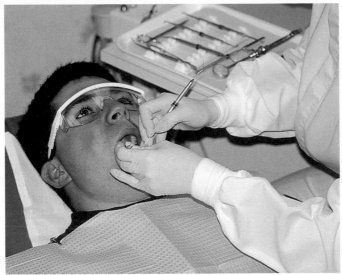

FIGURE 1.5 Expanded-functions dental assistant (EFDA).

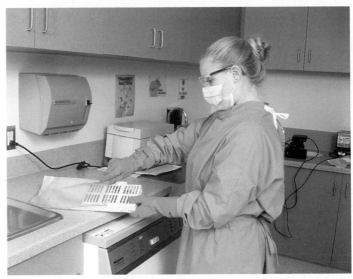

FIGURE 1.7 A sterilization assistant is an important member of the dental team

FIGURE 1.6 Chairside dental assistant is supported by a circulating assistant (six-handed dentistry).

FIGURE 1.8 The business assistant.

The **sterilization assistant** efficiently and safely processes all instruments and disinfection procedures and manages biohazardous waste. The responsibility for infection control procedures can be delegated to a specific individual or fall on all clinical staff to share this important responsibility. Other tasks include weekly monitoring of sterilizers and the maintaining of sterilization monitoring reports (Fig. 1.7). The sterilization assistant is often responsible for the selection of infection control products and for performing quality assurance procedures (see Chapters 7 and 8).

The **business assistant**, also referred to as the **administrative assistant** or **receptionist**, is primarily responsible for the smooth and efficient operation of the business office (Fig. 1.8). Two or more assistants may work in the business area of a dental office. It is not uncommon for a chairside dental assistant to move into a business office position. It is immensely helpful when the individual at the desk has an excellent understanding of how the clinical practice functions.

Roles and Responsibilities of the Dental Assistant (Chairside, Circulating, Infection Control, Business)

- Seating and preparing patients for clinical care
- Collecting and recording medical and dental history and patient vital signs
- Assisting the dentist in managing medical and dental emergencies
- Providing patient information on oral health care
- Assisting the dentist in a range of restorative and specialty procedures
- Preparing and delivering dental materials throughout a dental procedure
- Providing postoperative patient instructions
- Managing infection control throughout the office, such as by preparing and sterilizing instruments and equipment and developing an infection control protocol
- Performing radiographic procedures

- Performing basic laboratory procedures (e.g., pouring impressions to create diagnostic casts)
- Providing assurance and support for the patient, which includes patient instructions
- Performing expanded function procedures that are legal in the state in which they practice
- Recording a treatment in the patient's record
- Greeting patients and answering the telephone
- Making and confirming appointments.
- Managing patient records, payroll, insurance billing, and financial arrangements
- Ensuring that patient privacy measures are in place and followed
- Overseeing patient relations

Registered Dental Hygienist

A **registered dental hygienist (RDH)** is a licensed oral health professional whose attention is on preventing and treating oral diseases to protect the teeth and gums (Fig. 1.9). The functions delegated to the dental hygienist vary from state to state. A thorough understanding of the laws of the state in which they practice is important for dental hygienists. Employment opportunities for dental hygienists are available in private and specialty dental offices, health clinics, school systems, research facilities, public health departments, educational programs, and marketing and sales of dental products.

The minimal education required for a dental hygienist is 2 academic years of college study and an associate degree in an ADA-accredited dental hygiene program. Dental hygiene is also offered in bachelor's and master's degree programs. The RDH must pass both written national or regional board examinations and clinical state board examinations to be licensed by the state in which they plan to practice. In most states, the RDH is required to work under the supervision of a licensed dentist.

Dental hygienists may be members of their professional organization, the **American Dental Hygienists Association (ADHA)**. For additional information on dental hygiene, visit the Web site at http://www.adha.org.

Roles and Responsibility of the Dental Hygienist

- Performing an oral health care assessment that includes a review of the patient's health history, dental charting, oral cancer screening, and an evaluation of gum disease
- Educating patients on proper oral hygiene techniques to maintain healthy teeth and gums
- Performing dental prophylaxis (e.g., removing plaque from crowns and root surfaces)
- Removing plaque and calculus from above and below the gumline with the use of dental instruments
- Applying cavity-preventive agents, such as fluoride and sealants
- Exposing, processing, and interpreting dental radiographs
- Assessing the periodontal status of patients and measuring the depth of periodontal pockets and the condition of oral tissues
- Exposing, processing, and evaluating the quality of radiographs
- Performing additional procedures, such as administering local anesthetic and administering nitrous oxide if allowed by the state.

Dental Laboratory Technician

The dental laboratory technician uses both the science and art of dentistry to create tooth replacements that are both aesthetically pleasing and functional. Although some dental offices have "in-house" laboratories, the **dental laboratory technician** usually does not work in the dental office with the other team members. Many dental technicians choose to be employed in private laboratories, and others choose to own and operate their own laboratory (Fig. 1.10). In either case, the dental laboratory

FIGURE 1.9 Registered dental hygienist performing an oral prophylaxis. (From Darby M, Walsh M: *Dental hygiene: theory and practice,* ed 4, St. Louis, 2015, Elsevier.)

FIGURE 1.10 Dental lab technician.

technician works under the direction of a licensed dentist by following a detailed **written prescription** to create crowns, bridges, implants, and dentures from impressions taken by the dentist and sent to the dental laboratory. The dental assistant often communicates with the dental laboratory technician to discuss the length of time needed to return a case or to relay special instructions from the dentist about a case. Maintaining a good working relationship with the dental laboratory is important.

Dental laboratory technicians can receive their training through apprenticeship, commercial schools, or CODA-accredited programs. Many have received their training in CODA-accredited programs that are 2 years in length. Dental laboratory technicians have extensive knowledge of dental anatomy and materials and excellent manual dexterity.

To become a **certified dental technician (CDT)**, the dental laboratory technician must pass a written examination. Dental technicians may be members of their professional organization, the **National Association of Dental Laboratories.** For additional information on dental laboratories, visit the Web site at **http://www.nadl.org**.

FIGURE 1.11 Reception area of a dental office. (Courtesy Dr. Peter Pang, Sonoma, California.)

Roles and Responsibilities of the Dental Laboratory Technician

- Working with a variety of materials, such as waxes, plastics, alloys, stainless steel, porcelains, composites, and polymer glass
- Fabricating partial and full dentures
- Fabricating fixed bridges
- Fabricating veneers and crowns
- Fabricating orthodontic appliances

Overview of the Dental Office

The types and sizes of dental offices vary greatly, and the interior design and decor usually reflect the dentist's personal style. Nevertheless, certain areas are found in every dental office; these include the reception area, the business office, treatment rooms, nonclinical areas, an instrument-processing area, and the dental laboratory.

Reception Area

The reception area is where patients are received, pleasantly greeted, and made to feel welcome. The reception area should not be a "waiting room"; with proper scheduling, patients can be seen on time for their appointments.

Patients often judge the quality of their care by the appearance of the office. Therefore the reception area and all areas of the dental office must always be kept neat and clean (Fig. 1.11).

Business Office

The business office is the hub for the management of the business aspect of the dental practice (Fig. 1.12). It includes a **scheduling area,** where patients can make future appointments; an area where patients can make **financial arrangements;** and an area for **record storage**, where patient records can be safeguarded,

FIGURE 1.12 Business office.

and privacy can be maintained. It is not uncommon for a dental office to have two or more staff members working in this important area.

Treatment Rooms

Dental treatment rooms, also known as the **dental operatory**, are the heart of the clinical area of the dental practice. Patients receive treatment in the treatment rooms. Most practices have several treatment rooms (Fig. 1.13).

It is common to have at least one treatment room for the dental hygienist. In some practices, separate treatment rooms serve as an extra room for emergencies or short procedures, such as a postoperative checkup after surgery.

Nonclinical Areas

The dentist will usually have a **private office** for personal use. Other staff members should respect the privacy of this area.

The dentist discusses the proposed treatment plans with patients in the **consultation room.** When no consultation area is available, the dentist's private office is used for this purpose.

FIGURE 1.13 Dental treatment area. (Courtesy Patterson Dental, St Paul, Minnesota.)

FIGURE 1.14 Sterilization area. (Copyright luckyracoon/iStock.)

The **staff lounge** is an area where the staff may rest, eat, and hold meetings. Contaminated clothing or items must not be brought into this area. Staff members are responsible for keeping this area clean and neat at all times.

FIGURE 1.15 Private dental laboratory. (Courtesy Dental Masters Laboratory, Santa Rosa, California.)

Sterilization Area

The sterilization is also referred to as the instrument-processing area and is where contaminated instruments are cleaned, packaged, sterilized, and stored for reuse (Fig. 1.14). For more information, see Chapters 7 and 8.

Dental Laboratory

The dental laboratory in the dental office is used by the staff to pour impressions, prepare study models, and polish removable items, such as dentures or space maintainers (Fig. 1.15). The entire laboratory must always be kept clean and neat. Food or drink should never be present in the laboratory area because it is considered an area of potential contamination.

Ethical Implications

Dental assisting is a rewarding career. It offers you pride and professional opportunities. You may decide to pursue a career in general dentistry, specialty practices, public health clinics, or dental schools. Someday, you may even choose to become a dental assisting educator.

Always remember to maintain an attitude of professionalism and cooperative teamwork with other staff members, and never forget that the patient is the most important person in the office.

Multiple Choice

Circle the letter next to the correct answer.

1. The dental specialty in which the patient is the entire community is _____.
   a. periodontics
   b. orthodontics
   c. public health dentistry
   d. pediatric dentistry

2. A patient who needs a root canal treatment might be referred to a(n) _____.
   a. periodontist
   b. oral surgeon
   c. endodontist
   d. oral pathologist

3. The MOST important person in the dental practice is the _____.
   a. dentist
   b. dental hygienist
   c. dental assistant
   d. patient

4. Contaminated dental instruments should be returned to the _____.
   a. dental laboratory
   b. reception area
   c. sterilization center
   d. dental operatory

5. The newest dental specialty is _____.
   a. oral and maxillofacial surgery
   b. oral medicine
   c. dental public health
   d. endodontics

6. The member of the dental health team who is licensed to scale and polish teeth is the _____.
   a. dental hygienist
   b. dental assistant
   c. dental laboratory technician
   d. all of the above

7. Model trimmers and dental lathes are found in the _____.
   a. business office area
   b. staff lounge
   c. dental laboratory
   d. operatories

8. The dentist explains the treatment plan to the patient in the _____ of the practice.
   a. staff lounge
   b. business office
   c. consultation room
   d. dental laboratory

9. The head of the dental health care team is the _____.
   a. dentist
   b. dental hygienist
   c. dental assistant
   d. patient

10. The dentist recognized as having used the first dental assistant was _____.
    a. Dr. C. Edmund Kells
    b. Dr. Louis Pasteur
    c. Dr. W.C. Roentgen
    d. Dr. G.V. Black

Apply Your Knowledge

1. Visit the Web page of your state's Dental Board and search "dental assisting" to learn what functions a dental assistant in your state may legally perform. Are there any special credentialing or licensing requirements for dental assistants in your state?

2. Think about your own dental office where you receive care. Does your office resemble what was discussed in the chapter? If not, what are the differences that stand out in your mind. How many people make up the dental health care team, and what is their role?

CHAPTER 2

Professional and Legal Aspects of Dental Assisting

http://evolve.elsevier.com/Robinson/essentials/

LEARNING OBJECTIVES

1. Pronounce, define, and spell key terms.
2. Discuss the following topics related to the professional dental assistant:
   - The concept of professionalism
   - The characteristics of a professional dental assistant
   - The personal qualities of a professional dental assistant
3. Give the types of credentialing for the dental assistant.
4. Know the role of the regulatory and professional organizations:
   - Organizations for dentists, dental assistants, and dental hygienists
   - Government agencies
5. Explain the differences between ethics and law and discuss the five principles of ethics.
6. Discuss risk management, including the steps necessary to help avoid malpractice suits.
7. Discuss the guidelines and types of informed consent.
8. Discuss the purpose of a state's Dental Practice Act and the legal aspects of dentistry.
9. Describe the levels of dental supervision for the dental assistant.

KEY TERMS

act of commission
act of omission
breach of contract
certified dental assistant (CDA)
civil law
contract law
dental auxiliary
direct supervision

ethics
general supervision
HIPAA
implied consent
indirect supervision
informed consent
legal
licensure

patient of record
professionalism
reciprocity
registered dental assistant (RDA)
res gestae
risk management
tort law

You have chosen an exciting and challenging career as a professional dental assistant. A career in dental assisting offers diversity, job satisfaction, opportunity for service, and financial reward. Dental assisting is a career that requires dedication, personal responsibility, integrity, and a commitment to continuing education.

A highly skilled dental assistant is a vital member of the dental health care team. Reducing patient anxiety, making decisions, simplifying treatment procedures, and improving the quality of patient care are all part of a dental assistant's day.

Characteristics of a Professional Dental Assistant

Becoming a dental assistant involves more than acquiring the knowledge and skills necessary to perform a variety of responsibilities. Becoming a dental assistant is about becoming a **professional**.

Professionalism is an attitude that is apparent in everything you do and say, in and out of the dental office. Professionalism is what distinguishes people who "have a job" from those who "pursue a career." The public's expectations of health care workers are higher than the expectations of individuals in other occupations. The dental assistant must demonstrate patience and compassion when communicating with patients and other team members. When you demonstrate professionalism, you earn respect and acknowledgment from your colleagues and patients as a valued member of the dental health care team.

Professional Appearance

The professional appearance of a dental assistant should promote a confidence that represents the entire office. Essential aspects of a professional appearance include (1) good health, (2) good grooming, and (3) appropriate dress.

Good health requires getting an adequate amount of rest, eating well-balanced meals, and exercising enough to keep your mind and body fit. Dental assisting is a mentally and physically demanding profession.

For **good grooming**, your hair should be neat and away from your face. Your fingernails should be clean and not extend beyond your fingertips. Long nails and ornate jewelry can cause tears in your gloves. Also, avoid the use of artificial fingernails, which can harbor bacteria.

Personal cleanliness involves taking a daily bath or shower, using a deodorant, and practicing good oral hygiene. Perfume or cologne should not be used. You are working in close personal proximity to coworkers and patients who may be allergic to or irritated by some scents. Avoid the use of tobacco products because the odor lingers on your hair and clothing and is offensive, especially in a professional setting.

Appropriate dress involves wearing clothing appropriate for the type of position in which you are working. Regardless of the type of professional wear, it must be clean, wrinkle-free, and worn over appropriate undergarments (Fig. 2.1). Personal protective clothing is discussed in greater detail in Chapter 6. In any position in a dental office, excessive makeup and jewelry are not considered appropriate for a professional appearance. Infection control requirements must also be considered when clinical clothing and jewelry are selected.

FIGURE 2.1 The attire of a professional dental assistant may vary, depending on the duties performed. *Left,* Scrubs are acceptable at times. *Center,* Full personal protective wear is indicated for chairside procedures. *Right,* Surgical gowns may be indicated for surgery or hospital dentistry.

Teamwork

Teamwork is essential in a dental office. Think of the letters in the word **team,** "**T**ogether, **E**veryone **A**ccomplishes **M**ore." Dental assistants should step in to do the work of an absent colleague and be willing to help coworkers when other tasks are completed. When several assistants are in an office, each should be able and willing to substitute for the others in an emergency.

Attitude

Patients, employers, and coworkers appreciate the dental assistant who has a good attitude. Showing a willingness to get along by avoiding criticism of others, showing appreciation for what others have done, and being willing to pitch in and help are important attributes. The dental office can be a stressful place for patients and staff, so maintaining a positive attitude is important.

Dedication

Professional dental assistants are dedicated to their dental practice, their patients, and the profession of dental assisting. Dedication is possible only if the assistant genuinely cares for people, is empathetic to their needs, and maintains a positive attitude.

Remember. … Patients do not care how much you know until they know how much you care.

Responsibility and Initiative

The dental assistant can demonstrate work responsibility by (1) arriving on time, (2) staying for their full shift, (3) being a cooperative team member, and (4) not asking to leave early. Assistants should understand what is expected in their regular job and, if time permits, should be willing to help others who may be overworked.

You can show a willingness to learn additional skills through continuing education. Finding tasks to perform without being asked shows initiative. Calling the office when you are ill or unavoidably late shows responsibility. Personal problems should never be discussed in the dental office with your patients or with other staff members. Using your cell phone in a dental office for personal use sends a message to your patients and coworkers that you are more interested in your personal life than in your professional life.

Personal Qualities

A visit to the dentist can bring up feelings of anxiety, stress, and intimidation. The dental assistant should (1) demonstrate sensitivity to the patient's needs, (2) show empathy, (3) say "the right thing at the right time," and (4) be sincere.

Types of Personal Qualities

- Am I friendly? Do I have a pleasant attitude?
- Do I listen more than I speak?
- Am I courteous?
- Am I considerate, respectful, and kind?
- Do I control my temper?
- Do I try to see the other person's point of view?
- Am I dependable?
- Am I attentive to details?
- Am I calm in an emergency?
- Am I responsible for my own actions?
- Do I offer to help others without being asked?

By learning to be a good listener, you will develop sensitivity for the opinions and concerns of others. Building rapport (good relations) with the patients in your office is nearly impossible if they do not trust you. Nonverbal signals such as a reassuring smile or a pat on the arm can be very comforting to a nervous patient.

Credentialing of Dental Assistants

Credentialing is the process of obtaining, verifying, and evaluating the qualifications of a practitioner to provide care or services in a health care environment. The types of credentials that a dental assistant can obtain will vary based on their training, academic background, allowed functions, and the state in which they are practicing. The purpose of credentialing is to protect the public from unqualified or incompetent practitioners.

Upon completion of your training and education, you will prepare to sit for your national and/or state-recognized knowledge-based competence exam. After successfully completing the exam, you will receive a credential.

Certified Dental Assistants

A **certified dental assistant** (**CDA**) is an individual who has taken and passed a *national examination* administered by the Dental Assisting National Board (DANB). To remain currently certified, the CDA must complete a specified number of continuing education hours, take a review course of cardiopulmonary resuscitation (CPR), and pay a yearly renewal fee. Some states require a dental assistant to either be a CDA or have an additional credential to perform certain expanded functions. Additional information regarding certification can be obtained by visiting the DANB Website.

DANB offers five national certifications to meet the needs of essential knowledge and state-specific needs.

DANB National Certifications

- National Entry Level Dental Assistant (**NELDA**) – This exam has three components: Radiation Health and Safety (RHS); Infection Control (ICE); and Anatomy, Morphology, and Physiology (AMP).
- Certified Dental Assistant (**CDA**) – This exam contains three components: General Chairside (GC), Radiation Health and Safety (RHS), and Infection Control (ICE).
- Certified Orthodontic Assistant (**COA**) – This exam has two components: Orthodontic Assistant (OA) and Infection Control (ICE).
- Certified Preventive Functions Dental Assistant (**CPFDA**) – This exam has four components: Coronal Polish (CP), Sealants (SE), Topical Anesthetic (TA), and Topical Fluoride (TF).
- Certified Restorative Functions Dental Assistant (**CRFDA**) – This exam has six components: Anatomy, Morphology, and Physiology (AMP); Impressions (IM); Temporaries (TPM); Isolation (IS); Sealants (SE); and Restorative Functions (RF).

Registered Dental Assistant

A **registered dental assistant (RDA)** is an individual who has taken and passed an examination required by a specific state to perform functions allowed only in that state. States that require registration generally require periodic (annual or biannual) renewal, a specified number of hours of continuing education credits, CPR renewal, and a yearly fee. Registration of dental assistants is not practiced in all states.

Licensed Dental Assistant

The requirements for licensure vary from state to state for dentists and dental hygienists, and, in some states, registered dental assistants must be licensed by the state in which they practice. Licensure is one method of supervising individuals who practice in the state.

An increasing number of states are requiring either licensing or registration for dental assistants. Some states have assigned various titles to dental assistants that allow them to perform specific functions. Understanding the requirements for practice in a state is essential.

Regulatory and Professional Organizations

Recognizing and understanding the roles of the government agencies and professional organizations that have a direct influence on the practice of dentistry are important for the dental assistant (Table 2.1). As you begin your education, and as a practicing dental assistant, these agencies are excellent resources for information for you and are easily accessed online.

Ethics and Law

Throughout life, our values and morals may be modified because of increased knowledge, improved understanding, and life experiences. In addition to the law, each of us has our own personal values, morals, and standards of behavior. Ethics refers to what you *should* do, whereas the law deals with what you *must* do.

Understanding Ethics

Ethics is about moral conduct—right and wrong behavior, "good" and "evil." Ethics includes values, high standards of conduct, and personal obligations in our interactions with other professionals and patients. Ethical issues are subject to individual interpretation as to the right or wrong of a situation. A behavior can be unethical and still be legal, but it cannot be illegal and still be ethical.

Most professions will have a written code of ethics. The code of ethics states the ideal behavior, which is always higher than the minimum standard set forth by the law. Ethical behavior is important to dental health care professionals as they provide dental care and privacy to their patients.

Basic Principles of Ethics

The following five basic principles of ethics have been developed by the American Dental Association (ADA) for dentists and the profession to follow as a high ethical standard in providing care.

TABLE 2.1

Functions of Professional Organizations and Government Agencies in Dentistry

Professional Organization	Function
American Dental Association (**ADA**)	Professional organization for dentists to serve the public and profession of dentistry. The ADA does not regulate or mandate guidelines; it sets standards of practice for dentists. Dental schools, dental assisting, dental hygiene, and dental laboratory technology programs are accredited by the Commission on Dental Accreditation through the ADA. See www.ada.org
American Dental Assistants Association (**ADAA**)	Professional organization for dental assistants. It encourages education, registration, and certification for dental assisting professionals and provides a network of personal services for its members. ADAA membership gives the dental assistant a voice in national affairs. See www.adaausa.org
Dental Assisting National Board (**DANB**)	Nationally recognized certification board for dental assistants recognized by the ADA. Founded in 1948, DANB administers the Dental Assisting Board Examination and issues the credential of Certified Dental Assistant (CDA). See www.danb.org
Organization for Safety, Asepsis and Prevention (**OSAP**)	Dentistry's resource for infection control and safety information. OSAP is a nonprofit organization made up of all members of the dental health team, dental manufacturers, researchers, educators, and dental consultants. Its mission is to promote infection control and related health and safety policies and practices. See www.osap.org
Government Agencies	**Function**
Occupational Safety & Health Administration (**OSHA**)	Agency of the U.S. government under the Department of the U.S. Department of Labor. OSHA's mission is to ensure safety at work and a healthful work environment and to prevent work-related injuries, illnesses, and deaths. See www.osha.gov
Centers for Disease Control and Prevention (**CDC**)	The primary mission of the CDC is to track, investigate, and report the spread, virulence (strength), and incidence of specific diseases affecting the U.S. population. The CDC publishes treatment guidelines and provides information on disease prevention and education. See www.cdc.gov
U.S. Environmental Protection Agency (**EPA**)	The EPA is an agency of the U.S. federal government whose mission is to protect human and environmental health by having clean air, land, and water. The EPA is also responsible for reviewing chemicals used. See www.epa.gov
U.S. Food and Drug Administration (**FDA**)	The FDA is responsible for protecting public health by assuring human and veterinary drugs, vaccines, biologic products, and medical and dental devices are safe and effective. See www.fda.gov

Patient **autonomy** states that the professional has a duty to treat the patient according to the patient's desires, within the bounds of accepted treatment, and to protect the patient's confidentiality.

Everything that is said or completed in the dental office must remain confidential. The members of the dental team have access to a vast amount of personal and financial information about their patients. Such information must be held in strict confidence and not discussed with others. Breaches of confidentiality can result in a lawsuit against all parties involved.

HIPAA (the Health Insurance Portability and Accountability Act of 1996) is a set of federal privacy laws. These laws apply to all types of health care providers and are methods that must be used to ensure that patient privacy is protected when health information is shared between health care providers (Fig. 2.2).

The **patient record,** also referred to as the dental chart, is an important legal document that must be protected and handled with care. All examination records, diagnoses, radiographs, consent forms, updated medical histories, copies of medical and laboratory prescriptions, and correspondence to or about a patient are filed together in the patient's chart. Patient records

are acceptable in court and clearly show the dates and the details of services provided for each patient. Nothing should be left to memory. Incomplete or unclear records are damaging evidence in a malpractice case. Every entry in a chart should be made as if the chart will be seen in a court of law.

The dentist technically "owns" all patient records and radiographs. According to most state laws, however, the patient has the right to access (review) and retrieve (remove) their records and radiographs. In most situations, duplicate radiographs and a photocopy of the record will satisfy the patient's needs.

Nonmaleficence (which means "do no harm") is the most basic element in morality. It relates to all levels of interpersonal and professional behavior. It means that members of a dental team work to keep their knowledge and skills current but that they also know their limitations. This is especially vital when it comes to the use of auxiliary personnel. The dentist is accountable to protect the health of the patient by only delegating clinical functions to a qualified dental auxiliary (dental hygienist or dental assistant).

Beneficence (which means "do good") is based on the idea that actions are ethical if they benefit a person or a community.

HIPAA: Summary of the Health Insurance Portability and Accountability Act of 1996

The Health Insurance Portability and Accountability Act of 1996 (HIPAA) was signed into law by President Bill Clinton on August 21, 1996. Conclusive regulations were issued on August 17, 2000, to take effect by October 16, 2002. HIPAA requires that transactions of all patient healthcare information be formatted in a standardized electronic style. In addition to protecting the privacy and security of patient information, HIPAA includes legislation on the formation of medical savings accounts, the authorization of a fraud and abuse control program, the easy transport of health insurance coverage, and the simplification of administrative terms and conditions.

HIPAA encompasses privacy requirements that can be broken down into three types: privacy standards, patients' rights, and administrative requirements.

Privacy Standards

A central concern of HIPAA is the careful use and disclosure of protected health information (PHI), which generally is electronically controlled health information that is able to be distinguished individually. PHI also refers to verbal communication, although the HIPAA Privacy Rule is not intended to hinder necessary verbal communication. The U.S. Department of Health and Human Services (USDHHS) does not require restructuring, such as soundproofing, architectural changes, and so forth, but some caution is necessary when health information is exchanged through conversation.

An Acknowledgment of Receipt of Notice of Privacy Practices, which allows patient information to be used or divulged for treatment, payment, or healthcare operations (TPO), should be procured from each patient. A detailed and time-sensitive authorization can also be issued, which allows the dentist to release information in special circumstances other than TPO. A *written consent* is also an option. Dentists can disclose PHI *without* acknowledgment, consent, or authorization in very special situations, for example, perceived child abuse, public health supervision, fraud investigation, or law enforcement with valid permission (e.g., a warrant). When divulging PHI, a dentist must try to disclose only the *minimum necessary* information to help safeguard the patient's information as much as possible.

It is important that dental professionals adhere to HIPAA standards because healthcare providers (as well as healthcare clearinghouses and healthcare plans) who convey *electronically* formatted health information via an outside billing service or merchant are considered *covered entities*. Covered entities may be dealt serious civil and criminal penalties for violation of HIPAA legislation. Failure to comply with HIPAA privacy requirements may result in civil penalties of up to $100 per offense with an annual maximum of $25,000 for repeated failure to comply with the same requirement. Criminal penalties resulting from the illegal mishandling of private health information can range from $50,000 and/or 1 year in prison to $250,000 and/or 10 years in prison.

Patients' Rights

HIPAA allows patients, authorized representatives, and parents of minors, as well as minors, to become more aware of the health information privacy to which they are entitled. These rights include, but are not limited to, the right to view and copy their health information, the right to dispute alleged breaches of policies and regulations, and the right to request alternative forms of communicating with their dentist. If any health information is released for any reason other than TPO, the patient is entitled to an account of the transaction. Therefore it is important for dentists to keep accurate records of such information and to provide them when necessary.

The HIPAA Privacy Rule ensures that the parents of a minor have access to their child's health information. This privilege may be overruled, for example, in cases where child abuse is suspected, or the parent consents to a term of confidentiality between the dentist and the minor. Parents' rights to access their child's PHI also may be restricted in situations where a legal entity, such as a court, intervenes and the law does not require a parent's consent. For a full list of patients' rights provided by HIPAA, be sure to acquire a copy of the law and to read it well.

Administrative Requirements

Complying with HIPAA legislation may seem like a chore, but it does not need to be so. It is recommended that you become appropriately familiar with the law, organize the requirements into simpler tasks, begin compliance early, and document your progress in compliance. An important first step is to evaluate the information and practices currently in place in your office.

Dentists will need to write a *privacy policy* for their office, a document for their patients that details the office's practices concerning PHI. The *HIPAA Privacy Kit* of the American Dental Association (ADA) includes forms that you (the dentist) can use to customize your privacy policy. It is useful to try to understand the role of healthcare information for your patients and the ways in which they deal with this information while they are visiting your office. Train your staff; make sure they are familiar with the terms of HIPAA and your office's privacy policy and related forms. HIPAA requires that you designate a *privacy officer,* a person in your office who will be responsible for applying the new policies in your office, fielding complaints, and making choices involving the minimum necessary requirements. Another person in the role of *contact person* will process complaints.

A *Notice of Privacy Practices*—a document that details the patient's rights and the dental office's obligations concerning PHI—also must be drawn up. Further, any role of a third party with access to PHI must be clearly documented. This third party is known as a *business associate* (BA) and is defined as any entity who, on behalf of the dentist, takes part in any activity that involves exposure of PHI. The *HIPAA Privacy Kit* provides a copy of the USDHHS "Business Associate Contract Terms," which presents a concrete format for detailing BA interactions.

The original HIPAA privacy compliance date, including all staff training, was April 14, 2003, although many covered entities that submitted a request and a compliance plan by October 15, 2002, were granted 1-year extensions. Contact your local branch of the ADA for details. It is recommended that dentists prepare their offices ahead of time for all deadlines pertaining to preparation of privacy policies and forms and business associate contracts, as well as employee training sessions.

For a comprehensive discussion of all of these terms and requirements, a complete list of HIPAA policies and procedures, and a full collection of HIPAA privacy forms, contact the American Dental Association for a *HIPAA Privacy Kit.* The relevant ADA Web site is www.ada.org/goto/hipaa. Other Web sites that may provide useful information about HIPAA are the following:

- USDHHS Office of Civil Rights: www.hhs.gov/ocr/hipaa
- Work Group on Electronic Data Interchange: www.wedi.org/SNIP
- Phoenix Health: www.hipaadvisory.com
- USDHHS Office of the Assistant Secretary for Planning and Evaluation: http://aspe.os.dhhs.gov/admnsimp/

Data from HIPAA Privacy Kit and American Dental Association (www.ada.org).

FIGURE 2.2 HIPAA: Summary of the Health Insurance Portability and Accountability Act of 1996.

Specific areas of service include engaging in community service, becoming familiar with signs of abuse and neglect in patients, and reporting suspected cases of abuse or neglect to the proper authorities (consistent with state laws). See Chapter 27 for additional discussion regarding child abuse.

Justice (which also means "fairness") indicates that the dentist has a duty to treat people fairly and give people what they deserve and are entitled to receive. This concept is demonstrated in the philosophy that all patients should receive the same quality of dental care, regardless of their race, creed, color, gender, sexual orientation, gender identity, national origin, or disability.

Veracity is the principle involving "truthfulness." The professional has a duty to be honest and trustworthy in their relationship with patients. It is in the patient's best interest to know the truth about their care. For example, if a professional tells a child that a specific treatment will not hurt, when in fact it may, that professional is not adhering to the principle of veracity.

Types of Law

Today, we have laws that enforce certain standards of behavior. **Criminal law** seeks to punish the offender, and civil law seeks to compensate the victim. In criminal law, a governmental agency, such as law enforcement or the board of dentistry, begins the legal action. For example, a dental assistant who performs a procedure that is not legal for them to perform is in violation of criminal law. Insurance fraud is another example of a criminal offense that may be committed in a dental office. Civil law involves crimes against an individual with another individual initiating legal action (i.e., a lawsuit). For example, a patient sues a dentist because they are dissatisfied with the treatment or were injured during treatment. A civil action against a dentist may involve either contract law or tort law.

For a contract or agreement to be binding, it must be established between two competent people. This eliminates mentally incompetent persons, those under the influence of alcohol or drugs, and minors. A tort is a civil wrong that can bring harm to a person or damage to property. It can be either intentional or unintentional. For example, a breach of confidentiality is an intentional tort. In addition, a tort can be an act of omission, which is something that should have been done but was not, like not taking radiographs as part of the exam.

Requirements for Contract Law to Apply

- Consideration is when each party (dentist and patient) agrees to a fee for treatment.
- A contract needs to be valid, understandable, and specific, with acceptance from both parties.
- The contract must have a legal purpose that does not break any law.
- Both parties must enter the contract willingly and not be forced to do so.
- Both parties must have agreed on the terms and are bound by the contract.

Risk Management

Risk management refers to concepts and techniques that members of the dental team can use to help prevent malpractice lawsuits. The major areas of risk management (prevention of malpractice lawsuits) involve (1) maintaining accurate and complete records, (2) obtaining **informed consent**, and (3) doing everything possible to maintain the highest standards of clinical excellence. Most patients who take legal action are angry and believe they have been wronged. When patients become angry or frustrated and believe they are not being heard, they are more likely to file a lawsuit.

The primary factor in avoiding legal entanglements with patients is maintaining good rapport and open communication with all patients.

Avoiding Malpractice Lawsuits

Prevention and good communication with the patient are the best defenses against malpractice (Fig. 2.3). Patients are less likely to initiate a lawsuit when they have a clear understanding of the following:

- Planned treatment
- Reasonable treatment results
- Potential treatment complications
- Financial obligations

The dental assistant plays an important role in the prevention of malpractice litigation by being aware of the signs of patient dissatisfaction and alerting the dentist.

"Silence Is Golden"

The dental assistant must never make critical remarks about dental treatment rendered by an employer or another dentist. The dental assistant should never discuss other patients and should avoid discussing the dentist's professional liability insurance.

Under the concept of **res gestae** ("part of the action"), statements spontaneously made by anyone (including the dental assistant) at the time of an alleged negligent act are admissible

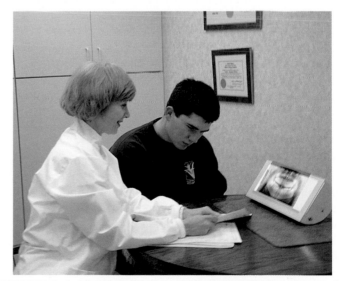

FIGURE 2.3 An important role of the dental assistant is to help maintain good communication with the patient.

as evidence and may be damaging to the dentist and the dental assistant in a court of law. Comments such as "whoops" or "uh-oh" may unnecessarily frighten the patient and should be avoided.

Guidelines for Informed Consent

Informed consent is permission that has been granted by the patient after having received full knowledge of the possible risks and benefits from the dentist. The patient has the right to know all of the important facts about the proposed treatment.

Informed Patient Consent

Two things must occur for the patient to give informed consent: (1) **being informed** and (2) **giving consent**. This means that the dentist must provide the patient with enough information about their condition and explain all available treatment options. The patient and the dentist must first discuss these options, and then the patient can choose the most suitable treatment option.

When a patient has traveled to a dental practice and entered a dentist's office, it is reasonable to assume that the patient has given implied consent to proceed with a dental examination or any additional procedure. Provided the patient is capable, implied consent is given when the patient agrees to treatment or at least does not object to treatment. In a court of law, implied consent is a less reliable form of consent in a malpractice suit. **Written consent** is the preferred means of obtaining and documenting the patient's consent and understanding of the procedure.

Informed Refusal

If a patient refuses the proposed treatment, then the dentist must inform the patient about the likely consequences and must obtain the patient's informed refusal.

Nevertheless, obtaining the patient's informed refusal does not release the dentist from the responsibility of providing the standard of care. A patient may not consent to substandard care, and the dentist may not legally or ethically agree to provide such care. For example, if a patient refuses radiographs, then the dentist may refer the patient to another provider because the dentist believes radiographs are a necessary standard of care. Another dentist, however, may be willing to treat the patient without radiographic images and may request that the patient sign a written and dated informed refusal for radiographs. This statement is then filed with the patient's record.

Informed Consent for Minors

The parent, custodial parent, or legal guardian must give consent for treating minor children. When parents live separately, the child's personal information form should indicate which parent is the custodial parent. When separated parents share custody, the child's record should contain letters from each parent providing consent and authorization to treat. Asking in advance for a parent's or a custodial parent's *blanket* consent for emergency treatment avoids confusion and delays should the child require emergency care when a parent or guardian is not present.

Documenting Informed Consent

Most states do not require a specific means for documenting discussions on informed consent. At minimum, the patient's record should indicate that the patient received information about the risks, benefits, and alternatives and consented to or refused the proposed treatment.

When dental treatment becomes extensive, invasive, or risky, a written informed consent document is recommended. The patient, the dentist, and a witness should sign the written consent form. The patient should receive a copy of the form, and the original should be kept with the patient's chart.

Legal Regulations in Dentistry

Each state has a right to regulate the practice of dentistry within that state. To protect the public from incompetent dental health care providers, each state has established a **Dental Practice Act.** The Dental Practice Act specifies the legal requirements for the practice of dentistry within each state. It may be a single law or a compilation of laws that regulate the practice of dentistry. The Dental Practice Act also defines the responsibilities of the dental hygienist and dental assistant and what is legal for them to perform in that state. Each state's Dental Practice Act is now accessible on the Internet. You can learn about your state's Dental Practice Act online by going to their website.

State Board of Dentistry

A state board of dentistry is responsible for enforcing a state's Dental Practice Act within their state. The members of the state board of dentistry are appointed by the governor of the state. In addition to licensed dentists, some state boards have members that are dental assistants, dental hygienists, and public members. The state board of dentistry has the authority to not only issue licenses but also revoke, suspend, or deny renewal of a license. Most states will take action if the licensed person has a felony conviction or a misdemeanor involving drug addiction, moral corruptness, incompetence, or mental or physical disability that may cause harm to patients.

Some states have a reciprocity agreement with another state. Reciprocity is an agreement between two or more states that allows a dentist or a dental hygienist who is licensed in one state to receive, usually without further examination, a license to practice in any of the other states in the reciprocity agreement. Reciprocity agreements are usually made between states with adjoining borders and similar testing requirements. States without reciprocity agreements require dentists and dental hygienists licensed in another state to take their state board examination.

Expanded Functions and Levels of Supervision

Expanded functions are specific intraoral tasks delegated to qualified dental auxiliaries. When these functions are included in a Dental Practice Act, the dentist may delegate them to the dental assistants that have met the additional education, certification, or registration qualifications needed to perform these functions. Regulations regarding dental assistants vary greatly from state to state. It is important to have a clear understanding of the law in your state as it relates to dental assisting and the practice of dentistry. You must always practice within the laws of your state.

In states that allow the dentist to delegate intraoral functions to a dental auxiliary (dental assistant or dental hygienist), the rules in the state's Dental Practice Act are usually specific regarding the types of auxiliary supervision that the dentist must provide. The following terms are often used in Dental Practice Acts:

Direct supervision means that the dentist has delegated a specific procedure to be performed for a patient of record by a legally qualified dental auxiliary, who meets the requirements of the state board of dentistry. The dentist must examine the patient before delegating the procedure and again when the procedure is complete. *The dentist must be physically present in the office at the time the procedure is performed.*

General supervision (indirect supervision) generally means that the dentist has authorized and delegated specific procedures that may be performed by a legally qualified dental auxiliary for a patient of record. Exposing a radiograph or recementing a temporary crown that has become dislodged are examples of functions that are often delegated under general supervision.

Illegal Practice of Delegated Functions

Performing procedures that are not legal is the same as practicing dentistry without a license and is a **criminal act**. Ignorance of the Dental Practice Act is no excuse for illegally practicing dentistry. *If the dentist asks you to perform an expanded function that is not legal in your state and you choose to do so, then you are committing a criminal act.*

Ethical Implications

Having a clear understanding of the Dental Practice Act in your state, especially as it relates to the duties assigned to the dental assistant, is especially important. If you move to another state, be certain to check with the state board of dentistry regarding the laws of that state before you begin to practice there. Remember that your personal and professional ethics are the basis of your dental assisting career.

Multiple Choice

Circle the letter next to the correct answer.

1. The aspect of dentistry that deals with codes of behavior, values, and morals is _____.
   a. ethics
   b. legal

2. A violation of licensing regulations or an inappropriate use of drugs would be regulated under _____.
   a. civil law
   b. criminal law
   c. tort law
   d. contract law

3. The agency in each state that is responsible for regulating the practice of dentistry is the _____.
   a. American Dental Association
   b. state dental association
   c. state board of dentistry
   d. none of the above

4. Reciprocity occurs when _____.
   a. the fees are the same in two dental offices
   b. one state recognizes the dental license of an individual from another state
   c. a dental assistant practices dentistry without a license
   d. all patients are treated equally

5. The type of supervision that requires the dentist to be in the office while the dental auxiliary performs certain functions is _____.
   a. direct supervision
   b. general supervision

6. The credential of a certified dental assistant (CDA) is awarded by the _____.
   a. American Dental Assistants Association
   b. Dental Assisting National Board
   c. state board of dentistry
   d. American Dental Association

7. The methods of preventing lawsuits in a dental office are called _____.
   a. tort law
   b. risk management
   c. liability prevention
   d. risk assessment

8. Another term for malpractice is _____.
   a. professional negligence
   b. risk management
   c. liability
   d. none of the above

9. When a dentist fails to recognize a dental disease and the patient's condition worsens, this scenario is known as _____.
   a. an act of commission
   b. reciprocity
   c. an act of omission
   d. risk management

10. When a patient is given specific information about a dental procedure and any possible risks involved and then signs a form that states that they understand the risks and agree to the dental procedure about to be performed, this process is called _____.
    a. implied consent
    b. informed consent
    c. general consent

Apply Your Knowledge

1. You are a new dental assisting graduate beginning your first job in a beautiful new office with an excellent salary and great benefits. Dr. Morris is impressed with your clinical skills and is anxious to have you be a part of the team. On a busy morning, Dr. Morris asks you to take on a specific procedure that is not a legal function for dental assistants in your state. What should you do? You do not want to lose this job.

2. Mrs. Weirs has called your office and has asked you to send her records to another dentist because she is unhappy with the treatment she received in your office. When you check her clinical record, you notice that the last entry is not as complete as it should be. You remember that appointment very well, however, and could "adjust" the record to make the entry more complete. Should you send the patient's chart to another dentist and how should you update the patient's chart to be more complete?

3. Your patient is a 78-year-old gentleman who does not speak English very well. The dentist is explaining the reasons he should have a crown on one of his molars. He seems to understand because he is smiling and nodding his head. Is this informed consent? Why or why not? What would you do?

CHAPTER 3

Anatomy and Physiology

http://evolve.elsevier.com/Robinson/essentials/

LEARNING OBJECTIVES

1. Pronounce, define, and spell the key terms.
2. Name and describe the terms used to designate directions, planes, and sections of the body.
3. List and describe the organizational levels of the human body.
4. Name each body system and identify its major function.
5. Discuss the structures of the head and neck and explain why a dental assistant should be familiar with these structures.
6. Identify the major muscles of mastication and facial expression and state the function of each.
7. Name and locate the landmarks of the face and oral cavity.

KEY TERMS

ala of the nose	innervation	philtrum
alveolar socket	lateral	physiology
anatomy	lingual	posterior
angle of the mandible	mandibular	proximal
anterior	masticatory mucosa	sagittal plane
anterior naris	maxillary	septum
attached gingivae	medial	superior
buccal	mental protuberance	tissues
canthus	midsagittal plane	tragus
cells	mucogingival junction	transverse plane
distal	mucous membrane	trigeminal nerve
frontal plane	nasion	zygomatic arch
glabella	organs	
inferior	palate	

The human body is an incredible living creation. It has 11 body systems that function together more smoothly than the world's greatest computers. Having entered a health care field, the study of **anatomy** (study of the structure of the human body) and **physiology** (study of how the human body functions) is important for so many reasons when providing health and dental care to your patients. The following chapter will help you gain knowledge about how the various aspects of the human body work together so that you can communicate effectively as a dental health care professional.

Anatomic Directions and Planes

To be able to identify the locations of the organs that contribute to vital functions, you need some points of reference for description.

Directions in the Body

In the study of anatomy, the human body is described as if it were dissected. Terms used to describe directions in relation to the whole body are easier to understand if you think of them as pairs of opposite directions, such as up and down, left and right, or front and back (Table 3.1).

TABLE 3.1
Directional Terms for the Body

Term	Definition	Example
Superior	Above another part or closer to head	Nose is superior to mouth.
Inferior	Below another part or closer to feet	Heart is inferior to neck.
Proximal	Closer to a point of attachment or closer to the trunk of the body	Elbow is proximal to wrist.
Distal	Farther from a point of attachment or farther from the trunk of the body	Fingers are distal to wrist.
Lateral	The side or away from the midline	Ears are lateral to eyes.
Medial	Toward or nearer the midline	Nose is medial to ears.
Dorsal	On the back	Spine is on the dorsal side of the body.
Ventral	On the front	Face is on the ventral side of the body.
Anterior	Toward the front	Heart is anterior to spine.
Posterior	Toward the back	Ear is posterior to nose.

FIGURE 3.1 Body in anatomic position. (From Patton K: *Structure and function of the body*, ed 16, St Louis, 2020, Elsevier.)

Planes and Sections of the Body

Imaginary planes are used to help visualize the spatial relationships of internal body parts. These planes are used to describe the location of an organ or a problem (Fig. 3.1).

1. The **sagittal plane** is any vertical plane parallel to the midline dividing the body into right and left portions. If the plane divides the body into two equal parts, then it is called the **midsagittal plane**.

2. The **transverse plane**, also known as the horizontal plane, is positioned to divide the body into **superior** (top) and **inferior** (bottom) portions. This type of view is also referred to as a cross section.

3. The **frontal plane**, also known as the coronal plane, divides the body into **anterior** (front) and **posterior** (back) sections and is perpendicular to both the sagittal plane and the transverse plane.

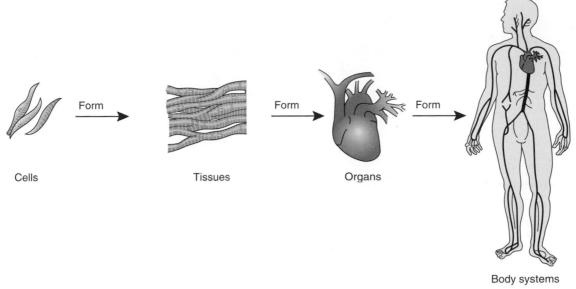

FIGURE 3.2 Organizational levels of the body.

Cells

Tissues

Organs

Body systems

Structural Units of the Body

The human body has four organizational levels or units. From the simplest to the most complex, they include cells, tissues, organs, and **body systems** (Fig. 3.2).

Cells

Cells are the smallest units in the human body. The structure of a cell is based on the function of that cell. Cells have a specific make-up that include the nucleus, which is the control center of the cell; cytoplasm, which is a gel-like fluid making up the major portion of the cell; and the cell membrane, which is the form of the cell or its physical/chemical property.

Tissues

Four primary types of tissues are found in the human body: **epithelial, connective, muscle,** and **nervous.** Like cells, each type of tissue is designed to perform a specific function.

> **Tissue Types and Functions**
> * Epithelial tissue forms the covering of all body surfaces and lines body cavities and hollow organs. It includes the skin, intestines, lungs, tubes of the reproductive system, and the lining of the oral cavity.
> * Connective tissue binds structures together. It forms the framework and support for organs and the entire body, stores fat, transports substances, and helps repair tissue damage. It includes fat, tendons and ligaments, cartilage, blood, and bone.
> * Muscle tissue produces the movement of body parts. It includes body movements, the pumping action of the heart, food movement through the digestive process, and urine movement through the bladder.
> * Nervous tissue is found in the brain, spinal cord, and nerves. It coordinates and controls many body activities, stimulates muscle contraction, creates awareness of the environment, and plays a major role in emotions, memory, and reasoning.

Organs

Organs work together as a team to keep each body system functioning. Organs are formed when several types of tissues group together to perform a single function. For example, the stomach is an organ that contains four tissue types (nerve, connective, muscle, and epithelial) and performs the digestive functions of the body.

Body Systems

Body systems are made up of organs. Occasionally, the same organ belongs to more than one system. For example, ovaries and testes clearly belong to the reproductive system, but because one of their functions is to produce hormones, they are also part of the endocrine system. Body systems do not function independently. For example, when you exercise hard, your muscular system needs extra oxygen. Your respiratory system meets this need by supplying additional oxygen.

There are 11 major systems in the human body (Fig. 3.3). Although each system has its own specific function, all systems work together as a team to support life (see Fig. 3.3).

Digestive System

The functions of the digestive system are to ingest food, process it into molecules that can be used by the body, and then eliminate the residue. The main organs that make up the digestive system (in order of function) are the **mouth, esophagus, stomach,** small and large **intestines, rectum,** and **anus.** Helping the food along the way is the teeth, **salivary glands, pancreas,** and **liver.**

Nervous System

The nervous system causes muscles to contract, stimulates glands to secrete, and regulates many other systems of the body. The nervous system also allows sensations such as pain, pressure, and touch to be perceived. The two primary divisions of the nervous system are the **central nervous system,** which consists of the spinal cord and brain, and the **peripheral nervous system,** which consists of the cranial and spinal nerves.

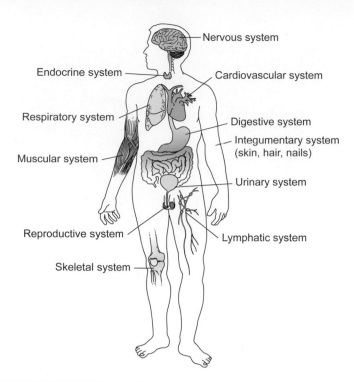

Nervous system

Endocrine system

Cardiovascular system

Respiratory system

Digestive system

Integumentary system
(skin, hair, nails)

Muscular system

Urinary system

Reproductive system

Lymphatic system

Skeletal system

Body System	Components	Major Functions
Skeletal	206 bones	Protection, support, and shape; hematopoietic; storage of certain minerals
Muscular	Striated, smooth, and cardiac muscle	Holding body erect, locomotion, movement of body fluids, production of body heat, communication
Cardiovascular	Heart, arteries, veins, and blood	Respiratory, nutritive, excretory
Lymphatic and immune	White blood cells; lymph fluid, vessels, and nodes; spleen and tonsils	Defense against disease, conservation of plasma proteins and fluid, lipid absorption
Nervous	Central and peripheral nervous systems, special sense organs	Reception of stimuli, transmission of messages, coordinating mechanism
Respiratory	Nose, paranasal sinuses, pharynx, epiglottis, larynx, trachea, bronchi, and lungs	Transportation of oxygen to cells, excretion of carbon dioxide and some water wastes
Digestive system	Mouth, pharynx, esophagus, stomach, intestines, and accessory organs	Digestion of food, absorption of nutrients, elimination of solid wastes
Urinary system	Kidneys, ureters, bladder, and urethra	Formation and elimination of urine, maintenance of homeostasis
Integumentary system	Skin, hair, nails, sweat glands, and sebaceous glands	Protection of body, regulation of body temperature
Endocrine system	Adrenals, gonads, pancreas, parathyroids, pineal, pituitary, thymus, and thyroid	Integration of body functions, control of growth, maintenance of homeostasis
Reproductive system	Male: testes and penis Female: ovaries, fallopian tubes, uterus, and vagina	Production of new life

FIGURE 3.3 The 11 body systems.

Cardiovascular System

The cardiovascular system is made up of the heart, blood vessels, and blood. The functions of the cardiovascular system is to carry oxygen, nutrients, and hormones in the blood to the cells and to remove waste products, such as carbon dioxide. **Arteries** carry blood away from the heart and **veins** carry blood back to the heart. There are two major subdivisions of this system. **Pulmonary circulation** is the flow of blood from the heart, through the lungs (where it receives oxygen), and back to the heart. **Systemic circulation** includes blood flow to all parts of the body except to the lungs.

Endocrine System

The endocrine system consists of glands and organs that produce hormones that regulate the rate of metabolism, energy level, reproduction, growth, sexual development, and response to injury, stress, and mood. Hormones are directly secreted into the bloodstream (not through a duct). The following are integral parts of the endocrine system: **hypothalamus, pineal body, pituitary gland, thyroid** and **parathyroid glands, thymus, adrenal gland, pancreas, ovaries,** and **testes.**

Respiratory System

Your respiratory system is a system of organs and tissues that help you breathe. The respiratory system helps your body absorb oxygen from the air so your organs can work. It also cleans waste gases, such as carbon dioxide from your blood. Your airway includes the **mouth** and **nose, paranasal sinuses, pharynx, trachea, bronchial tubes,** and **lungs.**

Lymphatic System

The lymphatic system is part of the immune system and plays an important role in the defense of the body against infection and disease, the maintaining of body fluid levels, the absorption of digestive tract fats, and the removal of cellular waste. The lymphatic system includes the **thymus, spleen, tonsils, lymph vessels, lymph nodes,** and **lymphatic nodules** located in the digestive system.

Muscular System

The muscular system consists of three basic types of muscles: **striated** (striped), **smooth,** and **cardiac.** These types of muscle are described according to their appearance and function (Fig. 3.4).

Types of Muscle

Striated muscles are known as the skeletal or voluntary muscles. Skeletal muscles attach to the bones of the skeleton and make bodily motions possible.

Smooth muscle fibers move the internal organs, such as the digestive tract, blood vessels, and secretory ducts leading from the glands.

Cardiac muscle forms most of the wall of the heart and is the contraction of the muscle that causes the heart to beat.

Skeletal System

The skeletal system works as a support structure for your body. It gives the body its shape, allows movement, makes blood cells, provides protection for organs, and stores minerals. There are 206 bones in an adult human skeleton. It also includes connective tissue, cartilage, tendons, and ligaments, which is referred to as the musculoskeletal system.

Urinary System

The urinary system function is to filter blood and create urine as a waste by-product. The organs of the urinary system include: two **kidneys,** with the function of removing waste products from the body, balance the body's fluids, release hormones to regulate blood pressure and control production of red blood cells; two **ureters** to carry urine from kidney to bladder; the **bladder,** which stores the urine; and the **urethra,** through which the bladder is emptied to the outside through the process of urination.

Integumentary or Skin System

The integumentary system consists of the skin, hair, nails, and exocrine glands. It has many important functions. It helps regulate body temperature, keeps bacteria from entering the body, excretes liquids and salts, and provides sensitivity to touch. The

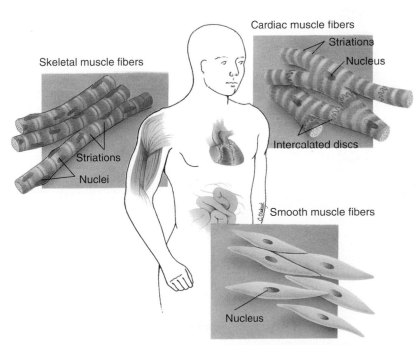

FIGURE 3.4 Types of muscle. (From Thibodeau GA, Patton KT: *The human body in health and disease,* ed 5, St. Louis, 2010, Mosby.)

skin also absorbs ultraviolet rays from the sun and uses them to convert chemicals into vitamin D, which is necessary for the absorption of calcium.

Reproductive System

The reproductive system is a collection of internal and external organs in both females and males that work together for the purpose of reproducing. The female reproductive system consists of the **ovaries, fallopian tubes, uterus,** and **vagina.** Fertility begins at puberty (the onset of menstruation) and ceases at the time of menopause. The male reproductive system includes the **testes, prostate,** and **seminal vesicles.**

Structures of the Head and Neck

As a dental assistant, your knowledge and understanding of the structures of the head and neck will be useful for almost every task you perform.

Types of Bone

Bone is the hard connective tissue that makes up most of the human skeleton. There are two types of bone.

Cortical bone, also known as compact bone, is hard, dense, and strong. It forms the outer layer of bones where it is needed for strength. For example, the outer layer of the mandible (lower jaw) is made of compact bone (Fig. 3.5A).

Cancellous bone, also known as **spongy bone,** is found in the interior of bones and is lighter in weight and not as strong as compact bone. For example, the inner layer of the maxillary bones (upper jaw) is made of cancellous bone (see Fig. 3.5B).

The **periosteum** is the specialized connective tissue covering of all bones in the body.

FIGURE 3.5 A, Cortical bone appears hard and dense. **B,** Cancellous bone appears spongy. (From Haring JI, Lind LJ: *Radiographic interpretation for the dental hygienist,* Philadelphia, 1993, Saunders.)

Anatomy of the Skull

The human skull is divided into two sections: the cranium and the face. The **cranium** is composed of eight bones that cover and protect the brain; the face consists of 14 bones (Table 3.2).

Specific landmarks for the skull are illustrated in Figs. 3.6 through 3.9. For the maxilla, hard palate, and mandible, landmarks are illustrated in Figs. 3.10 and 3.11.

Paranasal Sinuses

The paranasal sinuses are part of the upper respiratory tract. They are a group of air-filled spaces located within the bones of the skull and facial bones. Their functions include lightening the weight of the head, humidifying inhaled air, increasing the resonance of speech, and protecting vital structures (Fig. 3.12).

Types of Paranasal Sinuses
- The maxillary sinuses are located inferior to the nasal cavities and are the largest sinuses.
- The frontal sinuses are triangular in shape and are found under the forehead just above the eyes.
- The ethmoid sinuses are a mass of small cavities that are located between the eyes.
- The sphenoid sinuses lie posterior to the ethmoid sinuses and nasal cavity.

Temporomandibular Joint

The temporomandibular joint (TMJ) is a hinge joint that allows for jaw movement. It is located on each side of the head where the temporal bone and the mandible join. The TMJ makes it possible for the lower jaw to move so that we can speak and chew. The dental professional must understand the anatomy of the TMJ and the normal movements of the joint because this is part of the extraoral exam completed for the patient.

The **capsular ligament** is a dense fibrous capsule that surrounds the TMJ. It is attached to the neck of the condyle and to the nearby surfaces of the temporal bone. The ligaments of the TMJ attach the mandible to the cranium.

The **articular space** is the area between the capsular ligament and the surfaces of the glenoid fossa and the condyle. The **articular disc,** also known as the meniscus, is a cushion of dense connective tissue that divides the articular space into fluid-filled upper and lower compartments. The structure of these compartments and the presence of fluid make smooth movement of the joint possible (Fig. 3.13).

The movement of the TMJ is produced by the muscles of mastication and the hyoid muscles, causing the following functions:
- Depression – opening the mouth
- Elevation – closing the mouth
- Protrusion – protraction of the chin
- Retrusion – retraction of the chin
- Lateral – side-to-side movement in chewing or grinding

TABLE 3.2
Bones of the Skull

Bone	Number	Location
Eight Bones of the Cranium		
Frontal	1	Forms the forehead, most of the orbital roof, and the anterior cranial floor
Parietal	2	Form most of the roof and upper sides of the cranium
Occipital	1	Forms the back and base of the cranium
Temporal	2	Form the sides and base of the cranium
Sphenoid	1	Forms part of the anterior base of the skull and part of the walls of the orbit
Ethmoid	1	Forms part of the orbit and the floor of the cranium
Fourteen Bones of the Face		
Zygomatic	2	Form the prominence of the cheeks and part of the orbit
Maxillary	2	Form the upper jaw
Palatine	2	Form the posterior part of the hard palate and the floor of the nose
Nasal	2	Form the bridge of the nose
Lacrimal	2	Form part of the orbit at the inner angle of the eye
Vomer	1	Forms the base for the nasal septum
Inferior conchae	2	Form part of the interior of the nose
Mandible	1	Forms the lower jaw
Six Auditory Ossicles		
Malleus, incus, stapes	6	Bones of the middle ear

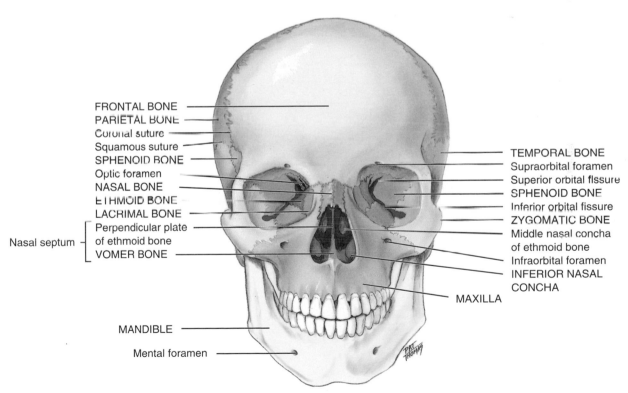

FIGURE 3.6 Frontal view of the skull. (From Applegate E: *The anatomy and physiology learning system,* ed 4, St. Louis, 2011, Saunders.)

Major Muscles of Mastication and Facial Expression

Mastication "chewing" is the initial step in the digestion process. Mastication breaks down food so that it can be digested.

The muscles of mastication are responsible for closing the jaws, bringing the lower jaw forward and backward, and shifting the lower jaw from side to side. The muscles of mastication work with the TMJ to accomplish a number of movements.

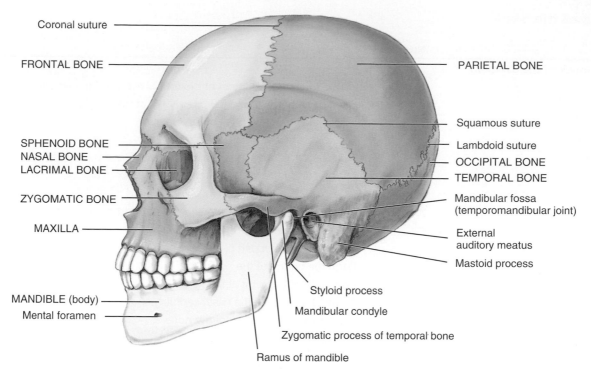

FIGURE 3.7 Lateral view of the skull. (From Applegate E: *The anatomy and physiology learning system,* ed 4, St. Louis, 2011, Saunders.)

FIGURE 3.8 Base of the skull. (From Applegate E: *The anatomy and physiology learning system,* ed 4, St. Louis, 2011, Saunders.)

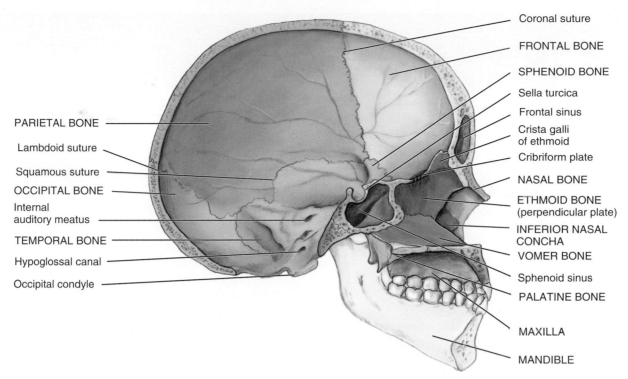

FIG. 3.9 Midsagittal view of the skull. (From Applegate E: *The anatomy and physiology learning system,* ed 4, St. Louis, 2011, Saunders.)

Muscles Involved in Mastication and Facial Expression

- Buccinator – compresses the cheeks and holds food in contact with the teeth.
- External (lateral) pterygoid – depresses, protrudes, and moves the mandible from side to side.
- Internal (medial) pterygoid – closes and aids in sideways movement.
- Masseter – raises the mandible, closes the jaws, and occludes the teeth.
- Montalis – raises and wrinkles the skin of the chin and pushes up the lower lip.
- Orbicularis oris – closes and puckers the lips and aids in chewing by pushing the food against the teeth.
- Temporal – raises the mandible, closes the jaw, and occludes the teeth.
- Zygomatic major – draws the angles of the mouth upward and backward, as in laughing.

FIGURE 3.10 Bones and landmarks of the hard palate. (©Elsevier Collection.)

Blood Supply to the Face and Mouth

Arteries carry oxygenated blood away from the heart to all parts of the body with a pulsing motion. Veins carry blood back to the heart (Fig. 3.14).

Lymph Nodes

Lymph nodes, also called lymph glands, play a vital role in your body's ability to fight off infections. They are small, round, or oval structures located in the lymph vessels. With some infections and immune disorders, the lymph nodes become swollen and tender. During the examination, the dentist examines the nodes of the neck to detect signs of swelling or tenderness. The lymph nodes of the face and neck are shown in Fig. 3.15.

Nerve Supply to the Mouth

Sensory **innervation** of the oral cavity is supplied by the branches of the **trigeminal nerve,** which is a branch of the fifth cranial nerve, the primary source of the nerve supply for the mouth. Innervation is another term for nerve supply. The trigeminal nerve divides into **maxillary** and **mandibular** branches to serve the mouth (Fig. 3.16).

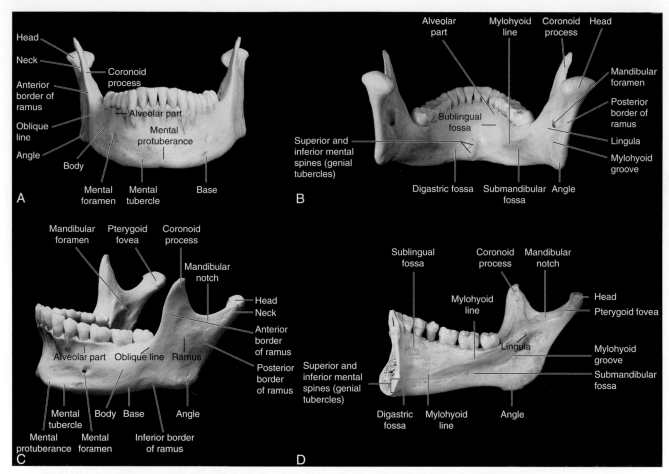

FIGURE 3.11 Views of the mandible. **A,** From the front. **B,** From behind and above. **C,** From the left and front. **D,** Internal view from the left. (From Malamed SF: *Handbook of local anesthesia,* ed 6, St. Louis, 2013, Mosby. Data from Abrahams PH, Boon J, Spratt J: *McMinn's clinical atlas of human anatomy,* ed 6, St. Louis, 2008, Mosby.)

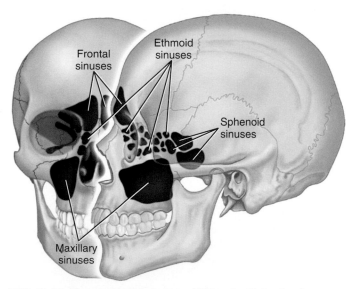

FIG. 3.12 The paranasal sinuses. (©Elsevier Collection.)

Maxillary Innervation

The maxillary division of the trigeminal nerve supplies the maxillary (upper) teeth, periosteum, mucous membrane, maxillary sinuses, and soft palate. The mucous membrane is the specialized tissue that lines the inside of the mouth.

The maxillary division further subdivides to provide the following routes of the nerve supply:

- The **nasopalatine nerve,** which passes through the incisive foramen, supplies the tissue palatal to the maxillary anterior teeth. (Anterior means *toward the front.* A **foramen** is an opening in a bone through which blood vessels, nerves, and ligaments pass.)
- The anterior palatine nerve, which passes through the posterior palatine foramen and forward over the palate, supplies the **mucoperiosteum** (mucoperiosteum is periosteum that has a mucous membrane surface).

The anterior superior alveolar nerve supplies the maxillary central, lateral, and cuspid teeth plus their periodontal membrane and gingivae. This nerve also supplies the maxillary sinus.

- The middle superior alveolar nerve supplies the maxillary first and second premolars, the mesiobuccal root of the maxillary first molar, and the maxillary sinus.
- The posterior superior alveolar nerve supplies the other roots of the maxillary first molar and the maxillary second and third molars. This nerve also branches forward to serve the lateral wall of the maxillary sinus.
- The buccal nerve supplies branches to the buccal mucous membrane and to the mucoperiosteum of the maxillary and mandibular molar teeth. (**Buccal** means *pertaining to* or *directed toward the cheek.*)

Capsular ligament • Glenoid fossa • Meniscus • Articular eminence

Condyloid process

Jaw Closed

Jaw Open (Hinge Action)

Jaw Wide Open (Glide-and-Hinge Action)

FIGURE 3.13 Lateral view of the joint capsule of the temporomandibular joint and its lateral temporomandibular ligament. (©Elsevier Collection.)

Posterior superior alveolar

Infraorbital

Middle superior alveolar

Anterior superior alveolar

Maxillary

Inferior alveolar

Facial

Mylohyoid

Internal carotid

External carotid

Lingual

Common carotid

ARTERIES

Pterygoid plexus • Maxillary

Superficial temporal

Facial

Buccal

Deep facial

Mental

Submental

Inferior alveolar

Anterior facial

Lingual

Posterior auricular

Rotromandibular

Common facial

External jugular

Internal jugular

VEINS

FIGURE 3.14 Major arteries and veins of the face and oral cavity. (©Elsevier Collection.)

Mandibular Innervation

The mandibular division of the trigeminal nerve subdivides into the buccal, **lingual**, and **inferior** alveolar nerves (Fig. 3.17).

- The buccal nerve supplies branches to the buccal mucous membrane and to the mucoperiosteum of the maxillary and mandibular molar teeth.

- The lingual nerve supplies the anterior two thirds of the tongue and gives off branches to supply the lingual mucous membrane and mucoperiosteum. (Lingual means of, or pertaining to, the tongue.)
- The inferior alveolar nerve subdivides into the following:
  - The mylohyoid nerve supplies the mylohyoid muscles and the anterior belly of the digastric muscle.

A

B

FIGURE 3.15 **A,** Superficial lymph nodes of the head and associated structures. **B,** Deep cervical lymph nodes and associated structures. (©Elsevier Collection.)

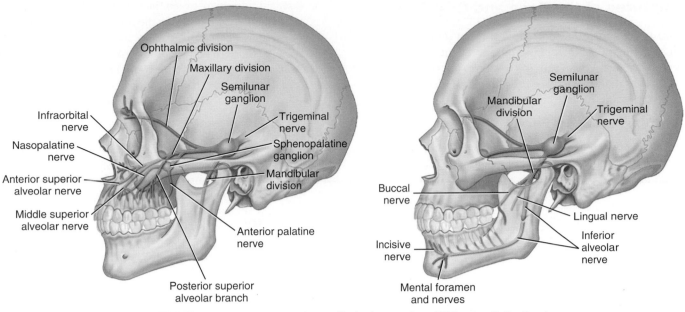

FIGURE 3.16 Maxillary and mandibular innervation. (©Elsevier Collection.)

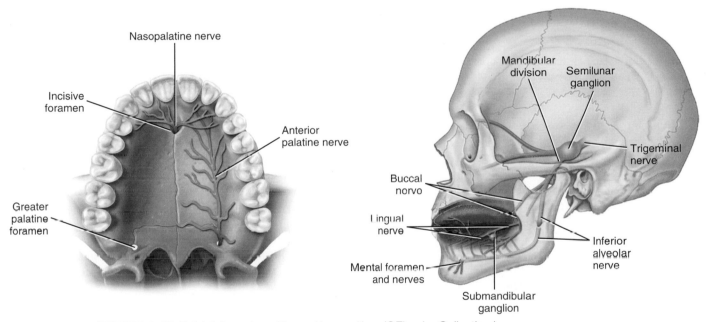

FIGURE 3.17 Palatal, lingual, and buccal innervation. (©Elsevier Collection.)

Major Arteries and Veins of the Face and Mouth

- Facial expression – Branches and small arteries from maxillary, facial, and ophthalmic arteries
- Maxilla – Anterior, middle, and posterior alveolar arteries
- Maxillary teeth – Anterior, middle, and posterior alveolar arteries
- Mandible – Inferior alveolar arteries
- Mandibular teeth – Inferior alveolar arteries
- Tongue – Lingual artery
- Muscles of mastication – Facial arteries

- The small dental nerves supply the molar teeth and premolar teeth, alveolar process, and periosteum of the mandible.
- The mental nerve moves outward through the mental foramen and supplies the chin and mucous membrane of the lower lip.
- The incisive nerve continues interiorly and gives off small branches to supply the cuspid, lateral, and central teeth.

Structures of the Face and Oral Cavity

Before you begin your studies in advanced dental procedures, such as radiographic imaging or intraoral dental functions, it is imperative to learn the terms and locations of various structures of the face and oral cavity. See Procedure 3.1: Identify the Major Landmarks and Structures of the Face.

Landmarks of the Face

The face is defined as the part of the head visible in a frontal view that is anterior to the ears and that lies between the hairline and the chin.

Regions of the Face

The facial region can be subdivided into nine areas (Fig. 3.18):
1. Forehead, extending from the eyebrows to the hairline
2. Temples, or temporal area posterior to the eyes
3. Orbital area, containing the eye and covered by the eyelids
4. External nose
5. Zygomatic (malar) area, the prominence of the cheek
6. Mouth and lips
7. Cheeks
8. Chin
9. External ear

Features of the Face

The dental assistant should be able to identify the following important facial landmarks (Fig. 3.19):
1. Outer **canthus** of the eye: Fold of tissue at the outer corner of the eyelids
2. Inner canthus of the eye: Fold of tissue at the inner corner of the eyelids
3. **Ala of the nose**: Winglike tip on the outer side of each nostril
4. **Philtrum**: Rectangular area between the two ridges running from under the nose to the midline of the upper lip
5. **Tragus** of the ear: Cartilaginous projection anterior to the external opening of the ear

6. **Nasion**: Midpoint between the eyes just below the eyebrows; on the skull, the point where the two nasal bones and frontal bone join
7. **Glabella**: Smooth surface of the frontal bone; also the anatomic area directly above the root of the nose
8. **Root**: Commonly called the *bridge* of the nose
9. **Septum**: Tissue that divides the nasal cavity into two nasal fossae
10. **Anterior naris**: Nostril
11. **Mental protuberance**: Part of the mandible that forms the chin
12. **Angle of the mandible**: Lower posterior of the ramus
13. **Zygomatic arch**: Prominence of the cheek

Oral Cavity

The oral cavity is also referred to as the mouth and includes all its parts, such as the lips, tongue, teeth, and the roof and floor of the mouth.

The oral cavity consists of the following two areas:
1. Oral cavity proper: Space on the tongue side within the upper and lower dental arches
2. Vestibule: Space between the teeth and the inner mucosal lining of the lips and cheeks

Tongue

The tongue is primarily made up of muscle. It is covered on top with a thick layer of mucous membrane and thousands of tiny projections called *papillae*. Inside the papillae are the sensory organs and the nerves for both taste and touch. On a healthy tongue, the papillae are usually pinkish-white and velvety smooth.

The tongue is one of the body's most versatile organs and is responsible for a number of functions: (1) speech, (2) positioning food while eating, (3) tasting and tactile sensations, (4) swallowing, and (5) cleansing the oral cavity. After eating, notice how your tongue moves from crevice to crevice, seeking out and removing bits of retained food in your mouth.

The anterior two thirds of the tongue, called the *body,* is found in the oral cavity. The root of the tongue is the posterior part that turns vertically downward to the pharynx. The dorsum consists of the superior (upper) and posterior roughened

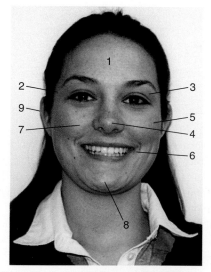

FIGURE 3.18 Regions of the face.

FIGURE 3.19 Features of the face.

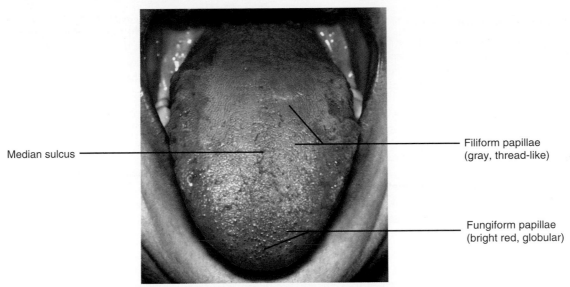

FIGURE 3.20 Dorsum of the tongue. (From Liebgott B: *The anatomic basis of dentistry*, ed 3, St. Louis, 2010, Mosby.)

FIGURE 3.21 Sublingual aspect of the tongue. (From Liebgott B: *The anatomic basis of dentistry*, ed 3, St. Louis, 2010, Mosby.)

aspects of the tongue and is covered with small papillae of various shapes and colors (Fig. 3.20).

The sublingual surface of the tongue is covered with thin, smooth, transparent mucosa through which many underlying vessels can be seen (Fig. 3.21). Two small papillae are present on either side of the lingual frenulum (frenum) just behind the central incisors. Through these papillae are the openings of the submandibular ducts. The saliva enters the oral cavity through these ducts. On either side of the lingual surface are two smaller fimbriated folds. The lingual frenum is the thin fold of mucous membrane that extends from the floor of the mouth to the underside of the tongue.

Frenum

A frenum is a narrow band of tissue that connects two structures. The maxillary labial frenum passes from the oral mucosa at the midline of the maxillary arch to the midline of the inner surface of the upper lip. The mandibular labial frenum passes from the oral mucosa at the midline of the mandibular arch to the midline of the inner surface of the lower lip.

In the area of the first maxillary permanent molar, the buccal frenum passes from the oral mucosa of the outer surface of the maxillary arch to the inner surface of the cheek. The lingual frenum passes from the floor of the mouth to the midline of the ventral border of the tongue.

Salivary Glands

The salivary glands produce saliva that lubricates and cleans the oral cavity and helps with digestion. The nervous system controls these glands. The salivary glands have ducts (openings) to help drain the saliva directly into the oral cavity where the saliva is used. The salivary glands may become enlarged, tender, and possibly firm as the result of various disease processes. Certain medications or disease processes may result in decreased or increased production of saliva by these glands (Fig. 3.22).

Hard and Soft Palates

The hard and soft palates serve as the roof of the mouth. The hard palate is the bony part of the roof closer of the teeth, and the soft palate is at the back of the roof (Fig. 3.23). The structure of the hard and soft palate includes:

- The hard palate, which forms the anterior aspect of the palate and is covered with masticatory mucosa
- The soft palate, which is the posterior portion of the palate that is mobile for swallowing and speech. It is made up of muscle fibers and covered by a mucous membrane
- The palatine rugae, which are irregular ridges or folds in the mucosa on the palate just behind the maxillary central incisors
- The incisive papilla, which is the pear-shaped pad of tissue located directly behind the maxillary central incisors
- The uvula, which is a fleshy extension at the back of the soft palate that hangs above the throat and helps in swallowing and speaking

Gag Reflex

The gag reflex is an involuntary protective mechanism located in the posterior region of the mouth. This overly sensitive area includes the soft palate, the uvula, the surrounding tissue, and the posterior portion of the tongue.

When a foreign body encounters the membranes of this area, it causes gagging. This is important to know when taking impressions or working in that area of the mouth.

Alveolar Process

The alveolar process is the alveolar bone made up of hard compact bone. It is the part of the maxilla and mandible that supports the roots of the teeth and keeps them in place. The teeth are firmly held in place within the bone of the alveolar process.

Cortical Plate

The cortical plate, also known as the *cribriform plate,* is the dense outer layer of bone covering the alveolar process that provides strength and protection. The cortical plate of the mandible is dense with few openings. The cortical plate of the maxilla is not as dense.

The Alveolar Crest

The alveolar crest is the highest point of the alveolar ridge. In an unhealthy mouth, the alveolar crest can be destroyed.

Alveolar Socket

The **alveolar socket** is the space within the alveolar process in which the root of a tooth is held in place by the periodontal ligament.

Oral Mucosa

The oral mucosa is the mucous membrane lining inside your mouth (Fig. 3.24). Two types of oral mucosa are known as:

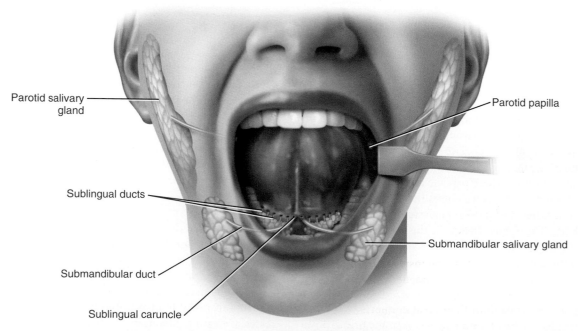

FIGURE 3.22 Major salivary glands. (©Elsevier Collection.)

Parotid salivary gland

Parotid papilla

Sublingual ducts

Submandibular duct

Sublingual caruncle

Submandibular salivary gland

Palatal rugae

Lingual (palatal) gingiva

Incisive papilla

Median palatine raphe

Ducts for palatal glands

Soft palate

Anterior faucial pillar

Uvula

Posterior faucial pillar

Palatine tonsil

Posterior wall of pharynx

FIGURE 3.23 A, Surface features of the hard palate. **B,** Surface features of the soft palate. (From Liebgott B: *The anatomic basis of dentistry,* ed 3, St. Louis, 2010, Mosby.)

FIGURE 3.24 A, Dense masticatory mucosa makes up the gingiva. **B,** Delicate lining mucosa covers the vestibule.

- The **lining mucosa,** which covers the inside of the cheeks, vestibule, lips, ventral surface of the tongue, and soft palate and is delicate, thin, and easily injured.
- The **masticatory mucosa,** which covers the gingivae (gums), hard palate, and dorsum of the tongue and is attached to the bone, very dense, and designed to withstand the vigorous activity of chewing and swallowing food.

Gingivae

Gingiva (plural, *gingivae*), commonly referred to as the *gums,* is masticatory mucosa that covers the alveolar processes of the jaws and surrounds the necks of each tooth (Fig. 3.25).

Location and Structures of Gingiva

- The epithelial attachment is healthy gingiva that covers the alveolar bone and attaches to the teeth on the enamel surface just above the neck of the tooth.
- The free gingiva extends from the base of the gingival sulcus to the gingival margin. It is not attached to the surface of the tooth.
- The gingival sulcus is the space between the free gingiva and the tooth. A normal, healthy gingival sulcus is 3 mm or less in depth.
- The gingival margin is the upper edge of the gingiva. Its shape follows the curvatures of the cervical line of the tooth.
- The free gingival groove is a shallow groove that extends from the base of the sulcus to the mucogingival junction. It is a stippled, dense tissue that is firmly bound to the underlying bone.
- The attached gingivae extend from the base of the sulcus to the mucogingival junction.
- The mucogingival junction is the line that separates the attached gingivae from the alveolar mucosa.

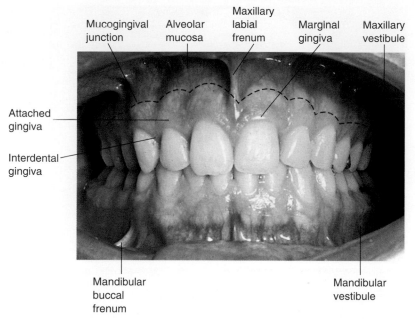

FIGURE 3.25 View of the gingivae and associated anatomic structures.

Epithelial Attachment

Healthy gingivae cover the alveolar bone and attach to the teeth on the enamel surface just above the neck of the tooth. This structure is known as the *epithelial attachment*.

Free Gingivae

The free gingivae are the parts of the gingiva that extend higher than the epithelial attachment. They are made up of tissue from the gingival margin to the base of the gingival sulcus and are normally light pink and coral in color in light-skinned people. The gingival sulcus is the space between the free gingivae and the tooth. See Procedure 3.2: Identify the Major Landmarks, Structures, and Normal Tissues of the Mouth.

Teeth

The types of teeth, their structures, and their tissues are discussed in Chapter 4.

Procedure 3.1

Identify the Major Landmarks and Structures of the Face

Goal

To identify the major landmarks and structures of the face correctly.

Procedural Steps

Identify each of the following:
1. Ala of the nose
2. Inner canthus and outer canthus of the eye
3. Commissure of the lips
4. Location of the frontal sinuses
5. Location of the maxillary sinuses
6. Location of the parotid glands
7. Philtrum
8. Tragus of the ear
9. Vermilion border
10. Zygomatic arch

Procedure 3.2

Identify the Major Landmarks, Structures, and Normal Tissues of the Mouth

Goal

To identify and correctly locate the major landmarks, structures, and normal tissues of the mouth.

Procedural Steps

Identify/locate each of the following:
1. Locate the dorsum of the tongue.
2. Locate the area of the gag reflex.
3. Identify the hard and soft palates.
4. Identify the gingival margin.
5. Locate the incisive papilla.
6. Identify the mandibular labial frenum.
7. Identify the maxillary labial frenum.
8. Locate the sublingual frenum.
9. Identify the vestibule of the mouth.
10. Locate Wharton duct.

Chapter Exercises

Multiple Choice

Circle the letter next to the correct answer.

1. The simplest organizational level in the human body is the _____.
   a. cell
   b. organ
   c. tissue
   d. body system

2. The body system that absorbs nutrients and eliminates solid wastes is the _____.
   a. digestive
   b. nervous
   c. cardiovascular
   d. endocrine

3. The white blood cells, spleen, and tonsils are components of the _____ system.
   a. respiratory
   b. muscular
   c. lymphatic
   d. nervous

4. The type of movements made by the TMJ is _____.
   a. protrusion
   b. lateral
   c. corrective
   d. a and b

5. What nerve supplies the upper back teeth in the mouth?
   a. anterior superior alveolar
   b. middle superior alveolar
   c. posterior superior alveolar
   d. buccal

6. The structures that carry blood back to the heart are _____.
   a. arteries
   b. lymph nodes
   c. veins
   d. trigeminal nerve

7. The top of the tongue is called the _____ surface.
   a. lateral
   b. ventral
   c. dorsal
   d. facial

8. Which of the following is (are) functions of the salivary glands?
   a. Provide lubrication.
   b. Clean the oral cavity.
   c. Aid in digestion.
   d. All of the above are functions.

9. Which type of oral mucosa covers the inside of the cheeks, vestibules, lips, and ventral surface of the tongue?
   a. Lining mucosa
   b. Masticatory mucosa
   c. Gingiva
   d. Epithelial attachment

10. The _____ is the cavity within the alveolar process that holds the tooth.
    a. alveolar crest
    b. alveolar socket
    c. cortical plate
    d. periodontal ligament

Apply Your Knowledge

1. A patient comes into your office complaining that when he bit into a hot piece of pizza, he burned the front part of the roof of his mouth. Which oral landmark was most likely affected?

2. The dentist asks you to place a cotton roll over the Stensen duct to help control the flow of saliva during a procedure. Where in the mouth would this be?

3. The dentist is performing a restorative procedure on the mandibular teeth. Which nerve would be involved in being anesthetized?

4. When placing an x-ray sensor, which area of the mouth would be of concern of the patient gagging?

CHAPTER 4

Dental Anatomy

http://evolve.elsevier.com/Robinson/essentials/

LEARNING OBJECTIVES

1. Pronounce, define, and spell the key terms.
2. Identify the anatomic parts of the tooth and explain the makeup of each of the tissues of a tooth.
3. Complete the following related to describing the teeth and associated structures:
   - Identify the different types of teeth.
   - Describe the two dental arches.
   - Describe the differences between anterior and posterior teeth.
   - Use the correct terminology when describing the teeth.
4. Identify the locations of all surfaces of the teeth, name the tooth surfaces, and describe the anatomic features of each tooth.
5. Complete the following related to dentition:
   - Identify the number of teeth in the primary dentition.
   - Discuss mixed dentition.
   - Identify the number of teeth in the permanent dentition.
6. Use the Universal National System, International Standards Organization System, or Palmer Notation System to designate and name the surfaces of each tooth and to identify the correct location of each permanent tooth.

KEY TERMS

anatomic crown	dentinal tubules	morphology
apex	embrasure	numbering systems
apical	enamel	occlusion
bifurcation	enamel prisms	Palmer Notation System
cementoenamel junction	exfoliation	periapical
cementum	Federation Dentaire Internationale	periodontal ligament
clinical crown	(FDI) System	periodontium
contact point	fossae	permanent dentition
cusp	International Standards	primary dentition
dentin	Organization (ISO) System	pulp
dentinal fiber	mixed dentition	trifurcation
		Universal National System

Dental anatomy is a branch of gross anatomy focused on the makeup of teeth, which includes the study of the **morphology**, location, and identification of each tooth in the human dentition.

Dentition

The term *dentition* refers to the natural teeth in the mouth. The term *edentulous* means without natural teeth and is used to describe the condition when the permanent teeth have been lost. The normal human has two complete sets of teeth in a lifetime:

primary dentition and **permanent dentition**. The transition from one dentition state to the other is known as the **mixed dentition** period. During this period, both primary teeth and permanent teeth are in the mouth.

Primary Dentition

All 20 teeth of the primary dentition should erupt and be in place shortly after the age of 2 years. **Eruption** is the movement of a tooth through the bone and gingival tissue (Fig. 4.1). All primary teeth, also known as *deciduous teeth,* are exfoliated to make way for their replacements. **Exfoliation** is the normal

FIGURE 4.1 Facial and buccal view of a primary dentition. From Fehrenbach MJ, Popowics T: *Illustrated dental embryology, histology, and anatomy,* ed 4, St. Louis, 2016, Saunders.

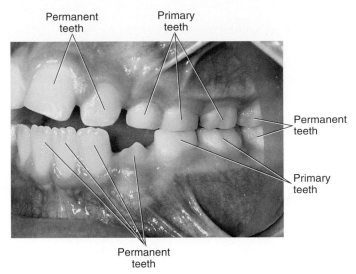

FIGURE 4.2 An example of the oral cavity during the mixed dentition period. (From Fehrenbach MJ, Popowics T: *Illustrated dental embryology, histology, and anatomy*, ed 4, St Louis, 2016, Saunders.)

TABLE 4.1
Primary Dentition in Order of Eruption

Dentition	Date of Eruption	Date of Exfoliation
Maxillary Teeth		
Central incisor	6–10 months	6–7 years
Lateral incisor	9–12 months	7–8 years
First molar	12–18 months	9–11 years
Canine	16–22 months	10–12 years
Second molar	24–32 months	10–12 years
Mandibular Teeth		
Central incisor	6–10 months	6–7 years
Lateral incisor	7–10 months	7–8 years
First molar	12–18 months	9–11 years
Canine	16–22 months	9–12 years
Second molar	20–32 months	10–12 years

FIGURE 4.3 Facial and buccal view of a permanent dentition.

process by which primary teeth are shed. During this process, the root of the primary teeth is **resorbed** (removed by a normal body process). Table 4.1 shows the average ages for eruption and exfoliation of the primary dentition.

Mixed Dentition

When primary teeth no longer meet the needs of the growing child, they are lost and replaced by the permanent teeth, which are larger, stronger, and more numerous.

The exfoliation, or shedding process, of the primary teeth takes place between the ages of 5 and 12 years. During the time of this mixed dentition, the child has some permanent and some primary teeth (Fig. 4.2).

Permanent Dentition

The permanent dentition period begins when the last primary tooth is shed, after approximately 12 years of age, and includes the eruption of all 32 of the permanent teeth (Fig. 4.3). The jaws have nearly completed their growth when the stages of puberty pass.

Dental Arches

There are two dental arches—the maxillary and the mandibular—found in the human mouth. The lay person may refer to the maxillary arch as the upper jaw and the mandibular arch as the lower jaw. The **maxillary arch,** which is part of the skull, is fixed and not capable of movement. The **mandibular arch** is capable of movement through the action of the temporomandibular joint (see Chapter 3).

It is important to remember when looking into the patient's oral cavity that the directions are reversed (your right will be the patient's left side, and your left will be the patient's right side).

Quadrants and Sextants

An imaginary midline divides each dental arch into mirror halves. The two arches, each divided into halves, create four sections, which are called **quadrants.**

Quadrants

When the maxillary and mandibular arches are each divided into halves, the following four sections, called *quadrants,* result:

Maxillary right quadrant
Maxillary left quadrant
Mandibular left quadrant
Mandibular right quadrant

Each quadrant of the primary dentition contains five teeth, and each quadrant of the permanent dentition contains eight permanent teeth (Fig. 4.4).

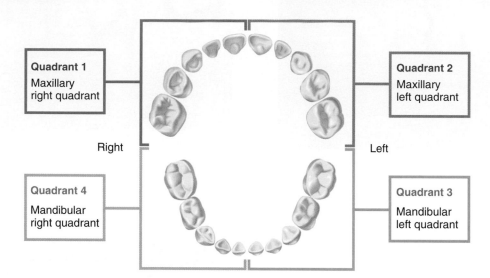

Quadrant 1
Maxillary right quadrant

Quadrant 2
Maxillary left quadrant

Right

Left

Quadrant 4
Mandibular right quadrant

Quadrant 3
Mandibular left quadrant

A **Primary Dentition**

Quadrant 1
Maxillary right quadrant

Quadrant 2
Maxillary left quadrant

Right

Left

Quadrant 4
Mandibular right quadrant

Quadrant 3
Mandibular left quadrant

B **Permanent Dentition**

FIGURE 4.4 Permanent dentition in quadrants. (©Elsevier Collection.)

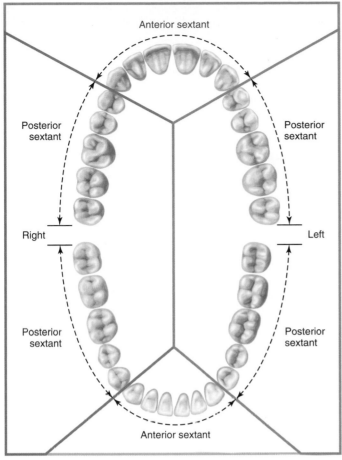

Maxillary

Anterior sextant

Posterior sextant

Posterior sextant

Right

Left

Posterior sextant

Posterior sextant

Anterior sextant

Mandibular

FIGURE 4.5 Permanent dentition in sextants. (©Elsevier Collection.)

Sextants

Each arch can also be divided into sextants rather than quadrants. A sextant is one sixth of the dentition. There are three sextants in each arch. The dental arch is divided as follows (Fig. 4.5):
1. Maxillary right posterior sextant
2. Maxillary anterior sextant
3. Maxillary left posterior sextant
4. Mandibular right posterior sextant
5. Mandibular anterior sextant
6. Mandibular left posterior sextant

Types of Teeth

Humans eat a diet that includes meats, vegetables, grains, and fruit. To accommodate this variety in our diet, our teeth are designed for cutting, shearing or incising, tearing, and grinding different types of food. There are four types of teeth in the human dentition: **incisors, canines, premolars,** and **molars**. Each quadrant of the primary dentition contains one central incisor, one lateral incisor, one canine, and two molars, whereas each quadrant of the permanent dentition contains one central incisor, one lateral incisor, one canine, two premolars, and three molars (Fig. 4.6).

Types of Teeth
- **Incisors** are single-rooted teeth with a sharp and thin edge; they are located at the front of the mouth. Their function is to cut food without heavy force.
- **Canines** are also referred to as the *cuspids* and are located at the "corner" of the dental arch. The crown is thick, with one pointed cusp. Canines have the longest root and are the most stable teeth in the mouth. Their function is cutting and tearing food with force.
- **Premolars** are known as *bicuspids* because of their broader chewing surface. There are no premolars in the primary dentition. Their function is for grasping and tearing food.
- **Molars** are the largest teeth in the mouth and have the largest chewing surface. Their function is to chew or grind up food.

Anterior and Posterior Teeth

To assist in describing their locations and functions, the teeth are classified as being **anterior** (toward the front of the mouth) or **posterior** (toward the back of the mouth). The anterior teeth are the incisors and canines and are usually visible when people smile. The anterior teeth are aligned in a gentle curve. The posterior teeth are the premolars and molars and are aligned with little or no curvature; they appear to be in an almost straight line.

Anatomic Parts of the Tooth

Each tooth consists of the crown of a tooth and one or more roots. The size and shape of the crown and the size and number of roots vary according to the type of the tooth.

Crown

The **anatomic crown** is the portion of the tooth covered with enamel. The size of the anatomic crown remains the same throughout the life of the tooth, regardless of the position of the gingiva (also referred to as your gums).

The **clinical crown** is the portion of the tooth that is visible in the mouth. The length of the clinical crown can vary during the life cycle of the tooth, depending on the location of the gingiva. The clinical crown is shortest when the tooth erupts into position and becomes longer as the surrounding gingiva recedes (Fig. 4.7).

Root

The root is the portion of the tooth that is normally embedded in the alveolar process and is covered with cementum. Depending on the type of tooth, one, two, or three roots may be present. **Bifurcation** means division into two roots, and **trifurcation** means division into three roots. The tapered end of each root tip is known as the **apex**. Anything that is located at the apex is referred to as **apical**, and anything surrounding the apex is said to be **periapical**.

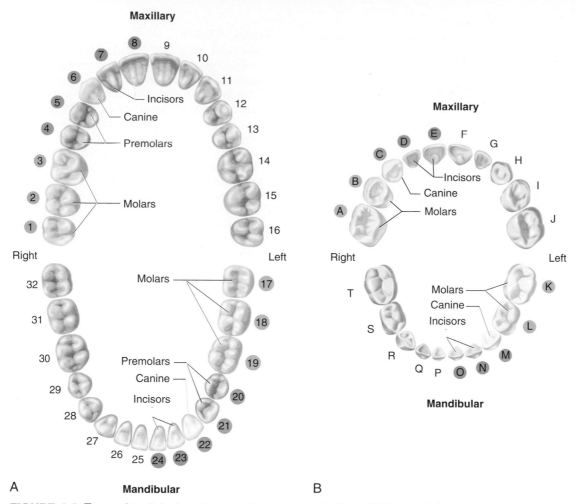

FIGURE 4.6 Types of teeth in the primary and permanent dentition. (©Elsevier Collection.)

FIGURE 4.7 The anatomic and clinical crown.

Cervix

The cervix is the narrow area of the tooth where the crown and the root meet. (**Cervix** means *neck*.) The **cementoenamel junction** is formed by the enamel of the crown and the cementum of the root. This area is also known as the *cervical line* or the *cementoenamel junction (CEJ)*.

Tissues of the Tooth

Your teeth are composed of four different types of tissues: enamel, dentin, cementum, and the pulp (Fig. 4.8)

Enamel

Enamel, which makes up the anatomic crown of the tooth, is the hardest material of the body. This hardness is important because enamel forms the protective covering for the softer underlying dentin. It also provides a strong surface for tearing, crushing, grinding, and chewing food.

Enamel is translucent and ranges in color from yellow-white to gray-white. (*Translucent* means that the substance allows some light to pass through it.)

Enamel is similar to bone in its hardness and mineral content. Unlike bone, mature enamel does not contain cells that can repair themselves. Nevertheless, some remineralization is possible (see Chapter 17).

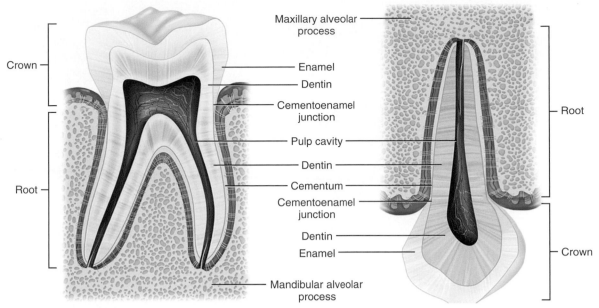

Labels on the figure:

Maxillary alveolar process
Enamel
Dentin
Cementoenamel junction
Pulp cavity
Dentin
Cementum
Cementoenamel junction
Dentin
Enamel
Mandibular alveolar process
Crown
Root
Root
Crown

FIGURE 4.8 Tissues of the teeth. (©Elsevier Collection.)

Structure of Enamel

Enamel is composed of millions of calcified **enamel prisms**, which are also known as *enamel rods*. These extend from the surface of the tooth to the dentinoenamel junction.

The enamel prisms tend to be grouped into rows that follow a course that is approximately perpendicular to the surface of the tooth.

Dentin

Dentin makes up the main portion of the tooth structure and extends almost the entire length of the tooth. It is covered by enamel on the crown and by cementum on the root.

In the primary teeth, dentin is light yellow. In the permanent teeth, it is light yellow and somewhat transparent. The color of the dentin tends to darken as we age.

Structure of Dentin

Dentin is a mineralized tissue that is not as hard as enamel. Dentin is a very porous tissue made up of microscopic canals called **dentinal tubules** that extend from the exterior surface, where the dentin joins the enamel or cementum, to the interior surface, which forms the pulp chamber. If the dentin is not protected by enamel, then these tubules form a direct passage for invading bacteria into the pulp to cause decay.

Each tubule contains a **dentinal fiber** that can transmit pain into the pulp. Dentin is a sensitive living tissue; therefore it must be protected against dehydration (excessive drying) and thermal shock (sudden temperature changes) during dental treatment.

Because dentin is capable of some repair, the dentist can use dental materials that will help encourage the repair process when restoring the tooth.

Pulp

The **pulp** is the inner portion of the tooth. The portion of the pulp that lies within the crown portion of the tooth is called

the *coronal pulp;* this includes the pulp horns, which are extensions of the pulp that project toward the **cusp** tips and incisal edges.

The other portion of the pulp is more apically located and is referred to as *radicular* or *root pulp*. The radicular pulp of each root is continuous with the tissues of the periapical area via an apical foramen.

In young teeth, the apical foramen is not yet fully formed, and this opening is wide. With increasing age, the pulp chamber becomes smaller.

Structure of the Pulp

The pulp is made up of connective tissue, blood vessels, and nerves that enter the pulp chamber through the apical foramen. The blood supply is derived from branches of the dental arteries and from the periodontal ligament.

The nerves in the pulp receive and transmit pain stimuli. When a stimulus such as hot or cold is strong, the reaction is greater, and the patient feels pain. When the stimulus is weak, the response by the pulpal system is weak, and the interaction goes unnoticed.

Cementum

Cementum, which is not as hard as either enamel or dentin, protects the root of the tooth and joins the enamel at the CEJ. Cementum is of a light yellow shade that is somewhat lighter than the color of dentin and darker than enamel. Cementum also lacks the luster and translucent qualities of enamel.

Structure of the Cementum

Cementum is similar in chemical composition to bone but more porous to help the periodontal ligaments attach to the tooth. If cementum becomes exposed because of gingival recession and bone loss, then cementum becomes sensitive and susceptible to decay.

FIGURE 4.9 Periodontium of the tooth. (©Elsevier Collection.)

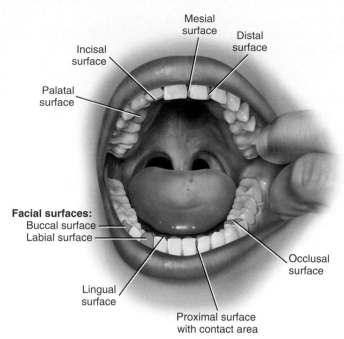

FIGURE 4.10 Surfaces of the teeth. (©Elsevier Collection.)

Periodontium

The **periodontium** supports the teeth in the alveolar bone and consists of cementum, alveolar bone, and the periodontal ligaments. These tissues also protect and nourish the teeth.

Periodontal Ligament

The **periodontal ligament** is dense connective tissue organized into groups of fibers that connect the cementum covering the root of the tooth with the alveolar bone of the socket wall. At one end, the fibers are embedded in cementum; at the other end, they are embedded in bone. These embedded portions become mineralized and are known as *Sharpey fibers*. The periodontal ligament ranges in width from 0.1 to 0.38 mm, with the thinnest portion around the middle third of the root. As we age, a gradual progressive decrease in the width of these fibers occurs (Fig. 4.9).

Tooth Surfaces

Each tooth has five surfaces: facial, lingual, incisal/occlusal, mesial, and distal (Fig. 4.10).

Additional terms related to surfaces within the mouth are **interproximal** space, which refers to the space where two teeth are touching each other (between the teeth), and **palatal** surfaces, which are surfaces of the teeth that are near the palate. See Procedure 4.1: Identify the Teeth and Name the Tooth Surfaces.

Anatomic Features of the Teeth

The anatomic features of the teeth—contours, contacts, and embrasures—help maintain the positions of the teeth in the dental arch and protect the tissues during chewing.

Surfaces of the Teeth

- The **facial** surface is the surface of the tooth closest to the face. The facial surfaces closest to the lips are termed the labial surfaces, and the facial surfaces closest to the cheeks are the buccal surfaces.
- The **lingual** surface of the tooth is the surface of the tooth closest to the tongue.
- The **incisal** surface of the tooth is the chewing surface of anterior teeth.
- The **occlusal** surface of the tooth is the chewing surface of posterior teeth.
- The **mesial** surface of the tooth is the surface closest to the midline.
- The **distal** surface of the tooth is the surface away from the midline.

Contours

All teeth have a curved surface except when the tooth is fractured or worn. Some surfaces are convex (curved outward); others are concave (curved inward). Although the general contours vary, the general principle that the crown of the tooth narrows toward the cervical line is true for all types of teeth.

Facial and Lingual Contours

The curvatures found on the facial and lingual surfaces provide natural passageways for food. This action protects the gingiva from the impact of foods during mastication. The normal contour of a tooth provides the gingiva with adequate stimulation for health and still protects it from being damaged by food (Fig. 4.11A).

When a tooth is restored, returning it to a normal contour is important. With inadequate contour, the gingiva may be traumatized by food pushing against it (see Fig. 4.11**B**). With overcontouring, the gingiva will lack adequate stimulation and will be difficult to clean (see Fig. 4.11**C**).

Contacts

The contact area of the mesial or distal surface of a tooth is the area that touches the adjacent tooth in the same arch. The contact point is the exact spot at which the teeth touch each other. The terms *contact* and *contact area* are frequently used interchangeably to refer to the contact point (Fig. 4.12).

The crown of each tooth in the dental arches should be in contact with its adjacent tooth or teeth. A proper contact relationship between adjacent teeth serves the following three purposes:

1. It prevents food from being trapped between the teeth.
2. It stabilizes the dental arches by holding the teeth in either arch in positive contact with each other.
3. It protects the interproximal gingival tissue from trauma during mastication.

Embrasures

An embrasure is a triangular space near the gingiva between the proximal surfaces of two adjoining teeth. Embrasures are continuous with the interproximal spaces between the teeth. All tooth contours, including contact areas and embrasures, are important in the function and health of the oral tissue (Fig. 4.13).

Occlusion

Occlusion is the relationship between your maxillary teeth and mandibular teeth and how they come together when you bite down. The occlusal surfaces consist of cusps (raised areas) and fossae (indentations or grooves). The cusps of the teeth in one arch fit into the fossae of the teeth in the opposing arch, which produces a highly effective grinding action for chewing food.

A patient is considered to have "normal occlusion" when the mesiobuccal cusp of the upper first molar occludes with the buccal grove of the lower first molar (Fig. 4.14). Any deviation from the alignment of normal occlusion would be considered malocclusion. Refer to Chapter 28 for the definition and images of malocclusion.

Tooth Numbering Systems

Numbering systems are used as a simplified means of identifying the teeth for charting and descriptive purposes (Table 4.2).

Universal National System

The Universal National System, which is approved by the American Dental Association, is used throughout the United States. In the Universal National System, the primary teeth are lettered with capital letters from A to T. Lettering begins with the upper-right second primary molar (tooth A), works around to the upper-left second primary molar (tooth J), drops to the lower-left second primary molar (tooth K), and works around to the lower-right second primary molar.

The permanent teeth are numbered from 1 to 32. Numbering begins with the upper-right third molar (tooth #1), works around to the upper-left third molar (tooth #16), drops to the lower-left third molar (tooth #17), and works around to the lower-right third molar (tooth #32).

International Standards Organization System

The International Standards Organization (ISO) System is based on the Fédération Dentaire Internationale (FDI) System and is used in most other countries.

The ISO/FDI System uses a two-digit, tooth-recording system. The first digit indicates the quadrant, and the second digit indicates the tooth within the quadrant, with numbering from

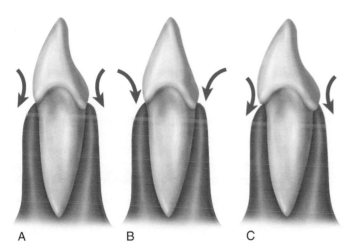

FIGURE 4.11 Facial and lingual contours. **A,** normal contour, **B,** Inadequate contour, **C,** Overcontouring contour. (©Elsevier Collection.)

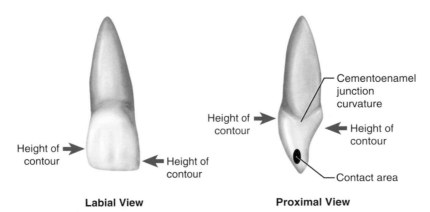

Labial View

Proximal View

Cementoenamel junction curvature

Height of contour

Height of contour

Height of contour

Height of contour

Contact area

FIGURE 4.12 Contact area. (©Elsevier Collection.)

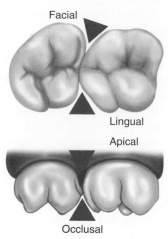

FIGURE 4.13 Embrasures. (©Elsevier Collection.)

FIGURE 4.14 Normal occlusion. (From Graber LW, Vanarsdall RL, Vig KWL: *Orthodontics: current principles and techniques,* ed 5, Philadelphia, 2012, Mosby.)

the midline toward the posterior. The digits should be separately pronounced. For example, the permanent canines are teeth #1-3 ("number one-three"), #2-3 ("number two-three"), #3-3 ("number three-three"), and #4-3 ("number four-three").

To avoid miscommunication internationally, the ISO/FDI System also provides designation of areas in the oral cavity. A two-digit number designates these, and at least one of the two digits is zero (0). In this system, for example, 00 ("zero-zero") designates the whole oral cavity, and 01 ("zero-one") indicates the maxillary area only.

Palmer Notation System

In the **Palmer Notation System**, each of the four quadrants is given its own tooth bracket made up of a vertical line and a horizontal line. This method is often used by orthodontists in their practice. The Palmer method is a shorthand diagram of the teeth as if the patient's teeth are viewed from the outside. The teeth in the right quadrant would have the vertical midline bracket to the right of the tooth numbers or letters, as when looking at the patient. The midline is to the right of the teeth in the right quadrant.

For example, if the tooth is a maxillary tooth, the number or letter should be written above the horizontal line of the bracket, thus indicating an upper tooth. Conversely, a mandibular tooth symbol should be placed below the line, indicating a lower tooth.

The number or letter assigned to each tooth depends on its position relative to the midline. For example, central incisors, the teeth closest to the midline, have the lowest number 1 for

permanent teeth and the letter A for primary teeth. All central incisors, maxillary and mandibular, are given the number 1. All lateral incisors are given the number 2, canines are given the number 3, premolars are numbers 4 and 5, molars are 6 and 7, and third molars are number 8. See Procedure 4.2: Identify the Primary and Permanent Teeth Using the Universal National System, the Fédération Dentaire Internationale System, and the Palmer Notation System.

Tooth Diagrams

The diagrams used for dental charting have the teeth in the right quadrants arranged on the left side of the page and the teeth in the left quadrants arranged on the right side of the page. The purpose of this layout is to simulate looking into the patient's mouth. The skills you have learned in this chapter will be used when you study dental charting in detail in Chapter 12.

Ethical Implications

Your understanding of dental terminology and dental anatomy is fundamental to a variety of clinical procedures you will be performing every day in the dental setting. In addition, your ability to use the proper terminology when communicating with patients and dental professionals demonstrates your level of training and education and enhances your role as a dental professional.

TABLE 4.2

A and B Tooth Designation Systems for Primary and Permanent Dentition

	Molars		Canine	Incisors				Canine	Molars	
					Maxillary Arch					
I	A	B	C	D	E	F	G	H	I	J
II	55	54	53	52	51	61	62	63	64	65
III	E⌋	D⌋	C⌋	B⌋	A⌋	⌊A	⌊B	⌊C	⌊D	⌊E

	Molars		Canine	Incisors				Canine	Molars	
III	E⌉	D⌉	C⌉	B⌉	A⌉	⌈A	⌈B	⌈C	⌈D	⌈F
II	85	84	83	82	81	71	72	73	74	75
I	T	S	R	Q	P	O	N	M	L	K
				Mandibular Arch						
	Right					Left				

I   Universal tooth numbering system

II   International Standards Organization

III   Palmer Method

From Fehrenbach MJ, Popowics T: *Illustrated dental embryology, histology, and anatomy*, ed 4, St. Louis, 2016, Saunders.

	Molars			Premolars		Canine	Incisors				Canine	Premolars		Molars		
							Maxillary Arch									
I	1	2	3	4	5	6	7	8	9	10	11	12	13	14	15	16
II	18	17	16	15	14	13	12	11	21	22	23	24	25	26	27	28
III	8	7	6	5	4	3	2	1	1	2	3	4	5	6	7	8

	Molars			Premolars		Canine	Incisors				Canine	Premolars		Molars		
III	8	7	6	5	4	3	2	1	1	2	3	4	5	6	7	8
II	48	47	46	45	44	43	42	41	31	32	33	34	35	36	37	38
I	32	31	30	29	28	27	26	25	24	23	22	21	20	19	18	17
							Mandibular Arch									
	Right							Left								

I   Universal tooth numbering system

II   International Standards Organization

III Palmer Method

From Fehrenbach MJ, Popowics T: *Illustrated dental embryology, histology, and anatomy*, ed 4, St. Louis, 2016, Saunders

Procedure 4.1

Identify the Teeth and Name the Tooth Surfaces

Goal

To identify the teeth and name the tooth surfaces correctly.

Equipment and Supplies

- Study model or typodont.

Procedural Steps

Identify each of the following:

1. Maxillary central incisors
2. Mandibular central incisors
3. Maxillary lateral incisors
4. Mandibular lateral incisors
5. Maxillary canines
6. Mandibular canines
7. Maxillary premolars
8. Mandibular premolars
9. Maxillary molars
10. Mandibular molars
11. Occlusal surfaces
12. Incisal surfaces
13. Lingual surfaces
14. Facial surfaces
15. Mesial surface of the maxillary central incisors
16. Distal surface of the mandibular central incisors

Procedure 4.2

Identify the Primary and Permanent Teeth Using the Universal National System, the Fédération Dentaire Internationale System, and the Palmer Notation System

Goal

To identify the teeth correctly using each numbering system.

Equipment and Supplies

- Study model or typodont
- Worksheet from student workbook or Evolve (or create your own worksheet by dividing a piece of paper into three columns labeled with the three numbering systems and a row to fill in the name of each tooth)

Procedural Steps

Identify each of the following:

1. Primary teeth in each arch using the Universal National System.
2. Primary teeth in each arch using the Fédération Dentaire Internationale System.
3. Primary teeth in each arch using the Palmer Notation System.
4. Permanent teeth in each arch using the Universal National System.
5. Permanent teeth in each arch using the Fédération Dentaire Internationale System.
6. Permanent teeth in each arch using the Palmer Notation System.

Chapter Exercises

Multiple Choice

Circle the letter next to the correct answer.

1. The chewing surfaces of the posterior teeth are called _____ surfaces.
   a. incisal
   b. lingual
   c. buccal
   d. occlusal

2. How many teeth are in the permanent dentition?
   a. 28
   b. 32
   c. 16
   d. 20

3. In the Universal National System, tooth #9 is the _____.
   a. maxillary left central incisor
   b. maxillary right central incisor
   c. mandibular left central incisor
   d. mandibular right central incisor

4. In the Fédération Dentaire Internationale (FDI) System, tooth #11 is the _____.
   a. maxillary right third molar
   b. maxillary right central incisor
   c. maxillary left central incisor
   d. maxillary left canine

5. The surfaces of the teeth that are nearest to the tongue are the _____ surfaces.
   a. buccal
   b. lingual
   c. occlusal
   d. incisal

6. *Occlusion* refers to the _____.
   a. contact area on the proximal surfaces of the teeth
   b. contact of the maxillary and mandibular arches
   c. space between the proximal surfaces of the teeth
   d. contours of the teeth

7. When the arches are divided into six parts, each part is called a(n) _____.
   a. quadrant
   b. sextant
   c. arch
   d. embrasure

8. The primary dentition contains four premolars.
   a. True
   b. False

9. The teeth that are sometimes called the "corner" of the arch are the _____.
   a. lateral incisors
   b. premolars
   c. canines
   d. first permanent molars

10. The proximal surface that is located farthest away from the midline is the _____ surface.
    a. distal
    b. mesial
    c. facial
    d. lingual

Apply Your Knowledge

1. Provide the professional terminology for each of the following dental terms: front tooth, back tooth, top teeth, bottom teeth, and chewing surfaces.
2. In which area of the mouth is tooth #19 located?
3. The parent of a 3-year-old asks you to tell her about the process of her daughter losing her "baby" teeth and wants to know when she will get her permanent teeth. How would you reply?

CHAPTER 5

Microbiology and Disease Transmission

http://evolve.elsevier.com/Robinson/essentials/

LEARNING OBJECTIVES

1. Pronounce, define, and spell the key terms.
2. Compare and contrast the types of pathogens, and provide examples of each.
3. Explain the concept of the chain of infection.
4. Explain the differences between acute, chronic, latent, and opportunistic infections.
5. Identify the various modes in which disease transmission can occur in the dental office setting.
6. Name and describe the viral diseases that are of major concern to dental health care professionals.
7. Name and describe the bacterial diseases that are of major concern to dental health care professionals.

KEY TERMS

acute infection
aerosols
bacteria
bacterial endocarditis
bloodborne diseases
chronic infection
coronavirus
cross-contamination
direct transmission
fungi
hepatitis A

hepatitis B
hepatitis C
hepatitis D
HIV
host
host susceptibility
human papillomavirus
indirect transmission
infectious disease
latent infection
microbiology

mists
opportunistic infection
parenteral transmission
pathogen
portal of entry
spores
tuberculosis
virulence
viruses

The dental assistant is at risk for exposure to infectious diseases through occupational exposure. In this chapter, you will learn about the organisms that cause infectious diseases and how to recognize the diseases that are of concern to dental professionals. You will learn how these diseases can spread in the dental office and the steps you can take to protect yourself, other staff members, and patients from disease transmission in the dental office.

Microbiology is the study of microorganisms (with *micro* meaning microscopically small and *bio* meaning living organisms). Because of their microscopic size, the existence of microorganisms usually goes unnoticed unless they cause illness. Most people experience common colds in the winter months, and others may experience life-threatening illnesses caused by microorganisms.

Pathogens

A **pathogen** is any small organism such as a virus, bacteria, or other microorganism that can cause disease. These microorganisms are so small that they can be seen only under a microscope.

Bacteria

Bacteria (singular bacterium) are a large group of one-celled microorganisms that can be found in all environments, such as soil, water, organic matter, and the bodies of animals. Most bacteria can live independently under favorable environmental conditions and can be spread by many means of transmission.

Humans naturally **host** a variety of bacteria. The skin, respiratory tract, and gastrointestinal tract are inhabited by a variety of harmless bacteria called normal flora. They are beneficial and protect the human host by aiding in metabolism and preventing entrance of harmful bacteria. An infection occurs when bacteria occurring naturally in one part of the body invade another part of the body and become harmful. The discovery of the first true antibiotic penicillin in 1928 for bacterial infections is considered one of the most important breakthroughs in medical history.

When viewed under a microscope, bacteria have three shapes: spherical, rod shaped, and spiral (Fig. 5.1 and Table 5.1).

Spores

Under unfavorable conditions, some bacteria change into a highly resistant form called **spores**. Spores are one-cell units that can grow into new organisms with the right conditions. Tetanus is an example of a disease caused by a spore-forming bacillus.

Bacteria can remain alive in the spore form but be inactive to reproduce or cause disease. When conditions are favorable, the bacteria can become active and then capable of causing disease.

TABLE 5.1

Shapes of Bacteria and Diseases in Which They Occur

Shape	Name	Disease
Spherical	Streptococci	"Strep" throat, pneumonia, tonsillitis
	Staphylococci	Boils, skin infections, MRSA
Rod-shaped	Bacilli	Urinary tract infections, food poisoning, meningitis. Tuberculosis
Spiral-shaped	Spirochetes	Syphilis, Lyme disease

MRSA, Methicillin-resistant Staphylococcus aureus.

Spores represent the most resistant form of life. They can survive in extremes of heat and dryness, as well as in the presence of disinfectants and radiation. Because of this incredible resistance, spore testing is now used to test the effectiveness of sterilization of instruments used in dentistry (see Chapter 8).

Viruses

Viruses are microorganisms smaller than bacteria that live and multiply only inside an appropriate host cell. Host cells may be human, animal, plant, or bacteria. A virus invades a host cell, replicates (produces copies of itself), and then destroys the host cell, releasing the virus into the body. A virus can spread

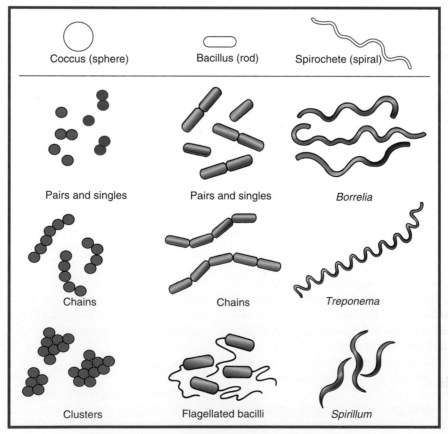

FIGURE 5.1 Three basic shapes of bacteria.

through touch, exchange of saliva, coughing or sneezing, sexual contact, contaminated food or water, and insects.

Despite their tiny size, many viruses cause fatal diseases. New and increasingly destructive viruses are being discovered and have resulted in the creation of a special area within microbiology called *virology* (the study of viruses and their effects).

The various forms of viruses are discussed in greater detail later in this chapter.

Latency

Some viruses establish a latent (dormant) state in host cells. A latent virus can be reactivated in the future and can produce more infective viral particles, followed by signs and symptoms of the disease.

Stress, infection with another virus, and exposure to ultraviolet light can reactivate a virus. Some patients with human immunodeficiency virus (HIV) infection have experienced prolonged periods of latency and have remained in good health for many years. For example, hepatitis C virus (HCV) is known to have a latency period of 15 to 25 years.

Treatment of Viral Diseases

Viruses cause many clinically significant diseases in humans. Unfortunately, most viral diseases can only be symptomatically treated (i.e., by treating the symptom, not the infection itself).

General antibiotic medications are not effective in preventing or shortening viral infections. Even the few drugs that are effective against specific viruses have limitations because viruses often produce different types of infection, have different host cells, or can cause serious side effects.

Vaccines are being developed against viruses, but because a virus is capable of mutation (changing), they can be very difficult to develop. Viruses can change to become better suited to survive current conditions and to resist efforts to kill them.

Fungi

Fungi are organisms that eat organic material, such as plants, yeasts, and molds that lack chlorophyll. (Chlorophyll is the substance that makes plants green.) Athlete's foot, ringworm (which is not a worm), and candidiasis are examples of diseases caused by fungi.

Oral candidiasis is caused by the yeast *Candida albicans.* Oral candidiasis is characterized by white membranes on the surface of the oral mucosa, on the tongue, and elsewhere in the oral cavity. The lesions may resemble thin cottage cheese; wiping reveals a raw, red, and sometimes bleeding base (Fig. 5.2). All forms of candidiasis are opportunistic infections, especially affecting the young, elderly, and patients who are extremely ill. Candidiasis is frequently seen in patients who wear dentures or in patients with HIV infection.

Candidiasis is treated with topical antifungal preparations such as nystatin in the form of lozenges.

Chain of Infection

To understand how infections can occur, imagine a chain that has six links. Each link is a condition that *must be present* before infection or disease can occur. Infection control practices are

FIGURE 5.2 Pseudomembranous candidiasis. (From Ibsen OAC, Phelan JA: *Oral pathology for the dental hygienist,* ed 6, St. Louis, 2014, Saunders.)

designed to break one or more of the links. The links in the chain of infection include: (1) infectious agent, (2) reservoir, (3) portal of exit, (4) method of transmission, (5) portal of entry, and (6) susceptible host (Fig. 5.3).

An **infectious agent** is a pathogen (e.g., bacterium, virus, fungus) and must be present in sufficient numbers to cause infection. In addition to the numbers, the organism must be **virulent**. Virulence means the degree, or the strength, of an organism's ability to cause disease. If an organism is not very potent, then it may not be capable of causing disease.

A **reservoir** is the place where the organisms normally live and reproduce. Examples of reservoirs include humans, animals, water, food, contaminated surfaces, and bioburden. *Bioburden* refers to organic materials such as blood and saliva. Handwashing and cleaning contaminated surfaces will minimize reservoirs for microorganisms.

Portal of exit refers to the method the pathogen uses to leave the reservoir. It could be from contaminated hands, surfaces or instruments, or body fluids such as a sneeze.

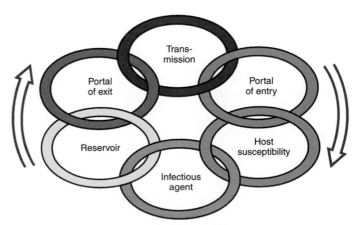

FIGURE 5.3 At least one link must be removed to break the chain of infection. (From Potter PA, Perry AG, Stockert P, et al: *Mosby's basic nursing,* ed 7, St. Louis, 2013, Mosby.)

TABLE 5.2

Portals of Entry for Disease Transmission

Portal	Examples	Means of Prevention
Inhalation	Breathing aerosols generated from handpieces or the air-water syringe or from uncovered ultrasonic cleaning devices	Wear face masks for chairside procedures and when processing contaminated instruments and surfaces. Note: Face shields protect against splatter but not against inhalation.
Ingestion	Swallowing droplets of blood or saliva spattered into the mouth; bare hands coming into contact with contaminated surfaces or items, then handling food items	Wear personal protective equipment (PPE), frequently wash hands, and keep surfaces free from contamination by using barriers or surface disinfectants.
Mucous membrane	Droplets of blood or saliva spattering into the eyes, nose, or mouth	Wear face masks and safety glasses with side and bottom shields during chairside procedures and when processing contaminated instruments and surfaces.
Breaks in skin	Cuts or sticks from contaminated sharps; instrument punctures; cuts or cracks on ungloved hands or torn gloves	Develop and practice safe work habits. Replace torn or punctured gloves as soon as possible. Protect hands from becoming chapped or cracked. Wash hands.

Transmission is the mechanism the pathogen uses to spread from one host to another.

Portal of entry refers to the method by which the pathogen enters the body. The portals of entry for airborne pathogens are through the mouth and nose. Bloodborne pathogens must have access to the blood supply as a means of entry into the body. The portal of entry into the blood supply can occur through a break in the skin caused by a needlestick, a cut, or even a human bite. It can also occur through the mucous membranes of the nose and oral cavity (Table 5.2).

Host susceptibility is the ability of the human body (host) to resist a pathogen. The healthier you are, the better your resistance to disease. Low resistance resulting from fatigue, physical or emotional strain, poor nutrition, injury, surgery, or the presence of other diseases can weaken a person's immunity. The more pathogens that are present, the better their chances of overwhelming the host and producing disease.

Infection control efforts are aimed at preventing the transmission of disease and reducing the number of pathogens that are present.

Factors Affecting Resistance to Infection

- Patient's immune status
- Patient's age
- Patient's nutritional status
- Medications taken
- Allergies
- Alcohol consumption
- Psychologic state

Types of Infections

An infection occurs when a pathogenic microbe can multiply in the tissue within which it is lodged. An **infectious disease** is one that is communicable or contagious. This term means that the disease can be transmitted (spread) in some way from one host to another.

Acute Infection

In an **acute infection**, symptoms are often severe and usually appear soon after the initial infection occurs. Acute infections are short in duration. For example, with a viral infection, such as the common cold, the body's defense mechanisms usually eliminate the virus within 2 to 3 weeks.

Chronic Infection

A **chronic infection** is one during which the microorganism is present for a long duration; in some chronic infections, microorganisms may persist for life. The person may be asymptomatic (not showing symptoms of the disease) but may still be a carrier of the disease, such as with **hepatitis B** virus (HBV), HCV, or HIV infection.

Latent Infection

A **latent infection** is a persistent infection during which the symptoms "come and go." Cold sores (oral herpes simplex) and genital herpes are latent viral infections.

The virus first enters the body and causes the original lesion. It then lies dormant away from the surface in a nerve cell until certain conditions, such as illness with fever, sunburn, or stress, cause the virus to leave the nerve cell and again seek the surface. Once the virus reaches the surface, it becomes detectable for a short time and causes another outbreak at that site.

Opportunistic Infection

An **opportunistic infection** is normally caused by non-pathogenic organisms and occurs in individuals whose resistance is decreased or compromised. For example, an individual diagnosed with the flu may develop pneumonia or an ear infection. Opportunistic infections are common in patients with autoimmune disease or diabetes and in older adults.

Modes of Disease Transmission

Before you can prevent disease transmission in the dental office, you must first understand how infectious diseases are spread (Fig. 5.4).

Direct Transmission

Pathogens can be transferred through direct transmission by coming into direct contact with an infectious lesion or infected body fluids, including blood, saliva, semen, and vaginal secretions. Many viruses and pathogenic bacteria are directly transmitted and cause hepatitis, herpes infection, HIV infection, and tuberculosis.

Exposure to blood and saliva is of concern for dental professionals during dental treatment. Although blood may not be visible in the saliva, it is often present.

Indirect Transmission

Indirect transfer of organisms to a susceptible person can occur by handling contaminated instruments or by touching contaminated surfaces and then touching the face, eyes, or mouth. Frequently washing your hands to avoid indirect transmission of microorganisms is important. Indirect transmission is also known as cross-contamination.

In the dental office, diseases may be indirectly transmitted via soiled hands and towels, contaminated instruments, and even dust. In addition, anything that is touched during patient care—faucet handles, switches, handpieces, instrument drawer handles, dental materials, the patient record, protective eyewear, and even the pen used to make an entry—is considered contaminated and potentially capable of spreading disease.

Splash or Spatter

Blood, saliva, or nasopharyngeal (nasal) secretions can be sprayed or spattered during dental procedures. Diseases can be transmitted during a dental procedure by splashing the mucosa (mouth or eyes) or nonintact skin with blood or blood-contaminated saliva.

Intact skin, which is not broken in any way, acts as a natural protective barrier. Nonintact skin, in which a cut, scrape, or needlestick injury has occurred, provides an entrance for pathogens to enter the body.

Airborne Transmission

Airborne transmission, also known as **droplet infection**, is the spread of disease through droplets of moisture containing bacteria or viruses. Most of the contagious respiratory diseases are caused by pathogens carried in droplets of moisture. Some of these pathogens are carried long distances through the air and ventilation systems. Airborne transmission can also occur when someone coughs or sneezes.

Aerosols containing saliva, blood, and microorganisms are created with the use of the high-speed handpiece, air-water syringe, and ultrasonic scaler during dental procedures (Fig. 5.5). Inhaling bacteria and debris in the aerosol (without the protection of a face mask) is comparable to having someone sneeze in your face twice a minute at a distance of 1 foot.

Mists are droplet particles larger than those generated by the aerosol spray. Mists, such as those from coughing, can transmit respiratory infections. Nevertheless, mists do not appear to transmit HBV or HIV infection, despite being inhaled.

Spatter consists of large droplet particles contaminated with blood, saliva, and other debris. Spatter is created during all restorative and hygiene procedures involving rotary and ultrasonic dental instruments. The use of the air-water syringe may also produce spatter.

Spatter droplets travel farther than the aerosol mist and tend to land on the upper surfaces of the wrist and forearms, upper arms, and chest. Droplets may also reach the collar area of the dentist, dental assistant, or hygienist.

Parenteral Transmission

Parenteral means through the skin, as with cuts or punctures. Parenteral transmission of bloodborne pathogens (disease-causing organisms transferred through contact with blood or other bodily fluids) can occur through needlestick injuries, human bites, cuts, abrasions, or any break in the skin.

Bloodborne Transmission

Certain pathogens, referred to as *bloodborne*, are carried in the blood and body fluids of infected individuals and can be

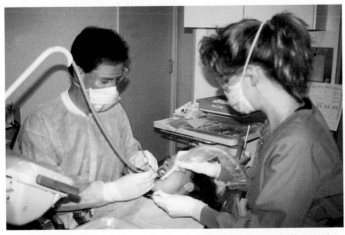

FIGURE 5.4 Pathogens can be transferred from staff member to patient, from patient to staff member, or from patient to patient through contaminated equipment.

FIGURE 5.5 Aerosol from an ultrasonic scaler. (Courtesy Hu-Friedy Manufacturing, Chicago, Illinois.)

transmitted to others. Bloodborne transmission occurs through direct or indirect contact with blood and other body fluids. Saliva is of concern during dental treatment because it is frequently contaminated with blood. Remember, although blood is not visible in the saliva, it may be present.

Improperly sterilized instruments and equipment can transfer all **bloodborne diseases**. Individuals who share needles when using illegal drugs easily transmit these diseases to each other. Unprotected sex is another common method of transmitting a bloodborne disease.

Common bloodborne microorganisms of concern in dentistry include HCV, HBV, and HIV. Because dental treatment often involves contact with blood and always with saliva, bloodborne diseases are of major concern in the dental office.

Food and Water Transmission

Many diseases are transmitted by contaminated food that has not been properly cooked or refrigerated and by water that has been contaminated with human or animal fecal material. For example, contaminated food or water spread tuberculosis, botulism, and staphylococcal and streptococcal infections.

Fecal-Oral Transmission

Many pathogens are present in fecal matter. If proper sanitation procedures, such as handwashing after using the toilet, are not followed, then these pathogens may be directly transmitted by touching another person or may be indirectly transmitted by contact with contaminated surfaces or food.

Fecal-oral transmission occurs most often among health care and daycare workers (who frequently change diapers) and in irresponsible food handlers.

Transient Bacteremia

Bacteria entering the bloodstream and causing the temporary presence of bacteria in the blood is called *transient bacteremia*. (**Transient** means *temporary* or *moving*, and **bacteremia** means the *presence of bacteria in the blood*.)

For most healthy patients, transient bacteremia is not a problem because the body is able to destroy the bacteria quickly. Nevertheless, even the temporary presence of bacteria in the blood is dangerous for high-risk patients, such as those with a history of congenital heart disease, rheumatic fever, or open heart surgery; those with certain forms of heart disease; those wearing pacemakers; and those with an artificial joint, such as a hip replacement.

For high-risk patients, the danger of **bacterial endocarditis** (bacterial infection of the lining of the heart) or a bacterial infection at the site of the implant exists. The administration of prophylactic (preventive) antibiotic medications for these patients is discussed in Chapter 9.

Viral Diseases of Major Concern to Dental Health Care Workers

A viral disease is an illness or health condition caused by a virus. Many viruses are spread from person to person.

Respiratory Viral Diseases

This type of flu or viral infection attacks your respiratory system (nose, throat, and lungs). For most individuals, the flu will run its course on its own, but sometimes the flu and its complications can affect a higher risk population.

The virus will travel through the air in droplets through a cough, sneeze, or just talking. You can also inhale the droplets directly or pick up the germs from an object that you have touched then transmitted to your eyes, nose, or mouth.

The Centers for Disease Control and Prevention (CDC) recommends an annual flu vaccination for everyone 6 months of age or older. The vaccine is a yearly vaccine and most health care providers are encouraged or even required to receive the flu vaccine.

Coronavirus is an upper respiratory virus that infects humans. The virus is spread through the air by coughing and sneezing, close personal contact, and touching an object or surface. The two most known coronaviruses to date are the SARS-CoV (severe acute respiratory syndrome) and the most recent COVID-19 (2019 novel coronavirus). The World Health Organization designated SARS as a global health threat in 2003 and the epidemic killed approximately 774 people worldwide before it was contained.

COVID-19 was recently deemed a pandemic and has a confirmed 4.9 million cases diagnosed, with 5 million world wide deaths. People with COVID-19 have had a wide range of symptoms reported, ranging from mild to severe illness to death. Because this virus is ever-changing, it is important to keep up to date by visiting the CDC at www.cdc.gov/coronavirus/2019-ncov.html.

Gastrointestinal Viral Diseases

This virus, also referred to as the "stomach flu," affects your digestive tract. A gastrointestinal virus initiates in food or water that has been contaminated by feces. The virus can also be transmitted when sharing utensils or personal objects with someone who has the virus.

Exanthematous Viral Diseases

Also known as infectious diseases of childhood, the exanthematous viral diseases include measles, rubella, German measles, and mumps. The term *exanthem* describes a rash type of reaction to something. Most of these viruses are spread through respiratory droplets from a cough or sneeze but can also be transmitted by coming into contact with fluid from broken skin lesions. The incidence of these diseases, which were once endemic among childhood populations, is now prevented by the administration of a vaccine.

Hepatic Viral Diseases

The hepatic viral diseases cause inflammation of the liver, also known as viral hepatitis. There are at least five types of viral hepatitis, each of which is caused by a different virus: **hepatitis A** virus (HAV), **HBV**, **HCV**, **hepatitis D** virus (HDV), and **hepatitis E** virus (HEV) (Table 5.3).

Hepatitis A

HAV can affect anyone. It is spread from person to person by putting something in the mouth that has been contaminated with the stool of a person with HAV. This type of transmission is

TABLE 5.3
Primary Types of Hepatitis

	A (HAV)	B (HAV)	C (HCV)	D (HDV)	E (HEV)
Source of the virus	Fecal-oral	Blood and body fluids	Blood and body fluids	Blood and body fluids	Fecal-oral
Route of transmission	Fecal-oral	Percutaneous and mucosal tissues	Percutaneous and mucosal tissues	Percutaneous and mucosal tissues	Fecal-oral
Chronic infection	No	Yes	Yes	Yes	No
Prevention	Vaccine	Immunization	Perform blood donor screening; modify risky behavior	Hepatitis B vaccine	Ensure safe drinking water

From Bird D, Robinson D: *Modern dental assisting,* ed 11, St. Louis, 2015, Elsevier.

called *fecal-oral.* Good personal hygiene and proper sanitation can help prevent HAV. Always wash your hands after changing a diaper or using the bathroom. HAV is the least serious form of viral hepatitis. A vaccine is available that provides long-term prevention in persons older than 2 years.

Hepatitis B

HBV is transmitted when blood, semen, or another body fluid from a person infected enters the body. HBV is the leading cause of broad-spectrum liver diseases such as liver cancer, cirrhosis of the liver, liver failure, and even death. HBV is a bloodborne disease that may also be transmitted by other body fluids, including saliva.

Anyone who has ever had HBV and some who have been exposed but have not actually been ill may be carriers of HBV, which means that patients who appear to be healthy and have no history of the disease may actually be spreading the infection to others. HBV is responsible for 34% of all types of acute viral hepatitis, which presents a high risk for dental personnel because dental treatment brings them into contact with saliva and blood. In addition, dental personnel may unknowingly be carriers of the disease. In this situation, the risk for transmitting the infection to the patient during treatment is always present.

Hepatitis B immunization. A highly effective vaccine is available to prevent HBV. All dental personnel with a chance of occupational exposure should be vaccinated against HBV. The Occupational Safety & Health Administration (OSHA) Bloodborne Pathogens (BBP) Standard (see Chapter 6) requires that an employer offer the HBV vaccination at no cost to an employee within 10 days of initial assignment to a position in which the chance of occupational exposure to blood and/or other body fluids exists. The employee has the right to refuse the offer of vaccination; however, that employee must sign a release form indicating that the employer offered the vaccine and that the employee understands the potential risks of contracting HBV.

Postvaccination testing is recommended 1 to 6 months after the third injection to ensure that the individual has developed the antibodies necessary for immunity. Should antibodies not be present, the three-dose series should be repeated. The HBV vaccine is considered safe for pregnant women.

Hepatitis C

HCV is a bloodborne viral infection. The primary concern of occupational exposure to HCV is needlesticks or other percutaneous injuries. *Percutaneous* means performed through the skin and can occur from an accidental needlestick to an employee in a dental office, from sharing contaminated needles among injection drug users, or from contaminated tattoo needles. The carrier rate associated with HCV is higher than that associated with HBV. Unfortunately, no vaccine against HCV exists, nor has a cure for the disease been found. The U.S. Food and Drug Administration (FDA) approved two new direct-acting antiviral drugs to treat chronic HCV infection.

Hepatitis D

HDV is a viral infection that only occurs with HBV and causes liver inflammation and damage. Persons with coinfection of HBV and HDV often have more severe acute disease and a higher risk for death compared with those infected with HBV alone. Vaccination against HBV will also prevent infection with HDV.

Hepatitis E

HEV is a virus that affects the liver. It is not transmitted through bloodborne contact and is most frequently transmitted via the fecal-oral route through contaminated food or water. The disease is most frequently seen in the form of an epidemic in developing countries, and transmission is not a major concern in a standard dental setting.

Human Immunodeficiency Virus

HIV infection is a bloodborne viral disease. The virus attacks and weakens or destroys the immune system. A blood test can be used to determine the presence of antibodies to HIV before symptoms appear.

A **positive test**, also known as a *seropositive result,* indicates that the individual is infected with HIV, is a carrier, and can transmit the virus to others. (As used here, *sero-* refers to serum, which is the liquid portion of blood.)

A **negative test**, also known as a *seronegative result,* means that no infection was present at the time of the test. This result does not, however, suggest immunity to the virus.

A person with HIV infection may remain healthy for many years. People who are HIV positive develop acquired immunodeficiency syndrome (AIDS) when they become sick with serious illnesses and infections that can occur with HIV infection. Several oral conditions are frequently associated with HIV infection.

Routes of Human Immunodeficiency Virus Transmission

HIV infection is spread by sexual contact with an infected person or by needle sharing among drug users. Before blood donor screening for HIV, the virus was also transmitted by blood transfusions. Now that blood is screened for HIV antibodies, the blood supply in this country is safe. Babies born to HIV-infected mothers may become infected before or during birth or through breastfeeding after birth.

In (nondental) health care settings, workers have been infected with HIV by being stuck with needles containing HIV-infected blood or, less frequently, after infected blood has gotten into the worker's bloodstream through an open cut or splashes into a mucous membrane (e.g., eyes, inside of the nose).

Transmission of HIV itself is a concern but is not a major threat in the dental setting. Nevertheless, patients who are HIV positive often have other diseases that can be transmitted more easily through dental treatment. Transmission of these diseases, particularly tuberculosis and HBV, pose a threat to dental personnel (Table 5.4).

Herpes Viruses

The herpes virus is a viral infection. Infections are categorized based on the part of the body infected.

Herpes Simplex Virus Type 1

Herpes simplex virus (HSV)-1, also referred to as *oral herpes*, is a viral infection that causes recurrent sores on lips. Because these sores frequently develop when the patient has a cold or fever of another origin, the disease has become commonly known as *fever blisters* or *cold sores.*

Primary Herpes

Primary herpes, which is highly contagious, makes its first appearance in young children (1 to 3 years of age).

The child may have a slight fever, pain in the mouth, increased salivation, bad breath, and a general feeling of illness. The inside of the mouth becomes swollen, and the gingivae are inflamed.

Natural healing begins within 3 days, and the illness is usually over in 7 to 14 days. During this time, supportive measures can be taken to make the child more comfortable, to relieve the pain, and to prevent secondary infection.

Recurrent Herpes Labialis

After an initial herpes labialis infection during childhood, the HSV lies dormant and reappears later in life as the familiar recurring fever blister or cold sore (Fig. 5.6).

Recurrences tend to take place when the patient's general resistance is lowered because of stress, fever, illness, injury, and exposure to the sun. Use of sunscreen with a sun protection factor (SPF) of 15 helps prevent sun-induced recurrences of herpes.

Attacks may recur as infrequently as once a year or as often as weekly or even daily. As in the case of primary herpes, recurrent herpes labialis sores heal by themselves in 7 to 10 days, leaving no scar.

Herpes Simplex Virus Type 2

HSV-2, also known as *genital herpes,* is one of the most common sexually transmitted diseases (STDs) in the United States. Initial symptoms, which generally appear 2 to 10 days after infection, include tingling, itching, and a burning sensation during urination.

Once a person is infected with HSV-2, outbreaks will recur. The disease can be transmitted only during these recurrences.

A mother with active vaginal or cervical herpetic lesions at the time of delivery can pass HSV-2 to her newborn. Approximately 50% of such newborns will be infected as they pass through the birth canal. At least 85% of infected infants will be severely damaged or killed by the virus.

Herpes Zoster Virus

Herpes zoster virus (HZV; human herpesvirus type 3) causes both varicella (chickenpox) and herpes zoster (shingles). Although these are two different diseases, both are caused by the same organism. Chickenpox is the primary infection, and herpes zoster is the reactivation of illness. HZV is a highly contagious infection in individuals who have not been previously exposed to the virus. Transmission occurs by direct contact with skin lesions or by droplet infection from infectious saliva.

Cytomegalovirus

Cytomegalovirus (CMV; human herpesvirus type 5) rarely causes disease unless other factors, such as a compromised immune system, are present. Nevertheless, CMV can infect the fetus during pregnancy. In some cases, infants will be born deaf or will suffer mental retardation. The route of transmission of CMV is unclear.

Epstein-Barr Virus

Epstein-Barr virus (EBV; human herpesvirus type 4) is responsible for several infections, including infectious mononucleosis, nasopharyngeal cancer, lymphoma, and oral hairy leukoplakia

TABLE 5.4

Routes of Human Transmission of the Human Immunodeficiency Virus (HIV)

Routes of Transmission	Comments
Sexual contact	Is most easily transmitted through blood, semen, and vaginal secretions during sexual intercourse; women are 10 times more likely than men to become infected in this manner
Shared needles	Is transmitted through exposure to shared needles during illegal drug use and through tattoo needles
Exposure to blood	Is transmitted through accidental exposure to blood that occurs in the health care setting
Organ donation Blood or blood product transfusions	Transmission can also occur in rituals during which commingling of blood occurs, such as becoming "blood brothers"
During birth During breastfeeding	An infected mother can transmit the HIV infection to her child

FIGURE 5.6 Herpes labialis. **A,** 12 hours after onset. **B,** 48 hours after onset. (From Ibsen OAC, Phelan JA: *Oral pathology for the dental hygienist,* ed 6, St. Louis, 2014, Saunders.)

FIGURE 5.7 Hairy leukoplakia. (From Ibsen OAC, Phelan JA: *Oral pathology for the dental hygienist,* ed 6, St. Louis, 2014, Saunders.)

(a condition commonly seen in patients with HIV) (Fig. 5.7). Infectious mononucleosis is an acute infectious disease that primarily affects people between 15 and 20 years of age. EBV is present in the saliva and is transmitted by kissing; thus it is often called the "kissing disease."

Herpes Transmission

The major transmission route for the herpesvirus is through direct contact with lesions or with infectious saliva. When oral lesions are present, the patient may be asked to reschedule their appointment for a time after the lesions have healed. Even when no active lesions are present, viral transmission through saliva or through the aerosol spray from the dental handpiece is still a possibility.

Because no preventive vaccine is available to protect against herpes, taking precautions to prevent exposure is essential.

Protective eyewear for the dental professional is particularly important because a herpes infection in the eye may cause blindness. Gloves protect the dental professional against infection through lesions or abrasions on the hands.

Human Papillomavirus

Human papillomavirus (HPV) is the most common sexually transmitted disease (STD) in the United States. The population most affected are in their late teens and early 20s. A person can get HPV by having vaginal, anal, or oral sex with someone who has the virus. The virus can be transmitted even when an infected person has no signs or symptoms.

The most common symptoms are skin or mucous membrane growths (warts), but some types of the genital HPV can cause cancer. The risk factors for the infection include multiple sexual partners, age, weakened immune system, and personal contact.

The HPV two-dose vaccination is recommended for all boys and girls at age 11 to 12, and then 6 to 12 months after the first dose. If a person did not receive the vaccine at that age, it is recommended for everyone through the age of 26 years.

Bacterial Diseases of Major Concern to Dental Health Care Workers

Tuberculosis

Tuberculosis, which is caused by the bacterium *Mycobacterium tuberculosis,* is the leading cause of death worldwide from infectious diseases.

Because patients infected with HIV have a weakened immune system, they are highly susceptible to tuberculosis; therefore HIV and tuberculosis are often present together. Of the two, tuberculosis presents a greater health risk for health care workers. One reason for this is that the rod-shaped tubercle bacillus can withstand disinfectants that kill many other bacteria. Surface disinfectants are further discussed in Chapter 7.

Transmission of Tuberculosis

Infection with active disease. A patient who is diagnosed with the signs described is in the active stage.

Signs of Tuberculosis
- Productive cough lasting longer than 3 weeks (Sputum, a thick mucus from the lungs, is productive and expelled in the cough)
- Unexplained fever, fatigue, or night sweats
- Unexplained weight loss and loss of appetite
- Member of a high-risk group

This patient may easily spread the disease through prolonged close contact. Tuberculosis is primarily spread when the individual coughs and the tubercle bacilli, which are present in the sputum, are expelled through the mouth. These bacteria are inhaled by others and carried to their lungs. A healthy individual is generally able to fight off the infection; however, someone who is already weakened with other illnesses may become infected.

Transmission of the disease can also occur through the consumption of contaminated milk and through contact with infected cattle.

Infection without active disease. Of all people who are exposed to tuberculosis, 90% are infected without active disease; that is, they carry the disease but never have active symptoms. Although they do not transmit the disease at this stage, if resistance is weakened, then the tubercle bacilli may become active.

After a patient has had the active disease and seems to be well, they will always be a carrier for the disease.

Legionnaires' Disease

The *Legionella pneumophila* bacterium (named after an epidemic of this disease during an American Legion convention in Philadelphia) is responsible for two acute bacterial diseases: Pontiac fever and legionnaires' disease. Bacteria are transmitted through aerosolization and aspiration of contaminated water (see Chapter 7 for a discussion on dental unit water lines).

No person-to-person transmission occurs. *L. pneumophila* bacteria have been found to thrive in lakes, creeks, hot tubs, spas, air-conditioning systems, shower heads, water distillation systems, and the biofilm found in dental unit water lines (Fig. 5.8). Dental personnel have higher antibodies against *L. pneumophila* than the public, indicating occupational exposure and a resistance to this organism.

Pontiac fever is the least serious form of infection, causing acute flulike symptoms with headache, high fever, dry cough, chills, diarrhea, chest pain, and abdominal pain.

Legionnaires' disease is the more serious form of infection, causing very severe pneumonia. In those who are immunocompromised or in older adults, the disease can be fatal.

Tetanus

Tetanus, which is also known as *lockjaw,* is a dangerous and often fatal disease that is caused by a spore-forming bacillus

FIGURE 5.8 Bacteria in biofilm taken from dental unit water lines. (Courtesy Dr. Shannon Mills.)

FIGURE 5.9 Chancres on the tongue and lip seen in a person with primary syphilis. (From Schachner LA, Hansen RC, eds: *Pediatric dermatology,* ed 4, London, 2011, Mosby.)

found in soil, dust, or animal or human feces. This microbe is usually introduced into the body through a wound or break in the skin (as in a puncture wound from a soiled instrument).

The organism causing tetanus produces the severe muscle spasms and rigidity that give the disease its popular name of lockjaw. The disease can be prevented by the administration of a vaccine; however, immunity must be kept current through booster doses. (It is important that dental personnel keep all immunizations current.)

Syphilis

Syphilis, an STD, is caused by *Treponema pallidum* spirochetes. Although these bacteria are fragile outside of the body, the danger of direct cross-infection exists in the dental operatory through contact with oral lesions.

The first stage of syphilis involves the presence of a painless ulcerating sore, known as a *chancre,* which is infectious on contact. When it occurs on the lip, it may resemble herpes, but the crusting is darker (Fig. 5.9).

Oral Signs of Syphilis

- Split papules at the corners of the mouth
- Grayish-white, moist mucous patches on the tongue, roof of mouth, tonsils, or inner surfaces of the lips (These patches are highly infectious.)
- Generalized rash resembling a measles rash, poxlike pustules, oozing sores, and hair falling out of the scalp

---

The second stage of syphilis is also infectious, and immediate infection may occur through contact with an open sore. The third stage, known as *latent syphilis,* is usually fatal and may occur after the disease has been dormant for 20 years.

☐ Ethical Implications

Regardless of whether your state has established minimum standards for infection control in the dental setting, doing everything possible to prevent the transmission of disease to patients, to other staff members, and to yourself is your ethical responsibility.

Chapter Exercises

Multiple Choice

Circle the letter next to the correct answer.

1. A microorganism that can cause disease is called a(n) _____.
   a. pathogen
   b. host
   c. virulence
   d. autogenous

2. A large group of one-celled microorganisms capable of causing a disease are _____.
   a. pathogens
   b. bacteria
   c. viruses
   d. all of the above

3. The forms of life that are most resistant to extremes of heat and dryness are _____.
   a. bacteria
   b. viruses
   c. fungi
   d. spores
   e. all of the above

4. Another term for the disease often called *lockjaw* is _____.
   a. hepatitis
   b. Pontiac fever
   c. tetanus
   d. bacterial endocarditis

5. The serious disease that can be transmitted from contaminated dental water in dental lines is _____.
   a. hepatitis
   b. tuberculosis
   c. legionnaires' disease
   d. herpes

6. The sexually transmitted form of herpes is _____.
   a. HSV-1
   b. HSV-2
   c. HZV
   d. EBV

7. The virus that enters the human body and attacks the immune system is _____.
   a. HBV
   b. HCV
   c. HZV
   d. HIV

8. Which of the following types of hepatitis is *NOT* a bloodborne disease?
   a. HAV
   b. HBV
   c. HCV
   d. HDV

9. Which of the following types of hepatitis is *NOT* capable of replicating itself?
   a. HAV
   b. HBV
   c. HCV
   d. HDV

10. An infection resulting from bacteria that are normally present in the patient's mouth is called _____.
    a. coinfection
    b. autogenous infection
    c. transient bacteremia
    d. carrier transmission

Apply Your Knowledge

1. Your patient today, Mr. Jerry Davis, informs you that he is recovering from shingles. What is shingles? Will this affect his dental care today. What additional precautions will you take?

2. Mrs. Jones brings her 7-year-old son, Stanley, for a fluoride treatment. Stanley shows you several yellowish-colored sores inside his mouth. What could these sores be, and what should you do?

3. Mrs. Robinson accompanies her 87-year-old mother (who resides in a nursing home) for her dental visit. The older woman appears weak and is coughing into a handkerchief. What questions should you ask regarding the potential medical condition of this patient?

4. A newly hired dental assistant in your office confides in you that she is against all vaccines because they cause more harm than good. What are your thoughts on this, and how would you advise her?

CHAPTER 6

Management of Infection Control and Hazardous Materials

http://evolve.elsevier.com/Robinson/essentials/

LEARNING OBJECTIVES

1. Pronounce, define, and spell the key terms.
2. Provide an overview of the roles and responsibilities of the Centers for Disease Control and Prevention (CDC) and Occupational Safety & Health Administration (OSHA) when it comes to workplace safety and infection control in dentistry.
3. Complete the following related to OSHA's Bloodborne Pathogens Standard (BBP):
   * Explain the components of the OSHA BBP Standard.
   * Name the components of an exposure control plan.
   * Explain Standard Precautions.
   * Categorize tasks and procedures according to occupational exposure risks.
   * Discuss employee training in relation to the BBP Standard.
   * Describe the importance of vaccinations for dental personnel.
   * Discuss the maintenance of employee personal medical records.
   * Describe and demonstrate the proper disposal of contaminated sharps.
   * State how to prevent needle sticks.
   * Describe postexposure management and how to provide first aid after an exposure incident.
4. Describe and demonstrate the proper technique of handwashing.
5. Describe and demonstrate the appropriate use of alcohol-based hand rubs.
6. Explain the requirements for personal protective equipment (PPE), including the steps to putting on PPE and removing PPE.
7. Describe the types of dental waste and the management of each.
8. Identify and discuss the five components of the OSHA Hazard Communication Standard.

KEY TERMS

alcohol-based hand rubs
Bloodborne Pathogens (BBP) Standard
Centers for Disease Control and Prevention (CDC)
Globally Harmonized System (GHS) of Classification and Labeling of Chemicals
hazard class

Hazard Communication Standard (HCS)
hazard statement
hazardous waste
infectious waste
occupational exposure
Occupational Safety & Health Administration (OSHA)
percutaneous

per mucosal
personal protective equipment (PPE)
pictogram
regulated waste
safety data sheets (SDSs)
sharps
signal word
Standard Precautions
Universal Precautions

Within the dental office, there are necessary infection preventive and control measures that must be put into place and followed. This chapter reviews the basic concepts and the step-by-step procedures required to prevent the transmission of disease and to manage hazardous materials safely in the dental office.

Roles and Responsibilities of the CDC and OSHA

There are two federal agencies that play an important role in workplace safety and infection control for dentistry: the **Centers for Disease Control and Prevention (CDC)** and the **Occupational Safety & Health Administration (OSHA)**.

The CDC's role is to issue specific recommendations based on sound scientific evidence on health-related matters. Although these recommendations are not law and the CDC cannot regulate their practice, the CDC Guidelines for Infection Control in Dental Health Care Settings are now the standard of care.

Guidelines for Infection Control in Dental Health Care Settings

- Use of Standard Precautions rather than Universal Precautions
- Work restrictions for health care personnel infected with infectious diseases
- Postexposure management of occupational exposure to bloodborne pathogens (hepatitis B virus [HBV], human immunodeficiency virus [HIV], hepatitis C virus [HCV])
- Selection of devices with features to prevent sharps injuries
- Hand hygiene products and surgical hand asepsis
- Contact dermatitis and latex hypersensitivity
- Sterilization of unwrapped instruments
- Dental unit water line concerns
- Dental radiology infection control
- Aseptic technique for injectable medications
- Preprocedural mouth rinses for patients
- Oral surgical procedures
- Laser and electrosurgery plumes
- Tuberculosis
- Creutzfeldt-Jakob disease and other prion-related diseases
- Evaluation of infection control program
- Research considerations

OSHA is a regulatory agency. Its role is to issue specific regulations, also called *standards*, to protect the health of employees in the United States. Failure to comply with OSHA requirements can have serious consequences, including a monetary fine. As a dental assistant, following the guidelines and recommendations is essential.

OSHA's Bloodborne Pathogens Standard

OSHA's Bloodborne Pathogens (BBP) Standard is the most important infection control law in dentistry. It is designed to protect employees against health hazards related to bloodborne pathogens, such as the hepatitis B virus (HBV), hepatitis C virus (HCV), and human immunodeficiency virus (HIV).

The BBP Standard requires employers to protect their employees from exposure to blood and other potentially infectious material (OPIM) in the workplace and to provide proper care to the employee if an exposure should occur. The Standard applies to any type of facility in which employees might be exposed to blood and other body fluids, including dental and medical offices, hospitals, funeral homes, emergency medical services, and nursing homes.

OSHA requires that a copy of the BBP Standard be present in every dental office and clinic. A copy of the OSHA BBP Standard may be obtained by visiting osha.gov and searching for "Bloodborne Pathogens Standard."

Exposure Control Plan

Each dental office must have a written exposure control plan that clearly describes how that office complies with the BBP Standard. The exposure control plan must be reviewed and updated at least annually. A copy must be accessible to all employees.

Written Exposure Control Plan Required by OSHA

- Use of Standard Precautions
- Required use of personal protective equipment
- Standardized housekeeping
- Laundering of contaminated protective clothing
- Standardized policy on cleaning and disinfecting
- Policy on general waste disposal
- Labeling procedure (secondary labeling)
- Policy on sterilization (including monitoring) and disinfection
- Use of sharps containers and disposal system
- Standardized handwashing protocol
- HBV vaccination
- Postexposure evaluation and medical follow-up

HBV, Hepatitis B virus; *OSHA*, Occupational Safety & Health Administration.

Universal and Standard Precautions

The term Universal Precautions was initially introduced by the CDC and means that all human blood and body fluids are to be treated as infectious because patients with bloodborne infection can be asymptomatic or unaware they are infected.

The CDC later expanded the concept and changed the term to Standard Precautions. Standard Precautions apply not only to contact with blood but also to contact with (1) all body fluids, secretions, and excretions (except sweat), regardless of whether they contain blood; (2) nonintact skin, which can include an abrasion or open wound; (3) mucous membranes; and (4) saliva.

Categories of Employees

OSHA's BBP Standard requires members of the dental team to be categorized into three subgroups, according to their tasks and the procedures during which they might have an occupational exposure (Table 6.1).

TABLE 6.1
Occupational Exposure Determination

Category	Exposure	Dental Team Member
I	Routinely exposed to blood, saliva, or both	Dentist, dental hygienist, dental assistant, sterilization assistant, dental laboratory technician
II	May, on occasion, be exposed to blood, saliva, or both	Receptionist or office manager who may, on occasion, clean a treatment room or handle instruments or impressions
III	Never exposed to blood, saliva, or both	Financial manager, insurance clerk, computer operator

The BBP Standard defines an occupational exposure as "any reasonably anticipated skin, eye, [or] mucous membrane contact, or percutaneous injury, with blood or any other potentially infectious materials." Percutaneous (through the skin, such as needlesticks, cuts, and human bites) and permucosal (contact with mucous membranes, such as the eyes or mouth) exposures to blood, saliva, and other body fluids pose the greatest risk for the transmission of an infectious disease

Employee Training

The BBP Standard requires the dentist and/or employer to provide training in infection control and safety issues to all personnel who may encounter blood, saliva, or contaminated instruments or surfaces. Employee training must be provided at the time of initial assignment to tasks during which occupational exposure may occur. Annual training is required within 12 months of the previous training. The training is tailored to the education and language level of the employee and offered during the normal work shift. The record of each training session must include the date of the session, the name of the presenter, the topic, and the names of all employees who attended.

OSHA's Bloodborne Pathogens Standard Training Requirements

Employee training is required in each of the following areas:
- Epidemiology, modes of transmission, and prevention of HBV and HIV
- Possible risks to the fetus from HIV and HBV
- Location and proper use of all protective equipment
- Proper work practices using Standard Precautions
- Meaning of color codes, biohazard symbol, and precautions to follow in handling infectious waste
- Procedures to be followed if a needlestick or other exposure incident occurs

---

HBV, Hepatitis B virus; *HIV,* human immunodeficiency virus; *OSHA,* Occupational Safety & Health Administration.

Hepatitis B Immunization

The BBP Standard requires the dentist and/or employer to offer the HBV vaccination series to all employees whose assignments include category I and II tasks. If the employee does not have documented evidence of a complete HBV vaccine series, or an up-to-date blood test showing immunity to hepatitis B, then it is recommended for the employee to get: (1) a three-dose series of the vaccine (initial, 1 month out, and 5 months out), and (2) an anti-HBs serologic test 1 to 2 months after the final dose. To document compliance, the dentist or employer must obtain proof from the physician who administered the vaccination to the employee.

The employee has the right to refuse the HBV vaccine for any reason. If this is the case, the employee is required to sign an informed refusal form that is kept on file in the dental office. Although the employee originally signed the refusal form, they always have the right to reverse the decision and receive the vaccine later at no charge.

Influenza Immunization

It is recommended by the CDC that all personnel within a health care setting receive an annual flu vaccine. This is imperative to protect the employee, their patients, and their family members.

Employee Medical Records

The dentist or employer must keep a confidential medical record for each employee. The employer must store these in a secure place for the duration of employment, plus 30 years after the employee has left.

Requirements for Employee Medical Records

- Employee's name and Social Security number
- Proof of employee's hepatitis B virus (HBV) vaccination or signed refusal
- Circumstances of any exposure incident (e.g., needlestick) involving the employee and the name of the source individual (patient whose blood or bodily fluid is involved in the incident)
- Copy of the postexposure follow-up procedures for any injuries sustained by that employee

---

Managing Contaminated Sharps

Contact with contaminated needles and other disposable sharps, such as scalpel blades, orthodontic wires, and broken glass, may expose dental personnel to blood that contains pathogens. The sharps container is puncture resistant, closable, leakproof, and color-coded or labeled with the biohazard symbol (Fig. 6.1).

Sharps containers must be located as close as possible to the place of immediate disposal. Needles should not be cut, bent, or broken before disposal, and a needle should never be removed from a disposable-type device.

FIGURE 6.1 A puncture-resistant sharps disposal container should be located as close as possible to the area where the disposal of sharps takes place.

Preventing Needlesticks

Needlestick injuries remain as one of the most serious hazards in health care. There are syringes on the market made with needles that have safety guards to prevent accidental needlesticks (Fig. 6.2). Another means of prevention is to use a single-handed scoop technique or the use of a safety device for recapping (Fig. 6.3).

Postexposure Management

Despite efforts to prevent occupational exposure incidents, accidents happen. The employer must provide training to employees on the proper response to an exposure incident. Therefore, before an accident occurs, the BBP Standard requires the employer to have a written plan. This plan explains exactly what steps the employee must follow after the exposure incident occurs and the type of medical follow-up that will be provided to the employee at no charge. An employee has the right to refuse testing, and no adverse actions can be taken against them. Nevertheless, the employee will be required to sign an informed refusal form. Procedure 6.1 reviews first-aid steps after an exposure incident.

Postexposure Follow-up for an Exposed Worker

The following services must be offered to the employee without charge:

- Confidential medical counseling
- HIV test series (immediately and at 6-week, 12-week, and 6-month intervals)
- HBV immunoglobulin (if the employee has not been vaccinated for HBV)
- Tetanus booster
- Documentation of the incident on the appropriate OSHA form

HBV, Hepatitis B virus; *HIV*, human immunodeficiency virus; *OSHA*, Occupational Safety & Health Administration.

FIGURE 6.2 Ultra Safety Plus XL aspirating syringe. **A,** Ready for injection. **B,** Needle sheathed to prevent a needlestick injury. (From Logothesis DD: *Local anesthesia for the dental hygienist,* St. Louis, 2012, Mosby.)

FIGURE 6.3 Recapping devices.

Handwashing and Hand Care

Hand Hygiene

Keeping the skin of your hands intact and healthy is key to infection control. Hand hygiene is important as the first line of defense against the spread of infectious diseases. If you have just started your day at your dental office, are preparing to apply or remove gloves from a dental procedure, or are working in the sterilization or laboratory area, it is imperative that you follow a routine handwashing procedure (see Procedure 6.2: Handwashing).

Washing before gloving reduces the number of microorganisms to begin with and washing after glove removal reduces the number of organisms that have increased. Washing your hands after you remove your gloves is important because the growth of bacteria on your skin will increase because of the warm, moist environment under the glove.

A liquid soap is a recommended hygiene product used for handwashing. To minimize cross-contamination, treatment room sinks equipped with *hands-free* faucets that are electronically activated or are activated with foot pedals are preferable (Fig. 6.4).

Alcohol-Based Hand Rubs

Waterless antiseptic agents are alcohol-based products that are available in gels, foams, or rinses (Fig. 6.5). They do not require the use of water. The product is simply applied to the hands, which are then rubbed together to cover all surfaces.

FIGURE 6.4 Sensing device automatically turns the water on and off with hands-free operation.

FIGURE 6.5 Alcohol-based hand rub agents are available for refillable wall-mounted containers, in counter size, and in purse size. (Courtesy Crosstex International, Inc., Hauppauge, New York.)

These products are more effective at reducing microbial flora than plain soap or even an antimicrobial hand wash. Concentrations of 60% to 95% are the most effective. In addition, these products are good for your skin. They contain emollients that reduce the incidence of chapping, irritation, and drying of the skin.

Alcohol-based hand rubs are NOT indicated if your hands are visibly soiled or are contaminated with organic matter, such as blood or saliva. In this case, your hands need to be washed first with soap and water and then followed with the alcohol-based product.

See Procedure 6.3: Applying Alcohol-Based Hand Rubs.

Hand-Hygiene Recommendations

Healthy skin is better able to withstand the damaging effects of repeated washing and of wearing gloves. Drying your hands well is important before donning gloves.

Dental personnel with open sores or weeping dermatitis must avoid activities involving direct patient contact and handling contaminated instruments or equipment until the condition on the hands is healed.

Because rings and long fingernails can harbor pathogens and damage gloves, nails should be kept short and well manicured. Rings, long nails, and artificial nails are likely to puncture examination gloves. In addition, microorganisms can enter the body through any break in the skin. CDC guidelines recommend that rings, fingernail polish, and artificial nails not be worn at work.

Lotions

You can use lotions to prevent skin dryness caused by frequent handwashing. Nevertheless, you must use caution when selecting a product. Lotions with a base of petroleum, lanolin, mineral oil, palm oil, or coconut oil have a negative effect on latex gloves. Use these products only at the end of the workday.

FIGURE 6.6 Appropriate personal protective equipment (PPE) at chairside includes long-sleeved gowns, gloves, and eyewear.

Lotions containing aloe vera, glycerin, vitamin E, or vitamin A are a good choice throughout the workday.

Personal Protective Equipment

OSHA's BBP Standard requires the employer to provide employees with appropriate **personal protective equipment (PPE)** (Fig. 6.6) without charge to the employee. Examples of PPE include protective clothing, masks, protective eyewear, face shields, disposable patient treatment gloves, and heavy-duty utility gloves.

Chairside dental assistants must wear PPE whenever they are performing tasks that could encounter blood and body fluids. It is just as essential to wear appropriate PPE when performing other clinical activities that require handling items contaminated with patient secretions. Examples include instrument trays, laboratory cases, dentures, and other prosthetic appliances or contaminated equipment and surfaces.

See Procedure 6.4: Placing on Personal Protective Equipment and Procedure 6.5: Removing Personal Protective Equipment.

Protective Clothing

The purpose of protective clothing is to protect the skin and underclothing from exposure to saliva, blood, aerosol, and other contaminated materials. Types of protective clothing can include reusable gowns, disposable gowns, and surgical gowns that are sterile and prioritized for surgical procedures. Additional items can include scrub (surgical) hats and shoe covers.

The decision as to the type of protective clothing you should wear is based on the degree of anticipated exposure to infectious materials. For example, assisting in a dental procedure that includes aerosol and spatter from a dental handpiece or air/water syringe carries a high risk for exposure to contaminated aerosol. Recording clinical information in a patient record during an oral examination, on the other hand, carries a low risk for exposure because it does not involve contaminated aerosol (Fig. 6.7).

FIGURE 6.7 Depending on the task, the dental assistant's attire might be scrubs, laboratory coats, or surgical gowns. *Left,* Dental assistant in scrubs. *Center,* Dental assistant in a laboratory coat. *Right,* Dental assistant in surgical gown.

Protective Clothing Requirements

Protective clothing should be made of fluid-resistant material. Cotton, cotton-polyester mix, or disposable jackets or gowns are satisfactory for routine dental procedures.

To minimize the amount of uncovered skin, clothing should have long sleeves and a high neckline. The design of the sleeve should allow the cuff to be tucked inside the band of the glove. Buttons, trim, zippers, and other ornamentation (which may harbor pathogens) should be kept to a minimum.

Guidelines for Wearing Protective Clothing

- Protective clothing should not be worn out of the office for any reason; it can spread contamination.
- Protective clothing should be changed at least daily or more often if it becomes visibly soiled.
- Protective clothing should be IMMEDIATELY changed if it becomes soiled or saturated with body fluids or chemicals.
- Protective clothing must NEVER be worn in the staff lounge areas or where coworkers are eating or consuming beverages.

Handling Contaminated Laundry

The BBP Standard prohibits an employee from taking protective clothing home to be laundered. Laundering contaminated protective clothing is the responsibility of the employer, and many offices have a laundry service that will pick up contaminated laundry from the dental office. Some dental offices have chosen to

FIGURE 6.8 Containers of contaminated laundry must be labeled with the universal biohazard symbol.

install washers and dryers for PPE within the office. In this situation, any employee responsible for laundering contaminated PPE must be trained in the proper handling of contaminated PPE and must wear PPE when handling contaminated items.

Contaminated linens that are removed from the office for laundering should be in a leakproof bag with a biohazard label or an appropriately color-coded label (Fig. 6.8). Disposable gowns must be discarded daily and more often if visibly soiled.

Protective Masks

A face mask is worn over the nose and mouth to protect the person from inhaling infectious organisms spread by the aerosol spray of the handpiece or air-water syringe and by accidental splashes. Selecting a mask that fits your face well is important. Masks should be changed between patients or during patient treatment if the mask becomes wet.

The American Dental Association (ADA) recommends that the chairside dental team wear two types of masks depending on the level of risk. Table 6.2 provides a better understanding of the types of masks recommended and their use. The two most common types of surgical masks are the dome-shaped and flat types. Some operators prefer the dome-shaped type, particularly during lengthy procedures, because it conforms or "molds" more effectively to the face and creates an air space between the mask and the wearer (Figs. 6.9 and 6.10).

Guidelines for Using Protective Masks

- Change masks for every patient or more often, particularly if heavy spatter is generated during treatment or if the mask becomes damp.
- Handle masks ONLY by touching the side edges and avoid contact with the more heavily contaminated body of the mask.
- Conform the mask to your face.

- Do not allow the mask to contact your mouth when being worn. The moisture will reduce the mask filtration efficiency. A damp or wet mask is not an efficient mask.
- Change your mask approximately once each hour during a long procedure.
- Remember, a face shield is not a substitute for a mask because it provides no protection from aerosols.
- Never wear your face mask below your nose or on your chin. The outer surface of the mask is highly contaminated (Fig. 6.11).

Protective Eyewear

Eyewear is worn to protect the eyes against damage from aerosolized pathogens, such as herpes simplex viruses and staphylococci, and from flying debris, such as scrap amalgam and tooth fragments. Protective eyewear also prevents injury from splattered solutions and caustic chemicals. Such damage may be irreparable and may lead to permanent visual impairment or blindness.

The BBP Standard requires the use of eyewear with both front and side protection (solid side shields) for use during exposure-prone procedures. If you wear prescription glasses, you must add protective side and bottom shields. Protective eyewear that can be worn over prescription glasses is also available. If you wear contact lenses, then you must also wear protective eyewear with side shields or a face shield.

The CDC guidelines recommend that you clean your eyewear with soap and water or, if visibly soiled, clean and disinfect reusable facial protective wear between patients.

The two types of protective eyewear used during patient care are (1) glasses with protective side shields and (2) clear face shields.

Face Shields

A chin-length plastic face shield may be worn as an alternative to protective eyewear; however, a shield cannot replace a face mask because the shield does not protect against the inhalation of contaminated aerosols (Fig. 6.12).

When splashing or spattering of blood or other body fluids is likely during a procedure such as surgery, a face shield is often worn in addition to a protective mask.

TABLE 6.2
Understanding Masks Types

Understanding Mask Types

	SURGICAL (LEVEL 3) MASK	N95 EQUIVALENT MASK KN/KP95, PFF2, P2, DS/DL2, KOREAN SPECIAL 1ST*
Testing and Approval	Cleared by the U.S. Food and Drug Administration (FDA)	FDA Emergency Use Authorization (EUA)
Sizing	No	Yes. The sizing differs with each mask model. Some of the sizing options include small, small/medium, medium, medium/large, and large.
Intended Use and Purpose	Fluid resistant and provides the wearer protection against large droplets, splashes, or sprays of bodily or other hazardous fluids. Protects the patient from the wearer's mask emissions	Reduces wearer's exposure to particles including small particle aerosols and large droplets (non-oil aerosols). Manufactured in compliance with standards of other countries and considered equivalent to NIOSH approved N95 masks.
Face Seal Fit+	Loose-fitting	Tight-fitting**

*OSHA video on mask seal check: https://www.youtube.com/watch?v=pGXiUyAoEd8 .
Facial hair may affect the fit of the mask: https://www.cdc.gov/niosh/npptl/pdfs/FacialHairWmask11282017-508.pdf

+Note: A seal test is a user test performed by the wearer every time the mask is put on to insure that the mask is properly seated to the face. If not, it needs to be adjusted. A fit test is used to determine appropriate mask size for the individual.

**A mask that does not fit does not protect you, meaning that you should not rely on it to protect you from infection.

From the ADA website. https://www.ada.org/-/media/project/ada-organization/ada/ada-org/files/resources/coronavirus/covid-19-safety-and-clinical-resources/ada_covid19_understandingmasks.pdf. © American Dental Association. All rights reserved. Reprinted with permission.

FIGURE 6.9 Types of face mask. **A,** Flat. **B,** Dome-shaped or molded. (**A,** Courtesy Practicon Dental, Greenville, North Carolina. **B,** Courtesy Crosstex International, Inc., Hauppauge, New York.)

FIGURE 6.10 Face mask and safety glasses. (Courtesy Crosstex International, Inc., Hauppauge, New York.)

Patient Eyewear

Patients should be provided with protective eyewear because they may also be subject to eye damage from (1) handpiece

spatter; (2) spilled or splashed dental materials, including caustic chemical agents; and (3) airborne bits of acrylic or tooth fragments (Fig. 6.13).

When laser treatments are performed, patients must be supplied with special filtered-lens glasses.

Gloves

The types of gloves used in a dental practice vary by the various types of procedures that are performed in the practice.

Examination Gloves

Examination (*exam*) gloves are made from one of three materials: nitrile, latex, or vinyl. Latex gloves are the most common and they provide flexibility and comfort and act as a good barrier protection and resistant to chemicals. The one drawback is that some people are allergic to latex (Fig. 6.14). The person who is sensitive to latex can wear gloves made from vinyl, nitrile, or other non–latex-containing materials. If you think you may be developing an allergy to latex, you should have a blood test to confirm the diagnosis.

Examination gloves are inexpensive, available in a range of sizes from extra-small to extra-large, and fit either hand. These gloves are nonsterile and strictly serve as a protective barrier for the wearer.

Gloves Damaged during Treatment

Gloves are effective only when they are intact (not damaged, torn, ripped, or punctured). If gloves are damaged during treatment, immediately change them and wash your hands before regloving. The steps for regloving are: (1) excuse yourself and leave the chairside; (2) remove and discard the damaged gloves; (3) thoroughly wash your hands; and (4) reglove before returning to the chairside to resume the dental procedure.

Overgloves

Overgloves, also referred to as *food handler gloves,* are made of lightweight, inexpensive, clear plastic. They may be worn

FIGURE 6.11 Face masks should never be worn below the nose or on the chin. (From Bird DL, Robinson DS: *Modern dental assisting,* ed 11, St. Louis, 2015, Saunders.)

FIGURE 6.12 Face shields provide adequate eye protection, but a face mask is still required when assisting with aerosol-generating procedures.

FIGURE 6.14 Examination gloves. (Courtesy Crosstex International, Inc., Hauppauge, New York.)

FIGURE 6.13 Protective eyewear should be provided to patients.

FIGURE 6.15 Overgloves worn over examination glove. (Courtesy Certol International, Commerce City, Colorado.)

over contaminated treatment gloves (overgloving) to prevent contamination of clean objects handled during treatment (Fig. 6.15) .

Sterile Surgical Gloves

Sterile gloves, the type used in hospital surgical units, should be worn for invasive procedures involving the cutting of bone or significant amounts of blood or saliva, such as oral surgery, implant, and periodontal treatment.

Sterile gloves are supplied in prepackaged units to maintain sterility before use. They are provided in specific sizes and are fitted to the left or right hand. The procedure of donning sterile gloves is described in Chapter 26.

Utility Gloves

Utility gloves are not used for direct patient care. Utility gloves are worn (1) when the treatment room is cleaned and disinfected between patients, (2) where contaminated instruments are being cleaned or handled, and (3) for surface cleaning and

disinfecting (Fig. 6.16). Utility gloves may be washed, disinfected, or sterilized and reused. Utility gloves must be discarded, however, when they become worn and no longer can provide barrier protection. After use, utility gloves must be considered contaminated and must be appropriately handled until they have been properly disinfected or sterilized. Each staff member responsible for cleanup procedures must have their own designated pair of utility gloves.

Medical Waste Management

Waste within a dental practice must be disposed of according to applicable federal, state, and local regulations. Although the term **medical waste** is commonly used, more accurate terms are **contaminated waste** and **infectious waste** or **regulated waste**.

FIGURE 6.16 Utility gloves are used when preparing instruments for sterilization.

Classifications of Waste

The handling, storing, labeling, and disposing of waste depends entirely on the type of waste. For example, when reprocessing a treatment room, the waste will be separated into different containers. You must understand the types of waste to know what goes into which container (Table 6.3).

OSHA's Hazard Communication Standard

OSHA issued the Hazard Communication Standard (HCS) to require employers to inform their employees about the identity and hazards of chemicals that they use in the workplace. The HCS, also known as the "Employee Right-to-Know Law," requires employers to implement a hazard communication program.

Revision of the Hazard Communication Standard

In 2012 OSHA revised the HCS and adopted the **Globally Harmonized System (GHS) of Classification and Labeling of Chemicals** (Fig. 6.17). Although most of the standard remains unchanged, some modifications to the terminology have been made. For example, the term *hazard determination* has been changed to hazard classification, and *material safety data sheet* has been changed to safety data sheet.

Under the new international system, each chemical will be classified and labeled the same, regardless of where in the global market the chemical is manufactured or used, thus ending confusion and eliminating the need for different labels.

The three major areas of change are in **hazard classification, labels**, and safety data sheets (SDSs).

The revised HCS will still require chemical manufacturers and importers to evaluate the chemicals they produce or import and provide hazard information to employers and workers by applying specific labels on containers and preparing SDSs. The new system is being implemented throughout the world by

TABLE 6.3

Classification of Waste

Type	Examples	Handling Requirements
General waste	Paper towels, paper mixing pads, empty food containers	Discard in covered containers made of durable materials, such as plastic or metal.
Hazardous waste	Waste that presents a danger to humans or the environment (e.g., toxic chemicals)	Follow your specific state and local regulations.
Contaminated waste	Waste that has been in contact with blood or other body fluids (e.g., used barriers, patient napkins)	In most states, contaminated waste is disposed of with the general waste.
Infectious or regulated waste (biohazard)	Waste that can transmit an infectious disease	Follow your specific state and local regulations. Containers for all three types of infectious waste must be labeled with the biohazard label.
Blood and blood-soaked materials	Blood or saliva that can be squeezed out, or dried blood that may flake off of an item	Follow your specific state and local regulations.
Pathologic waste	Soft tissue and extracted teeth	Follow your specific state and local regulations. Never dispose of extracted teeth with amalgam restorations with waste that will be incinerated.
Sharps	Contaminated needles, scalpel blades, orthodontic wires, endodontic instruments (e.g., reamers files)	Containers should be closeable, leakproof, and puncture resistant. Containers should be color coded red and marked with the biohazard symbol. Sharps containers should be located as close as possible to the work area.

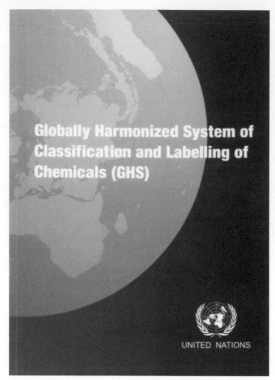

FIGURE 6.17 Globally Harmonized System of Classification and Labeling of Chemicals. (From https://www.osha.gov/dsg/hazcom/global.html. Accessed April 26, 2013.)

countries including Canada, China, Australia, and Japan, as well as in the European Union.

Hazard Communication Standard

The hazard communication program has the following five parts:
1. Written program
2. Chemical inventory
3. Safety data sheets (SDSs)
4. Labeling
5. Employee training

Written Program

The written program must identify, by name, all employees in the office who are exposed to hazardous chemicals. It must also identify the individual who is responsible for the program. The program describes (1) staff training; (2) how chemicals are handled in the office, including all labeling and safety measures; and (3) how to respond to chemical emergencies, such as spills or exposures.

If several dentists are working in one clinic or practice, then all employers must be aware of the hazards and protective measures so that they can train their employees.

Chemical Inventory

The chemical inventory is a list of every product used in the office that contains chemicals and includes amalgam, composites, bonding materials, etching agents, disinfectants, and impression materials, among others. Each time a new product containing any chemical is brought into the office, it must be added to the chemical inventory list. The dentist will often appoint the dental assistant to be the program coordinator and to be responsible for maintaining the chemical inventory and updating the SDS file.

Safety Data Sheet

In the revised HCS, SDSs have replaced Material Safety Data Sheets (MSDSs). The SDSs contain health and safety information about every product in the office that contains chemicals. The SDSs provide comprehensive technical information and are a resource for employees working with chemicals. They describe the physical and chemical properties of a chemical, its health hazards, routes of exposure, and precautions for safe handling and use, as well as emergency and first-aid procedures and spill control measures.

The manufacturer of a product that contains chemicals is required to supply the dental office with an SDS for the product; however, the program coordinator for the dental office is responsible for ensuring that the office has an SDS for every chemical used. An SDS is often enclosed in the package with the product. SDSs should be organized in binders, providing employees ready access to be able to locate a particular SDS easily. The SDS now has a specified 16-section format (Table 6.4).

Labeling

As of 2015, all labels are required to have a harmonized signal word, pictogram, and hazard statement for each hazard class and category (Fig. 6.18).

When a chemical is transferred to a different container, the new container must also be labeled. For example, when a concentrated chemical disinfectant is mixed fresh and placed into a spray bottle or tub (secondary containers), the spray bottle or tub must be labeled. Other examples of secondary containers that hold chemicals and require labeling are automatic x-ray film processors and manual processing tanks, ultrasonic cleaning tanks, and chemical vapor sterilizers.

Hazard Classification

Specific criteria for hazards have been developed, and chemicals are classified into categories that compare hazard severity within a hazard class. Once a chemical is classified, warnings are automatically assigned so that each chemical in the same category will have the same label requirements and language. This consistency helps ensure that evaluations of the hazardous effects are consistent for all manufacturers and that labels and SDSs are also consistent.

The two most important considerations are that (1) OSHA HCS labels are used and (2) all employees are trained to understand and read the label.

Employee Training

Employee training is essential for a successful hazard communication program. Staff training is required (1) when a new employee is hired, (2) when a new chemical product is added to the office, and (3) once a year for all continuing employees. Records of each training session must be kept on file for a minimum of 5 years.

TABLE 6.4
Sections of Hazard Communication Safety Data Sheets

The Hazard Communication Standard (HCS) requires chemical manufacturers, distributors, or importers to provide Safety Data Sheets (SDSs) (formerly known as Material Safety Data Sheets or MSDSs) to communicate the hazards of hazardous chemical products. As of June 1, 2015, the HCS will require all new SDSs to be in a uniform format and include the section numbers, the headings, and associated information under the headings listed:

Section	Description	Explanation
1	Identification	Includes product identifier; manufacturer or distributor name, address, and telephone number; emergency telephone number; recommended use; and restrictions on use.
2	Hazard(s) identification	Includes all hazards regarding the chemical and required label elements.
3	Composition and information on ingredients	Includes information on chemical ingredients and trade secret claims.
4	First-aid measures	Includes important symptoms and effects, acute and delayed effects, and required treatment(s).
5	Fire-fighting measures	Lists suitable extinguishing techniques and equipment and chemical hazards from fire.
6	Accidental release measures	Lists emergency procedures, protective equipment, and proper methods of containment and cleanup.
7	Handling and storage	Lists precautions for safe handling and storage, including incompatibilities.
8	Exposure controls and personal protection	Lists OSHA's permissible exposure limits (PELs), threshold limit values (TLVs), appropriate engineering controls, and personal protective equipment (PPE).
9	Physical and chemical properties	Lists the chemical's characteristics.
10	Stability and reactivity	Lists chemical stability and possibility of hazardous reactions.
11	Toxicologic information	Includes routes of exposure; related symptoms and acute and chronic effects; and numerical measures of toxicity.
12	Ecologic information[a]	
13	Disposal considerations[a]	
14	Transport information[a]	
15	Regulatory information[a]	
16	Other information	Includes the date of preparation or the date of the last revision.

[a]Because other agencies regulate this information, OSHA will not be enforcing Sections 12 through 15(29 CFR 1910.1200(g)(2)).

OSHA, Occupational Safety & Health Administration

For more information: www.osha.gov; (800) 321-OSHA (6742); U.S. Department of Labor.

Although the dentist is responsible for providing the training, the dental assistant is responsible for routinely following safety precautions.

Outline for Hazard Communication Training Program*
- Requirements of the Hazard Communication Standard (HCS)
- Written communication plan for the office (e.g., location, use)
- Understanding of the hazards of the chemicals with which the employees work
- Ability to interpret warning labels and safety data sheets (SDSs)

*On completion, employees are asked to sign a training record that will remain in the personnel file.

Responsibilities of the Dental Assistant as Coordinator of the Hazard Communication Program
- Read and understand OSHA's Hazard Communication Standard (HCS).
- Implement the written hazard communication program.
- Compile a list (chemical inventory) of products in the office that contain hazardous chemicals.
- Obtain safety data sheets (SDSs).
- Update the SDS file as new products are added to the office inventory.
- Inform other employees of the location of the SDSs.
- Label appropriate containers.
- Provide training to other employees.

OSHA, Occupational Safety & Health Administration.

A

Hazard Communication Standard Labels

OSHA has updated the requirements for labeling of hazardous chemicals under its Hazard Communication Standard (HCS). As of June 1, 2015, all labels will be required to have pictograms, a signal word, hazard and precautionary statements, the product identifier, and supplier identification. A sample revised HCS label, identifying the required label elements, is shown on the right. Supplemental information can also be provided on the label as needed.

For more information:

 Occupational
Safety and Health
Administration
www.osha.gov

(800) 321-OSHA (6742)
www.osha.gov

SAMPLE LABEL

CODE_____
Product Name_____ } **Product Identifier**

Company Name_____
Street Address_____
City_____State_____
Postal Code_____Country_____
Emergency Phone Number_____ } **Supplier Identification**

Hazard Pictograms

**Signal Word
Danger**

Keep container tightly closed. Store in a cool, well-ventilated place that is locked.
Keep away from heat/sparks/open flame. No smoking. Only use non-sparking tools.
Use explosion-proof electrical equipment.
Take precautionary measures against static discharge.
Ground and bond container and receiving equipment.
Do not breathe vapors.
Wear protective gloves.
Do not eat, drink or smoke when using this product.
Wash hands thoroughly after handling.
Dispose of in accordance with local, regional, national, international regulations as specified.

In Case of Fire: use dry chemical (BC) or Carbon Dioxide (CO₂) fire extinguisher to extinguish.

First Aid
If exposed call Poison Center.
If on skin (or hair): Take off immediately any contaminated clothing. Rinse skin with water.

Precautionary Statements

Highly flammable liquid and vapor.
May cause liver and kidney damage. } **Hazard Statements**

Supplemental Information
Directions for Use
_____
_____
_____

Fill weight:_____ Lot Number:_____
Gross weight:_____ Fill Date:_____
Expiration Date:_____

OSHA 3492-02 2012

B

FIGURE 6.18 **A,** Hazard Communication Standard (HCS) pictograms. **B,** Sample label. (From http://www.osha.gov/dsg/hazcom/standards.html. Accessed April 26, 2013.)

Exemptions to Labeling Requirements

Certain chemicals are exempted from the standard, including tobacco and tobacco products, wood and wood products, food, drugs, cosmetics, and alcoholic beverages sold and packaged for consumer use. Drugs dispensed by a pharmacy to a health care provider for direct administration to a patient also are exempt from the labeling requirement, as are over-the-counter drugs, such as aspirin and first-aid supplies, and drugs intended for personal consumption by employees while in the workplace.

- Maintain good ventilation.
- Do not eat, drink, smoke, apply lip balm, or insert contact lenses in areas in which chemicals are used.
- Keep chemicals away from open flames and heat sources.
- Always have an operational fire extinguisher on hand.
- Know and use proper cleanup procedures.
- Keep neutralizing agents available for strong acid and alkaline solutions.
- Dispose of all hazardous chemicals according to safety data sheet (SDS) instructions.

Guidelines for Minimizing Exposure to Chemical Hazards in the Dental Office

- Keep a minimum of hazardous chemicals in the office.
- Read the labels and use only as directed.
- Store each chemical according to the manufacturer's directions.
- Keep containers tightly covered.
- Avoid mixing chemicals unless consequences are known.
- Wear appropriate personal protective equipment (PPE) when handling hazardous substances.
- Immediately wash hands after removing gloves.
- Avoid skin contact with chemicals; immediately wash skin that has come in contact with chemicals.

Ethical Implications

Infection control and management of **hazardous waste** can present legal and ethical issues for dental assistants. Taking shortcuts can lead to the transmission of disease or accidents. Always following proper infection control and chemical management procedures is a matter of personal commitment and integrity.

Patients should have absolute confidence that infection control procedures followed in the office are never compromised. This confidence is as important for the protection of the dental team as it is for your patients.

First Aid After an Exposure Incident

Goal

To perform appropriate first aid after an exposure incident.

Equipment and Supplies

- Soap and water
- Paper towels
- Antiseptic cream or ointment
- Adhesive bandage
- Exposure incident report form

Procedural Steps

Immediately stop operations.

1. Remove your gloves.
2. Thoroughly wash your hands using antimicrobial soap and warm water.
3. Dry your hands.
4. Apply a small amount of antiseptic to the affected area.
   Note: Do not apply caustic agents, such as bleach or disinfectant solutions, to the wound.
5. Apply an adhesive bandage to the area.
6. Complete applicable postexposure follow-up paperwork.
   Note: The employer should be immediately notified of the injury after initial first aid is provided.

Handwashing Before Gloving

Goal

To wash hands properly before gloving.

Equipment and Supplies

- Sink with running water
- Liquid soap in a dispenser
- Nailbrush or orange stick
- Paper towels in a dispenser

Procedural Steps

1. Remove all jewelry, including watches and rings.
   Purpose: Jewelry is difficult to clean, can harbor microbes, and can puncture the gloves.
2. Use the foot or electronic control to regulate water flow. If this is not available, then use a paper towel to grasp the faucets to turn them on and off. Discard the towel after use. Allow your hands to become wet.
   Purpose: Faucets may have been contaminated by being touched with soiled or contaminated hands.
3. Apply soap; lather using a circular motion with friction while holding your fingertips downward. Rub well between your fingers. If this is the first handwashing of the day, then use a nailbrush or an orange stick. Inspect and clean under every fingernail during this step.
   Purpose: Friction removes soil and contaminants from your hands and wrists.

4. Vigorously rub the lathered hands together under a stream of water to remove surface debris.
Purpose: Scrubbing the first time removes gross debris.

5. Apply more soap, and vigorously rub the lathered hands together for a minimum of 10 seconds under a stream of water.
Purpose: Secondary scrubbing removes residual debris and tenacious microorganisms, which thrive under the free edges of the fingernails.

6. Rinse the hands with cool water.
Purpose: Cool water closes the pores.
7. Use a paper towel to dry the hands thoroughly, and then dry the forearms.

Purpose: Reusable cloth towels remain moist, contribute to microbial growth, and spread contamination.

8. If water faucets are not foot operated, turn off the faucet with a clean paper towel.
Purpose: The faucet is dirty and will contaminate your clean hands.

Illustrations from Proctor DB, Adams AP: *Kinn's the medical assistant: an applied learning approach*, ed 12, St. Louis, 2014, Saunders.

Applying Alcohol-Based Hand Rubs

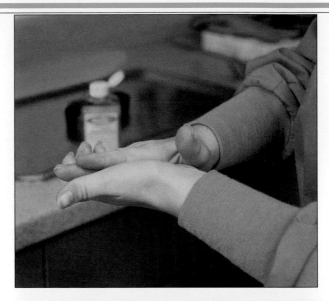

Goal

To apply an alcohol-based hand rub.

Equipment and Supplies

• Alcohol-based hand rub (60% to 95% concentration)

Procedural Steps

1. Check your hands to be sure they are not visibly soiled or contaminated with organic matter, such as blood or saliva. If necessary, wash your hands with soap and water and dry them thoroughly.

   Purpose: Alcohol-based hand rubs are not effective in the presence of organic matter.

2. Carefully read directions to determine the proper amount to dispense.

   Purpose: These products are dose sensitive. If you use a smaller amount than is recommended, then their effectiveness will be seriously decreased.

(Courtesy Crosstex International, Inc., Hauppauge, New York.)

3. Dispense the proper amount of the product into the palm of one hand.

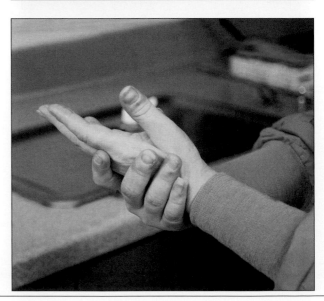

4. Rub the palms of your hands together.
5. Rub the product between your fingers.
6. Rub the product over the backs of your hands.

   Purpose: Thoroughly covering both of your hands is important.

Putting on Personal Protective Equipment

Goal

To put on personal protection equipment (PPE) before patient care.

Equipment and Supplies

- Protective clothing
- Surgical mask
- Protective eyewear
- Gloves

Procedural Steps

1. Put your protective clothing over your uniform, street clothes, or scrubs.
   Note: Protective clothing can be long-sleeved laboratory coats, clinic jackets, or gowns.

2. Put on your surgical mask and adjust the fit.
3. Put on your protective eyewear.
   Note: Eyewear should be impact resistant and have side protection. Goggles or face shields are also acceptable.
4. Thoroughly wash and dry your hands.
   Note: If your hands are not visibly soiled, then you may use an alcohol-based hand rub.
5. Hold one glove at the cuff, place your opposite hand inside the glove, and pull it onto your hand. Repeat with a new glove for your other hand.
   Important Note: Regarding the sequence of putting on PPE, putting on the gloves last to avoid contaminating them before your hands are placed in the patient's mouth is the most important step.

Modified from Organization for Safety Asepsis and Prevention: *Policy to practice: OSAP's guide to the guidelines*, Annapolis, Md, 2004, OSAP.

Removing Personal Protective Equipment

Goal

To remove personal protective wear.

Equipment and Supplies

- Protective clothing
- Surgical mask
- Protective eyewear
- Gloves

Procedural Steps

Gloves

1. Use your gloved hand to grasp the other glove at the outside cuff. Pull downward, turning the glove inside out as it pulls away from your hand.
2. For the other hand, use your ungloved fingers to grasp the inside (uncontaminated area) of the cuff of the remaining glove. Pull downward to remove the glove, turning it inside out. Discard the gloves into the waste receptacle.

Eyewear

1. Remove eyewear by touching it only on the ear rests (which are not contaminated).
2. Place the eyewear on a disposable towel until it can be thoroughly cleaned and disinfected.

Wash and thoroughly dry your hands.

Protective Clothing

1. Pull the gown off, turning it inside out as it comes off.
   Note: Be careful not to allow the gown to touch underlying clothes or skin.

Masks

1. Slide the fingers of each hand under the elastic strap in front of your ears and remove the mask. Discard the mask into the waste receptacle.
   Note: Be sure your fingers contact only the mask's ties or elastic strap.

Note: If no visible contamination exists and if the gloves have not been torn or punctured during the procedure, then you may use an alcohol-based hand rub in place of handwashing. If your hands are damp from perspiration or have glove powder, however, then you may prefer to wash them with antimicrobial soap and water.

Modified from Organization for Safety Asepsis and Prevention: *Policy to practice: OSAP's guide to the guidelines*, Annapolis, Md, 2004, OSAP.

Chapter Exercises

Multiple Choice

Circle the letter next to the correct answer.

1. The goal of an infection control program is to prevent disease transmission to the _____.
   a. patient from the staff
   b. staff from the patient
   c. patient from another patient
   d. a, b, and c

2. Which of the following could result in a percutaneous injury?
   a. Splash to the eyes
   b. Cut from an instrument
   c. Splash to the mouth
   d. Needlestick
   e. b and d

3. As a dental assistant, when should you wash your hands?
   a. Before you glove
   b. After you remove your gloves
   c. Both before and after wearing your gloves

4. Which of the following are considered PPE?
   a. Protective clothing
   b. Mask
   c. Eyewear or chin-length face shield
   d. Disposable gloves
   e. All of the above

5. Which of the following statements is NOT true regarding the use of face masks?
   a. They should be changed between patients.
   b. They should be changed if they become damp.
   c. The inside of the mask should contact your mouth when worn.
   d. The mask should conform to your face.

6. Which type of glove should be used when cleaning and disinfecting the treatment room?
   a. Latex examination gloves
   b. Overgloves
   c. Sterile surgical gloves
   d. Utility gloves

7. Safety data sheets (SDSs) should be supplied by the _____.
   a. manufacturer of the material
   b. sales person
   c. delivery person
   d. all of the above

8. Which of the following items are exempt from the chemical labeling laws?
   a. Tobacco and tobacco products
   b. Foods
   c. Cosmetics and drugs for employees' personal use in the workplace
   d. All of the above

9. Wearing jewelry under latex gloves is considered a safe practice.
   a. True
   b. False

10. Waste that presents a danger to humans or the environment (e.g., toxic chemicals) is classified as _____ waste.
    a. general
    b. hazardous
    c. contaminated
    d. pathologic

Apply Your Knowledge

1. While preparing instruments for sterilization, you accidentally stick the palm of your hand with a contaminated surgical instrument. What is your first step for postexposure follow-up?

2. During Ms. Parish's first visit to your office, she asks you why everyone is wearing such "elaborate garb" as masks and face shields. She seems annoyed and tells you that her previous dentist knew she did not have any disease and that he did not feel that those items were necessary. How would you respond to Ms. Parish?

3. Pamela Leong is a new employee hired to work at the front desk and, on occasion, clean up an operatory or process instruments; however, Pamela has not had formal dental assisting training. According to the OSHA BBP Standard, what would be her category of risk?

4. You are a clinical dental assistant and accidentally spill a chemical used for cleaning instruments in the sterilization area. Where would you be able to find information on how to clean up and dispose of that chemical?

CHAPTER 7

Surface Disinfection and Treatment Room Preparation

http://evolve.elsevier.com/Robinson/essentials/

KEY TERMS

alcohol
antiseptic
bioburden
biofilm
chlorine dioxide
critical instruments

disinfection
glutaraldehyde
iodophors
noncritical instruments
ortho-phthalaldehyde (OPA)
precleaning

semicritical instruments
sodium hypochlorite
surface barriers
synthetic phenol

During patient treatment, the equipment and treatment room surfaces become contaminated with saliva and aerosol, which can contain saliva and/or blood. Another primary source of contamination occurs when a member of the dental team touches surfaces with contaminated gloves. Cleaning and disinfecting these surfaces are important components in an effective infection control program.

The Occupational Safety & Health Administration (OSHA) Bloodborne Pathogens (BBP) Standard requires that contaminated work surfaces be disinfected between patient visits. Three methods can be applied to protect surface contamination. One method is to prevent the surface from becoming contaminated by using a surface barrier. The second method is to use single use/disposable items to prevent cross-contamination, and the third method is to preclean and disinfect the surface between patients. There are advantages and disadvantages of all methods, but most dental offices will use a combination of the three methods (Table 7.1).

Surface Barriers

Surface barriers are used to prevent contamination on the surface and do not need to be cleaned and disinfected between patients.

A wide variety of surface barriers are available today. All should be resistant to fluids to keep microorganisms in saliva, blood, and other liquids from soaking through to contact the surface underneath (Fig. 7.1). Plastic fluid-resistant coverings

TABLE 7.1

Comparison of Surface Barriers versus Precleaning and Disinfection

	Advantages	Disadvantages
Surface barrier	Protects surfaces that are not easily cleaned and disinfected. Prevents contamination when properly placed. Is less time-consuming. Reduces handling and storage of chemicals. Provides patient with visual assurance of cleanliness. Does not damage equipment or surfaces.	Adds plastics to the environment after disposal. May be more expensive than precleaning and disinfecting. Requires a variety of sizes and shapes. May become dislodged during treatment.
Precleaning and disinfecting	May be less expensive than surface barriers. Does not add plastic to the environment. Some dentists do not like the appearance of plastic barriers.	Requires more time; therefore cleaning and disinfecting are sometimes not properly performed. Not all surfaces can be adequately precleaned. Over time, some chemicals are destructive to dental equipment surfaces. Chemical containers must be properly labeled, and safety data sheets must be on file in the office. No method is available to determine whether the microbes have been removed or killed. Some disinfectants must be prepared fresh daily. Chemicals are added to the environment upon disposal.

are especially designed to fit the shape of items in the dental operatory (Fig. 7.2). Plastic barrier sticky tape is frequently used to protect smooth electrical surfaces, such as touch pads on equipment or electrical switches on chairs or x-ray equipment (Fig. 7.3). Aluminum foil can also be used because it is easily formed around any shape. See Procedure 7.1: Placing and Removing Surface Barriers.

Surfaces Typically Protected with Barriers

Headrest on dental chair
Control button on dental chair
Light handles
Light switches
Evacuator hoses and controls
X-ray control switches
Air-water syringe handles
Dental unit control touch pads
Patient mirror handles
Handle on light-curing device
Switch on amalgamators or other automatic mixing devices
Drawer handles
Adjustment handles on operator and assistant stools
Bracket table

Single-use items, also referred to as disposable devices, are another way to provide infection control measures. A single-use item is designed to be used on one patient and then discarded, not cleaned (Fig. 7.4). Using disposable items improves patient safety by eliminating the risk for patient-to-patient contamination.

Example of Single-Use Only Items

Air-water syringe tips
Burs
Evacuator tips
Impression trays
Prophy cups and brushes
Scalpel blades
Syringe needles
Orthodontic brackets

FIGURE 7.1 An example of water on a fluid-resistant material. (Courtesy Crosstex International, Inc., Hauppauge, New York.)

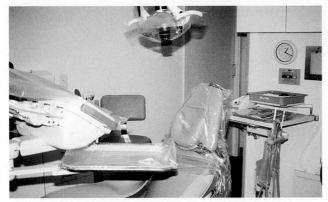

FIGURE 7.2 Surfaces touched during patient care should be covered with protective barriers. If not protected, then the surfaces should be cleaned and disinfected.

FIGURE 7.4 Examples of disposable items. (From Miller CH: *Infection controls and management of hazardous materials for the dental team,* ed 6, St Louis, 2018, Elsevier.)

FIGURE 7.3 Tube socks provide barrier protection for difficult-to-clean areas. (From Miller CH: *Infection controls and management of hazardous materials for the dental team,* ed 6, St Louis, 2018, Elsevier.)

Precleaning and Disinfection

Precleaning and disinfecting techniques are most effective on smooth and easily accessible contaminated treatment room surfaces. Always wear your utility gloves, mask, protective eyewear, and protective clothing when precleaning and disinfecting.

Precleaning

Precleaning means to clean before disinfecting (Fig. 7.5). All contaminated surfaces **must** be precleaned before they can be disinfected. This sequence reduces the number of microbes and removes the blood and/or saliva (also called **bioburden**). Not all types of disinfectants contain a precleaning agent.

Regular soap and water may be used for precleaning but selecting a disinfectant that contains detergents for both the precleaning step and the disinfecting steps is more efficient. Remember—if a surface is not clean, it cannot be disinfected.

Disinfection

Disinfection is intended to kill disease-producing microorganisms that remain on the surface after precleaning. Spores are *not* killed during disinfection procedures. Do not confuse disinfection with sterilization. **Sterilization** is the process during which all forms of life are destroyed. Sterilization techniques are discussed in Chapter 8.

The term **disinfectant** is used with chemicals that are applied to inanimate surfaces, such as countertops and dental equipment, and the term **antiseptic** is used for antimicrobial agents that are applied to living tissue. Disinfectants and antiseptics should never be interchangeably used because tissue toxicity and damage to equipment can result.

See Procedure 7.2: Performing Treatment Room Cleaning and Disinfection.

Levels of Disinfectants

The **U.S. Environmental Protection Agency (EPA)** registers and regulates disinfectants and chemical sterilants and places them in a specific classification (Table 7.2). In dentistry, only those products that are registered with the EPA as hospital disinfectants with tuberculocidal claims (kills the organism *Mycobacterium tuberculosis*) should be used to disinfect dental treatment areas. *M. tuberculosis* is highly resistant to disinfectants (Fig. 7.6).

Characteristics of Surface Disinfectants

Ideally, the perfect surface disinfectant would be one that rapidly kills all types of pathogenic organisms, is odorless, gentle to dental equipment surfaces, nontoxic, and economical to use. There are several types of low-level and intermediate disinfectants available for use on floors, walls, and surfaces that have pros and cons about their elements (Table 7.3).

Many manufacturers of dental equipment will recommend specific surface disinfectants that are most appropriate for their dental equipment and unit accessories.

Types of Chemical Disinfectants

Alcohol. Ethyl alcohol and isopropyl alcohol are the most common types of low to intermediate level disinfectant, having been used as skin antiseptics and surface disinfectants. Because of their rapid evaporation, however, alcohols are not effective in the

FIGURE 7.5 Surface precleaning and disinfection by the wipe-discard-wipe technique. Precleaning consists of **A,** obtaining a fresh surface wipe, **B,** wiping the surface to clean it, and **C,** discarding the wipe. Disinfection is **D,** obtaining a fresh surface wipe and **E** is wiping the surface again, followed by the appropriate contact time. (From Miller CH: *Infection controls and management of hazardous materials for the dental team*, ed 6, St Louis, 2018, Elsevier.)

TABLE 7.2

Chemical Classification of Disinfecting and Sterilizing Chemicals

Category	Definition	Examples	Use
Sterilant	Destroys all microorganisms, including high numbers of bacterial spores	Glutaraldehyde, glutaraldehyde phenate, hydrogen peroxide, hydrogen peroxide with peracetic acid, peracetic acid	Heat-sensitive reusable items: immersion only
High-level disinfectant	Destroys all microorganisms but not necessarily high numbers of bacterial spores	Glutaraldehyde, glutaraldehyde phenate, hydrogen peroxide, hydrogen peroxide with peracetic acid, peracetic acid, ortho-phthalaldehyde	Heat-sensitive reusable items: immersion only

TABLE 7.2

Chemical Classification of Disinfecting and Sterilizing Chemicals—cont'd

Category	Definition	Examples	Use
Intermediate-level disinfectant	Destroys vegetative bacteria, most fungi, and most viruses; inactivates *Mycobacterium tuberculosis* var. *bovis* (is tuberculocidal)	EPA-registered hospital disinfectant with label claim of tuberculocidal activity (e.g., chlorine-based products, phenolics, iodophors, quaternary ammonium compounds with alcohol, bromides)	Clinical contact surfaces; noncritical surfaces with visible blood
Low-level disinfectant	Destroys vegetative bacteria, some fungi, and some viruses; does not inactivate *M. tuberculosis* var. *bovis* (is not tuberculocidal)	EPA-registered hospital disinfectant with no label claim of tuberculocidal activity (e.g., quaternary ammonium compounds)	Housekeeping surfaces (e.g., floors, walls); noncritical surfaces without visible blood; clinical contact surfaces

EPA, U.S. Environmental Protection Agency.

Adapted from Kohn WG, Collins AS, Cleveland JL, et al: Centers for Disease Control and Prevention: guideline for infection control in dental health-care settings—2003, *MMWR Recomm Rep* 52 (No. RR-17):66, 2003.

presence of bioburden, which limits their antimicrobial activity. In addition, alcohols are damaging to certain materials, such as plastics and vinyl, which are prevalent in the dental environment.

The American Dental Association (ADA), the Centers for Disease Control and Prevention (CDC), and the Organization for Safety and Asepsis Procedures (OSAP) do not recommend alcohol as an environmental surface disinfectant.

Iodophors. Iodophors are EPA-registered, intermediate-level hospital disinfectants with tuberculocidal action. Iodophors are recommended for disinfecting surfaces that have been soiled with potentially infectious patient material. When used according to the manufacturer's instructions, iodophors are usually effective within 5 to 10 minutes. Iodophors are inactivated by hard water; consequently, they must be mixed with soft or distilled water. Because they contain iodine, iodophors may corrode or discolor certain metals or may temporarily cause red or yellow stains on clothing and other surfaces.

Synthetic Phenol Compounds. Synthetic phenol compounds are EPA-registered, intermediate-level hospital disinfectants with broad-spectrum activity, meaning that they can kill a wide range of microbes. When properly diluted, phenols are used for surface disinfection, provided the surface has first been thoroughly cleaned.

Phenols can be used on metal, glass, rubber, or plastic. They also can be used as a holding solution for instruments; however, phenols leave a residual film on treated surfaces. A synthetic phenol compound is prepared daily. Phenols may also be used to disinfect impressions; however, always check with the manufacturer of the impression material.

Sodium Hypochlorite. Sodium hypochlorite, also referred to as bleach, is classified as an intermediate-level disinfectant with the primary active ingredient ortho-phenylphenol. Sodium hypochlorite is a fast acting, economical, and broad spectrum disinfectant. EPA-approved disinfectant products that contain sodium hypochlorite or other chlorine compounds are available on the market. Always check the product label for the EPA registration number.

> **Disadvantages of Sodium Hypochlorite**
> * Unstable and needs daily preparation.
> * Has a strong odor and is corrosive to some metals.
> * Is destructive to fabrics and eventually may cause plastic chair covers to crack.
> * Is irritating to the eyes and skin.

Liquid Chemical Sterilants and High-Level Disinfectants. Liquid chemical sterilants are chemicals on the market that are classified for use as a sterilant or high-level disinfection. When used as sterilants, they destroy all microbial life, including bacterial endospores. Depending on the type of sterilant, the time for sterilization to work can range from 6 to 30 hours. At weaker dilutions or at shorter contact times, these chemicals provide high-level disinfection, which inactivates all microorganisms except endospores (Table 7.4). In the dental office, however, monitoring for microbial kill is not possible, as it is

FIGURE 7.6 Intermediate-level surface disinfectant. (Courtesy Biotrol, Earth City, Missouri.)

TABLE 7.3
EPA-Registered Surface Disinfectants for Dentistry

Category and Active Ingredient	Pros	Cons
Chlorines: Sodium hypochlorite diluted in-office, chlorine dioxide, and commercial preparations of sodium hypochlorite with added surfactants	Economical Rapid, broad-spectrum activity Tuberculocidal action Effective in diluted solutions	Diluted solutions must be prepared daily; they cannot be reused. Corrosive to some metals and may destroy fabrics. May irritate skin and other tissue. Chlorine dioxide is a poor cleaner.
Complex phenols: Synthetic phenols containing multiple phenolic agents	Broad-spectrum activity Residual activity Effective cleaner and disinfectant Tuberculocidal action Compatible with metal, glass, rubber, and plastic	Extended exposure may degrade some plastics or leave etchings on glass. Many preparations are limited to 1 day of use. May leave a residual film on treated surfaces.
Dual and synergized quaternary ammonium compounds: Alcohol and multiple quaternary ammonium compounds	Broad-spectrum activity Tuberculocidal action Hydrophilic virus claims Low toxicity Contains detergent for cleaning	Are readily inactivated by anionic detergents and organic matter. Can damage some materials.
Iodophors: Iodine, combined with a surfactant	Broad-spectrum activity Tuberculocidal action Relatively nontoxic Effective cleaner and disinfectant Residual biocidal action	Are unstable at higher temperatures; may discolor some surfaces. Inactivated by alcohol and hard water. Must be prepared daily. Dilution and contact times are critical.
Phenol-alcohol combinations: Phenolic agent in an alcohol base	Tuberculocidal action Fast-acting Residual activity Some inhibit the growth of mold, mildew, and other fungi	May cause porous surfaces to dry and crack. Have poor cleaning capabilities.
Other halogens: Sodium bromide and chlorine	Fast-acting Tuberculocidal action Supplied in tablet form for simple dilution Requires minimal storage space	Are for use on hard surfaces only. Have a chlorine smell.

Note: Glutaraldehydes and simple quaternary ammonium compounds should not be used for surface disinfection in dentistry. High-concentration alcohols (ethyl alcohol or isopropyl alcohol of at least 70%) should be used on precleaned surfaces.

Note: Always follow manufacturer's recommendations regarding surface contact time.

EPA, U.S. Environmental Protection Agency.

From Organization for Safety, Asepsis and Prevention: *Infection control in practice,* vol 1, no 3, Annapolis, MD, 2002, OSAP.

TABLE 7.4
FDA-Cleared Instrument Immersion Disinfectants for Dentistry

Category or Active Ingredient	Steriliant Contact Time	High-Level Disinfectant Time
Glutaraldehyde 2.4%–3.4% alkaline and acidic formulations*	6–10 hr at 20°C, 22°C, or 25°C*	20–90 min at 20°C, 22°C, or 25°C*
Hydrogen peroxide, 7.3%	6 hr at 20°C	30 min at 20°C
Ortho-phthalaldehyde, 0.55%	Not indicated for sterilization	12 min at 20°C

FDA, U.S. Food and Drug Administration.

with heat sterilization. Spore tests for biologic monitoring have not yet been developed for office testing.

Most of these chemicals are toxic and can irritate the eyes, skin, and lungs. Personal protective equipment (PPE) must always be worn when using these chemicals. They are to be used for immersion (soaking) of heat-sensitive items and should never be used as surface disinfectants.

Always keep the container lid closed to minimize fumes.

Glutaraldehyde. Glutaraldehyde is classified as a high-level disinfectant and sterilant. It can be used as a liquid sterilant when the immersion time is greatly increased (see Chapter 8). Times for disinfection range from 10 to 90 minutes; always read the manufacturer's recommendations. Glutaraldehyde products are useful for plastics or other items that cannot withstand heat sterilization. Some glutaraldehyde products are effective for only 28 days after activation.

Glutaraldehyde is very toxic and should be carefully handled to avoid the fumes. Glutaraldehyde-treated instruments should never be used on patients unless the items have been thoroughly rinsed with water. Prolonged contact of certain types of instruments with glutaraldehyde solutions can lead to discoloration and corrosion of instrument surfaces and cutting edges.

Chlorine Dioxide. Chlorine dioxide is classified as a high-level disinfectant and sterilant. Products containing chlorine dioxide can be used as effective, rapid-acting, environmental surface disinfectants (3 minutes) or as chemical sterilants (6 hours). Nevertheless, chlorine dioxide products do not readily penetrate organic debris and must be used with a separate cleaner.

Other disadvantages of chlorine dioxide include the following: (1) it must be prepared fresh daily, (2) it must be used with good ventilation, and (3) it is corrosive to aluminum containers.

Ortho-Phthalaldehyde. Ortho-phthalaldehyde (OPA) is a chemical used in high-level disinfectant and is effective in achieving high-level disinfection within 12 minutes at room temperature. OPA is more expensive than glutaraldehyde solutions, but it may be a good alternative for health care workers with sensitivity to glutaraldehyde. OPA has little odor and does not require activation or mixing.

Disadvantages of an OPA solution include that it: (1) has a high cost, (2) can only be used half as long as most glutaraldehyde products in dentistry, (3) may stain skin and fabrics, (4) turns plastics a blue-green color where proteins have not been removed, and (5) does not have a sterilization claim.

Classifications of Instruments, Equipment, and Surfaces

Instruments, equipment, and surfaces used during patient care are divided into three classifications: critical, semicritical, and noncritical items. These classifications are used to determine the type of posttreatment processing (Table 7.5).

Critical Instruments

Critical items *must be* **heat sterilized**. Critical instruments are items used to penetrate soft tissue or bone. They have the greatest risk for transmitting infection and must be sterilized by heat. Examples of critical instruments include forceps, scalpels, bone chisels, scalers, and burs.

Semicritical Instruments

Semicritical items *should be* **heat sterilized**. Semicritical instruments are those instruments that do not penetrate soft tissue or bone but contact oral tissues and have a lower risk for transmission. Most semicritical items in dentistry are heat tolerant and should be sterilized. If the item will be damaged by heat, then it should receive, at a minimum, high-level disinfection (see Chapter 8).

Examples of semicritical items include mouth mirrors, high-volume evacuator (HVE) tips, rubber dam forceps, X-ray film holders, and amalgam carriers. Items manufactured for single use should be disposed, not disinfected.

In dental offices today, most items used intraorally can withstand the heat of sterilization. A fundamental rule of infection control states, "If an item can be heat sterilized, it should be heat sterilized."

TABLE 7.5
CDC Classification of Instruments and Procedures

Category	Functions and Examples	Intraoral Use	Risk of Disease Transmission	Procedure
Critical	**Function:** To touch bone or to penetrate soft tissue **Examples:** Surgical and dental instruments used to penetrate soft tissue or bone, including forceps, scalpels, bone chisels, scalers, and burs	Yes	Very high	Sterilization
Semicritical	**Function:** To touch mucous membranes but will not touch bone or penetrate soft tissue **Examples:** Mouth mirrors and amalgam carrier	Yes	Moderate	Sterilization or high-level disinfection
Noncritical	**Function:** Contact only with intact skin **Examples:** External dental X-ray head	No	Very low or none	Intermediate-to low-level disinfection or basic cleaning

Note: Always follow manufacturer's recommendations regarding surface contact time.

CDC, Centers for Disease Control and Prevention.

Noncritical Instruments

Noncritical instruments pose the least risk for transmission of infection because they contact only intact skin, which is an effective barrier to microorganisms. These items should be cleaned and processed with an EPA-registered, intermediate-level or low-level disinfectant after each patient use.

Noncritical clinical devices include the position indicator device (PID) of the x-ray unit tube head, the lead apron, and the curing light that comes into contact only with intact skin.

Additional Aseptic Techniques

In addition to precleaning and disinfecting equipment and surfaces, several additional steps can be taken to reduce the spread of microorganisms in the dental office.

Steps to Reduce the Spread of Microorganisms

- Avoid unnecessary touching of surfaces.
- Use high-volume evacuation.
- Use a dental dam.
- Use preprocedural mouth rinses.
- Use disposable items.
- Reduce dental unit water line contamination.

Unnecessary Touching of Surfaces

During patient care procedures, gloves become contaminated with blood and saliva, and that contamination is easily transferred when members of the dental team touch items or surfaces with their gloved hands. By planning ahead and having all needed items present at chairside before the procedure begins, you will reduce the need for leaving chairside or reaching into drawers with contaminated gloves. If you must leave chairside, then use an overglove to reach for necessary items. Remember not to touch or rub your eyes, nose, or skin or touch your hair with gloved hands.

High-Volume Evacuation

The use and proper placement of the HVE greatly reduces the quantity of salivary aerosols and spatter emitted from the patient's mouth (see Chapter 14). The HVE system should be cleaned at the end of the day by running a detergent or a water-based detergent-disinfectant through the system. In addition, the disposable trap should be periodically replaced. Remember to always wear masks, protective eyewear, and protective clothing when cleaning the HVE system or replacing traps.

Dental Dam

Using a dental dam with simultaneous use of the HVE provides the best approach to minimize dental aerosols and spatter emitted from the patient's mouth (see Chapter 14).

Preprocedural Mouth Rinse

Some dentists will have their patients rinse with an antimicrobial mouth rinse before dental procedures are begun. This procedure is intended to reduce the number of microorganisms released in the form of aerosol or spatter. In addition, preprocedural mouth rinsing can decrease the number of microorganisms introduced into the patient's bloodstream during invasive dental procedures. Preprocedural mouth rinses are especially useful before procedures during which a rubber dam cannot be used (e.g., ultrasonic scaler).

Use of Disposables

Disposable items, typically made of plastic and not heat tolerant, are made for a single use. A disposable item must be properly disposed of after use, and you *should not attempt* to preclean and disinfect or sterilize it for reuse on another patient.

Dental Unit Water Line Contamination

Bacteria capable of causing disease can be found in dental unit waterlines, which is reason for concern (Fig. 7.7). As water and debris lay in the dental unit water lines, bacteria will attach to and accumulate on the inside walls, forming a **biofilm** (Fig. 7.8). (Bacteria in dental plaque serve as an excellent example of biofilm formation.) When bacteria are embedded in the protective biofilm, it becomes difficult to remove. As water flows through the lines, bacteria from the biofilm not only can potentially contaminate patients but also can contaminate the dental team through aerosols and spatter generated using the high-speed handpiece, ultrasonic scalers, and air-water syringes.

Although eliminating biofilm from dental unit water lines is not yet entirely possible, methods have been found to greatly reduce the level of bacterial contamination.

FIGURE 7.7 Close-up of dental tube opening.

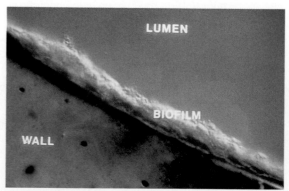

FIGURE 7.8 Magnification of a cross section of a dental unit water line showing biofilm formation.

Cleaning and Disinfection of the Laboratory Area

In contrast to the dental treatment room, the laboratory area in the dental office is often overlooked when infection control practices are implemented. Steps should be taken to prevent cross-contamination between patients and dental team members or to other patients. Standard precautions should always be observed in the dental laboratory.

The counter surfaces should be covered with impervious paper or cleaned and disinfected on a regular basis. All case pans should be cleaned and disinfected before they are used for another case. You should not eat, drink, smoke, apply cosmetics or lip balm, handle contact lenses, or store food in the laboratory area because it is an area of contamination.

A wide variety of dental items, such as impressions, crown and bridges, dentures, and orthodontic retainers, are brought into the lab from the dental treatment area. Remember, items brought into the laboratory from the treatment area are contaminated, and exposure control is just as important here as when you are with the patient.

Equipment used in the laboratory setting should be cleaned and disinfected with an intermediate-level disinfectant. All powder products should be dispensed using the unit dose concept (just enough for one patient). All brushes, rag wheels, and other laboratory tools should be sterilized or disinfected between patients (Fig. 7.9).

Cleaning and Disinfecting the Radiology Area

Cross-contamination can occur during an oral radiographic procedure. That is why it is just as important that the surfaces that the operator touches while producing radiographs are considered noncritical and must be cleaned and disinfected with a low-level or intermediate-level disinfectant after the patient is dismissed. An alternative to surface disinfection is to cover the noncritical surfaces with removable plastic barriers.

Plastic wrap and plastic bags are commonly used as barriers. Barriers should be placed over the chair headrest, countertops, extension arm, tube head, PID of the x-ray machine, control panel, and exposure button (Fig. 7.10).

FIGURE 7.9 Impression trays are heat sterilized in individual bags.

FIGURE 7.10 **A,** Exposure control protected with barrier. **B,** Radiography operatory with barriers in place.

As a dental assistant, you play an especially important role in organizing, managing, and implementing the infection control program in the office. Infection control is a rapidly expanding and changing area within dentistry. New diseases continue to emerge, and familiar pathogens have become resistant to antibiotics. Your employer, fellow staff members, and your patients depend on you to have a solid understanding of the basic concepts of infection control and the ability to perform step-by-step procedures.

Today, more than at any other time in history, patients are concerned about the risk for disease transmission in the dental office. From a legal and ethical aspect, malpractice lawsuits have occurred because of disease transmission to patients caused by improper infection control techniques. Everyone in the dental office must understand the importance of good infection control and must follow all infection control procedures.

Procedure 7.1

Placing and Removing Surface Barriers

Goal

To place surface barriers before patient treatment and to remove the barriers at the end of the procedure.

Equipment and Supplies

- Liquid antimicrobial hand soap
- Utility gloves
- Plastic surface barriers
- Noncontaminated surfaces in dental treatment room

Procedural Steps

1. Wash and dry hands.
2. Select the appropriate surface barrier to be placed over the clean surface.
   Note: If the surfaces to be covered have been previously contaminated, then put on utility gloves and preclean and disinfect the surface. Then wash, disinfect, and remove your utility gloves. Wash and dry your hands before applying the surface barriers.
3. Place each barrier over the entire surface to be protected. Check to ensure that the barrier is secure and will not come off.
   Purpose: If the barrier slips out of position, then the underlying surface will become contaminated and will require precleaning and disinfecting, negating the barrier's purpose.

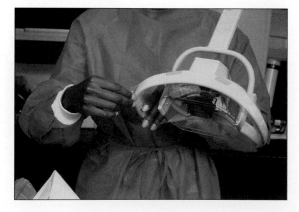

4. Wear utility gloves to remove contaminated surface barriers after dental treatment.
   Purpose: Utility gloves protect the skin from contamination.

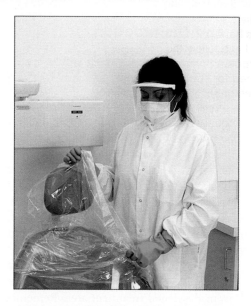

5. Very carefully remove each cover without touching the underlying surface with either the utility glove or the contaminated outside surface of the barrier.
   Purpose: If a surface is accidentally touched during removal of the cover, then the surface must be precleaned and disinfected.
6. Discard the used covers in the regular waste trash. (Check disposal laws in your state.)
   Purpose: Most states do not consider barriers to be regulated waste (requiring special disposal) unless an item is soaked or caked with blood or saliva that would be released if the item were to be compressed.
7. Wash, disinfect, and remove your utility gloves. Wash and dry your hands, then apply fresh surface covers for the next patient.
   Purpose: Your utility gloves are contaminated from handling the used barriers. By washing, drying, and disinfecting your utility gloves, you will know they are ready for their next use.

Goal

To clean and disinfect dental treatment rooms effectively.

Equipment and Supplies

- Personal protective equipment (PPE), including utility gloves, goggles, and mask
- Intermediate-level surface cleaner and/or disinfectant
- Paper towels

Procedural Steps

1. Put on utility gloves, protective eyewear, and protective clothing.

   Purpose: To prevent contact with contaminated surfaces and chemicals.

   Note: The latex examination gloves used in patient care should not be used for precleaning and disinfecting procedures. The chemicals will degrade the latex glove and allow chemicals and contaminants to penetrate to the skin.

2. Make sure that the precleaning and/or disinfecting products have been correctly prepared and are fresh. Always read and follow the manufacturer's instructions.

   Purpose: Some products are concentrated and must be diluted for use. In addition, some products must be prepared daily.

3. To preclean, spray the paper towel or gauze pad with the product and vigorously wipe the surface. You may use a small brush for surfaces that do not become visibly clean from wiping. If you are cleaning a large area, then use several towels or gauze pads.

   Purpose: Overspray is reduced by spraying the product onto the towel or gauze pad. Large areas require more towels or pads to avoid spreading bioburden instead of removing it.

4. To disinfect, spray a fresh paper towel or gauze pad with the product. Let the surface remain moist for the manufacturer's recommended time for tuberculocidal action (usually 10 minutes).

5. If the surface is still moist after the kill time and you are ready to seat another patient, then you may wipe the surface dry. Use water to rinse any residual disinfectant from surfaces that will come in contact with the patient's skin or mouth.

   Purpose: The chemicals used for precleaning and disinfecting may irritate the patient's skin or damage the patient's clothing.

Multiple Choice

Circle the letter next to the correct answer.

1. A mouth mirror is an example of a _____ instrument.
    a. critical
    b. semicritical
    c. noncritical
2. A dental bur is an example of a _____ instrument.
    a. critical
    b. semicritical
    c. noncritical
3. Which of the following PPE should NOT be worn while precleaning and disinfecting a treatment room?
    a. Mask
    b. Eyewear
    c. Gown
    d. Latex examination gloves
4. Surface barriers are NOT necessary to place on _____.
    a. electrical outlets
    b. x-ray control switches
    c. drawer handles
    d. control button on dental chair
5. The best way to manage surface asepsis is with the use of _____.
    a. surface disinfectants only
    b. surface barriers only
    c. a combination of surface barriers and surface disinfectants
6. Laboratory items used on a patient's denture should be changed _____.
    a. daily
    b. weekly
    c. after each use
7. Which of the following items can produce contaminated dental unit water?
    a. High-speed handpieces
    b. Air-water syringes
    c. Ultrasonic handpieces
    d. All of the above
8. When placing surface barriers on a clean and disinfected, you should use _____.
    a. clean bare hands
    b. latex examination gloves
    c. utility gloves
    d. sterile gloves
9. _____ instruments *must* be heat sterilized between patients.
    a. Semicritical
    b. Critical
    c. Noncritical
    d. All of the above
10. Which of the following types of disinfectants may not necessarily have tuberculocidal action?
    a. High level
    b. Intermediate level
    c. Low level

Apply Your Knowledge

1. While seating your next patient in the dental treatment, you notice that the surface barrier on the light handle has become dislodged and is barely hanging on. Although you do not see any visible contamination on the light handle, you are not sure if you replaced the barrier. What should you do?
2. A patient has baked some cookies for everyone in your dental office. As she enters the hallway en route to the treatment room, she offers to put the cookies in the laboratory for you so you can enjoy them later. What would you do?
3. After seeing a recent news story about COVID-19, a patient expresses his concern about the possibility of disease transmission in your dental office. How would you reassure this patient?
4. You are preparing a dental treatment room for your next patient. Where would surface barriers be placed and why?

CHAPTER 8

Instrument Processing

http://evolve.elsevier.com/Robinson/essentials/

LEARNING OBJECTIVES

1. Pronounce, define, and spell the key terms.
2. List the seven steps of processing contaminated dental instruments.
3. Describe the "ideal" instrument-processing area.
4. Complete the following related to precleaning and packaging instruments:
   - List and describe the three ways to preclean instruments.
   - Describe how to operate an ultrasonic cleaner.
   - Explain the steps in packaging instruments.
   - Discuss the various types of packaging materials used for sterilization.
5. Complete the following related to methods of sterilization:
   - Identify the three methods of heat sterilization and give the advantages and disadvantages of each.
   - Describe the process of using an autoclave.
   - Describe the process of using chemical vapor, dry heat, and chemical liquid.
6. Complete the following related to sterilization monitoring:
   - Give the three types of sterilization monitoring currently used.
   - Explain the differences between process indicators and process integrators.
7. Describe the purpose and steps in biologic monitoring.
8. Give the reasons for sterilization failure.

KEY TERMS

autoclave	dry heat sterilization	process integrators
biologic monitoring	forced air sterilizer	static air sterilizer
chemical vapor sterilization	holding solution	ultrasonic cleaner
clean areas	instrument processing	
contaminated area	process indicators	

Appropriate sterilization procedures are essential to a dental practice and one of the most important responsibilities of the dental team.

To prevent disease agents from being transferred to you, to another member of the dental team, or to the next patient, **instrument processing** procedures must be performed in a consistent and disciplined seven-step process (Table 8.1). Although the seven steps are not difficult to understand, having a clear knowledge of how and why each step is performed is especially important.

Processing the procedure tray setup begins in the treatment area at the completion of the patient visit by discarding disposable needles, scalpels, and other contaminated sharp items into a puncture-resistant sharps disposal container. Waste, such as used cotton rolls, gauze squares, and additional disposal items from your setup, is discarded.

The contaminated instruments are then transferred to the sterilization center (processing area). To prevent injury, the following personal protection equipment (PPE) is required when handling soiled instruments: nitrile utility gloves, protective clothing, mask, and protective eyewear.

Sterilization Center

The sterilization area should be centrally located in the office to allow easy access from all patient care areas. An ideal instrument-processing center should be dedicated only to instrument processing, physically separated from the dental treatment areas and dental laboratory and not be a part of a common pathway for patients (Fig. 8.1).

TABLE 8.1

Seven Steps for Instrument Processing

Step		Technique
1.	Transport	Transport contaminated instruments to the processing area in a manner that minimizes the risk for exposure to persons and the environment. Use appropriate PPE and a rigid, leakproof container.
2.	Cleaning	Clean instruments using a hands-free, mechanical process, such as an ultrasonic cleaner or instrument washer. If instruments cannot be immediately cleaned, use a holding solution.
3.	Packaging	In the clean area, wrap and/or package instruments in appropriate types of materials. Place a chemical indicator inside the package next to the instruments. If an indicator is not visible on the outside of the package, then place an external process indicator on the package.
4.	Sterilization	Load the sterilizer according to the manufacturer's instructions. Label the packages. Do not overload the sterilizer. Place the packages on their edges in single layers or on racks to increase circulation of the sterilizing agent around the instruments. Operate the sterilizer according to the manufacturer's instructions. Allow packages to cool before removing them from the sterilizer. Allow packages to cool before handling.
5.	Storage	Store instruments in a clean, dry environment in a manner that maintains the integrity of the package. Rotate packages so that those with the oldest sterilization dates will be used first.
6.	Delivery	Deliver packages to the point of use in a manner that maintains sterility of the instruments until they are used. Inspect each package for damage. Aseptically open each package.
7.	Quality assurance program	An effective quality assurance program should incorporate training, record keeping, maintenance, and the use of biologic indicators.

PPE, Personal protective equipment.

Data from the Organization for Safety, Asepsis and Prevention (OSAP).

The size of the area should accommodate all the equipment and supplies necessary for instrument processing, with multiple outlets and proper lighting, water, and an air-line and vacuum line for flushing high-speed handpieces. A deep sink should have hands-free controls for instrument rinsing and a foot-operated or other hands-free trash receptacle. The flooring should be an uncarpeted, seamless, and hard surface.

Workflow Pattern

Regardless of the size or shape of the sterilization center, the area needs to be subdivided into well-defined areas with the

intent of moving instruments from the "dirty side" to a "clean side." Instruments that are being processed should proceed in a single direction—from contaminated to precleaning to sterilization to storage—without ever *doubling back* (Fig. 8.2). The Centers for Disease Control and Prevention (CDC) recommends the processing areas include the following sections:

- Contaminated (Receiving, cleaning, and decontamination)
- Preparation and packaging
- Sterilization/Storage

This method works well to prevent mixing contaminated and sterile items in a small sterilization area.

Contaminated Area

All soiled instruments that are brought into the **contaminated area** are received, cleaned, and decontaminated. Any disposable items not already discarded in the treatment room are removed from the instrument tray and disposed of as contaminated waste (Fig. 8.3).

The contaminated area contains clean PPE, a counter space, a sink, a waste disposal container, a **holding solution**, an **ultrasonic cleaner**, an eyewash station, and supplies for wrapping instruments before sterilization.

Note: Soiled and clean instruments are never stored in the same cabinet.

Holding Solution

In a busy practice, you may not always be able to clean dental instruments immediately after a procedure. This can present a problem because biologic debris (blood, saliva) left on instruments can dry and harden, which can make it difficult

FIGURE 8.1 The clean area includes the sterilizer and space to store prepared trays. (From iStock.com/luckyraccoon.)

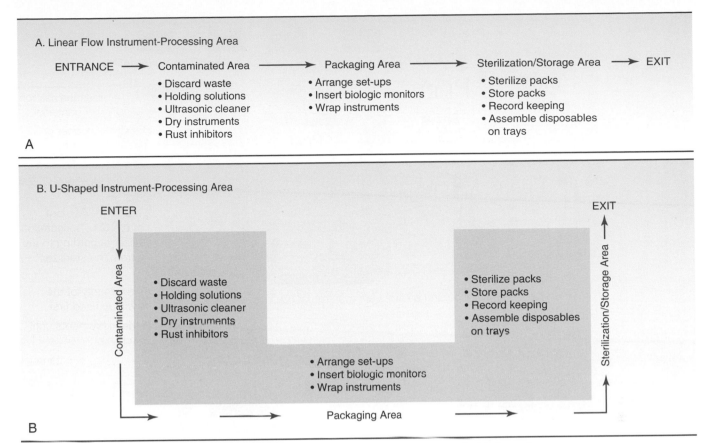

A. Linear Flow Instrument-Processing Area

ENTRANCE → Contaminated Area → Packaging Area → Sterilization/Storage Area → EXIT

Contaminated Area
- Discard waste
- Holding solutions
- Ultrasonic cleaner
- Dry instruments
- Rust inhibitors

Packaging Area
- Arrange set-ups
- Insert biologic monitors
- Wrap instruments

Sterilization/Storage Area
- Sterilize packs
- Store packs
- Record keeping
- Assemble disposables on trays

A

B. U-Shaped Instrument-Processing Area

ENTER

EXIT

Contaminated Area
- Discard waste
- Holding solutions
- Ultrasonic cleaner
- Dry instruments
- Rust inhibitors

Sterilization/Storage Area
- Sterilize packs
- Store packs
- Record keeping
- Assemble disposables on trays

- Arrange set-ups
- Insert biologic monitors
- Wrap instruments

Packaging Area

B

FIGURE 8.2 Instrument processing area. **A,** Linear. **B,** U-shaped.

FIGURE 8.3 Waste items are properly discarded.

to remove, like food left on your dishes at home. Instruments that cannot be cleaned immediately should be placed in a holding solution to prevent blood and debris from drying on the instruments.

The holding solution can be a detergent or a commercial solution that helps dissolve organic debris (Fig. 8.4). Dishwasher detergent makes a good holding solution because it is low cost, low foaming, and readily available. If you are using a manufactured product, follow the manufacturer's instructions when choosing a solution.

The container must have a lid and be labeled with both a biohazard label (because of the contaminated instruments) and a chemical label (because of the cleaner and/or detergent). The holding solution should be changed at least twice daily and more frequently if it becomes clouded.

Precleaning and Packaging Instruments

Instruments may be precleaned in one of three ways: (1) hand scrubbing, (2) ultrasonic cleaning, or (3) instrument washing machines.

Hand Scrubbing

Hand scrubbing is the LEAST desirable method of cleaning instruments because it requires direct hand contact with the contaminated instrument. If you absolutely must hand-scrub instruments, then adhere to the following precautions:

- Wear goggle-type eyewear, puncture-resistant gloves, and protective clothing.
- Clean only one or two instruments at a time.
- Use only a long-handled brush, preferably one with a hand guard or a wide surface.
- Keep items above the water line; fully immersing them in a basin of soapy water interferes with the ability to see sharp ends.
- Allow the instruments to air dry, or carefully pat them with thick toweling. Never rub or roll the instruments inside the towel because of the risk for accidental injury.

Note: Some states have specific infection control guidelines or Occupational Safety & Health Administration (OSHA) plans that prohibit hand scrubbing of instruments. In these states, an ultrasonic cleaner or machine cleaning must be used.

FIGURE 8.4 Commercial holding solutions are available for use in precleaning. (Courtesy Biotrol, Earth City, Missouri.)

FIGURE 8.5 Ultrasonic cleaning. Instruments are placed in an ultrasonic cleaning basket, and the basket is placed in the cleaning solution. (From Miller CH: *Infection controls and management of hazardous materials for the dental team*, ed 6, St Louis, 2018, Elsevier.)

FIGURE 8.6 A commercial all-purpose ultrasonic cleaner. (Courtesy Certol, Commerce City, CO.)

Ultrasonic Cleaning

Ultrasonic cleaners are used to loosen and remove debris from instruments (Fig. 8.5). These cleaners also reduce the risk for hand injuries from cuts and punctures during the cleaning process.

Puncture-resistant utility gloves, a mask, protective eyewear, and a protective gown should always be worn when the ultrasonic cleaner is used. To further limit contact with contaminated instruments, keep a set of tongs near the ultrasonic unit for removing instruments after the cleaning cycle.

The ultrasonic cleaner works by producing sound waves beyond the range of human hearing. These sound waves, which can travel through metal and glass containers, cause cavitation (formation of bubbles in liquid). The bubbles, which are too small to be seen, burst by implosion (bursting inward, the opposite of an explosion). The mechanical cleaning action of the bursting bubbles combined with the chemical action of the ultrasonic solution removes the debris from the instruments.

Instruments should be processed in the ultrasonic cleaner until they are visibly clean. The time may vary from 5 to 15 minutes, depending on the amount and type of material on the instruments and the efficiency of the ultrasonic unit. Instruments in plastic or resin cassettes require slightly longer cleaning times because the cassette material absorbs some of the ultrasonic energy.

There are ultrasonic solutions that are specially formulated for use only in the ultrasonic cleaner. Some ultrasonic cleaning products have enzyme activity. Other ultrasonic cleaning products have antimicrobial activity, which reduces the buildup of microbes in solutions with repeated use. Antimicrobial activity does not disinfect the instruments; it merely prevents microorganisms from increasing in number (Fig. 8.6).

FIGURE 8.7 Aluminum foil test for ultrasonic cleaners. **A,** The lower half of the foil is submerged in the cleaning solution for 20 seconds of operation. **B,** Note the indentations and some holes evenly distributed over the submerged portion of the foil. (From Miller CH: *Infection controls and management of hazardous materials for the dental team,* ed 6, St Louis, 2018, Elsevier.)

Do not use other chemicals such as plain disinfectants in the ultrasonic cleaner. Some disinfectants can *affix* the blood and debris onto the instruments, making subsequent cleaning more difficult. Specific ultrasonic solutions are available that remove difficult materials, such as cements, tartar, stains, plaster, and alginate. Refer to the ultrasonic unit manufacturer's instructions regarding the specific solution to be used.

Like the holding solution, the ultrasonic cleaning unit should be labeled with both a chemical label and a biohazard label because it contains a chemical along with contaminated instruments. See Procedure 8.1: Operating the Ultrasonic Cleaner.

Care of the Ultrasonic Cleaner

The ultrasonic cleaner solution is highly contaminated and must be discarded at least once a day or sooner if it becomes visibly cloudy. When the solution is changed, the inside of the pan and lid should be rinsed with water, disinfected, rinsed again, and dried. All PPE should be worn for changing of solutions in the ultrasonic cleaner.

Testing the Ultrasonic Cleaner

If you notice that the instruments are not being completely cleaned after processing in the ultrasonic cleaner, then the unit may not be properly functioning.

To determine whether the ultrasonic cleaner is properly working, hold a 5 × 5-inch sheet of lightweight aluminum foil vertically (like a curtain) half-submerged in the fresh, unused solution. Run the unit for 20 seconds and then hold the foil up toward the light. The surfaces that were submerged in the solution should be evenly marked with a tiny pebbling effect over the entire surface (Fig. 8.7). An area on the foil that is greater than 1/2-inch without pebbling indicates that a problem with the unit exists and that it needs servicing by the manufacturer.

Automated Washers and Disinfectors

Automated instrument washers and disinfectors look and work like a household dishwasher, but the U.S. Food and Drug Administration (FDA) must approve them for use with dental instruments (Fig. 8.8).

FIGURE 8.8 Miele Dental Thermal Disinfector provides safe and thorough instrument cleaning, disinfecting, and drying. Instruments must be packaged and sterilized after the cycle.

Automated washing and disinfecting units use a combination of hot water recirculation and detergents to remove organic material, then the instruments are automatically dried. These units are classified as thermal disinfectors because they have a disinfecting cycle that subjects the instruments to a level of heat that kills most vegetative microorganisms.

Instruments processed in the automatic washers and disinfectors must be wrapped and sterilized before use on a patient.

Drying, Lubrication, and Corrosion Control

Certain instruments and burs made of carbon steel will rust in steam sterilization. Rust inhibitors, such as sodium nitrate or commercial products, are available as a spray or dip solution applied before the sterilization process and will help reduce rust and corrosion. Hinged instruments need to be lubricated to maintain proper opening. Take care to remove all excess lubricant before heat sterilization.

Thoroughly drying the instrument using dry heat or unsaturated chemical vapor sterilization (see the "Chemical Vapor Sterilization" section in this chapter) is an alternative to using rust inhibitors and does not cause rusting.

Clean Area

In the clean area, cleaned instruments and other dental supplies should be inspected, assembled into sets or trays, and wrapped or placed in packages for sterilization.

Remember, "clean" instruments *are not* sterile and can still harbor pathogens. Instruments must be packaged and sterilized before being used on a patient.

Packaging Instruments

Before sterilization, the instruments are wrapped or packaged to protect them from becoming contaminated after sterilization. When instruments are sterilized without being packaged, they are immediately exposed to the environment as soon as the sterilizer door is opened. They can be contaminated by aerosols in the air, dust, improper handling, or contact with nonsterile surfaces.

An additional advantage of packaging instruments is that they can be grouped into special setups according to the type of procedure they are to be used in.

Packaging Materials

Sterilization packaging materials and cassettes are medical devices and therefore must be FDA approved. Using only products and materials that are labeled as *sterilization packaging* is critical. Never substitute products such as plastic wraps, paper, or zipper-lock freezer bags that are not registered for this purpose. These products may melt or prevent the sterilizing agent from reaching the instruments inside.

Specific types of packaging material are available for each method of sterilization. You should use only the type of packaging material designed for the method of sterilization that you are using (Table 8.2).

A wide variety of sterilization packaging materials are available. Self-sealing or heat-sealed *poly bags* or tubes provide an excellent wrap (Fig. 8.9). In addition, paper wraps and cloth wraps are available. If the package is not the self-sealing type, then you should use only sterilization indicator tape to seal the package.

Never use safety pins, staples, paper clips, or other sharp objects that could penetrate the packaging material.

Reusing Wraps

Standard sterilization wraps are not to be reused; they are neither designed for reuse nor FDA registered for reuse. Reusing single-use sterilization wraps or bags can result in a loss of chemical indicator ability, insecure sealing of the package, and an inability of the package material to maintain sterility of the contents after processing.

Methods of Sterilization

Sterilization destroys all microbial forms, including bacterial spores. Sterile is an absolute term; there is no *partially* sterile or *almost* sterile.

All reusable items—critical and semicritical instruments—that come in contact with the patient's blood, saliva, or mucous membranes must be sterilized. The most common forms of heat sterilization in the dental office are (1) steam sterilization, (2) unsaturated chemical vapor sterilization, and (3) dry heat sterilization, (Table 8.3).

Although most reusable items can withstand heat processing, a few plastic items, such as rubber dam frames, shade guides, and X-ray film-holding devices, will be damaged by heat. For such items, a liquid sterilant must be used. A liquid sterilant is

---

TABLE 8.2

Packaging Materials and Types of Sterilization

Packaging Material	Tips
Steam Sterilization	
Paper wrap	Do not use closed containers.
Nylon tubing	Do not use thick cloth.
Paper or plastic peel pouches	Some plastics melt.
Thin cloth	
Wrapped perforated cassettes	
Dry Heat Sterilizers	
Paper wrap	Some paper may scorch.
Appropriate type of nylon *plastic* tube	Some plastics melt.
Closed containers (use biologic indicator)	Use only materials approved for dry heat.
Unsaturated Chemical Vapor	
Paper wrap	Do not use closed containers.
Paper or plastic peel pouches	Do not use cloth (absorbs too much chemical vapor).
Wrapped perforated cassettes	Some plastics melt.
	Use only materials approved for chemical vapor.

FIGURE 8.9 Instrument packing using a self-sealing, paper/plastic peel pouch. **A,** Packaged handpieces. **B,** Packaged instrument cassette. (From Miller CH: *Infection controls and management of hazardous materials for the dental team,* ed 6, St Louis, 2018, Elsevier.)

TABLE 8.3

Advantages and Disadvantages of Sterilization Methods

Method of Sterilization	Advantages	Disadvantages
Steam autoclave	Short time	Damages some plastic and rubber items
	No corrosion	Requires use of distilled water
	Instruments dry quickly after cycle	May rust non–stainless steel instruments and burs
		Cannot use closed containers
Unsaturated chemical vapor	Short time	Instruments must be dry
	Good penetration of steam	Damages some plastic and rubber items
	Commonly used in dental offices	Requires special solution
		Requires good ventilation
		Cannot sterilize liquids
		Cannot use closed containers
		Cloth wrap may absorb chemicals
Dry heat oven type (static air)	No corrosion	Long sterilization time
	Can use closed containers	Instruments must be predried
	Items are dry after cycle	Damages some plastic and rubber items
		Cannot sterilize liquids
Rapid heat transfer (forced air)	Very fast	Damages some plastic and rubber items
	No corrosion	Instruments must be predried
	Items are dry after cycle	Cannot sterilize liquids

not recommended for use on any item that can withstand heat sterilization or is disposable.

Be sure to have a Safety Data Sheet (SDS) for each product used in the sterilization of dental instruments. All employees should be trained on how to handle these products safely.

Autoclaving

An autoclave is used to sterilize dental instruments and other items by means of steam under pressure. The autoclave is used for sterilization of a variety of dental instruments and accessories, including heat-resistant plastics, dental handpieces, instruments, cotton rolls, and gauze (Fig. 8.10). Packaging material for autoclave sterilization must be porous enough to permit the steam to penetrate the packaging to the instruments inside. The packaging material may be fabric but most often is sealed film or paper pouches, nylon tubing, sterilizing wrap, or paper-wrapped cassettes.

Solid closed metal trays, capped glass vials, and aluminum foil cannot be used in an autoclave because they prevent the steam from reaching the inside of the pack.

A disadvantage of steam sterilization is that the moisture may cause corrosion on some high-carbon steel instruments.

FIGURE 8.10 Steam autoclave. (Courtesy SciCan Inc., Canonsburg, Pennsylvania.)

FIGURE 8.11 The unsaturated chemical vapor sterilizer. (From Miller CH: *Infection controls and management of hazardous materials for the dental team,* ed 6, St Louis, 2018, Elsevier.)

TABLE 8.4

Typical Steam Temperatures in Sterilizing Cycle

Temperature	Time
250°F (121°C)	30 minutes
250°F (121°C)	15 minutes
273°F (134°C)	10 minutes
273°F (134°C)	3 minutes

Distilled water should be used in autoclaves instead of tap water, which often contains minerals and impurities. Distilled water can minimize corrosion and pitting.

Operation Cycles

Dental office steam sterilizers operate through four cycles: (1) heat-up cycle, (2) sterilizing cycle, (3) depressurization cycle, and (4) drying cycle.

After water is added, the chamber is loaded, the door is closed, the unit is turned on, and the heat-up cycle begins to generate steam. The steam pushes out the air in the chamber, and when the set temperature is reached, the sterilizing cycle begins. The temperature is maintained for the set time, usually ranging from 3 to 30 minutes (Table 8.4).

All steam sterilizers operate in a similar manner, but different models and brands have different features. Various sizes of chambers and mechanisms of air removal, steam generation, drying, temperature displays, and recording devices are available.

Procedure 8.2 illustrates the use of an autoclave.

Chemical Vapor Sterilization

Chemical vapor sterilization is similar to autoclaving, except a combination of chemicals—alcohol, formaldehyde, ketone, acetone, and water—is used instead of water to create a vapor for sterilizing (Fig. 8.11 and Procedure 8.3). OSHA requires an SDS on the chemical vapor solution because of the chemicals' toxicity.

Advantages

The major advantage of the chemical vapor sterilizer is that it does not rust, dull, or corrode dry metal instruments. The low water content of the vapor prevents destruction of items such as endodontic files, orthodontic pliers, wires, bands, and burs. A wide range of items can be routinely sterilized without damage.

Other advantages include the short cycle time and the availability of a dry instrument after the cycle.

Disadvantages

The primary disadvantage of the chemical vapor sterilizer is that adequate ventilation is essential because residual chemical vapors containing formaldehyde and methyl alcohol can be released when the chamber door is opened at the end of the cycle. These vapors can temporarily leave an unpleasant odor in the area and may be irritating to the eyes.

Packaging

Standard packaging for chemical vapor sterilization includes film pouches or paper bags, nylon see-through tubing, sterilization wrap, and wrapped cassettes. Packages should not be too thick or tightly wrapped to ensure adequate contact with the chemical vapors.

As in autoclaving, closed containers (such as solid metal trays and capped glass vials) and aluminum foil cannot be used in a chemical vapor sterilizer because they prevent the sterilizing agent from reaching the instruments inside.

Pressure, Temperature, and Time

The three major factors in chemical vapor sterilization are pressure, which should measure 20 pounds per square inch (psi); temperature, which should measure 270°F (131°C); and time, which should measure 20 to 40 minutes.

Dry Heat Sterilization

Dry heat sterilization operates by heating up air and transferring that heat from the air to the instruments. This form of sterilization requires higher temperatures than steam or chemical vapor sterilization. Dry heat sterilizers operate at approximately

FIGURE 8.12 Example of a static air dry heat sterilizer. (From Miller CH: *Infection controls and management of hazardous materials for the dental team,* ed 6, St Louis, 2018, Elsevier.)

FIGURE 8.13 STATIM sterilizer. (Courtesy SciScan Inc. Canonsburg, Pennsylvania.)

320°F to 375°F (160°C to 190°C) and vary in the time of operation, depending on the manufacturer's instructions (Fig. 8.12). See Procedure 8.4: Sterilizing Instruments with Dry Heat.

The advantage of dry heat is that the instruments will not rust if they are thoroughly dry before they are placed in the sterilizer. Two types of dry heat sterilizers are static air and forced air.

Flash Sterilization

Rapid or flash sterilization of dental instruments is achieved by rapid heat transfer, steam, and unsaturated chemical vapor (Fig. 8.13).

Flash sterilization of instruments are placed in the chamber unwrapped, which presents a compromise because the sterility of the instruments is immediately defeated when the instruments are removed from the sterilizer.

Flash sterilization should be used only for instruments that are to be promptly used after removal from the sterilizer.

Chemical Liquid Sterilization

Not all items can withstand heat sterilization. Some types of plastics, such as some rubber dam frames, shade guides, and X-ray film-holding devices, are damaged by heat sterilization.

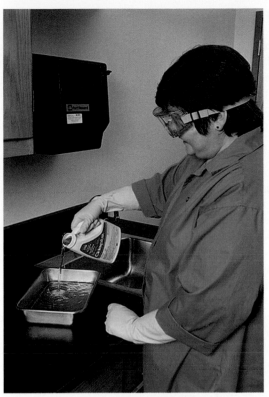

FIGURE 8.14 Preparing the high-level disinfectant/sterilizer used for immersion of instruments that cannot tolerate heat sterilization. (From Bonewit-West K, Hunt SA, Applegate E: *Today's medical assistant: clinical & administrative procedures,* ed 3, St Louis, 2016, Elsevier.)

Thus a liquid sterilant, such as 2% to 3.4% glutaraldehyde, may be used for sterilization of these items. Sterilization in glutaraldehyde requires a 10-hour contact time; anything less than 10 hours is disinfection, not sterilization (Fig. 8.14). Biologic monitoring is not possible when using chemical liquid sterilants. See Procedure 8.5: Sterilizing Instruments with Chemical Liquid.

Static Air Sterilizers

A static air sterilizer is similar to an oven; the heating coils are on the bottom of the chamber, and the hot air rises inside through natural convection. Heat is transferred from the static (nonmoving) air to the instruments in approximately 1 to 2 hours. The disadvantages of static dry heat are that the sterilization process is time-consuming. The wrapping material must be heat resistant. Aluminum foil, metal, and glass containers may be used. Paper and cloth packs should be avoided because they may burn or discolor from the intense heat.

Forced Air Sterilizers

A forced air sterilizer, also called a rapid heat transfer sterilizer, circulates hot air throughout the chamber at a high velocity. This action permits rapid transfer of heat energy from the air to the instruments, reducing the time needed for sterilization. After the sterilizing temperature has been reached, exposure time in forced air sterilizers ranges from 6 minutes for unpackaged items to 12 minutes for packaged items.

Sterilization Assurance

To ensure that the sterilization process is actually effective in achieving complete sterilization of all dental instruments, a comprehensive quality assurance program should be in place.

Currently, three types of sterilization indicators are used: physical, chemical, and biologic. All three processes are unique, have different functions, and must be consistently used to ensure sterility.

Physical Indicators

Physical indicators refer to the use of a checklist process that verifies certain factors for every sterilization cycle. The cycle factors to be monitored include:

- Level of solution
- Temperature (of chamber, not inside the pack)
- Pressure
- Time

Although correct readings do not guarantee sterilization, an incorrect reading is the first sign of a problem. Overloading or improper packaging would not be detected from the reading on the gauges.

FIGURE 8.15 **A,** Unprocessed instruments. **B,** Wrapped instruments after processing. Note the color change in the tape. (From Proctor DB, Adams AP: *Kinn's the medical assistant: an applied learning approach,* ed 12, St. Louis, 2014, Saunders.)

Chemical Indicators

Chemical indicators (external and internal) involve the use of a heat-sensitive chemical that changes color when exposed to certain conditions. The two types of chemical indicators are process indicators and process integrators.

Process Indicators

Process indicators (external) are placed outside the instrument packages before sterilization. Examples are autoclave tape and color change markings on packages or bags (Fig. 8.15).

Process indicators simply identify instrument packs that have been exposed to a certain temperature, but they do not measure the duration or the pressure. Process indicators are useful in distinguishing packages that were processed from those that were not. They can be used to prevent accidental use of unprocessed instruments.

Process Integrators

Process integrators (internal) are placed inside instrument packages. They respond to a combination of pressure, temperature, and time. Process integrators are also known as *multiparameter indicators.* All sterilization factors are integrated.

Examples of process integrators include strips, tabs, or tubes of colored liquid. The advantage of placing integrators inside each package is the guarantee that the sterilizing agent penetrated the packaging (Fig. 8.16).

Limitations

Process indicators and integrators provide immediate, visual control of sterilizing conditions. They do not indicate sterility and are not a replacement for biologic monitoring.

Biologic Monitoring

Biologic monitoring, or spore testing, is the only approved way to confirm whether sterilization has occurred and all bacteria and endospores have been killed. The CDC, the American Dental Association (ADA), and the Organization for Safety, Asepsis

FIGURE 8.16 Chemical indicators. The top of each pair shows appearance before being heat processed, and the bottom shows the color change after the processing. (From Miller CH: *Infection controls and management of hazardous materials for the dental team,* ed 6, St Louis, 2018, Elsevier.)

and Procedures (OSAP) recommend at least weekly biologic monitoring of sterilization equipment.

Several states also require routine biologic monitoring at weekly, monthly, or cycle-specific intervals, such as spore testing every 40 hours of use or every 30 days, whichever comes first. It is important to review your state regulations for biologic monitoring requirements. See Procedure 8.6: Performing Biologic Monitoring.

Biologic indicators (BIs), also known as spore tests, are vials or strips of paper that contain harmless bacterial spores (spores are highly resistant to heat).

Three BIs are used in testing. Two BIs are placed inside instrument packs, and the sterilizer is operated under normal conditions. The third strip is set aside as a control.

After the load has been sterilized, all BIs are cultured. If the spores survive the sterilization cycle (a positive culture), then a sterilization failure has occurred. If the spores are killed (a negative culture), then the sterilization cycle was successful.

Culturing of the spore test is usually handled through the use of a mail-in monitoring service (Fig. 8.17). If in-office culturing is performed, then the manufacturer's instructions must be carefully followed to avoid errors (Fig. 8.18). Maintaining accurate records of the results of each test is especially important.

Sterilization Failures

There can be several factors that can cause the sterilization process to fail. Table 8.5 provides the results of sterilization errors.

If using a biologic monitoring service, you will receive a report of a sterilization failure (a positive result) to the dental office immediately by telephone. (A positive report indicates that sterilization did not occur.) If the culture result is negative (sterilization did occur), then the monitoring service will mail

a report to the dental office to document that the cultures were read at 24, 48, and 72 hours.

Sterilizer Maintenance

A manufacturer will provide instructions for the operation and care of their product. Sterilization equipment must undergo daily and periodic maintenance to ensure accurate and reliable operation.

Essential Requirements for Sterilizer Maintenance

- Daily inspection and cleaning of door gaskets and internal and external surfaces
- Weekly preventive maintenance by draining solutions from reservoir; cleaning air traps, water sensor, and chamber; and lubricating parts
- Monthly cleaning of the chamber and calibration of pressure and temperature gauges, timers, recording devices, and control devices by running a sterilization cycle
- Yearly inspection of sterilizers during which they are cleaned thoroughly, tested, and calibrated
- Maintaining of documentation of maintenance

Ethical Implications

Federal, state, and local agencies have issued regulatory actions to protect patients and members of the dental team from the transmission of disease in the dental office. Proper instrument processing is an integral component in preventing microorganisms from being transferred to the next patient.

As a member of the dental team, performing the sterilization procedures described in this chapter in a thorough and careful manner is your ethical and legal responsibility.

FIGURE 8.17 Using a mail-in service is a convenient method of biologic monitoring. (Courtesy SPSmedical Supply Corporation, Rush, New York.)

FIGURE 8.18 In-office biologic monitoring system.

TABLE 8.5

Results of Sterilization Errors

Errors	Examples	Results
Inadequate instrument cleaning	Dried blood and/or cement remains on instruments	Organisms may be insulated from sterilizing agents.
Improper packaging	Excessive wrap (too thick)	Prevents sterilizing agent from reaching instruments.
	Packaging material is not compatible with type of sterilizer	Wrap may melt or sterilizing agent may not penetrate wrap.
	Closed container in chemical vapor or autoclave	Sterilizing agent cannot reach inside surfaces.
Improper loading of sterilizer	Overloading	Increases time to reach proper temperature and can slow the penetration to the center of the load.
	No separation between packages (too close together)	May prevent sterilizing agent from reaching all items and surfaces.
Improper timing	Operator error in timing	Insufficient time to sterilize.
	Timing started before reaching proper temperature (in nonautomatic units)	Insufficient time to sterilize.
	Dry heat sterilizer door opened during cycle without restarting time	Insufficient time to sterilize.
Improper temperature	Error in operation of sterilizer	Insufficient heat to sterilize.
	Malfunction of sterilizer	Insufficient heat to sterilize.

Goal

To prepare and use the ultrasonic cleaner effectively.

Equipment and Supplies

- Ultrasonic cleaning unit
- Instruments
- Ultrasonic solution
- Clean towel

Procedural Steps

1. Put on protective clothing, mask, eyewear, and utility gloves.
   Purpose: You will be handling sharps and contaminated instruments and using a chemical ultrasonic solution that could splash in your eyes.
2. Remove the lid from the container.
   Purpose: The lid should remain on the ultrasonic device when not in use to prevent evaporation of the solution and to minimize airborne contamination.
3. Be certain the container has been filled with solution to the level recommended by the manufacturer.
   Purpose: The instruments being cleaned must be completely submerged in the solution.
4. Place loose instruments in the basket or, if using cassettes, place the cassette in the basket.
5. Replace the lid and turn the cycle to "On." The time of the cycle may vary, depending on the efficiency of the ultrasonic unit. The time ranges from 5 to 15 minutes.
   Purpose: Instruments in resin or plastic cassettes require longer cleaning times because resin and plastic absorb some of the ultrasonic energy.
6. After the cleaning cycle, remove the basket and thoroughly rinse the instruments in a sink under tap water with minimal splashing. Hold the basket at an angle to allow water to run off into the sink to minimize splashing.

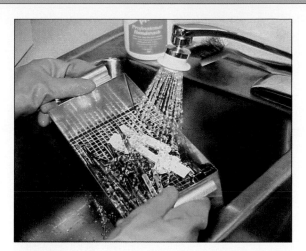

7. Gently turn the basket onto a towel and remove the instruments or cassettes. Replace the lid on the ultrasonic cleaner.

Goal

To prepare and autoclave instruments.

Equipment and Supplies

- Appropriate PPE
- Autoclaving wrapping materials
- Process integrator
- Corrosion inhibitor solution (1% sodium nitrate)
- Tape to seal packages
- Pen or pencil to label packages
- Oven mitt

Procedural Steps

Wrap the Instruments

1. Instruments must be clean, but not necessarily dry, before wrapping for autoclaving.
   Note: The exceptions are glass slabs and dishes, rubber items, and stones. These objects must be dry before being autoclaved.
2. Non–stainless steel instruments and burs may be dipped in a corrosion inhibitor solution (1% sodium nitrate) before being wrapped.

Continued

Note: An alternative for these instruments is sterilization by dry heat.

3. Insert the process integrator into the package.
4. Package, seal, and label the instruments.

Load the Autoclave

1. Place bagged and sealed items in the autoclave.
2. Separate articles and packs from each other by a reasonable space. Tilt glass or metal canisters at an angle.
   Purpose: A reasonable space between articles and packs permits the free flow of steam in and around all instrument packs.

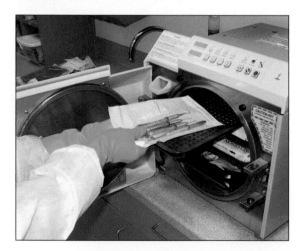

3. Place larger packs, which might block the flow of steam, at the bottom of the chamber.
   Purpose: Large loads prevent the autoclave from reaching the correct temperature and pressure and make it difficult for the steam to flow properly.
4. Never overload the autoclave.
   Purpose: Trapped air in the autoclave will inhibit the top-to-bottom flow of steam.

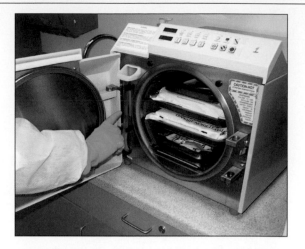

Operate the Autoclave

1. Read and follow the manufacturer's instructions. Most autoclaves require distilled water.
   Purpose: Tap water often contains minerals that can damage the autoclave by forming deposits on the chamber's inner surfaces and can corrode metals.
2. Ensure that an adequate supply of water is available. If not, add distilled water.
3. Set autoclave controls for the appropriate time, temperature, and pressure.
   Note: Pressure and temperature must be reached before timing begins. Duration of this warm-up time depends on the autoclave and the size of the load.
4. At the end of the sterilization cycle, vent the steam into the room. Allow the contents of the autoclave to dry and cool.
   Note: Most models automatically vent and cool. If the machine is not so equipped, then slightly open the door of the autoclave after the pressure has dropped within the chamber. Open the door with extreme caution because the contents and remaining steam are scalding. The contents should be allowed to dry and cool before they are removed.

Reassemble and Store the Trays

1. Wash your hands and put on clean examination gloves for handling sterile packs and reassembling trays.
2. Remove sealed packs from the sterilizer and place them in the clean area.
   Important Note: Work only in the clean area of the sterilization center.
3. Place the sealed packs on the tray, and add the supplies necessary to perform the procedure.
   Optional: In some practices, the necessary gloves and masks are added to the tray at this time. In other practices, these items are stored in the treatment room.
4. Store the prepared tray in the clean area until needed in the treatment room.

PPE, Personal protective equipment.

Sterilizing Instruments With Chemical Vapor

Goal

To prepare and sterilize instruments by chemical vapor sterilization.

Equipment and Supplies

- Appropriate PPE
- Chemical vapor wrapping materials
- Precleaned and dried instruments
- Process integrator
- Tape to seal packages
- Pen or pencil to label packages

Procedural Steps

Wrap the Instruments

1. Ensure that the instruments are clean and dry before wrapping them for chemical vapor sterilization.

Purpose: If instruments are not absolutely dry, they will rust.
2. Insert the appropriate process integrator into the test load instrument package.
3. Take care not to create packs that are too large to be sterilized throughout.

Purpose: Chemical vapor sterilization is not recommended for large loads or tightly wrapped instruments.

Load and Operate the Chemical Vapor Sterilizer

1. Read and follow the manufacturer's instructions.
   Important Note: Always follow the precautions in the SDS.
2. Load the sterilizer according to the manufacturer's instructions.
   Note: This step is similar to loading an autoclave.
3. Set the controls for the appropriate time, temperature, and pressure.
   Note: Pressure and temperature must be reached before timing begins.
4. Follow the manufacturer's instructions for venting and cooling.
5. When the instruments are cool and dry, reassemble and store the preset tray.

PPE, Personal protective equipment; *SDS*, safety data sheet.

Sterilizing Instruments With Dry Heat

Goal

To prepare and sterilize instruments by dry heat sterilization.

Equipment and Supplies

- Wrapping materials
- Precleaned instruments
- Process integrator for dry heat
- Tape to seal packages
- Pen or pencil to label packages

Procedural Steps

Wrap Instruments

1. Clean and dry instruments before wrapping.
   Purpose: Wet instruments can rust during dry heat sterilization.
2. Prepare hinged instruments, such as surgical forceps, hemostats, and scissors, with their hinges opened.
   Purpose: To allow heat to reach all areas during sterilization.

Load and Operate the Dry Heat Sterilizer

1. Read and follow the manufacturer's instructions.
2. Insert the process integrator into the test load package.
3. Load the dry heat chamber to permit adequate circulation of air around the packages.
   Purpose: Sterilization does not occur unless heat reaches all areas of the instruments.
4. Set the time and temperature according to the manufacturer's instructions. Allow time for the entire load to reach the desired temperature.

Purpose: Timing does not start until the desired temperature has been reached throughout the entire load.

5. Do not place additional instruments in the load once the sterilization cycle has begun.
   Purpose: Cooler instruments will significantly lower the temperature of the oven.
6. At the end of the sterilization cycle, allow the packs to cool and then handle them very carefully.
   Purpose: Packs are hot and can cause injury.

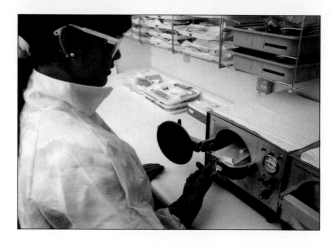

7. When the packs have cooled, remove them, and store the preset tray.

Sterilizing Instruments With Chemical Liquid

Goal

To prepare and sterilize instruments using a chemical sterilant.

Equipment and Supplies

- Appropriate PPE
- Precleaned and dried items that cannot be heat sterilized
- Liquid chemical sterilant
- Sterile instrument tongs
- Sterile rinse water

Procedural Steps

Prepare the Solution

1. Use utility gloves, mask, eyewear, and protective clothing when preparing, using, and discarding the solution.
   Purpose: Liquid sterilants are highly toxic and can lead to respiratory problems if not properly handled.
2. Follow the manufacturer's instructions for preparing and activating, using, and disposing of the solution.
   Purpose: In many areas, glutaraldehyde is considered a hazardous material, requiring special disposal methods; it may not be dumped down the sink.

3. Prepare the solution for use as a sterilant. Label the containers with the name of the chemical, the date of preparation (to indicate the use life), and any other information that relates to the hazards of this product. Use life is the period of time during which a germicidal solution is effective after having been prepared for use.
   Purpose: Some brands remain active for 30 days; others may have a longer or shorter use life.
4. Cover the container and keep it closed unless you are putting instruments in or taking them out.
   Purpose: Glutaraldehyde produces toxic fumes.

Use the Solution

1. Preclean, rinse, and dry the items to be processed.
2. Place the items in a perforated tray or pan. Place the pan in the solution and cover the container. An alternative method is to use tongs and avoid splashing.
3. Be certain that all items are fully submerged in the solution for the entire contact time.
   Purpose: The solution must be in contact with the items for the recommended contact time.

Sterilizing Instruments With Chemical Liquid—cont'd

4. Thoroughly rinse processed items with water and dry. Place the items in a clean package.
   Note: Sterility is best maintained by rinsing the processed items with sterile water, drying them with a sterile towel, and placing them in a sterile container.

Maintain the Solution

1. Periodically test the glutaraldehyde concentration of the solution with a chemical test kit (available from the manufacturer).

2. Replace the solution as indicated on the instructions or when the level of the solution is low or the solution is visibly dirty.

3. When you replace the used solution, discard all of the used solution, clean the container with a detergent, rinse with water, dry, and fill the container with a fresh solution.

PPE, Personal protective equipment.
Modified from Miller CH, Palenik CJ: *Infection control and management of hazardous materials for the dental team,* ed 4, St. Louis, 2010, Mosby.

Procedure 8.6

Performing Biologic Monitoring

Goal

To assess sterilization using BIs (spore tests).

Equipment and Supplies

- Appropriate PPE
- Instruments
- Pencil
- Dual-species BI
- Sterilization log
- Mail-in envelope

Procedural Steps

1. While wearing all PPE, place the BI strip in the bundle of instruments and seal the package.
   Purpose: Although the instruments have been pre-cleaned, they are still contaminated.

2. Place the pack with the BI in the center of the sterilizer load.
   Purpose: The center of the load is most difficult for the sterilizing agent to penetrate.

3. Place the remainder of the packaged instruments into the sterilizer and process the load through a normal sterilization cycle.

Purpose: The monitoring evaluates what is considered the *normal* cycle.

4. Remove utility gloves, mask, and eyewear. Wash and dry hands.
   Purpose: By removing all PPE and washing and drying hands, you prevent contamination of the sterilization log.

5. In the sterilization log, record the date of the test, type of sterilizer, cycle, temperature, time, and name of the person operating the sterilizer.
   Purpose: Maintaining records is part of the exposure control program, and specific information is necessary in the event of a sterilization failure.

6. After the load has been sterilized, remove the processed BI strip.
   Purpose: The BI strip has been exposed to the same sterilizing conditions as the instruments.

7. Mail the processed spore test strips and the control BI strip to the monitoring service.
   Purpose: Obtaining and maintaining the results as part of the exposure control program is important.

BI, Biologic indicator; *PPE,* personal protective equipment.

Chapter Exercises

Multiple Choice

Circle the letter of the correct answer.

1. How many steps are involved in instrument processing?
   a. 4
   b. 5
   c. 7
   d. 10

2. The only certain method to determine sterilization is with the use of _____.
   a. process indicators
   b. process integrators
   c. biologic monitoring
   d. none of the above

3. Contaminated instruments that cannot be cleaned after use should be placed in a(n) _____.
   a. ultrasonic cleaner
   b. thermal disinfector
   c. holding solution
   d. rapid heat transfer unit

4. The ultrasonic cleaner solution should be changed at least_____.
   a. after each patient
   b. three times daily
   c. once daily
   d. once monthly

5. The method of sterilization that uses glutaraldehyde over a long period of time is referred to as _____.
   a. dry heat sterilization
   b. chemical vapor sterilization
   c. autoclaving
   d. chemical liquid sterilization

6. The LEAST desirable method of precleaning instruments is _____.
   a. hand scrubbing
   b. ultrasonic cleaning
   c. thermal disinfector
   d. holding solutions

7. Which of the following can cause a sterilization failure?
   a. Improper cycle time
   b. Overloading the chamber
   c. Opening the door during the cycle
   d. All of the above

8. The fastest method of sterilization is the _____ method.
   a. autoclave
   b. chemical vapor
   c. dry heat static air
   d. dry heat forced air

9. The method of sterilization that produces the greatest risk for rust and corrosion on the instruments is the _____ method.
   a. autoclave
   b. chemical vapor
   c. dry heat static
   d. dry heat forced

10. The method of sterilization that produces unpleasant fumes is the _____ method.
    a. autoclave
    b. chemical vapor
    c. dry heat static
    d. dry heat forced

Apply Your Knowledge

1. Mrs. Hansen is a new patient and was referred by a patient in your office. Mrs. Hansen expressed concern about the sterilization procedures used in her previous dental office. What can you say and do to reassure Mrs. Hansen that your office takes instrument processing and sterilization very seriously?

2. There are days in the office that your schedule is so busy assisting in patient care that you are not able to clean contaminated instruments soon after their use. You have noticed that dried blood and cement is not always removed during the ultrasonic cleaning process. What step can you take to overcome this problem?

3. A new employee does not always wear her protective eyewear when in the sterilization center. How should the office manager/dentist help this new employee understand the importance of wearing all required PPE?

The Dental Patient

http://evolve.elsevier.com/Robinson/essentials/

LEARNING OBJECTIVES	

LEARNING OBJECTIVES

1. Pronounce, define, and spell the key terms.
2. Explain the role of the dental assistant in providing quality patient care.
3. Complete the following related to the patient record:
   - Give the types of forms in a patient record.
   - Describe how to register a new patient.
   - Discuss the importance of the patient's medical history when dental treatment is planned.
   - Describe the procedure for obtaining a medical-dental health history.
   - Explain how the Health Insurance Portability and Accountability Act (HIPAA) influences dental care.
4. Complete the following related to vital signs:
   - Define vital signs.
   - Give the four vital signs commonly taken in the dental office.
   - Describe the procedures for taking a patient's temperature, pulse, respiration, and blood pressure.

KEY TERMS

blood pressure
brachial
carotid
demographics
diastolic
Health Insurance Portability and Accountability Act (HIPAA)

medically compromised
patient record
pulse
respiration
sphygmomanometer
stethoscope
systolic

temperature
thermometer
vital signs

One of the key responsibilities of the dental team is to provide quality patient care. This includes making patients feel welcome, comfortable, and informed, along with maintaining the patient's safety and well-being during their treatment.

The Dental Assistant's Responsibilities to the Patient
- It is essential to be *alert* to the health status of your patients from the time they enter the office, to when they are escorted to the treatment area, during the course of treatment, when they are escorted to the reception area, and when they leave the practice.

- The better you are at *communicating* with your patients, the better assistant you will be at promoting respect and helping people feel comfortable.
- Make the effort to *understand* your patients. Recognize that your patient may be in pain, experiencing anxiety, or worried about payment for their dental care.
- Be *respectful* of your patient by paying attention to their needs and not leaving them unattended or ignored.

Patient Record

The **patient dental record** is the most important legal document maintained for each patient in a dental practice. Whether you are communicating with a patient by phone or in person, speaking to a pharmacy about a prescription, talking to an insurance company regarding payment, or referring a patient to a specialist, the dental record must be accessible for reference.

Personal and clinical information is obtained by asking the new patient to complete the printed or online forms before their first visit. Examples of the types of forms for the patient to complete include:

- Patient registration form
- Medical-dental health history form
- Medical alert information
- Health Insurance Portability and Accountability Act (HIPAA) Privacy Policy form

Circumstances can exist during which a patient may be unable to complete the forms, such as because of a language barrier, not being able to read, or being visually impaired. When this type of circumstance is apparent, assist the patient by helping them complete the forms and by answering any questions necessary to help the patient provide the required data.

Patient Registration

The **patient registration form** is primarily used for the business office in the management of the account. Information in the form must be complete and updated and must include the following (Fig. 9.1):

- Demographics: A patient must provide their full name, address, telephone number, employment information, and spousal information.
- **Responsible party:** Patients are not always responsible for payment of their own dental expenses. This section gathers information concerning the individual who accepts this responsibility. Information required here includes the responsible party's full name, address, home and work telephone numbers, and employment information. Be sure the responsible party signs the release of information and the assignment of benefits.
- **Insurance information:** This section gathers data required in completing dental insurance claims for the patient. The subscriber should provide specific insurance information, such as the group or policy number. Usually, the responsible party is also the insurance plan subscriber. Making a photocopy of the patient's insurance card is customary.

See Procedure 9.1: Registering a New Patient.

Medical History

Questions regarding the patient's medical history, present physical condition, chronic conditions, allergies, and medications are asked. Each new patient must complete a medical history form before treatment can begin (Fig. 9.2). The patient's signature on the form indicates that they have provided the information and takes responsibility for its accuracy.

A complete and up-to-date medical history is important because it:

- Alerts the dentist to medical conditions and medications that may affect the type of treatment provided.
- Aids the dentist in identifying any special treatment needs.
- Alerts the dentist to any allergies that could pose a potential medical emergency.

Returning patients are asked to **update** their medical history at each visit. The patient should sign the form to indicate that the information is accurate and up to date (Fig. 9.3).

The dentist may also wish to consult the patient's physician regarding health problems, particularly if the patient is medically compromised. (*Medically compromised* is defined as a patient with an illness or physical condition that may influence the way dental treatment is provided.)

Medication History

A medication history, which is an essential part of the medical history, is a record of all the medications a patient is currently taking. These include prescription medications, over-the-counter drugs, vitamins, and any other medicines. The medication history is particularly important in older patients, many of whom have chronic conditions and are taking several prescribed and over-the-counter medications.

The dentist needs to be aware of these medications because either the medicine or the condition for which it was prescribed may modify the selection of anesthetic, premedication, and procedures when providing dental treatment.

Allergies. If the patient has any known allergies, then making the dental team aware of these is extremely important. An allergic reaction could increase with severity each time the individual comes into contact with the substance. For this reason, asking about both known and suspected allergies is important.

Of particular concern in the dental setting are allergies to latex, antibiotics, pain medications, and local anesthetic solutions.

Substances Used in a Dental Practice That Could Cause an Adverse Reaction

Latex—Latex gloves and the dental dam are routinely used in patient care.

Antibiotics—Antibiotic medications may be prescribed for patients who are at high risk for bacterial endocarditis, which is a severe bacterial infection of the cardiac valves and supporting structures caused by bloodborne pathogens gaining entry to the bloodstream.

Pain medication—Pain medication may be prescribed to manage postoperative pain from dental treatment.

Topical and local anesthetic solutions—It will be necessary for the dentist to select an alternative anesthetic solution that does not cause an allergic reaction.

Medical Alert. If the patient has a predisposing medical condition that could affect decisions regarding dental treatment, then this information must be indicated on the inside cover of the patient record. Examples of this could include allergy to latex or has high blood pressure. A brightly colored "ALERT" sticker is placed for the attention of the dental team. An alert sticker should never be placed on the outside of a patient record; doing so would violate dentist–patient confidentiality and the privacy of the patient.

Dental History

The patient's dental history offers important clues in reference to previous dental care. Questions can include how recently the

FIGURE 9.1 Sample patient registration form. (From Gaylor LJ: *The administrative dental assistant,* ed 3, St. Louis, 2012, Saunders; form courtesy The Dental Record, Wisconsin Dental Association, Milwaukee, Wisconsin; Dentrix screenshot courtesy Henry Schein Practice Solutions, American Fork, Utah.)

Health History Form

Email: _____ Today's Date: _____

As required by law, our office adheres to written policies and procedures to protect the privacy of information about you that we create, receive or maintain. Your answers are for our records only and will be kept confidential subject to applicable laws. Please note that you will be asked some questions about your responses to this questionnaire and there may be additional questions concerning your health. This information is vital to allow us to provide appropriate care for you. This office does not use this information to discriminate.

Name:			Home Phone: *Include area code*	Business/Cell Phone: *Include area code*
Last	*First*	*Middle*	( )	( )

Address:	City:	State:	Zip:
Mailing address			

Occupation:	Height:	Weight:	Date of Birth:	Sex: M F

SS# or Patient ID:	Emergency Contact:	Relationship:	Home Phone: *Include area code* ( )	Cell Phone: *Include area code* ( )

If you are completing this form for another person, what is your relationship to that person?

Your Name _____ *Relationship* _____

Do you have any of the following diseases or problems: (*Check DK if you Don't Know the answer to the the question*) **Yes No DK**

Active Tuberculosis... ☐ ☐ ☐

Persistent cough greater than a 3 week duration .... ☐ ☐ ☐

Cough that produces blood.. ☐ ☐ ☐

Been exposed to anyone with tuberculosis .... ☐ ☐ ☐

If you answer yes to any of the 4 items above, please stop and return this form to the receptionist.

Dental Information *For the following questions, please mark (X) your responses to the following questions.*

Yes No DK

Do your gums bleed when you brush or floss? .... ☐ ☐ ☐

Are your teeth sensitive to cold, hot, sweets or pressure? .... ☐ ☐ ☐

Is your mouth dry? .... ☐ ☐ ☐

Have you had any periodontal (gum) treatments? .... ☐ ☐ ☐

Have you ever had orthodontic (braces) treatment? .... ☐ ☐ ☐

Have you had any problems associated with previous dental treatment? ... ☐ ☐ ☐

Is your home water supply fluoridated? .... ☐ ☐ ☐

Do you drink bottled or filtered water? .... ☐ ☐ ☐

If yes, how often? *Circle one:* DAILY / WEEKLY / OCCASIONALLY

Are you currently experiencing dental pain or discomfort? .... ☐ ☐ ☐

What is the reason for your dental visit today?

How do you feel about your smile?

Yes No DK

Do you have earaches or neck pains? .... ☐ ☐ ☐

Do you have any clicking, popping or discomfort in the jaw? .... ☐ ☐ ☐

Do you brux or grind your teeth? .... ☐ ☐ ☐

Do you have sores or ulcers in your mouth? .... ☐ ☐ ☐

Do you wear dentures or partials? .... ☐ ☐ ☐

Do you participate in active recreational activities? .... ☐ ☐ ☐

Have you ever had a serious injury to your head or mouth? .... ☐ ☐ ☐

Date of your last dental exam:

What was done at that time?

Date of last dental x-rays:

Medical Information *Please mark (X) your response to indicate if you have or have not had any of the following diseases or problems.*

Yes No DK

Are you now under the care of a physician? .... ☐ ☐ ☐

Physician Name: _____ Phone: *Include area code* ( )

Address/City/State/Zip:

Are you in good health? .... ☐ ☐ ☐

Has there been any change in your general health within the past year? ... ☐ ☐ ☐

If yes, what condition is being treated?

Date of last physical exam:

Yes No DK

Have you had a serious illness, operation or been hospitalized in the past 5 years? .... ☐ ☐ ☐

If yes, what was the illness or problem?

Are you taking or have you recently taken any prescription or over the counter medicine(s)? .... ☐ ☐ ☐

If so, please list all, including vitamins, natural or herbal preparations and/or dietary supplements:

_____

_____

_____

_____

A

FIGURE 9.2 Example of a medical-dental health history form. **A,** Dental history. **B,** Medical history. (Copyright 2012, American Dental Association. All rights reserved. Reprinted with permission.)

Medical Information

Please mark (X) your response to indicate if you have or have not had any of the following diseases or problems.

(Check DK if you Don't Know the answer to the question)

	Yes	No	DK
Do you wear contact lenses?	☐	☐	☐

Joint Replacement. Have you had an orthopedic total joint (hip, knee, elbow, finger) replacement? ☐ ☐ ☐

Date: _____ If yes, have you had any complications? _____

Are you taking or scheduled to begin taking an antiresorptive agent (like Fosamax®, Actonel®, Atelvia, Boniva®, Reclast, Prolia) for osteoporosis or Paget's disease? ☐ ☐ ☐

Since 2001, were you treated or are you presently scheduled to begin treatment with an antiresorptive agent (like Aredia®, Zometa®, XGEVA) for bone pain, hypercalcemia or skeletal complications resulting from Paget's disease, multiple myeloma or metastatic cancer? ☐ ☐ ☐

Date Treatment began: _____

	Yes	No	DK
Do you use controlled substances (drugs)?	☐	☐	☐
Do you use tobacco (smoking, snuff, chew, bidis)?	☐	☐	☐

If so, how interested are you in stopping?
Circle one: VERY / SOMEWHAT / NOT INTERESTED

Do you drink alcoholic beverages?	☐	☐	☐

If yes, how much alcohol did you drink in the last 24 hours? _____

If yes, how much do you typically drink i n a week? _____

WOMEN ONLY Are you:

	Yes	No	DK
Pregnant?	☐	☐	☐
Number of weeks: _____			
Taking birth control pills or hormonal replacement?	☐	☐	☐
Nursing?	☐	☐	☐

Allergies. Are you allergic to or have you had a reaction to:
To all **yes** responses, specify type of reaction.

	Yes	No	DK
Local anesthetics _____	☐	☐	☐
Aspirin _____	☐	☐	☐
Penicillin or other antibiotics _____	☐	☐	☐
Barbiturates, sedatives, or sleeping pills _____	☐	☐	☐
Sulfa drugs _____	☐	☐	☐
Codeine or other narcotics _____	☐	☐	☐

	Yes	No	DK
Metals _____	☐	☐	☐
Latex (rubber) _____	☐	☐	☐
Iodine _____	☐	☐	☐
Hay fever/seasonal _____	☐	☐	☐
Animals _____	☐	☐	☐
Food _____	☐	☐	☐
Other _____	☐	☐	☐

Please mark (X) your response to indicate if you have or have not had any of the following diseases or problems.

	Yes	No	DK
Artificial (prosthetic) heart valve	☐	☐	☐
Previous infective endocarditis	☐	☐	☐
Damaged valves in transplanted heart	☐	☐	☐
Congenital heart disease (CHD)			
Unrepaired, cyanotic CHD	☐	☐	☐
Repaired (completely) in last 6 months	☐	☐	☐
Repaired CHD with residual defects	☐	☐	☐

Except for the conditions listed above, antibiotic prophylaxis is no longer recommended for any other form of CHD.

	Yes	No	DK
Cardiovascular disease	☐	☐	☐
Angina	☐	☐	☐
Arteriosclerosis	☐	☐	☐
Congestive heart failure	☐	☐	☐
Damaged heart valves	☐	☐	☐
Heart attack	☐	☐	☐
Heart murmur	☐	☐	☐
Low blood pressure	☐	☐	☐
High blood pressure	☐	☐	☐
Other congenital heart defects	☐	☐	☐

	Yes	No	DK
Mitral valve prolapse	☐	☐	☐
Pacemaker	☐	☐	☐
Rheumatic fever	☐	☐	☐
Rheumatic heart disease	☐	☐	☐
Abnormal bleeding	☐	☐	☐
Anemia	☐	☐	☐
Blood transfusion	☐	☐	☐
If yes, date:			
Hemophilia	☐	☐	☐
AIDS or HIV infection	☐	☐	☐
Arthritis	☐	☐	☐

	Yes	No	DK
Autoimmune disease	☐	☐	☐
Rheumatoid arthritis	☐	☐	☐
Systemic lupus erythematosus	☐	☐	☐
Asthma	☐	☐	☐
Bronchitis	☐	☐	☐
Emphysema	☐	☐	☐
Sinus trouble	☐	☐	☐
Tuberculosis	☐	☐	☐
Cancer/Chemotherapy/ Radiation Treatment	☐	☐	☐
Chest pain upon exertion	☐	☐	☐
Chronic pain	☐	☐	☐
Diabetes Type I or II	☐	☐	☐
Eating disorder	☐	☐	☐
Malnutrition	☐	☐	☐
Gastrointestinal disease	☐	☐	☐
G.E. Reflux/persistent heartburn	☐	☐	☐
Ulcers	☐	☐	☐
Thyroid problems	☐	☐	☐
Stroke	☐	☐	☐

	Yes	No	DK
Glaucoma	☐	☐	☐
Hepatitis, jaundice or liver disease	☐	☐	☐
Epilepsy	☐	☐	☐
Fainting spells or seizures	☐	☐	☐
Neurological disorders	☐	☐	☐
If yes, specify: _____			
Sleep disorder	☐	☐	☐
Do you snore?	☐	☐	☐
Mental health disorders	☐	☐	☐
Specify: _____			
Recurrent Infections	☐	☐	☐
Type of infection: _____			
Kidney problems	☐	☐	☐
Night sweats	☐	☐	☐
Osteoporosis	☐	☐	☐
Persistent swollen glands in neck	☐	☐	☐
Severe headaches/ migraines	☐	☐	☐
Severe or rapid weight loss	☐	☐	☐
Sexually transmitted disease	☐	☐	☐
Excessive urination	☐	☐	☐

	Yes	No	DK
Has a physician or previous dentist recommended that you take antibiotics prior to your dental treatment?	☐	☐	☐

Name of physician or dentist making recommendation: _____

Phone: *Include area code* ( )

	Yes	No	DK
Do you have any disease, condition, or problem not listed above that you think I should know about?	☐	☐	☐

Please explain: _____

NOTE: Both doctor and patient are encouraged to discuss any and all relevant patient health issues prior to treatment.

I certify that I have read and understand the above and that the information given on this form is accurate. I understand the importance of a truthful health history and that my dentist and his/her staff will rely on this information for treating me. I acknowledge that my questions, if any, about inquiries set forth above have been answered to my satisfaction. I will not hold my dentist, or any other member of his/her staff, responsible for any action they take or do not take because of errors or omissions that I may have made in the completion of this form.

Signature of Patient/Legal Guardian: _____ Date: _____

Signature of Dentist: _____ Date: _____

FOR COMPLETION BY DENTIST
Comments:

B

FIGURE 9.2 Cont'd

```
┌─────────────────────────────────────────────────────────┐
│ MEDICAL HISTORY UPDATE                                   │
│                                                          │
│ GENERAL HEALTH: EXCELLENT ____  GOOD ____ FAIR ____ POOR ____ │
│                                                          │
│ YES ___ NO___ HAVE THERE BEEN ANY CHANGES IN YOUR HEALTH SINCE YOUR LAST │
│               DENTAL APPOINTMENT?                        │
│                                                          │
│ IF YES, PLEASE DESCRIBE: _____ │
│                                                          │
│ _____   │
│                                                          │
│                                                          │
│ YES ___ NO ___ HAS THERE BEEN ANY CHANGES IN YOUR MEDICATIONS? │
│                                                          │
│ IF YES, PLEASE DESCRIBE:                                 │
│                                                          │
│ _____   │
│                                                          │
│ _____   │
│                                                          │
│                                                          │
│ YES ___ NO ___ IS THERE ANY REASON THAT RECEIVING DENTAL CARE MIGHT POSE A │
│                RISK TO YOU, OUR STAFF, OR OTHER PATIENTS? │
│                                                          │
│ IF YES, PLEASE DESCRIBE:                                 │
│                                                          │
│ _____   │
│                                                          │
│ _____   │
│                                                          │
│ _____          _____ │
│      Date                         Patient Signature      │
│                                                          │
│ _____          _____ │
│      Date                         Dentist Signature      │
└─────────────────────────────────────────────────────────┘
```

FIGURE 9.3 Example of the medical-dental health history update form.

patient received dental treatment, the frequency of dental visits, and the patient's attitude concerning the importance of the appearance of their teeth and dental care.

See Procedure 9.2: Obtaining a Medical-Dental Health History.

Privacy Policy of the Health Insurance Portability and Accountability Act

HIPAA requires that all dental practices have a written privacy policy. This policy must inform the patient that the office will not use or disclose protected health information (PHI) for any purpose other than treatment, diagnosis, and billing. The privacy policy must be available for patients to review, and all patients (new and existing) must sign an acknowledgment of receiving these privacy practices established for the office. The signed acknowledgment must be kept in the patient's record for a minimum of 6 years (Fig. 9.4).

HIPAA states that additional authorization and consent from the patient would be required if the disclosure of documents were to be used for health care operations, research, or public need.

Being in a private or semiprivate area is necessary when reviewing a health history or any specific content of a patient record. Additional information about HIPAA can be found at: https://www.hhs.gov/hipaa/for-professionals/privacy/guidance/access/index.html.

Clinical Information

The patient record also includes forms that provide the dental team with updated information about the patient's medical and dental history, dental treatment completed, and dental treatment planned as dictated by the dentist. Forms that the dental team will refer to for clinical needs include:
- Clinical examination form
- Recall examination form
- Treatment plan form
- Progress notes form

The patient's radiographs, laboratory prescriptions, and any correspondence are also stored in the patient record. The patient must provide consent by signing a release-of-information form before a consultation between the dentist and the physician can take place.

Clinical Examination

The clinical examination form is the most comprehensive document in the patient record. This form provides all clinical data from the past, present, and future to the dental team. Each time a patient comes in for an appointment, this form is updated (Fig. 9.5).

Treatment Plan

The treatment plan for a patient refers to the dental problems that were identified during the examination and the diagnosis portion of the patient visit (Fig. 9.6).

ACKNOWLEDGEMENT OF RECEIPT OF NOTICE

As required by the Privacy Regulations, I hereby acknowledge that I have received a current copy of this practice's "NOTICE OF PRIVACY PRACTICES", revision date _____ .

As required by the Privacy Regulations, _____ from
Name of Staff Member
this practice has explained the "NOTICE OF PRIVACY PRACTICES" to my satisfaction.

As required by the Privacy Regulations, I am aware that this practice has included a provision that it reserves the right to change the terms of its notice and to make the new notice provisions effective for all protected health information that it maintains.

Requests:

☐ I wish to file a "Request for Restriction" of my Protected Health Information.

☐ I wish to file a "Request for Alternative Communications" of my Protected Health Information.

☐ I wish to object to the following in the "Notice of Privacy Practices":
_____
_____

I understand that this office may change their Notice of Privacy Practices and is not required to honor the terms of the original/previous version(s).

_____   _____
Signature   Date

_____
Print Name

_____

(OFFICE USE ONLY)

Signed form received by: _____ Date: _____

Good faith effort to obtain receipt: (Describe) _____
_____
_____

FIGURE 9.4 Example of a Notice of Privacy Practices form, acknowledging the receipt and understanding of the privacy practices established for a dental practice. (Courtesy Patterson Office Supplies, Champaign, Illinois.)

Progress Notes

At the conclusion of each visit, details of what was discussed, diagnosed, clinically completed, and to be completed at future appointments are entered in the progress notes of the patient chart (Fig. 9.7).

Vital Signs

Vital signs are indicators of a patient's overall health, and the most common readings taken in the dental office include the temperature, pulse, respiration rate, and blood pressure.

Vital signs of each new patient should be taken to obtain a baseline reading and then should be completed at each subsequent visit. Monitoring the patient's vital signs during an emergency is essential, and all staff members should be competent in these skills. As a dental assistant, you must:

- Always be accurate in your recordings. Never estimate! If you are unsure of your findings, then either repeat the procedure or ask someone else to check them.

- Never rely on your memory; immediately record your findings.

Temperature

The **temperature** of the human body is the measurement of body heat. Normal body temperature varies by person, age, activity, and time of day. The standard normal body temperature is 98.6° F (37° C). Some studies have shown that the normal body temperature can range from 97° F (36.1° C) to 99° F (37.2° C).

Temperature is taken with a **thermometer** (*thermo,* meaning heat, and *meter,* meaning measure). A patient's oral temperature is commonly taken using a digital thermometer, which displays the body temperature (Fig. 9.8).

Before taking an oral temperature, ask the patient if they have had anything hot or cold to drink, have been exercising, or have been smoking within the last 10 minutes. If the response is "yes," then wait before taking the temperature.

See Procedure 9.3: Taking an Oral Temperature Reading with a Digital Thermometer.

FIGURE 9.5 Example of a clinical examination form. (From Gaylor LJ: *The administrative dental assistant,* ed 3, St. Louis, 2012, Saunders; form courtesy The Dental Record, Wisconsin Dental Association, Milwaukee, Wisconsin; Dentrix screenshot courtesy Henry Schein Practice Solutions, American Fork, Utah.)

B

FIGURE 9.5 Cont'd

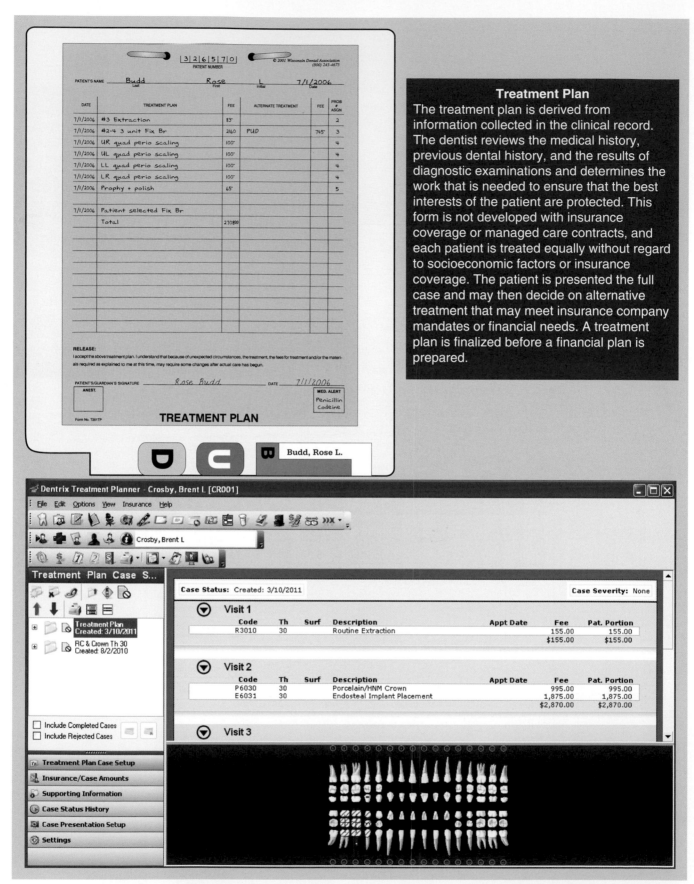

Treatment Plan

The treatment plan is derived from information collected in the clinical record. The dentist reviews the medical history, previous dental history, and the results of diagnostic examinations and determines the work that is needed to ensure that the best interests of the patient are protected. This form is not developed with insurance coverage or managed care contracts, and each patient is treated equally without regard to socioeconomic factors or insurance coverage. The patient is presented the full case and may then decide on alternative treatment that may meet insurance company mandates or financial needs. A treatment plan is finalized before a financial plan is prepared.

FIGURE 9.6 Example of a treatment plan form. (From Gaylor LJ: *The administrative dental assistant,* ed 3, St. Louis, 2012, Saunders; form courtesy The Dental Record, Wisconsin Dental Association, Milwaukee, Wisconsin; Dentrix screenshot courtesy Henry Schein Practice Solutions, American Fork, Utah.)

FIG. 9.7 Example of the progress notes form. (From Gaylor LJ: *The administrative dental assistant,* ed 3, St. Louis, 2012, Saunders; form courtesy The Dental Record, Wisconsin Dental Association, Milwaukee, Wisconsin; Dentrix screenshot courtesy Henry Schein Practice Solutions, American Fork, Utah.)

Pulse

A **pulse** is the rhythmic expansion of an artery each time the heart beats. By placing your index and middle fingers on a specific pulse location, it is possible to count the number of times the heart is beating per minute. The standard normal pulse rate in resting adults is between 60 and 100 beats per minute (bpm). For a child, the pulse rate is more rapid (70 to 110 bpm). Table 9.1 shows different pulse locations.

See Procedure 9.4: Taking a Patient's Pulse.

Respiration

Respiration is the process of inhaling and exhaling, or breathing, and is the way the body takes in oxygen and releases carbon dioxide as a waste product. The standard normal respiration rate for a relaxed adult is 10 to 20 breaths per minute. For children and teenagers, the rate ranges from 18 to

FIGURE 9.8 Digital thermometer. (Courtesy Welch Allyn, Inc., Skaneateles, New York.)

30 breaths per minute. To measure a patient's respiration rate, you observe the rise and fall of a patient's chest and assess the characteristics of their breathing. The characteristics of breathing include:

- *Rate,* which is the total number of breaths per minute
- *Rhythm,* which refers to the breathing pattern
- *Depth,* which is the amount of air inhaled and exhaled during a breath

See Procedure 9.5: Measuring a Patient's Respiration.

Blood Pressure

The term **blood pressure** refers to the amount of work the heart has to exert to pump blood throughout the body. Blood pressure is the most complex vital sign to obtain. Once you understand the steps and have practiced the procedure, it will become less difficult. Blood pressure readings for adults are classified according to normal values and stages of hypertension (Fig. 9.9).

There are varying types of sounds heard and referenced when taking a blood pressure reading. The two readings for blood pressure are the **systolic** and the **diastolic**. The systolic pressure involves the left chamber of the heart, which pumps oxygenated

TABLE 9.1
Pulse Locations

Pulse Point	Location	Description for Finding Pulse
Radial artery		Located on the inner surface of the wrist (thumb side). It is the most common site for taking a patient's pulse in the dental office. To take the pulse, place your index and middle fingers lightly on the patient's wrist between the radius (bone on the thumb side) and the tendon. This measures about 1 inch from the base of the thumb.
Brachial artery		Located on the inner fold of the arm, it is also referred to as the antecubital area of the elbow. This artery is used when a patient's blood pressure is taken.
Carotid artery		Locate alongside the patient's larynx (Adam's apple). Taking the carotid pulse is common when performing cardiopulmonary resuscitation (CPR; see Chapter 10). Because CPR is an emergency, it is important that you know how to find the carotid artery quickly. To detect the carotid pulse, place two fingers alongside the patient's larynx on the side of the neck nearest you. Move your fingers slowly down the groove to the soft area above the clavicle (collarbone), and then palpate this area gently to determine a pulse.
Temporal artery		Located just above the temple, on the sides of the head.
Femoral artery		Located in the inside front of the leg where it joins the pelvic.
Posterior tibial artery		Located on the foot behind the ankle.
Dorsalis pedis artery		Located on the top of the foot running along the vein from the large toe to the ankle.

Images ©Elsevier Collection.

Blood pressure category	Systolic mm Hg (upper number)		Diastolic mm Hg (lower number)
Normal	Less than 120	and	Less than 80
Elevated	120 – 129	and	Less than 80
High blood pressure (Hypertension) stage 1	130 – 139	or	80 – 89
High blood pressure (Hypertension) stage 2	140 or higher	or	90 or higher
Hypertensive crisis (consult your doctor immediately)	Higher than 180	and/or	Higher than 120

FIGURE 9.9 Blood pressure classifications from American Heart Association. (Reprinted with permission. https://www.heart.org/-/media/files/health-topics/high-blood-pressure/hbp-ranibowchart-english-pdf-ucm_4999220.pdf. Copyright 2017, American Heart Association, Inc.)

blood into the vessels. The diastolic pressure reflects the heart at rest when it is taking in blood to be oxygenated.

These readings are recorded as the **systolic pressure** (higher number) over the **diastolic pressure** (lower number). For example, 129/78 mm Hg indicates a systolic pressure of 129 mm Hg and diastolic pressure of 78 mm Hg.

An accurate reading is obtained with the use of a stethoscope and a sphygmomanometer. The stethoscope is used to amplify the sounds of the blood pumped within the artery (Fig. 9.10). These sounds heard are referred to as Korotkoff sounds, which are a series of sounds produced by the blood rushing back into the artery (Fig. 9.11). The sphygmomanometer is used to measure blood pressure (Fig. 9.12).

FIGURE 9.10 Stethoscope.

Korotkoff phases

Phase I   Blood is beginning to flow back into the artery and can be heard as a sharp tapping sound. This is the systolic blood pressure reading.

A sharp thump

Phase II   The cuff is deflated slowly, with blood flowing. A swishing sound may be heard. This sound is softened and becomes prolonged into a murmur.

A blowing or whooshing sound

Phase III   A large amount of blood is flowing into the artery. A distinct, sharp tapping sound returns and continues rhythmically.

A crisp, intense tapping

Phase IV   Blood is flowing easily, and the sound changes to a soft tapping. The sound becomes distinctly muffled and fainter.

A softer blowing sound that fades

Phase V   At this point, the artery is fully open, and the sound disappears. This is the diastolic blood pressure reading.

Silence

FIGURE 9.11 Five phases of Korotkoff sounds in blood pressure measurement. (Adapted from Potter PA, Perry AG, Stockert PA, et al: *Basic nursing,* ed 7, St. Louis, 2011, Mosby.)

A   B

FIGURE 9.12 Sphygmomanometer. (Courtesy Welch Allyn, Inc., Skaneateles, New York.)

The sphygmomanometer consists of a gauge attached to an inflatable rubber bladder enclosed in a cloth cuff. A closure, usually nylon tape (Velcro), is used to hold the cuff in place. A rubber bulb with a valve is used to inflate and deflate the bladder, which creates pressure to briefly control the blood flow in the artery. An **aneroid manometer** has a dial directly attached to the cuff.

See Procedure 9.6: Taking a Patient's Blood Pressure.

An **automated electronic blood pressure device** is used in many practices to simplify and speed the process (Fig. 9.13). It is important that you carefully follow the steps and practice using this type of device until you are able to both obtain an accurate reading and maintain patient comfort.

A   B

FIGURE 9.13 Automated electronic blood pressure devices. (Courtesy Welch Allyn, Inc., Skaneateles, New York.)

Procedure 9.1

Registering a New Patient

Equipment and Supplies

- Registration form
- Black pen
- Clipboard

Procedural Steps

1. Explain the need for the form to be completed. Give the registration form, along with a clipboard and a black pen, to the patient to be completed.
2. Review the completed form for the necessary information:
   a. Full name, birth date, and name of spouse or parent
   b. Home address and telephone number
   c. Occupation, name of employer, and business address and telephone number
   d. Name and address of person responsible for payment
   e. Method of payment (cash, check, or credit, assignment of benefits)
   f. Health insurance information (photocopy of both sides of the patient's insurance identification card)
   g. Name of the primary insurance carrier
   h. Group policy number
   Purpose: This information is necessary for processing financial arrangements and insurance claims.
3. Verify that the patient has signed and dated the form.

Procedure 9.2

Obtaining a Medical-Dental Health History

Equipment and Supplies

- Medical-dental health history form
- Black pen
- Clipboard

Procedural Steps

1. Explain the need for the information and the importance of fully completing the form.
2. Provide the patient with a black pen and the form on a clipboard.
3. Aid the patient in completing the form if needed.

Purpose: The patient may not understand the terminology or may have a language barrier.

4. Ask the patient to return the form and clipboard to you after answering all the questions.
5. Thank the patient for completing the form, and request that the patient take a seat in the reception area.
6. Review the form for blank areas and/or any questions that may arise before handing it to the dental assistant.
7. Use the information from the patient's medical-dental health history form to complete other documents. Remember that the information provided to you by the patient is confidential and must be maintained as such.

Procedure 9.3

Taking an Oral Temperature Reading With a Digital Thermometer

Equipment and Supplies

- Digital thermometer
- Probe cover
- Patient record for documenting temperature

Procedural Steps

1. Wash hands and don gloves.
2. Place a new sheath over the probe of the digital thermometer.
3. Turn on the thermometer. When the display indicates that it is ready, gently place the tip under the patient's tongue.
4. Tell the patient to close their lips over the thermometer and to refrain from talking or removing it from the mouth.

Purpose: Talking or removing the thermometer can alter the temperature reading.

5. Leave the thermometer in place until the display indicates a final reading; remove the thermometer from the patient's mouth.
6. Record the reading in the patient's record.
7. Turn off the thermometer, remove the sheath, and disinfect the thermometer as recommended by the manufacturer.

Date	Temp 99°F	
		Signature

Procedure 9.4

Taking a Patient's Pulse

Equipment and Supplies

- Watch with a second hand
- Patient record to document findings

Procedural Steps

1. Seat the patient in an upright position.
2. Extend the patient's arm, resting it on their leg or on the armrest of the chair. Have the arm at or below the heart level.
3. Place the tips of your index and middle fingers on the patient's radial artery.

Note: Indicate in the patient's record whether you are using the right or left arm.

4. Feel for the patient's pulse before beginning to count.

Purpose: This makes it easier to maintain one position during counting.

5. Count the pulse for 30 seconds, then multiply by 2 to compute the rate for a 1-minute reading.
6. Record the rate, along with any distinct changes in rhythm.

Date	Pulse rate— 77 bpm (strong)	
		Signature

Procedure 9.5

Measuring a Patient's Respiration

Equipment and Supplies

- Watch with a second hand
- Patient record to document findings

Procedural Steps

1. In keeping your position with taking the pulse, glance up at the patient's chest to count the respiration.

Purpose: If the patient is aware that you are observing their breathing, they may exaggerate the depth or rate.

2. Count the rise and fall of the patient's chest for 30 seconds, then multiply by 2 to compute the rate for a 1-minute reading.
3. Enter the rate, rhythm, and depth of breathing in the patient record.

Date	Respiration—14 breaths/min (slightly sighing, moderate depth)	
		Signature

Procedure 9.6

Taking a Patient's Blood Pressure

Equipment and Supplies

- Stethoscope
- Sphygmomanometer
- Patient record to document the findings

Procedural Steps

1. Seat the patient with their arm extended at heart level and supported on the chair arm or on a table.

Purpose: The patient's arm should be at the same level as the heart.

2. If possible, roll up the patient's sleeve.

Purpose: Tight clothing can interfere with an accurate measurement and reading.

3. If you are taking the patient's blood pressure for the first time and do not have a previous blood pressure reading to use for reference, then you will need to establish a basis to determine how high to inflate the cuff. To do this, first palpate the brachial artery to feel for the patient's pulse.

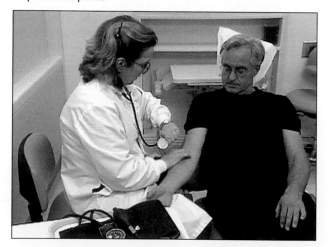

4. Take the patient's brachial pulse for 30 seconds, and then double the number for a 1-minute reading. Add 40 mm Hg to the reading to obtain your inflation level. For example, if the reading was 85, you would add 40, arriving at an inflation level of 125 mm Hg.

5. Expel any air from the cuff by opening the valve and gently pressing on the cuff.
6. Place the blood pressure cuff around the patient's arm approximately 1 inch above the antecubital space, making sure to center the arrow over the brachial artery.

Purpose: Pressure must be directly applied over the artery for a correct reading.

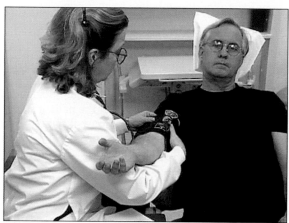

7. Tighten the cuff, using the Velcro closure to hold it in place.

Note: Make sure that the cuff is tight enough that you can squeeze only a finger between the cuff and the arm.

8. Place the earpieces of the stethoscope into your ears so that they are facing toward the front.
Purpose: This position of the earpieces is more comfortable and blocks out distracting noises while you are taking a blood pressure.
9. Place the stethoscope disc over the site of the brachial artery, using slight pressure with the fingers.

10. Grasp the rubber bulb with the other hand, locking the valve. Inflate the cuff to the noted reading.
Note: You need to inflate the bulb quickly.
11. Slowly release the valve and listen through the stethoscope.

12. Note the first distinct thumping sound as the cuff deflates. This is the systolic pressure reading.

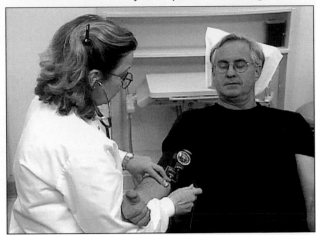

13. Slowly continue to release air from the cuff until you hear the last sound. This is the diastolic pressure reading.
14. Record the reading, indicating which arm was used.
15. Disinfect the stethoscope earpieces and diaphragm as recommended by the manufacturer. Return the setup to its proper place.

Date	Blood pressure 117/68 mm Hg R	
		Signature

Multiple Choice

Circle the letter next to the correct answer.

1. When recording the blood pressure in the patient record, the first number you record is the _____ pressure.
   a. diastolic
   b. systolic

2. A normal respiration rate for a relaxed adult is _____ breaths per minute.
   a. 10 to 20
   b. 15 to 25
   c. 20 to 26
   d. 25 to 30

3. Financial information gathered on the registration form is primarily for _____.
   a. collecting fees
   b. filing insurance claims
   c. making financial arrangements
   d. a, b, and c

4. A medication history is a record of _____ that the patient is currently taking.
   a. prescribed medications
   b. the type of anesthetic the dentist uses
   c. over-the-counter drugs
   d. a and c

5. A patient's medical health history form should be completed or updated _____.
   a. at each visit
   b. at the recall visit
   c. before initial treatment begins
   d. b and c

6. The person who has agreed to pay the fees associated with the patient's dental care is known as the _____.
   a. parent or guardian
   b. patient
   c. responsible party
   d. spouse

7. Routine pulse is measured by placing the index and middle fingers on the _____ artery.
   a. brachial
   b. carotid
   c. radial
   d. all of the above

8. When blood pressure is obtained, the patient's arm (at the elbow) should be _____.
   a. at the same level as their heart
   b. higher than their heart
   c. lower than their heart
   d. a or c

9. The patient record includes the _____.
   a. clinical examination form
   b. medical-dental health history form
   c. progress notes
   d. a, b, and c

10. The patient's signature on the medical health history questionnaire indicates that they _____.
    a. give permission for the use of this information
    b. are responsible for payment of the account
    c. personally completed the form
    d. take responsibility for the accuracy of the information

Apply Your Knowledge

1. A new patient has completed her medical-dental health history form and has handed it to the administrative assistant. When you review this material, you notice that several questions are unanswered. How would you handle this matter?

2. A patient is coming in tomorrow to have his remaining teeth extracted for the purpose of a full denture. What "paperwork" in the patient's dental record will you complete with the patient before beginning the procedure?

3. You have recorded a patient's vital signs in her record and notice that her blood pressure today is 148/70 mm Hg. At the patient's last visit, it was 122/60. Is there anything to be concerned about? If so, what steps should be taken?

CHAPTER 10

Medical Emergencies in the Dental Office

http://evolve.elsevier.com/Robinson/essentials/

LEARNING OBJECTIVES

1. Pronounce, define, and spell the key terms.
2. Give the standard of care for the dental assistant when handling medical emergencies in a dental setting.
3. Describe the assigned roles of dental office staff members during a medical emergency.
4. List the emergency telephone numbers considered essential during a medical emergency.
5. Provide the need for an emergency kit, and what drugs and supplies are standard in the kit.
6. Differentiate between a sign and a symptom of a medical emergency.
7. Discuss the protocol for emergency responses and demonstrate how to respond to specific types of emergencies that could occur in the dental office, such as:
   - An unconscious patient.
   - A patient with breathing difficulty.
   - A patient experiencing a seizure.
   - A patient experiencing a diabetic emergency.
   - A patient experiencing chest pain.
   - A patient experiencing a cerebrovascular accident (stroke).
   - A patient experiencing an allergic reaction.

KEY TERMS

acute myocardial infarction
allergen
anaphylaxis
angina pectoris
antigen
asthma

cerebrovascular accident (CVA)
diabetes
emergency
epilepsy
hyperglycemia
hyperventilation

hypoglycemia
postural hypotension
signs
symptoms
syncope

An **emergency** is a condition or circumstance that requires immediate action to be taken for a person who has become suddenly ill or injured. When a medical emergency occurs, there is no time to refer to a medical resource for answers. You must be prepared to respond immediately.

The population seen in the typical dental practice is diverse in age, with a wide range of medical conditions. For this reason, it is important for all personnel within the dental office to gain knowledge, confidence, and competency in:

- Understanding legal responsibilities when assisting in an emergency
- Assessing your patient to detect any change that might develop into a medical emergency
- Being prepared for a medical emergency

- Assessing a patient's condition throughout a medical emergency
- Having knowledge of the specific drugs readied for a medical emergency
- Having specific equipment for use in an emergency and knowing how to use it

Preventing Emergencies

The easiest way for the dental office staff to help in preventing a potential medical emergency is requesting that each patient complete an updated medical history. Knowledge of any chronic disorders, allergies, heart problems, and current medications allows the dentist to plan for an individual's dental treatment based on a patient's specific needs.

By having the patient update their health status and list of medications, the dental team can feel more confident in knowing a patient's health status. Once an update is completed, the patient is instructed to provide a signature to legally verify the information.

Legal Responsibilities

Handling a medical emergency is to be taken seriously but do not allow potential legal implications to intimidate or prevent you from doing your job.

In a professional situation, the law requires a health care worker to act or behave in a definable way known as the **standard of care**. A comparison of individuals with similar training and experience and how they would respond under similar circumstances, with similar equipment and in the same setting, determines the standard of care.

The standard of care for handling medical emergencies requires that the dental assistant become credentialed in:
- Obtaining and recording vital signs (see Chapter 9)
- Basic life support for the health care provider (cardiopulmonary resuscitation [CPR]) (see Procedure 10.1)
- Operation of the automated external defibrillator (AED) (see Procedure 10.2)
- Heimlich maneuver (see Procedure 10.3)

Emergency Preparedness

Every member of the dental team must be prepared for an emergency. A standardized procedure for the management of emergencies is established and observed.

Assigned Roles

In the management of an emergency, the combined efforts of trained staff members are most efficient when each person takes on a specific role. The dentist is responsible for defining these roles. Most commonly, staff members will take on roles related to where they are located in the office. Even though primary roles are assigned, staff members must be versatile and trained and prepared to fill other roles, if necessary.

Staff Roles During an Emergency
- Front desk staff member (business assistant) will call for help and remain on the telephone at all times to obtain appropriate medical assistance and to provide directions to the office.
- The dentist, clinical assistant, or dental hygienist will remain with the patient for assessment or to assist with basic life support.
- Additional clinical staff members (dental assistant or dental hygienist) will retrieve the oxygen and emergency drug kit.
- Additional dental team members will respond to the needs of other patients in the office.

Routine Drills

Training is kept current at all times. A mock emergency should be performed at a minimum of every 6 months in the dental office, allowing staff members to practice their roles, take part in cross-training, and be able to refine the emergency plan.

Emergency Telephone Numbers

A list of emergency telephone numbers should be posted next to each telephone throughout the office. Maintaining a current list of these telephone numbers is an important part of emergency preparedness. The list should include numbers for the local police, fire, and emergency medical service (EMS).

In areas of the United States and Canada, all three agencies can be reached by dialing 9-1-1. Nevertheless, emergency services vary widely, depending on the geographic area and the population served. An important part of emergency preparedness is to know:
- How quickly can the local EMS get to your office?
- What life support capabilities will they have? (Not all EMS services carry the same equipment or provide the same level of service.)
- What, if any, limitations and restrictions do they have? (Local restrictions may control the services the EMS is permitted to provide in a prehospital situation.)

Listing the telephone numbers of the nearest hospital, physicians, and oral surgeons is also essential. These professionals can offer the life support necessary when you are waiting for the EMS or another type of emergency response.

Emergency Supplies

In a dental office, a portable standardized emergency kit is maintained with emergency drugs and supplies. The clinical staff is assigned the task of maintaining and replacing outdated supplies on a routine schedule.

An emergency drug kit is to be readily accessible for retrieving for a medical emergency. There are seven essential medications to be included in a basic dental emergency medical kit. Fig. 10.1 lists the seven drugs, along with their use and route of administration.

Oxygen, being the most frequently used therapeutic agent, is considered a *drug* in a medical emergency. The ideal agent for resuscitation of a patient who is unconscious but still breathing is 100% oxygen.

Oxygen tanks (always color-coded green) must be checked weekly for any leaks. A portable unit of oxygen may be stored where it can be quickly moved into a treatment room, if necessary. *Note:* If the dental office is equipped with a nitrous oxide and oxygen unit, then oxygen from this unit can be used for emergency situations.

To maintain readiness in an emergency situation, it is necessary to:
- Routinely check supplies for their condition to determine whether they are properly working (rubber tubing, oxygen masks, intravenous [IV] needles and syringes, ventilation masks, and blood pressure equipment).
- Examine each drug in the emergency kit for its expiration date. (Drugs past the expiration date should be immediately replaced.)
- Perform weekly checks of the oxygen tank(s).

Patient Assessment

The dental staff needs to remain alert to a medical emergency occurring at any time. For this reason, ongoing

FIGURE 10.1 Basic dental emergency medical kit. (From HealthFirst https://www.healthfirst.com/blog/guidelines-for-emergency-medical-kits-for-dental-offices/).

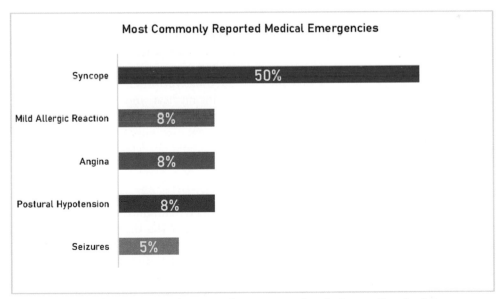

Most Commonly Reported Medical Emergencies

Syncope	50%
Mild Allergic Reaction	8%
Angina	8%
Postural Hypotension	8%
Seizures	5%

FIGURE 10.2 Most commonly reported emergences in private-practice dentistry. Percentages based on a total of 30,608 reported emergencies. (Data from Malamed SF: *Medical emergencies in the dental office,* ed 7, St. Louis, 2014, Elsevier.)

observation of the patient in the reception area, when moving to and from the dental treatment area, during a dental procedure, or when the patient is dismissed cannot be overemphasized. The ADA has provided a list of the most common types of medical emergencies seen in a dental office (Fig. 10.2).

Signs and Symptoms

When an emergency does occur, assessing the signs and symptoms of the patient is critical. A sign is what you observe in a patient, such as obtaining a rapid pulse rate or visually seeing a change in skin color. Because you actually observe these, signs are considered more conclusive than symptoms.

A symptom is what the patient tells you they are feeling or experiencing. The patient, for example, may say, "I feel dizzy," or "I am having difficulty breathing," or "My arm hurts." You would then at this point evaluate the symptom by taking their vital signs or inquiring for more information from the patient.

Vital Signs

By being alert and using your eyes, ears, and hands, you can obtain a significant amount of information about your patient. Monitoring vital signs (temperature, pulse, respiration, and blood pressure) is important. Observing the patient's skin color gives an indication of blood circulation and noticing the patient's face and eyes helps in assessing the patient's level of consciousness.

An accurate assessment of vital signs, also known as *diagnostic signs,* is essential for proper patient management during an emergency. During an emergency, vital signs should be reassessed every 10 to 15 minutes to determine whether the patient's condition is remaining constant, improving, or deteriorating. (How to obtain vital signs is discussed in Chapter 9.)

Emergency Responses

Diagnosis of a specific condition is not your job. Your responsibility is to recognize the symptoms and signs of a significant medical complaint, communicate this information to the dentist, and then assist with appropriate support and transportation procedures. Specific responses could include:

- "The patient's breathing is rapid and shallow [or slow and deep]."
- "The patient is perspiring."
- "The patient is pale."
- "The patient's skin is clammy."
- "The patient is confused."

When you assess a medical emergency situation, a primary factor in determining the mode of treatment is the consciousness of the patient. Medical emergencies described in this chapter and commonly encountered in the dental office are reviewed in Procedures 10.4 through 10.10.

Syncope

Syncope, commonly known as fainting, is one of the most frequent medical emergencies in the dental office. Syncope is the imbalance in the blood distribution of the brain and larger vessels within the body. This reduced blood flow to the brain causes the patient to lose consciousness. Both **psychologic** factors and **physical** factors can contribute to syncope.

Psychologic and Physical Factors Contributing to Syncope

Psychologic
- Stress
- Apprehension
- Fear
- Sight of blood or instruments

Physical
- Maintaining one position in the dental chair for a long period
- Being in a confined environment
- Skipping meals or being hungry
- Experiencing fatigue or exhaustion

Syncope is one emergency that can be prevented by closely observing the patient. A patient may complain of symptoms, and you may notice signs for several minutes before the patient actually loses consciousness.

Postural Hypotension

Postural hypotension, also known as *orthostatic hypotension,* is unconsciousness that can occur when the patient too quickly assumes an upright position. The lack of sufficient blood flow to the brain causes postural hypotension, and it may occur in a patient immediately after a sudden change in position, after receiving nitrous oxide and/or oxygen or IV sedation, or if the patient is pregnant.

The duration of unconsciousness is brief—usually only seconds to minutes. If unconsciousness persists longer, then there may be other causes, and appropriate action must be immediately taken.

See Procedure 10.3: Responding to the Unconscious Patient.

Hyperventilation

Hyperventilation is rapid or deep breathing. A person inhales oxygen and exhales carbon dioxide, but when hyperventilating, the excessive breathing creates low levels of carbon dioxide in the blood. The patient will usually remain conscious.

This medical emergency commonly occurs when a patient is extremely anxious or apprehensive before or during dental treatment. To prevent or reduce hyperventilation, the dental team should be alert at all times and be prepared to help the patient deal with severe apprehension in a positive manner.

Asthmatic Attack

Asthma is a chronic respiratory condition involving the airways of the lungs. This disorder can affect all ages. Asthma is characterized by a sudden onset of recurring periods of wheezing, chest tightness, shortness of breath, and coughing attacks. An allergic reaction, severe emotional stress, or respiratory infection can trigger an asthmatic attack.

Patients with asthma are aware of the sudden onset and should carry an inhaler that contains medication (a bronchodilator) used to relieve the first symptoms of an attack. Identifying asthma in the patient's medical history is especially important; the patient should bring the inhaler with them to each dental appointment.

See Procedure 10.4: Responding to the Patient with Breathing Difficulty.

Epilepsy

Epilepsy is a neurologic disorder characterized by clusters of nerve cells or neurons in the brain that abnormally signal and cause recurrent episodes of seizures. In most patients, epileptic seizures are controlled with medication; however, under stressful conditions, a seizure can occur.

Generally, seizures are categorized on the basis of what part of the brain is involved in a seizure. Seizures have been reclassified into three major groups: generalized onset seizures, focal onset seizures, and unknown onset seizures.

Major Groups of Seizures

Generalized Onset Seizures—Seizures that affect both sides of the brain or groups of cells on both sides of the brain at the same time.
- Tonic seizures cause stiffening of the muscles of the body, generally in the back, legs, and arms
- Clonic seizures can cause repeated jerking movements of muscles on both sides of the body.
- Atonic seizures cause a loss of muscle tone which leads to falling or a person's head dropping.

Focal Onset Seizures—Seizures that start in one area of group of cells on one side of the brain.
- Focal onset aware seizures are when a person is awake and aware during seizure.
- Focal onset Impaired Awareness is when a person is confused, or their awareness is affected

Unknown Onset Seizures—Seizures when the onset is not witnessed or seen by anyone, such as when a person is sleeping or lives alone.

See Procedure 10.5: Responding to the Patient Experiencing a Seizure.

Diabetes

Diabetes is a chronic disorder that affects how your body turns food into energy. With the help of a hormone called insulin, cells throughout the body absorb glucose and use it for energy. If you have diabetes, your body either does not make enough insulin or it cannot use the insulin it makes as well as it should; consequently, the blood glucose level, a type of sugar in the blood, becomes too high.

The disease is classified into two categories:
- **Type 1 diabetes**—Thought to be caused by an autoimmune reaction that stops your body from making insulin. It is usually diagnosed in children and young adults, which requires taking insulin daily to maintain a normal level of glucose.
- **Type 2 diabetes**—Develops over time and is when the body does not use insulin well and cannot keep blood sugar at normal levels. In the past, it was commonly diagnosed in adults, but because of an increase in obesity in children, type 2 diabetes is increasing in children and young adults. The patient is treated with lifestyle changes, oral medications (pills), and possibly insulin.

When the balance shifts, with too much or too little food ingested, insulin levels change, resulting in hyperglycemia (too much blood sugar) or hypoglycemia (too little blood sugar).

Hyperglycemia is a condition in which the glucose (sugar) level in the blood abnormally increases. (Hyperglycemia means blood sugar that is abnormally high.) If left untreated, hyperglycemia may progress to diabetic ketoacidosis and a life-threatening diabetic coma.

Hypoglycemia, also known as *insulin shock,* is an abnormal decrease in the glucose level in the blood. (Hypoglycemia means blood sugar that is abnormally low.) Hypoglycemia can rapidly manifest itself. The most common causes of hypoglycemia are missing a meal, taking an overdose of insulin without adequate food intake, or excessive exercising without an appropriate adjustment of insulin and food intake.

See Procedure 10.6: Responding to the Patient Experiencing a Diabetic Emergency.

Angina Pectoris

Angina pectoris, commonly referred to as *angina,* is a symptom of an underlying heart problem in which severe chest pain occurs when the heart muscle does not get enough oxygen-rich blood. Although painful, angina pectoris does not usually lead to the death of the patient or to permanent heart damage. It does, however, indicate that the person has some degree of coronary artery disease.

Because the signs and symptoms of angina and a myocardial infarction (MI) are similar, distinguishing between angina and MI is important.

Criteria for Distinguishing Angina from Myocardial Infarction
- Pain from angina will usually last from 3 to 8 minutes.
- Pain from angina is relieved or promptly eased with the administration of nitroglycerin.
- A patient with angina should include this information on their medical history.
- Although the patient has a history of angina, when an attack strikes, remembering that pain from angina could be myocardial infarction is important.

Acute Myocardial Infarction

During an acute MI, commonly known as a *heart attack,* the muscles of the heart are affected from insufficient oxygen. If this damage is severe, death can occur; however, prompt medical treatment can help limit damage to the heart.

It is crucial to call 911 or emergency medical help. Although other conditions exhibit similar symptoms, time is important, and the response of the dental team must be swift and prudent. Unexplained chest pain should be treated as a potential acute MI.

See Procedure 10.7: Responding to the Patient with Chest Pain.

Cerebrovascular Accident

A cerebrovascular accident (CVA) is the medical term for a *stroke,* which is an interruption of blood flow to the brain. If the interruption lasts long enough, it can cause damage to the brain, resulting in the loss of brain function. There are three types of strokes: (1) *ischemic stroke,* caused by an obstruction in a blood vessel that supplies blood to the brain; (2) *hemorrhagic stroke,* caused by a weakened blood vessel that bleeds into the brain; and (3) *transient ischemic attack (TIA),* caused by a temporary clot, often referred to as a "mini stroke." Prompt treatment is crucial. Early action can minimize brain damage and potential complications.

See Procedure 10.8: Responding to the Patient Experiencing a Cerebrovascular Accident (Stroke).

Allergic Reactions

An **allergy**, also known as *hypersensitivity,* is an altered state of reactivity in body tissue in response to specific antigens. An antigen is a foreign substance from the environment such as a chemical, bacteria, virus, or pollen that causes an immune response through the production of antibodies. An antigen that can trigger the allergic state is known as an allergen.

Although the patient's health history is the major factor in determining the risk for an allergic reaction, every new drug or dental material introduced to a patient can possibly produce a reaction. Of particular concern is the increasing incidence of allergic reactions to latex, which is used in examination gloves and dental dams.

The two most important factors to consider when managing an allergic reaction are the speed with which symptoms appear and the severity of the reaction.

A **localized allergic response**, also known as a *cellular response,* is usually slow to develop. Mild symptoms can include itching, erythema (redness of the skin), and large hives.

Anaphylaxis, also known as a *systemic reaction,* is a severe, potentially life-threatening allergic reaction. Your immune system will release chemicals that can cause a person to go into shock. Signs and symptoms include rapid pulse, drop in blood pressure, skin rash, nausea, and vomiting.

See Procedure 10.9: Responding to the Patient Experiencing an Allergic Reaction.

Documentation of an Emergency

When a medical emergency occurs in the dental office, the dentist will record all the events that transpired from the beginning of treatment through the crisis in the patient record. After such an emergency, the dentist will enter extensive notes in the patient's record explaining exactly what happened, the treatment provided, and the patient's condition at the time they left the office.

If an emergency is not fully resolved while the patient is in the office, then the dentist may telephone the patient, family, or patient's physician the next day to inquire about the patient's health.

Besides the patient record, the dentist is required to maintain records of office preparedness protocols and practices. These records are essential and could be used as valuable evidence if any legal problems arise.

Ethical Implications

As a health care professional, you are obligated to follow through and assist in a medical emergency. The *Good Samaritan* law tells us that we must ethically do all that we can do within our standards.

Because there are so many new drugs and procedures to follow with medical conditions, it is advantageous to update your medical emergency knowledge and skills by attending continuing education courses annually.

Remember to be alert to every patient who walks in the office. An emergency may take place when you least expect it.

Procedure 10.1

Performing Cardiopulmonary Resuscitation (CPR) (One Person)

Equipment and Supplies

Mannequin approved by the American Heart Association (AHA) and equipped with a printout for demonstration of proper technique (for instruction purposes and mock emergency drills).

Procedural Steps for Adult/Child/Infant CPR— Health Care Provider

Determine Unresponsiveness

Approach the victim and check for signs of circulation, such as normal breathing, coughing, or movement in response to stimulation. Pinch or tap the victim and ask, "Are you OK?"

Initiate Assistance

1. If there is no response, **call for assistance** and ask someone to call 911; obtain an AED/defibrillator if available.
2. If you are alone and your patient is an adult, phone 911 first and then begin compressions.
3. If the patient is a child, give 2 minutes of compression first, then call 911.

(Copyright American Heart Association.)

Initiate Compressions

1. Kneel at the victim's side opposite the chest. Move your fingers up the ribs to the point where the sternum and the ribs join. Your middle finger should fit into the area, and your index finger should be next to it across the sternum.
2. Place the heel of your hand on the chest midline over the sternum, just above your index finger. Place your other hand on top of your first hand and lift your fingers upward off the chest.

(From Sorrentino SA, Remmert LN: *Mosby's essentials for nursing assistants,* ed 5, St. Louis, 2014, Mosby.)

3. Bring your shoulders directly over the victim's sternum as you compress downward and keep your arms straight.

4. Provide 30 chest compressions at a rate of 100/minute with adequate depth. Specific techniques to remember during compressions are as follows:
   • Push hard and fast.
   • Allow complete chest recoil after each compression.
   • Minimize interruptions in compressions.
   • Avoid excessive ventilation.
   • If multiple rescuers are available, they should rotate the task of compressions every 2 minutes.
5. For adults and children over 8, compress the chest a depth of at least 2 inches (5 cm).
6. For infants compress the chest a depth of about 1 ½ inches (4 cm).

Airway and Ventilation

1. Opening the airway (followed by rescue breaths to improve oxygenation and ventilation) should be completed only if there are two rescuers and one of the rescuers is trained in cardiopulmonary resuscitation (CPR).
2. Once chest compressions have been started, a trained rescuer should deliver rescue breaths by mouth-to-mouth or bag-mask to provide oxygenation and ventilation, as follows:
   • Deliver each rescue breath over 1 second.
   • Give a sufficient tidal volume to produce visible chest rise.
   • Use a compression to ventilation ratio of 30 chest compressions to 2 ventilations.
   • Repeat ongoing cycles of CPR until emergency medical services (EMS) arrives, the person starts breathing, someone comes with an automated external defibrillator (AED), or another trained rescuer takes over.
3. Document emergency response in the patient record.

(From Sorrentino SA, Remmert LN: *Mosby's essentials for nursing assistants,* ed 5, St. Louis, 2014, Mosby.)

Operating the Automated External Defibrillator

Consider the following with this procedure: The procedure is to be documented in the patient record.

Equipment and Supplies

- Automated external defibrillator (AED)
- Electrode lines
- Paddles

Procedural Steps

1. Activate the emergency response system.
2. Begin providing compressions while the second responder readies the AED close to the victim's chest.
3. Turn on the power by lifting the top of the case and turning on the power switch.
4. Position the defibrillator machine on the left side of the patient's head, close to the ear. Turn on the power by lifting the top of the case or turning on the power switch.

5. Attach the electrode lines to the paddles.

6. Attach the paddles to the patient, one at the left sternal border and the second on the right side above the nipple area.

Operating the Automated External Defibrillator—cont'd

7. Clear the patient (i.e., make sure no one is in direct contact with the patient), and press the analyze button (or let the machine analyze automatically after the pads have been attached).

8. If the machine advises shock, confirm that everyone present is clear of the patient, and then deliver a shock.

9. After shock delivery, the rescuer should immediately begin chest compressions, followed by checking the pulse.
10. After 5 cycles of CPR, the AED should then analyze the cardiac rhythm and deliver another shock if indicated.
11. Document emergency response in the patient record.

Illustrations (except for the photo of the defibrillator) from Kostelnick C: Mosby's textbook for long-term care nursing assistants, ed 7, St Louis, 2015, Mosby.

Responding to a Patient with an Obstructed Airway

Signs and Symptoms

- Patient grasping at the throat (the universal sign of choking)
- Ineffective cough
- High-pitched breathing sound
- Respiratory difficulty
- Change in skin color

Procedural Steps

Care of the Patient

1. If the patient cannot speak, cough, or breathe, then the airway is completely blocked. Immediately call for assistance and begin administering the Heimlich maneuver.
2. Make a fist with one hand and place the thumb side of your hand against the patient's abdomen, just above the navel and below the xiphoid process of the sternum.

3. Grasp your fist with the other hand and forcefully thrust both hands into the abdomen, using an inward and upward motion.
4. Repeat these thrusts until the object is expelled.

Responding to the Conscious Seated Patient

1. Do not try to move the patient out of the dental chair before administering the Heimlich maneuver.
   Purpose: Patient movement may cause the lodged item to be swallowed.
2. Place the heel of one hand at the patient's abdomen above the navel and well below the xiphoid process.
3. Place your other hand directly over your first hand. Administer a firm, quick, upward thrust into the patient's diaphragm.
4. Repeat this maneuver 6 to 10 times as needed until the object is dislodged or until advanced emergency assistance arrives.

Responding to the Unconscious Patient

Syncope (Fainting)

Signs and Symptoms

- Feeling of warmth or flushing (flushed)
- Nausea
- Rapid heart rate
- Perspiration
- Pallor (pale skin color)
- Lower blood pressure

Response Steps

1. Place the patient in a subsupine position with the head lower than the feet.
   Purpose: This position causes blood to flow away from the stomach and back toward the brain and is frequently sufficient to revive the patient.
2. Call for emergency assistance (9-1-1).
3. Loosen any binding clothes on the patient.
4. Have an ammonia inhalant ready to administer by waving it under the patient's nose several times.
5. Have oxygen ready to administer.
6. Monitor and record the patient's vital signs.

(From Hupp JR, Ellis E III, Tucker M: *Contemporary oral and maxillofacial surgery*, ed 6, St. Louis, 2014, Mosby.)

Postural Hypotension

Signs and Symptoms

- Low blood pressure
- Altered state of consciousness to possible loss of consciousness

Response Steps

1. Place the patient in a subsupine position with the head lower than the feet.
   Purpose: This position causes blood to flow away from the stomach and back toward the brain and is frequently sufficient to revive the patient.
2. Establish an airway.
3. Slowly move the patient into an upright position.
4. If the patient does not immediately respond, then call for emergency assistance (9-1-1).
5. Monitor and record vital signs.

Responding to the Patient with Breathing Difficulty

Hyperventilation

Signs and Symptoms

- Rapid, shallow breathing
- Lightheadedness
- Tightness in the chest
- Rapid heartbeat
- Lump in the throat
- Panic-stricken appearance

Response Steps

1. Place the patient in a comfortable position.
2. Use a quiet tone of voice to calm and reassure the patient.
3. Have the patient breathe into their cupped hands.
   Note: Some sources recommend breathing into a paper bag, but a patient's cupped hands have been found to be quicker and more effective.

Asthma Attack

Signs and Symptoms

- Coughing
- Wheezing
- Increased anxiety
- Pallor
- Cyanosis (bluish skin around the nails)
- Increased pulse rate

Response Steps

1. Call for assistance.
2. Position the patient as comfortably as possible (upright is usually best).
3. Have the patient self-medicate with their inhaler.
4. Administer oxygen as needed.
5. Assess and record vital signs.

From Bird DL, Robinson DS: *Modern dental assisting,* ed 11, St. Louis, 2015, Saunders.

Responding to the Patient Experiencing a Seizure

Generalized Seizure

Signs and Symptoms

- Unconsciousness
- Increased body temperature
- Rapid heart rate
- Increased blood pressure

Response Steps

1. Call for emergency assistance (9-1-1).
2. If a seizure occurs while the patient is in the dental chair, quickly remove all materials from the mouth and place the patient in a supine position.
   Purpose: The patient could inflict self-harm if something is in their mouth. Do not place anything in the patient's mouth during a seizure.
3. Protect the patient from self-injury during movements of the convulsion.
4. Prepare to use an anticonvulsant medication (diazepam) from the drug kit.

5. Initiate basic life support (CPR), if needed.
6. Monitor and record vital signs.

Partial Seizure

Signs and Symptoms

- Intermittent blinking
- Mouth movements
- Blank stare
- Unresponsive to surroundings; seems to be in their "own world"

Response Steps

1. Call for emergency assistance (9-1-1).
2. Prevent injury to the patient.
3. Monitor and record vital signs.
4. Refer the patient for medical consultation.

CPR, Cardiopulmonary resuscitation.

Responding to the Patient Experiencing a Diabetic Emergency

Hyperglycemia

Signs and Symptoms

- Excessive urination
- Excessive thirst, dry mouth, and dry skin
- Acetone breath (fruity smell)
- Blurred vision and headache
- Rapid pulse
- Lower blood pressure
- Loss of consciousness

Response Steps

1. Call for emergency assistance (9-1-1).
2. If the patient is conscious, then ask when they last ate, whether the patient has taken their medication and/or insulin, and whether they have brought medication or insulin to their dental appointment.
   Purpose: If the patient has already eaten but has not taken insulin, then the patient may immediately need insulin.
3. Retrieve the patient's insulin if it is available. If able, the patient should self-administer the insulin.
4. Provide basic life support (CPR) if the patient becomes unconscious.
5. Monitor and record vital signs.

Hypoglycemia

Signs and Symptoms

- Mood changes
- Hunger
- Perspiration
- Increased anxiety
- Possible unconsciousness

Response Steps

1. Call for emergency assistance (9-1-1).
2. If the patient is conscious, then ask when they last ate, whether the patient has taken their medication and/or insulin, and whether they have brought medication or insulin to the dental appointment.
3. If the patient is conscious, then provide a glucose tablet, concentrated juice, or cake icing.
   Purpose: These substances will be rapidly absorbed into the bloodstream.
4. Provide basic life support (CPR) if the patient becomes unconscious.
5. Monitor and record vital signs.

CPR, Cardiopulmonary resuscitation.

Responding to the Patient with Chest Pain

Angina

Signs and Symptoms

- Tightness or squeezing sensation in the chest
- Sharp pain radiating to the left shoulder
- Sharp pain radiating to the left side of the face, jaws, and teeth

Response Steps

1. Call for emergency assistance (9-1-1).
2. Position the patient upright.
3. If possible, have the patient self-medicate with personal nitroglycerin supply (tablets, spray, or topical cream). If this is not possible, then obtain nitroglycerin from the office emergency kit.
4. Administer oxygen.
5. Monitor and record vital signs.

Acute Myocardial Infarction (Heart Attack)

Signs and Symptoms

- Chest pain ranging from mild to severe
- Pain in the left arm, jaw, and teeth
- Shortness of breath and sweating
- Nausea and vomiting
- Pressure, aching, or burning feeling of indigestion
- Generalized feeling of weakness

Response Steps

1. Call for emergency assistance (9-1-1).
2. Initiate basic life support (CPR) if the patient becomes unconscious.
3. Medicate with nitroglycerin from the office emergency kit.
4. Administer oxygen.
5. Monitor and record vital signs.

CPR, Cardiopulmonary resuscitation.

Procedure 10.9

Responding to the Patient Experiencing a Cerebrovascular Accident (Stroke)

Signs and Symptoms

- Paralysis
- Speech problems
- Vision problems
- Possible seizure
- Difficulty swallowing
- Headache
- Unconsciousness

Response Steps

1. Call for emergency assistance (9-1-1).
2. Initiate basic life support (CPR) if the patient becomes unconscious.
3. Monitor and record vital signs.

THINK YOU ARE HAVING A STROKE? CALL 9-1-1 IMMEDIATELY!

F.A.S.T. is an easy way to remember the sudden signs of stroke. When you can spot the signs, you'll know that **you need to call 9-1-1 for help right away.** *F.A.S.T. is:*

Face Drooping
Does one side of the face droop or is numb? Ask the person to smile. Is the person's smile uneven?

Arm Weakness
Is one arm weak or numb? Ask the person to raise both arms. Does one arm drift downward?

Speech Difficulty
Is speech slurred? Is the person unable to speak or hard to understand? Ask the person to repeat a simple sentence, like "The sky is blue." Is the sentence repeated correctly?

Time to call 9-1-1
If someone shows any of these symptoms, even if the symptoms go away, call 9-1-1 and get the person to the hospital immediately. Check the time so you'll know when the first symptoms appeared.

CPR, Cardiopulmonary resuscitation.

Procedure 10.10

Responding to the Patient Experiencing an Allergic Reaction

Localized Rash

Signs and Symptoms

- Itching
- Erythema (skin redness)
- Hives

Response Steps

1. Call for emergency assistance (9-1-1).
2. Prepare an antihistamine for administration.
3. Be prepared to administer basic life support (CPR), if necessary.
4. Refer the patient for medical consultation.
   Purpose: If the patient has an allergic reaction once, they may become increasingly hypersensitive and have a life-threatening response the next time.

Anaphylaxis

Signs and Symptoms

- Feeling physically ill
- Nausea and vomiting
- Shortness of breath
- Heart arrhythmia (irregular heartbeats)
- Sudden drop in blood pressure
- Loss of consciousness

Response Steps

1. Call for emergency assistance (9-1-1).
2. Place the patient in a supine position.
3. Start basic life support (CPR) if the patient becomes unconscious.
4. Prepare to assist in the administration of epinephrine (EpiPen) from emergency kit.
5. Administer oxygen.
6. Monitor and record vital signs.

CPR, Cardiopulmonary resuscitation.

Chapter Exercises

Multiple Choice

Circle the letter next to the correct answer.

1. An acute allergic reaction that can be life threatening is known as _____.
   a. acidosis
   b. anaphylaxis
   c. angina
   d. asthmatic attack

2. A sign of syncope is _____.
   a. tightness in the chest
   b. increased blood pressure
   c. rapid heart rate
   d. wheezing

3. The severe pain of _____ can be relieved by the administration of nitroglycerin.
   a. a cerebrovascular accident
   b. an acute myocardial infarction
   c. an asthmatic attack
   d. angina pectoris

4. The abbreviation EMS stands for _____.
   a. early medical station
   b. emergency medical service
   c. essential medical standards
   d. everything medically standard

5. A patient may _____ if they are extremely anxious about dental treatment.
   a. hyperventilate
   b. hypoventilate
   c. become hyperglycemic
   d. become hypoglycemic

6. The standard of care for handling medical emergencies requires that all dental personnel be certified in _____.
   a. basic first aid
   b. cardiopulmonary resuscitation (CPR)
   c. Heimlich maneuver
   d. b and c

7. An allergic reaction is caused by an _____.
   a. allergen
   b. analgesic
   c. antihistamine
   d. none of the above

8. Glucose can be administered in an emergency response to increase the level of blood sugar in the patient with _____.
   a. asthma
   b. hyperglycemia
   c. hypoglycemia
   d. postural hypotension

9. An ammonia inhalant is used to treat a patient who is experiencing _____.
   a. a CVA
   b. a mild allergic reaction
   c. an angina attack
   d. syncope

10. During an asthma attack, breathing can be eased by administering a(n) _____.
    a. bronchodilator
    b. insulin
    c. antihistamine
    d. a or c

Apply Your Knowledge

1. You are newly employed in a dental office, and, while assisting the dentist in a procedure, the dental hygienist calls out that she immediately needs assistance. What would be your role in this medical emergency?

2. You are currently certified in CPR but have been told that the American Red Cross has made changes to next year's protocol. How would you go about getting recertified and learning about the new changes you should follow?

3. You are assisting the dentist in a surgical procedure. It has been an exceptionally long procedure, and you are not used to standing. Your breathing becomes rapid, you can feel your pulse racing, and you are starting to perspire. What do you think is happening, and what should you do?

4. Your patient, Alice Jones, ran from her car into the office, knowing that she was 15 minutes late for her 11:30 appointment. You seat her and assist the dentist in administering the anesthetic. You notice that she is restless, perspiring, and complaining of hunger. What is going on, and how should you respond?

Delivering Dental Care

http://evolve.elsevier.com/Robinson/essentials/

LEARNING OBJECTIVES	**1.** Pronounce, define, and spell the key terms.
	2. Complete the following related to the clinical area of the dental office:
	• Give the four goals of team dentistry.
	• Identify the standard dental equipment located in the clinical area of the dental office.
	3. Describe the correct approach for admitting and seating a patient.
	4. Describe the ergonomically proper positioning of the dental team.
	5. Explain the clock concept for the dentist and dental assistant.
	6. List the operating zones for the right- and left-handed operator.
	7. Give the five basic principles of instrument transfer.
	8. Describe the dental assistant's role in expanded functions for restorative procedures.

KEY TERMS			
	carpal tunnel syndrome	ergonomics	operating zones
	cumulative trauma disorders	expanded function	subsupine
	dental operatory	grasp	supine

The way dental care is provided is one of the most important responsibilities of the dental team. For a typical day to run smoothly and still maintain the best patient care, the business assistant, clinical assistant, dental hygienist, and dentist must follow a specific routine. It is the responsibility of the entire team to ensure that the flow of patient care is maintained throughout the day.

By having advance groundwork in reviewing the patient record, having knowledge of the upcoming procedure, and setting out the required supplies and equipment, the dental team can prevent their daily routine from becoming hectic and stressful.

Clinical Area

The design of the clinical area depends on the physical size of the practice, the number of dentists associated with the practice, the number of dental assistants and dental hygienists on staff, and the number of patients seen daily.

The **dental treatment area,** also referred to as the dental operatory, is the center of the practice (Fig. 11.1). Patients receive their treatment in this designated area. Most practices

have two or more treatment areas for each dentist and then one additional treatment area for each dental hygienist.

Dental Treatment Area Equipment

A list of the standard dental equipment in a general dental office is provided in Table 11.1. Specific descriptions and features are provided to help you learn and be familiar with their use for each patient.

Care of Dental Equipment

Dental equipment is expensive, complex, and delicate. It must always be carefully maintained in accordance with the manufacturer's instructions. The clinical staff assumes the responsibility for the daily care of equipment throughout the dental office.

Standard Procedure Routine

No matter what type of dental procedure you are assisting in, a standard procedure routine must be followed when admitting a patient, seating a patient, and positioning the dental team.

FIGURE 11.1 Dental treatment area. (Courtesy Patterson Dental, St. Paul, Minnesota.)

Admitting the Patient

Attention to detail when admitting a patient into the clinical area is especially important in creating a positive experience for the patient. When entering the reception area, always greet the patient by their last name, make sure to establish eye contact, smile, and introduce yourself if this is the patient's first appointment.

When escorting your patient to the treatment area, place the patient's personal items in a safe and visible place, and initiate conversation to help the patient feel more comfortable and relaxed.

Positioning the Patient

The area of the mouth being treated and the type of procedure will determine the position of the patient chair. A patient can be placed in three different positions.

In the **upright position**, the back of the chair is placed at a 90-degree angle (Fig. 11.2). This position is used for patient entry and dismissal. It may also be used when radiographs are exposed and when impressions are taken.

TABLE 11.1
Dental Treatment Area Equipment

Type		Description	Features
Dental chair	(From iStock/Denes Farkas.)	Is designed to support the body with the patient's comfort in mind and to position the patient correctly for patient care.	• Adjustable headrest • Support for the arms • Controls to raise and lower the chair • Swivel chair • Adjustment controls to operate the chair
Operator's stool	(Courtesy A-dec, Newberg, Oregon.)	Is designed to be ergonomically sound to support the body for a long period.	• Five casters for movement and balance • Adjustable seat • Broad base • Adjustable back

TABLE 11.1

Dental Treatment Area Equipment—cont'd

Type		Description	Features
Assistant's stool	(Courtesy A-dec, Newberg, Oregon.)	Is designed to be ergonomically sound and to provide stability, mobility, and comfort.	• Broad base with platform base • Wide-base seat • Abdominal bar • Foot bar for support
Operating light	(From iStock/brightstars.)	Illuminates the oral cavity.	• Iridescent light • Track mounted
Air-water syringe	(From Boyd LRB: *Dental instruments: a pocket guide,* ed 4, St. Louis, 2012, Saunders.)	Is used in all procedures to rinse or dry a limited area or the complete mouth. Air is also used to keep the mouth mirror dry and clean.	• Provides a stream of water • Provides a stream of air • Provides a combined spray of air and water
Oral evacuation system	(From iStock/Peter Horrox.)	Removes excess water, saliva, blood, and debris from the patient's mouth.	• Saliva ejector • High-volume evacuator (HVE) (air and water syringe)

TABLE 11.1
Dental Treatment Area Equipment—cont'd

Type	Description	Features
Curing light 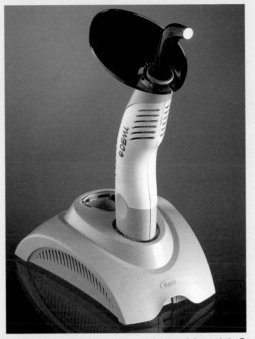 (From Boyd LRB: *Dental instruments: a pocket guide,* ed 4, St. Louis, 2012, Saunders.)	Electronically activated blue light polymerizes resins and composites.	• Lighted wand • Timer controlled
Amalgamator (Courtesy Ivoclar Vivadent, Inc., Amherst, NY.)	Electronically triturates encapsulated dental materials.	• Covered for hazardous substance management • Timer
Rheostat	Is used to operate the slow- and high-speed handpieces.	• Foot controlled • Attached to the dental unit • Speed control by foot pressure

TABLE 11.1
Dental Treatment Area Equipment—cont'd

Type		Description	Features
Dental unit		Provides electrical and air-operated mechanics to the equipment.	1. Saliva ejector 2. Air-water syringe 3. HVE 4. Light curing device 5. Bracket table 6. Chair adjustment advice

(From iStock/Zolnierek.)

FIGURE 11.2 Patient positioned in an upright position.

FIGURE 11.3 Patient positioned in a supine position.

In the **supine** position, the chair back is lowered until the patient is almost lying down (Fig. 11.3). Because of the contour of the chair, the patient will not appear flat. The patient's head and knees should be approximately at the same plane. The majority of dental procedures take place in this position.

FIGURE 11.4 The dental team correctly positions themselves for a procedure. (Courtesy A-dec, Newberg, Oregon.)

FIGURE 11.5 Ergonomic factors in dentistry.

The patient's head will be lower than the feet in the **subsupine** position, which is recommended during an emergency situation, especially if a patient becomes unconscious.

See Procedure 11.1: Admitting and Seating the Patient.

Positioning the Dental Team

The manner in which the dentist and the clinical assistant position themselves around the patient allows for smooth and efficient team interaction (Fig. 11.4). This concept was designed for the chairside assistant to work in close proximity with the dentist.

The rationale of this type of positioning of the dental team is to limit activities that can cause excessive reaching, bending, and twisting. **Ergonomics** is the science that seeks to adapt working conditions to suit the worker. If this model is not followed, then specific areas of the body can be afflicted with injury when working in a dental environment (Fig. 11.5).

FIGURE 11.6 Proper positioning for a seated operator.

Job-Related Injuries Associated with Dentistry

- **Carpal tunnel syndrome** (CTS)—problems associated with repetitive and forceful motion of the wrist
- **Cumulative trauma disorder** (CTD)—repetitive motion and overflexion and overextension of the wrist
- Shoulder and neck pain—strain or flexion of the shoulder for longer than 1 hour per day
- Neck and back pain—extension or elevation of the arm for an extended period
- Low back pain—twisting of the body over an extended period

Criteria for Proper Positioning of the Seated Operator (Fig. 11.6)

- The operator is seated in an unstrained position with back straight, feet flat on the floor, and thighs angled so that the knees are slightly lower than hip level.
- The operator should position elbows close to the sides, and the shoulders should be relaxed.
- The oral cavity should be positioned at the operator's elbow height.
- The operator's head should be positioned facing forward with eyes focused downward.

Criteria for Proper Positioning of the Clinical Assistant (Fig. 11.7)

- The clinical assistant is seated with a straight back and eye level approximately 4 to 5 inches higher than the operator.
  Purpose: This added height allows for better visibility and easier access.
- The clinical assistant is seated with the abdominal bar adjusted to provide back or abdominal support.
- The feet should be placed on the platform near the base of the stool.
- The body is positioned facing toward the patient's head, with the hips and thighs level to the floor and parallel to the patient's shoulders.

FIGURE 11.7 Proper positioning for a seated dental assistant.

Team Dentistry

Team dentistry, also referred to as **four-handed dentistry**, is a concept that describes the way the dentist and the dental assistant work together to perform clinical procedures in an ergonomically structured environment. The main goal of this concept is to:

- Increase patient comfort
- Provide quality dental care
- Increase productivity
- Reduce fatigue and stress

Treatment areas can vary considerably in their design from office to office, but the type and location of equipment and the basic concepts required for practicing efficient and comfortable four-handed dentistry should be applied.

The use of operating zones, based on a *clock concept,* is the best way to identify the working positions of the dental team. The locations of the zones vary, depending on whether the operator ("operator" and "dentist" are used interchangeably) is right- or left-handed.

Visualize a clock placed over the dental chair with the patient's face in the center of the circle and the top of the patient's head at the 12 o'clock position. The face of the clock is divided into four zones. Fig. 11.8 illustrates the zones for a right-handed and a left-handed operator.

Operating Zones

- Static Zone—Located directly behind the patient. A dental unit or a mobile cabinet is positioned in this area.
- Assistant's Zone—Located to the side of a patient, opposite from the operator. To minimize motion, a movable countertop can be positioned over the assistant's lap to hold the instrument tray, paper products, and dental materials.
- Transfer Zone—Located directly over the patient's chest. The instruments and dental materials are exchanged in this area. Special caution must be taken not to transfer anything over the patient's face.

- Operator's Zone—Located to the side of a patient, opposite of the assistant. This zone is larger in space because the operator requires additional access to the patient's mouth. The term "operator" generally refers to the dentist but can include the dental hygienist and dental assistant for certain procedures.

Instrument Transfer

The smooth, efficient transfer of instruments and dental materials is a team effort that requires coordination, communication, and practice between the dentist and the clinical assistant. The technique discussed is based on working with a right-handed dentist.

Basic Principles of Instrument Transfer

Instrument transfer, also referred to as *instrument exchange,* takes place in the transfer zone. The following principles are used to produce the most efficient instrument transfer:

- The clinical assistant understands the sequence of the procedure and is able to anticipate when a new instrument is required.
- A minimum of motion (involving only fingers, wrist, and elbow) should be used when transferring an instrument.
- Instruments are transferred in the **position of use**, which means that the working end of the instrument is directed toward the tooth being treated.
- The instrument is transferred so that the dentist can properly and firmly grasp the handle.
- The dentist must have a firm hold on the instrument.

Clinical Assistant's Transfer Technique

For transferring instruments throughout a procedure, a specific **single-handed technique** is designed to be used for its efficiency. This technique applies to hand instruments, dental handpieces, and the air-water syringe. Use the following basic principles to retrieve, transfer, and return instruments:

- The assistant will retrieve an instrument from the tray setup using the thumb, index finger, and middle finger of the left hand.
- The assistant retrieves the used instrument at the end of the handle or at the opposite end of the working end, using the last two fingers of the left hand.
- The assistant transfers the new instrument in the transfer zone and firmly positions it into the operator's grasp, making sure the working end of the instrument is directed toward the tooth surface or arch on which the operator is working.

See Procedure 11.2: Transferring Instruments Using the Single-Handed Technique.

Operator's Grasp in Receiving an Instrument

The manner in which the dentist holds an instrument is termed the grasp. The grasp is determined by the type of instrument, how it is used, and which arch is being treated. An understanding of these instrument grasps is essential for smooth instrument transfer and exchange of instruments (Fig. 11.9).

FIGURE 11.8 The clock concept for operating zones. **A,** Left zones for a right-handed dentist. **B,** Right zones for a left-handed dentist.

Variations of Instrument Exchange

Because of their design or their use, certain instruments will be transferred differently.

Mirror and Explorer

When beginning a procedure, the dentist will signal that the procedure is about to begin by placing one hand on each side of the patient's mouth ready to receive the mirror and explorer. The clinical assistant will simultaneously deliver the mirror and the explorer, using a two-handed exchange. The dentist uses the mouth mirror and the explorer to inspect the area to be treated (Fig. 11.10).

Hinged Instruments

Instruments with hinges, such as forceps, scissors, and pliers, are designed to have both open and closed use. For pickup and transfer, these instruments are held at the hinge of the instrument and are transferred by directing the handle of the instrument into the dentist's palm or by positioning the handle of the scissors over the dentist's fingers. See Procedure 11.3: Transferring Instruments Using the Two-Handed Technique.

Cotton Pliers

When cotton pliers are used to transfer small items to and from the oral cavity, a modification must be made to the single-handed technique. The pliers are delivered to the dentist while pinching together the beaks to prevent dropping the item being held (Fig. 11.11).

Dental Handpiece

The handpiece can be exchanged for an instrument through the same technique used when two instruments are transferred (Fig. 11.12). When you are exchanging the handpiece, take precaution not to tangle the hose.

Transfer of Dental Materials

Dental materials are generally delivered to the dentist in the transfer zone near the patient's chin.

Cements and liners are delivered on the mixing slab or pad along with the applicator instrument. Hold the mixing pad in the right hand and a 2 × 2 gauze sponge in the left hand. The dentist can access the material, and the tip of the instrument can be wiped with the gauze, as necessary.

FIGURE 11.9 Basic instrument grasps used by the operator. **A,** Pen grasp. **B,** Palm grasp. **C,** Palm-thumb grasp.

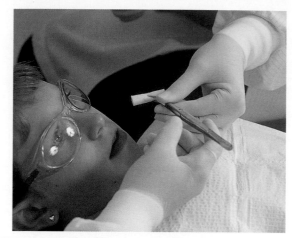

FIGURE 11.11 Transferring cotton pliers.

FIGURE 11.12 Transferring the dental handpiece.

FIGURE 11.10 Transferring the mirror and explorer.

Materials in syringes, such as etchants, composite resin materials, impression materials, and cements, are easily delivered directly to the dentist. The syringe is passed so that the dentist can grasp the syringe in the position of use with the tip turned upward for maxillary use and downward for mandibular use.

Restorative material is delivered to the dentist for placement into the prepared tooth. In some states, it is legal for the assistant to place the material into the prepared tooth.

Delegating this task may be a matter of the dentist's preference or simply one of convenience. The team member who can conveniently see and reach the preparation should place the material directly into the cavity, thus eliminating unnecessary instrument exchanges.

Expanded Functions for the Dental Assistant

An **expanded function** is a specific function of a clinical procedure in which the dentist delegates the task to a credentialed expanded function dental assistant (EFDA) or a registered dental assistant (RDA). For a function to be delegated, it must be legal in that state to do so. For the dental assistant to legally be delegated a function, training and credentialing is required from one of the following:
- Accredited dental assisting program
- Course, which includes a clinical or lab content, approved by the state dental board
- Continuing education course approved by the state dental board

Types of Expanded Functions

Expanded functions delegated to a dental assistant can take place in either a general dental office or specialty practice. As you take on the role of the operator for these functions, you are also taking on the responsibility of having the background knowledge and techniques used in the procedure. Listed is an overview of additional knowledge and skills required to practice as the operator for an expanded function.

Fundamentals When Working as the Operator When Practicing an Expanded Function

Operator Positioning Positioning yourself with the least amount of stress and strain on the body. This recommended position includes upright head position, straight back, elbows close to the body, and feet flat on the floor.

Dental Anatomy Detailed knowledge of dental anatomy is necessary when executing an expanded function. It is important to focus on the following:

- Occlusion of teeth to include proper form and function
- Structures of teeth to include enamel, dentin, cementum, and pulp
- Contours of each tooth
- Proximal contact and interproximal surfaces
- Pits and fissures of teeth
- Periodontium and its importance

Mirror Skills Learn how to use the mouth mirror for indirect vision, retraction, and light reflection.

Use of a Fulcrum Establish a finger rest when using an instrument intraorally. This stabilization will prevent the possibility of slipping.

Understanding Cavity Preparations Know specific cavity terms and classifications. This knowledge will help in the placement of matrix bands and wedges, application of dental materials, and fabrication and placement of temporary restorations.

Instrumentation Learn to adapt the working end of the instrument to each tooth surface, and then proceed by correctly moving the instrument to accomplish the task.

Application of Materials Each material is unique in how it is prepared and applied. Understand the application process for each type of restorative material.

Evaluate the Function An important aspect when acquiring an added responsibility as an EFDA/FDA is that you are accountable for your skills. It is important that the dentist and assistant have the same expectations and goals in the evaluation process of the delegated expanded function.

Ethical Implications

Each state has dental practice laws that permit the dental assistant to perform an expanded function. Be certain that you work in an office that maintains a current state-approved expanded-functions list and follows those guidelines. By displaying your credentials, your patients will feel more confident in your ability and your role in the dental practice.

Procedure 11.1

Admitting and Seating the Patient

Procedural Steps

1. Pleasantly greet the patient in the reception area by name. Introduce yourself and request that the patient follow you to the treatment area.
2. Place the patient's personal items, such as a jacket or handbag, in a safe place away from the procedure.
3. Initiate a conversation with the patient.
   Purpose: Chatting about things other than the treatment may help the patient feel more comfortable and relaxed.
4. Ask whether the patient has any questions that you can answer about the treatment for the day. If you do not know the answer, then say so and offer to discuss the question with the dentist.
   Purpose: Patients frequently ask the assistant questions about treatment that they are reluctant to ask the dentist. Willingness to answer these questions helps reassure the patient.
5. Ask the patient to sit on the side of the dental chair and then swing their legs onto the base of the chair.

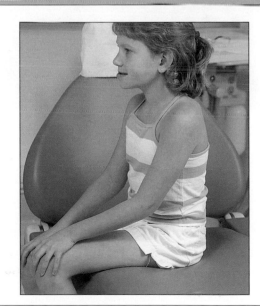

Admitting and Seating the Patient —cont'd

6. Lower or slide the chair arm into position.

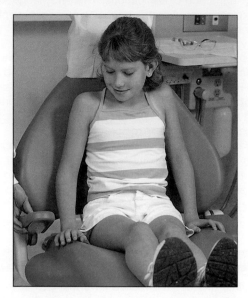

7. Place the disposable patient napkin over the patient's chest, and clasp the corners using a napkin chain.

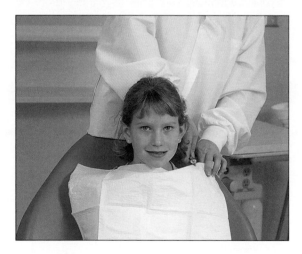

8. Inform the patient before adjusting the chair. Make the adjustments slowly until the patient and the chair are in the proper position for the planned procedure.
   Note: Remember that the most common position for dental procedures is the supine position.
9. Position the operating light over the patient's chest and turn it on.

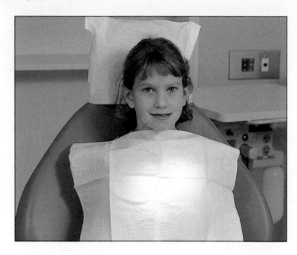

10. Once again, review the room to ensure that all treatment room preparations are organized and set out.
11. Wash your hands and put on your personal protective equipment.
12. You are now ready to position yourself and to begin the procedure.

Procedural Steps

1. Retrieve the instrument from the tray setup using the thumb, index finger, and middle finger of your left hand.
2. Grasp the instrument at the end of the handle or opposite

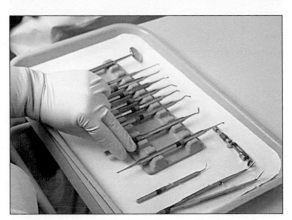

   the working end.
   Note: Most instruments have two ends (double-ended instruments).
3. Transfer the instrument from the tray into the transfer zone, ensuring that the instrument is parallel to the instrument in the dentist's hand.
4. Using the last two fingers of your left hand, retrieve the used instrument from the dentist, tucking in the instrument toward the palm.

5. Firmly position the new instrument into the operator's fingers.
   Note: When placing the instrument, make sure the working end is correctly positioned for the proper area of the mouth.

6. Place the used instrument back on the tray setup in its correct position of use.

Procedural Steps

1. Using your right hand, grasp the instrument on the tray setup closer to the working end with your thumb and first two fingers.
2. With your left hand, retrieve the used instrument from the dentist, using the reverse palm grasp to hold the instrument before placing it back on the tray.
3. Deliver the new instrument to the dentist so that it is oriented with the working end in the appropriate position.
4. Return the used instrument to its proper position on the tray.

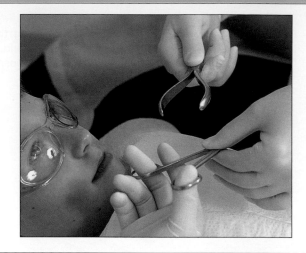

Chapter Exercises

Multiple Choice

Circle the letter next to the correct answer.

1. In the _____ position, the patient's head and knees are approximately on the same plane.
   a. supine
   b. subsupine
   c. upright
2. The operator's stool _____ have a ring near the base to support the feet.
   a. does
   b. does not
3. In preparing to seat a patient, the _____.
   a. arm on the patient chair is raised or moved out of the way
   b. chair is in the supine position
   c. headrest is removed
   d. patient napkin is placed before the patient is seated
4. The dental unit houses the _____.
   a. high-speed handpiece
   b. low-speed handpiece
   c. air-water syringe
   d. a, b, and c
5. The instrument tray and materials on the mobile unit are positioned in the _____ zone.
   a. static
   b. operator's
   c. assistant's
   d. a and b
6. The operator's zone for a right-handed dentist is from _____ o'clock.
   a. 2 to 4
   b. 4 to 7
   c. 7 to 12
   d. 12 to 2
7. When treating a tooth in the maxillary arch, the transfer of the next instrument should have the instrument's working end turned _____.
   a. downward
   b. upward
8. The assistant uses the _____ of the left hand when retrieving a used instrument from the dentist.
   a. last two fingers
   b. first three fingers
   c. thumb and index fingers
9. Surgical forceps are best transferred using a _____ transfer.
   a. single-handed
   b. two-handed
10. During instrument exchange, the handles of the two instruments should be parallel to prevent _____.
    a. injuring the patient
    b. injuring the dental team
    c. tangling
    d. a, b, and c

Apply Your Knowledge

1. Your dentist has agreed to *finally* update the clinical equipment in the treatment areas. You are asked to meet with the sales representatives from three companies and decide on the type of patient chair, operator's stool, and assistant's stool. What are some of the features that should be considered when choosing this equipment?
2. Dr. Allen is on vacation for the week, and a temporary dentist is filling in. She is left-handed. What changes must be made in (1) the operating zones and (2) the methods of instrument transfer?
3. During a team meeting, Dr. Allen expresses some concerns about the clinical procedures taking longer than they should. Everyone agrees that the clinical team could "fine tune" some of their team dentistry skills. What areas could be reviewed and possibly modified?

CHAPTER 12

Instruments, Handpieces, and Accessories

http://evolve.elsevier.com/Robinson/essentials/

LEARNING OBJECTIVES

1. Pronounce, define, and spell the key terms.
2. Give the three parts of a hand instrument design and define the function of each part.
3. Name the hand instruments used for the examination of a tooth and give their use.
4. Name the hand instruments used for the preparation of a tooth and give their use.
5. Name the hand instruments used for the restoration of a tooth and give their use.
6. Name the accessory instruments and items used in a restorative procedure and give their use.
7. Discuss the purpose of rotary instruments and their importance in restorative dentistry.
8. Identify dental handpieces by speed and/or type and give their use.
9. Identify dental burs by their basic shapes, materials, and number series.

KEY TERMS

burs	instruments	rotary
friction-grip	latch-type	torque
handpieces	manipulated	

There is a variety of dental instruments used in dental procedures today. This chapter is designed to provide you with an overview of the most frequently used dental hand **instruments**, handpieces, and accessories in restorative dentistry. Identifying and knowing their use will allow the dental assistant to prepare tray setups for a specific procedure, anticipate the transfer of instruments, and maintain inventory.

Hand Instruments

Dental hand instruments are so named because they are held and manipulated by the hand. (**Manipulated** is the method in which an instrument is managed and skillfully used.) Each hand instrument has a specific purpose and is applied for a specific technique. As you learn to identify new instruments, it is important to understand that manufacturers of instruments will design several styles of the same instrument to accommodate personal preferences.

Hand Instrument Design

Each hand instrument is made up of three parts (Table 12.1).

Parts of an Instrument

1. Handle—Portion of the instrument where the operator grasps or holds the instrument. It is designed in various shapes, sizes, and textures to accommodate the operator's needs.
2. Shank—Portion of the instrument that connects the handle with the working end. It can contain bends and angles to allow the operator better accessibility.
3. Working End—Portion of the instrument with a specific unction. The working end can include a "point," "blade," or "nib" for use in a procedure.

Types of Hand Instruments

Hand instruments are designed for and used in all types of dental procedures. The instruments discussed in this chapter are used in the setup for restorative procedures, such as the composite resin and amalgam procedure.

Restorative instruments can be assigned to one of four categories.

1. **Examination instruments** allow the dentist to examine the health status of the teeth and oral cavity (Table 12.2).

TABLE 12.1
Hand Instrument Design

Parts	Function
Handle	Portion of the instrument where the operator grasps or holds the instrument. The handle is designed in various shapes, sizes, and textures to accommodate handling the instrument.
Shank	Portion of the instrument that connects the handle and the working end. The shank may contain bends and angles to allow the operator better accessibility.
Working end	Portion of the instrument with a specific function. The working end can have a point, blade, or nib for use on the tooth structure or soft tissue.

TABLE 12.2
Examination Instruments

Instrument	Use
	The **mouth mirror** is designed to have a straight handle, a slight angle to the shank, and a working end, with a round metal disc and a mirror on one side. The mirror can have a flat or a concave (indented) surface. Mouth mirrors are used for a variety of purposes.
	Explorers are multifunctional instruments that are included in the setup for every procedure. Explorers are available in many shapes, but all explorers have a thin, flexible, wirelike working end with a sharp point at the tip. Common types of explorers are the *pig tail (1)*, *Shepherd's hook (2)*, and *right angle (3)*. The thin tip enables the operator to use **tactile** sensitivity to distinguish areas of calculus or decay from discrepancies on the surfaces of teeth.
	Cotton forceps (pliers) are used to carry, place, and retrieve small objects, such as cotton pellets, gingival retraction cord, matrix bands, and wedges, to and from the mouth. With *nonlocking* cotton forceps (pliers), the handles must be held closed with the fingers. With *locking* pliers, the handles can be locked in a closed position, and the tips do not open until the lock is released. The tips of the cotton forceps (pliers) are available with plain or serrated points, or *beaks.*

TABLE 12.2
Examination Instruments—cont'd

Instrument	Use
	The **periodontal probe** is used to measure the sulcus or pocket depth of the periodontium of each tooth. This measurement indicates to the clinician the overall gingival health of that area. The working end of the instrument has calibrated markings in millimeters, which are easier to read. Some probes are color coded to enhance reading (see Chapter 55).

Content from Bird DL, Robinson DS: *Modern dental assisting,* ed 11, St. Louis, 2015, Saunders. Photos from Boyd LRB: *Dental instruments: a pocket guide,* ed 5, St. Louis, 2015, Saunders.

See Procedure 12.1: Identifying Examination Instruments.

2. **Hand (manual) cutting instruments** allow the dentist to remove decay manually and to smooth, finish, and prepare the tooth structure in preparation for receiving a temporary or permanent restoration (Table 12.3).

See Procedure 12.2: Identifying Hand (Manual) Cutting Instruments.

3. **Restorative instruments** allow the dentist to place, condense, and carve a temporary or permanent restorative material back to the original anatomy of the tooth structure (Table 12.4).

See Procedure 12.3: Identifying Restorative Instruments.

4. **Accessory instruments and items** are added to the setup of a procedure for multipurpose functions. They can be used in preparation of an item used in a procedure, in carrying things to the mouth, or in the mixing or placement of a dental material (Table 12.5).

See Procedure 12.4: Identifying Accessory Instruments and Items.

Instrument Setup and Care

Having the necessary supplies, instruments, and dental materials readied before a procedure begins helps save time and creates a team approach to the procedure. Instruments are handled with care and organized according to the procedure and their uses.

TABLE 12.3
Tooth Preparation Instruments

Instrument	Instrument in Use	Use
		The **excavator** is one of the most versatile instruments on the tray setup. Excavators have a working end that is "spoon" shaped and circular or elongated. The two most used excavators are: 1. Spoon excavators, which are used for removal of soft dentin, debris, and decay from the tooth. 2. Black spoons, which have a flat appearance but are used for the same purposes.
		The **hoe** is similar in appearance to the garden tool. The blade is perpendicular to the handle. The *hoe* is used to prepare the tooth and plane the walls and floors of the tooth preparation with a push-pull action.

TABLE 12.3
Tooth Preparation Instruments—cont'd

Instrument	Instrument in Use	Use

The **chisel** has a straight or angled shank and a single-beveled cutting edge. Chisels are used to break down the enamel margin of the tooth preparation, to form sharp lines and point angles, and to place retention grooves.

Common types include the following:

(1) straight chisel

(2) bin-angle chisel

(3) Wedelstaedt chisel

(4) angle-formed chisel

Hatchets are similar in appearance to wood hatchets. The cutting edge is parallel to the long axis of the handle. Hatchets are used to cut enamel and to smooth the walls and floors of the tooth preparation.

The **gingival margin trimmer** is a type of chisel that has been modified so that the blade is curved slightly for mesial or distal access into the preparation. Gingival margin trimmers are used to cut enamel and to place bevels along the gingival enamel margins of the preparation

Photos from Boyd LRB: *Dental instruments: a pocket guide,* ed 6, St. Louis, 2018, Elsevier; Drawings ©Elsevier Collection.

A procedure tray is set up in a sequential order from left to right, starting with examination instruments, and followed by hand-cutting instruments, restorative instruments, and, finally, accessory instruments and items (Fig. 12.1). The rationale for this sequencing is based on how instruments are transferred and used throughout a dental procedure. Remember, as the clinical assistant, you will be using your left hand for the transfer of instruments with a right-handed dentist. Therefore the most frequently used instruments will be closer to the dentist for ready availability.

TABLE 12.4
Restorative Instruments

Instrument	Use
	An **amalgam carrier** is a double-ended instrument designed with wells on either end that is used to pack freshly mixed amalgam and carry it to the prepared tooth. Most amalgam carriers are designed to hold a large increment of amalgam at one end and a smaller increment at the opposite end. The dental assistant uses the amalgam carrier to carry an increment of amalgam, then transfers the carrier to the dentist or directly places the amalgam into the prepared tooth.
	Condensers have a flat working end that can be smooth or serrated; they come in varying sizes to accommodate the size of the preparation. To enable the operator to reach all areas of the preparation, the shank of the instrument is angled. The amalgam condenser, also known as a *plugger,* is used to condense (pack down) freshly placed amalgam into the preparation.
	A **burnisher** is an instrument with a smooth working end. The rounded working end is available in many shapes to accomplish different tasks. Common types include the 1. Football 2. Ball 3. Acorn 4. T-ball 5. Beavertail Routinely used to smooth the surface of a freshly placed amalgam restoration.

TABLE 12.4
Restorative Instruments—cont'd

Instrument	Use
	Carvers are designed with a sharp edge on the working end to remove excess material, to contour surfaces, and to carve anatomy back into the amalgam or intermediate restoration before it hardens. Various styles of carvers are available: 1. The **discoid-cleoid carver** is especially useful for carving of the occlusal surfaces. 2. The **Hollenback carver** is used to contour or remove excess material interproximally. 3, The **amalgam knife** is designed with a sharp edge for the removal of excess restorative material along the margin where the material and the tooth structure meet. The knife has several angles in the shank and working end that enable the operator to reach specific areas of a tooth (most often interproximal areas).
	A **composite placement instrument** is designed specifically for the placement of composite restorative materials. Composite placement instruments are made from anodized aluminum or Teflon. These materials prevent the composite material from being scratched. The instruments do not discolor the composite material, as do stainless steel instruments. 1. Teflon composite instrument 2. Aluminum composite instrument
	Woodson (FP–1) is a double-ended instrument that is made from hard plastic or stainless steel. 1. One end is a nib, which resembles a condenser. 2. The paddle on the other end is used for carrying dental materials to the prepared tooth structure.

Photos from Boyd LRB: *Dental instruments: a pocket guide,* ed 6, St Louis, 2018, Elsevier.

TABLE 12.5
Accessory Instruments

Instrument/Item	Use
	Spatulas are used for most procedures in which a dental material is involved. *Flexible mixing spatula* is single-ended; made of stainless steel; comes in two sizes (#15, #24); and is used to mix liners, bases, and cements.
	The **scissors** most often associated with restorative dental procedures are *crown and bridge* scissors, which are available with curved or straight blades. They are useful for many tasks, such as cutting dental dam material, retraction cords, and stainless-steel crowns.
	Amalgam well is made of metal and is weighted with a nonskid base. The newly mixed amalgam is placed in the well; it is then picked up in the carrier for transfer to the dentist.
	Howe pliers, also referred to as 110 pliers, are versatile pliers that can be used in many procedures for many tasks. Their design is straight and includes beaks that have a flat rounded end, making them useful for holding items. Howe pliers are useful for carrying cotton products to and from the oral cavity, for removing the matrix band, and for placing and removing the wedge.
	Articulating paper holder is used to hold and carry articulating paper to the mouth. This carbon paper material varies in thickness and color and is used to check a patient's "bite" after placement of a new restoration, crown, bridge, or denture. This mark must appear equal in distribution across the occlusal surface of the tooth. If one area appears lighter or darker, the patient's bite is incorrect and will need to be adjusted.

Photos of scissors, amalgam well, and Howe pliers from Boyd LRB: *Dental instruments: a pocket guide,* ed 5, St. Louis, 2015, Saunders. Photo of the spatula courtesy Hu-Friedy Manufacturing, Chicago, Illinois.

Steps to Instrument Setup and Care

Before Procedure

- Instruments are sterilized and remain wrapped until use.
- Complete setup of instruments should be organized and set up from left to right.
- Instruments should be placed in the order of their use.
- Instruments and accessory items should be already assembled, if necessary.

During Procedure

- Keep instruments in order of use.
- Transfer instruments in the transfer zone and for the proper grasp.
- Wipe off each instrument after its use using sterile 2 × 2 gauze.
- Disassemble an instrument or accessory after use. (This saves time when preparing the instruments for sterilization.)

After Procedure

- Discard sharps in a sharps container before taking the instruments to the sterilization center.
- Do not throw or toss instruments into a tub because of possible breakage, chips, and cracks.
- Place the instruments in a holding solution if not able to prepare for sterilization immediately.

Rotary Instruments

Rotary instruments are an essential part of restorative dentistry. The setup includes the dental handpiece and revolving mechanisms, which include cutting and finishing burs, polishing tips and points, and abrasive discs and stones that fit into the handpiece. The combination of the handpiece and mechanisms is a miniature representation of a power tool. Although many patients identify the handpiece as "the drill," it is important to educate your patients by making it seem less threatening.

FIGURE 12.1 Tray setup showing appropriate sequence of instruments. 1. Examination instruments. 2. Hand cutting instruments. 3. Restorative instruments. 4. Accessory instruments and items.

Common Uses of Handpieces and Burs in Restorative Dentistry

- Preparing a tooth for a new restoration
- Removing or excavating decay
- Finishing cavity walls of a tooth preparation
- Finishing restoration surfaces
- Removing old fillings
- Finishing the preparation of a tooth for a crown
- Separating crowns and bridges
- Adjusting and correcting temporary crowns

The handpiece provides power and rotary motion, whereas the dental bur, which is securely held in the handpiece, does the actual cutting or polishing. Handpieces and burs have a variety of uses in restorative dentistry. The two most commonly used handpieces are the low-speed handpiece and the high-speed handpiece.

Low-Speed Handpiece

The **low-speed handpiece**, often referred to as the **straight handpiece** because of its straight-line design, is the most versatile handpiece in dentistry. This handpiece operates at speeds from 6000 up to 30,000 revolutions per minute (rpm) and is used for finishing, polishing, and contouring procedures. On occasion, the low-speed handpiece is used for decay removal and fine finishing of the cavity preparation.

For this handpiece to be used for various procedures, a variety of attachments (sleeves) are adapted to fit onto the low-speed handpiece motor (Fig. 12.2).

The straight-line attachment slides onto the slow-speed motor and is locked into place (Fig. 12.3). This attachment is designed to hold larger burs for procedures completed outside of the mouth, such as denture adjustments and the finishing of temporary crowns.

FIGURE 12.2 Low-speed handpiece motor. (Courtesy KaVo Kerr, Orange, California.)

FIGURE 12.3 A straight attachment (2) slides onto the low-speed motor (1).

Contra-angle attachments slide onto the motor and have two different types of locking systems, the latch-type and friction-grip to hold the bur in place during use. The latch-type angle mechanically holds the bur in place by grasping a small notch on the end of the shank of the bur. The friction-grip angle holds the bur in place by grasping the shank of the bur with a friction chuck in the head of the contra-angle attachment (Fig. 12.4).

Prophy angles, also referred to as *prophylaxis angles,* are an attachment used for coronal polishing procedures. The most common type of prophy angle is the plastic **disposable prophy angle**, which is discarded after a single use. These angles are available with rubber cup attachments or bristle brushes already in place (Fig. 12.5). The **snap-on** type holds the polishing device in place by snapping over a smooth button.

FIGURE 12.4 Contra-angle attachment, showing both the friction-grip and the latch-type devices. 1. The contra-angle attachment. 2. The slow-speed motor. 3. Push button to secure bur when using a friction grip bur. 4. Latch-type closure. (Left photo courtesy DENTSPLY International, York, PA. Right photo from Boyd LRB: *Dental instruments: a pocket guide,* ed 5, St. Louis, 2015, Saunders.)

FIGURE 12.5 Disposable prophy cup (1) and brush (2). (From Boyd LRB: *Dental instruments: a pocket guide,* ed 5, St. Louis, 2015, Saunders.)

High-Speed Handpiece

The **high-speed handpiece** operates on air pressure and can operate at speeds from 250,000 to 450,000 rpm (Fig. 12.6). During restorative procedures, the bulk of the tooth structure is removed using the high-speed handpiece. Refinement of the preparation and removal of decay are accomplished with both the high-speed handpiece and hand-cutting instruments.

To protect the tooth against frictional heat caused by the high speed of the bur, high-speed handpieces are equipped with a water-spray device. The tooth and the bur are constantly sprayed with cool water during use. The water spray also helps remove debris from the cavity preparation.

High-speed handpieces are equipped with a fiberoptic light mounted in the head of the handpiece (Fig. 12.7). Light ports near the bur deliver the proper amount of light directly onto the site, which significantly reduces operator eyestrain and improves visibility.

Changing Burs in the Handpiece

With the large variety of handpiece designs available on the market, methods of inserting and removing burs from the handpiece vary according to the manufacturer's design. Regardless of the manufacturer, all high-speed handpieces use a friction-grip system to hold the burs, diamond stones, and polishing devices in place during use. Depending on the manufacturer, different styles for securing the bur are available, but they all operate on the same theory (Fig. 12.8).

See Procedure 12.5: Identifying and Attaching the Dental Handpiece.

Laboratory Handpiece

The **laboratory handpiece** is designed for use in the dental laboratory and not for the mouth. This type of handpiece operates at speeds of up to 20,000 rpm and uses laboratory burs of various shapes and sizes.

The laboratory handpiece provides greater torque than the intraoral handpiece. (**Torque** is the turning power of the

FIGURE 12.6 High-speed handpiece. (From Boyd LRB: *Dental Instruments: a pocket guide,* ed 7, St Louis, 2021, Elsevier.)

FIGURE 12.7 Fiberoptic light handpiece. (©iStock.com/jdpete05.)

FIGURE 12.8 Locking mechanisms for high-speed handpiece. Assembled handpiece **(A)**, lever **(B)**, push button **(C)**, and conventional chuck **(D)**. (From Boyd LRB: *Dental instruments: a pocket guide,* ed 5, St. Louis, 2015, Saunders.)

instrument when pressure is applied during the cutting procedure.) Increased torque is better suited to the heavier pressure required during laboratory grinding and polishing procedures.

Ultrasonic Handpiece

The **ultrasonic handpiece** uses mechanical radiant energy of water and sound vibrations to create a pulsating effect on a tooth surface. Uses for this handpiece include the removal of calculus and debris, stain on teeth surfaces, and bonding materials. Vibrations at the tip of an ultrasonic scaler range from 29,000 to 40,000 cycles per second. Water is needed to cool the friction created between the tip and the tooth surface. (The ultrasonic handpiece is a separate piece of equipment that is not connected to the dental unit; Fig. 12.9.)

Air Abrasion Handpiece

An **air abrasion handpiece** is a small version of a sandblaster and is most effective when used for sealant preparation, stain removal, class I and VI preparations, endodontic access, preparation of crown margins, and preparation of a tooth surface for cementation of a cast restoration. The air abrasion technique allows for the high-pressure delivery of aluminum oxide particles through a small probe to abrade the tooth surface (Fig. 12.10).

Laser Handpiece

The **laser handpiece** delivers energy in the form of light, which acts as a cutting instrument on hard tissue such as teeth and vaporizes soft tissue such as gingiva (Fig. 12.11). The introduction of lasers into dentistry is expanding from soft tissue procedures to removal of decay from tooth structure. This pain-free technique represents a promising addition to dental treatment.

Handpiece Maintenance

Problems with dental handpieces most often result from improper cleaning, sterilization, and lubrication. Inadequate cleaning of the handpiece before sterilization can result in the collection of debris in the internal parts of the handpiece, which creates wear similar to sludge within an automobile engine. If

FIGURE 12.9 The Swerv3 Ultrasonic Scaling Unit. (Courtesy Hu-Friedy Manufacturing, Chicago, Illinois.)

inappropriate cleaning solutions or techniques are used, then the working life of the handpiece is significantly shortened.

Some types of handpieces require lubrication before sterilization, some require lubrication after sterilization, and others require lubrication both before and after sterilization. Excessive lubrication can be as damaging as inadequate lubrication. Handpieces with ceramic bearings or heads require no lubrication at all.

FIGURE 12.10 Air abrasion handpiece. (Courtesy Danville Materials, San Ramen, California.)

FIGURE 12.11 Soft-tissue diode laser unit. (Courtesy Sirona Dental Systems, Charlotte, North Carolina.)

Following the manufacturer's directions for the maintenance of each handpiece is imperative. Failure to do so can result in voiding of the handpiece warranty.

Handpiece Sterilization

The dental handpiece is a critical instrument (one that comes in contact with blood, saliva, and tissue). Because of its use, it must be sterilized before reuse. Dental handpieces require special considerations for sterilization because blood and saliva can be sucked back into the internal portions of the handpiece.

Before the handpiece is removed from the dental unit, it should run for a minimum of 20 to 30 seconds to discharge water and air, which aids in physically flushing out bioburden that may have entered the turbine and air or water lines. Take care not to spread spray, spatter, and aerosols during this process. (**Bioburden** is visible organic debris; in dentistry, it is most often blood or saliva.)

See Procedure 12.6: Sterilizing the Dental Handpiece.

Dental Burs

There are many types of dental burs available, and each shape and makeup are designed for a specific use. Burs are made from a strong durable carbide material and are designed to have three basic parts: (1) shank, (2) neck, and (3) head (Fig. 12.12).

Parts of a Dental Bur

Shank

   Straight: Long, straight shank portion of the bur that fits into the straight attachment of the low-speed handpiece

   Latch type: Medium-length shank with a small notch at the end that mechanically locks into the contra-angle attachment of the low-speed handpiece

   Friction grip: Short and smooth shank that locks by a friction mechanism within the high-speed handpiece

   Neck Narrow portion of the bur that connects the shank to the head.

   Head Cutting, polishing, or finishing part of the bur.

Bur Shapes

Burs are manufactured in a variety of shapes and sizes. A number is assigned to a certain bur shape, and a sequence of numbers designates the size of a specific shape. Table 12.6 provides shapes, numbers associated with shapes, and uses of common bur shapes.

Bur Care

Burs must be sterilized before reuse. To minimize handling of contaminated burs, they should be placed in a bur block or holder before cleaning. This important step also prevents damage to the blades from rubbing or vibrating against each other or against any hard surface during cleaning. If a bur becomes dull or worn, it is to be discarded in the sharp's container.

Diamond Burs

Diamond burs, also referred to as **diamond stones,** have bits of industrial diamonds incorporated into their working surfaces. Many dentists use diamond accessories as an important part of restorative dentistry because of their cutting ability, which shortens preparation time and increases productivity. With multiple uses and sterilization, debonding of the diamond particles occurs, which decreases the cutting efficiency of the bur.

FIGURE 12.12 Bur parts and basic designs. **A,** Long-shank friction bur. **B,** Latch-type bur. **C,** Regular friction–type bur.

TABLE 12.6

Burs for Restorative Dentistry

Type of Bur	Series of Numbers	Uses	Example
Round	¼, ½, 1–8, 10	Initial entry into tooth structure Extends preparation Retention Removes decay	
Inverted cone	33½, 34–39, 36L, 37L	Removes decay Establishes retentive grooves	
Straight fissure plain cut	55–60, 57L, 58L	Initial entry into tooth Helps in forming the internal walls of the preparation	
Straight fissure cross-cut	556–560, 567L, 568L	Helps in forming the internal walls of the preparation	
Tapered fissure plain cut	169–172, 169L, 170L, 171L	Helps in providing angles to the walls of the prepared tooth	

Continued

TABLE 12.6
Burs for Restorative Dentistry—cont'd

Type of Bur	Series of Numbers	Uses	Example
Tapered fissure cross-cut	699–703, 699L, 700L, 701L	Helps in providing angles to the walls of the prepared tooth	
Pear	330–333, 331L	Initial entry into tooth structure Extends preparation	
End cutting	957, 958	Initial entry into tooth structure Creates a shoulder for the margin of a crown preparation	

Illustrations in the first column from Finkbeiner BL, Johnson CS: *Mosby's comprehensive dental assisting,* St. Louis, 1995, Mosby. Illustrations in the last column ©Elsevier Collection.

Indications for Using Diamond Burs

Round-end taper bur removes tooth structure and makes mechanical retention grooves.

Flat-end taper bur is used for crown preparation.

Cylinder bur smooths and finishes the walls in tooth preparations.

Flame-shaped bur makes bevels in crown preparations.

Round bur provides access to the pulp chamber for endodontic treatment and is used to adjust and shape occlusal surfaces.

Wheel-shaped bur is used for anterior crown preparations and can be used to adjust and shape occlusal surfaces.

Images courtesy DENTSPLY International, York, Pennsylvania.

To ensure that the diamond bur or stone is always working at its maximum cutting rate, single-use disposable diamond burs or stones are available prepackaged, sterile, and ready for use, and discarded after a single use.

The shapes of diamond burs are similar to those of carbide steel burs, and burs of most shapes are available in the diamond bur classification.

Trimming and Finishing Burs

Trimming and finishing burs are similar in appearance to carbide burs, but the blades or bevels on this type of bur are sharper and closer together. These instruments are ideal for finishing a composite-resin restoration. They are available only in the XF (super finisher) designation (Fig. 12.13).

Abrasive Rotary Accessories

Abrasive rotary accessories are the most varied of the rotary instruments (Fig. 12.14). **Polishing discs** and **wheels** are abrasives on a metal or paper backing. They are used during the finishing of a restoration and are available in four

FIGURE 12.13 Trimming and finishing burs. A, Round. **B,** Flame. **C,** Tapered fissure plain-cut. **D,** Pear. **E,** Tapered fissure cross-cut. **F,** End-cutting. (Courtesy Integra Miltex, York, Pennsylvania.)

FIGURE 12.14 Accessory abrasive attachments for rotary instruments. A, Silicon carbide produces a moderately rough surface and is available in wheels, points, and stones. The color varies from gray-green to black. Silicon carbide is used for polishing metal restorations. **B,** Rubber points come in varying colors, depending on their abrasiveness. The brown is the most abrasive, with green having less abrasiveness; white is a polishing point. **C,** Cuttlebone is most often adhered to discs and points and is used for final finishing and polishing of the restoration. **D,** Sandpaper discs refer to sand particles adhered to flexible paper discs or strips as a medium abrasive. They are used for finishing and polishing a restoration. Sandpaper discs snap on (1) or screw on (2) a metal center. **E,** Carborundum particles adhered to the disc. As with carborundum on burs, the bur is used to cut or separate one structure from another. (**B** and **D** from Boyd LRB: *Dental instruments: a pocket guide,* ed 5, St. Louis, 2015, Saunders.)

grits: coarse, medium, fine, and super fine. Coarser discs are used to remove excess filling material from the margins of a restoration. Finer discs are used to smooth and polish the completed restoration, similar to abrasive products used for finishing wood projects.

Abrasive discs and wheels are attached to a **mandrel** (metal shaft; Fig. 12.15). Mandrels are used to attach these accessories to the dental handpiece.

Stones are used when maximum abrasion is needed during a procedure, such as for adjusting the occlusion on an amalgam restoration or a gold crown.

Rubber points are embossed with a polishing agent and are used to polish the anatomic grooves of metallic restorations.

See Procedure 12.7: Identifying and Attaching Burs for Rotary Cutting Instruments.

HP   RA   FG

DM303–Huey's Screw Head

HP   RA

DM313–Moore Paper Disc

FIGURE 12.15 Types of mandrels. (Courtesy Integra Miltex, York, Pennsylvania.)

Ethical Implications

The sterilization of dental instruments and burs are no exception to your role in preventing the transmission of infectious diseases. The care you take in cleaning, packaging, and sterilizing these items is an essential step to decrease the risk that a patient may be injured or may acquire a disease because of a lack of sterilization methods. Sterilization helps to protect your office from a malpractice lawsuit.

Procedure 12.1

Identifying Examination Instruments

Equipment and Supplies
- Mouth mirror
- Explorer
- Cotton pliers
- Periodontal probe

Procedural Steps
1. Carefully examine each instrument.
2. Consider the general classification of each instrument.
3. Write the complete name of each instrument or item, correctly spell each name, and give the uses for each instrument.

Procedure 12.2

Identifying Hand (Manual) Cutting Instruments

Equipment and Supplies
- Excavators
- Hoe
- Chisels
- Hatchets
- Gingival margin trimmer

Procedural Steps
1. Carefully examine each instrument.
2. Consider the general classification of each instrument.
3. Write the complete name of each instrument or item, correctly spell each name, and give the uses for each instrument.

Procedure 12.3

Identifying Restorative Instruments

Equipment and Supplies

- Amalgam carrier
- Condensers
- Burnishers
- Carvers
- Amalgam knife
- Composite placement instruments
- Plastic instrument

Procedural Steps

1. Carefully examine each instrument.
2. Consider the general classification of each instrument.
3. Write the complete name of each instrument or item, correctly spell each name, and give the uses for each instrument.

Procedure 12.4

Identifying Accessory Instruments and Items

Equipment and Supplies

- Cement spatulas
- Impression spatulas
- Scissors
- Dappen dish
- Amalgam well
- Howe pliers

Procedural Steps

1. Carefully examine each instrument.
2. Consider the general classification of each instrument.
3. Write the complete name of each instrument or item, correctly spell each name, and give the uses for each instrument.

Procedure 12.5

Identifying and Attaching the Dental Handpiece

Equipment and Supplies

- Low-speed handpiece
- Straight attachment
- Contra-angle attachment
- Prophylaxis attachment
- High-speed handpiece

Procedural Steps

1. Identify and attach the low-speed handpiece to the dental unit, ensuring that the receptors are aligned and that the handpiece correctly fits onto the correct line.

2. Identify and attach the contra-angle attachment onto the straight attachment of the low-speed handpiece, ensuring that the attachment is locked.

Continued

Identifying and Attaching the Dental Handpiece—cont'd

3. Identify and attach the prophylaxis-angle attachment onto the straight attachment of the low-speed handpiece, ensuring that the attachment is locked.

5. Identify and attach the ultrasonic handpiece to the dental unit, ensuring that the receptors are aligned and that the handpiece correctly fits onto the correct line.

4. Identify and attach the high-speed handpiece to the dental unit, ensuring that the receptors are aligned and that the handpiece correctly fits onto the correct line.

Procedure 12.6

Sterilizing the Dental Handpiece

Consider the following with this procedure:
Personal protection equipment (PPE) is required for the health care team; the student is required to identify and prepare the instrument set-up and ensure appropriate safety protocols are followed.

Goal

To sterilize the dental handpiece according to the manufacturer's recommendations.

Equipment and Supplies

- Sterilizable handpiece
- Bur
- Ultrasonic cleaner (if recommended by the manufacturer)
- Lubrication (if recommended by the manufacturer)
- Cotton swab
- Alcohol
- Biologic indicators
- Chemical indicators
- Heat sterilizer

  Note: Always be certain to follow the manufacturer's instructions for cleaning, lubricating, and sterilizing dental handpieces.

Procedural Steps

1. With the handpiece still attached to the hose, and the bur still in the chuck, wipe away visible debris on the handpiece. Operate the handpiece for approximately 10 to 20 seconds to flush water and air into the lines.

   Purpose: This will remove any loose debris that has become lodged in the head.
2. Remove the bur from the handpiece and then the handpiece from the hose.
3. If the manufacturer recommends ultrasonic cleaning, follow those instructions, then thoroughly drain the handpiece, attach the hose, and briefly operate the handpiece to expel debris.
4. If ultrasonic cleaning is not expressly recommended, scrub the handpiece thoroughly under running water with a brush and soap/detergent cleaner.
5. If the handpiece requires presterilization lubrication, use a handpiece cleaner recommended by the manufacturer to remove internal debris, and lubricate the handpiece.
6. If the handpiece does not require presterilization lubrication, *do not* use a cleaner that contains a lubricant.
7. Follow the manufacturer's instructions for each type of handpiece used.

Sterilizing the Dental Handpiece—cont'd

Purpose: To avoid overlubricating the handpiece.

8. Reattach the handpiece to an air hose, and blow out the excess lubricant from the rotating parts. With most handpieces, a bur must be inserted before it is operated.
Purpose: Failure to do this can result in accumulation of excess lubricant in the head and "stickiness" of the excess during the heat cycle.

9. Use a cotton-tip applicator dampened (not soaked) with isopropyl alcohol to remove all excess lubricant from fiber optic interfaces and exposed optical surfaces. Never use strong solvents on fiber optics.
Purpose: Strong solvents can dissolve the epoxy binding between the fibers.

10. Be sure the handpiece is clean; then dry it and package it for sterilization. Sterilize according to the manufacturer's instructions. After the heat cycle, allow the bagged handpiece to cool and dry. Keep sterilization packaging sealed until the handpiece is to be prepared for use on a patient.

1. Flush water and air into the lines for 20 to 30 seconds before attaching the handpiece.
Purpose: To remove any residual debris and free-floating bacteria.

2. If the handpiece does not require poststerilization measures, open the sterilized bag at chairside in front of the patient to demonstrate that a fresh handpiece is being used.

3. If the handpiece requires poststerilization lubrication, keep a separate lubricant container for use on sterilized handpieces. Lubricate the handpiece as close as possible to the actual time of use.
Purpose: To reduce the risk of cross-contamination.

4. Open only the *end* of the sterilization packaging. Spray the lubricant into the handpiece air drive to reduce the amount of overspray and help control excess lubricant.
Note: The dental handpiece is now ready for use.

Identifying and Attaching Burs for Rotary Cutting Instruments

Equipment and Supplies

- Various types of dental rotary instruments, including carbide, diamond, finishing, abrasives, and laboratory burs
- Low-speed handpiece
- High-speed handpiece
- Contra-angle attachment
- Mandrel

Procedural Steps

1. Identify specific dental burs, such as carbide, diamond, finishing, and abrasion burs, by their name and number sequence.
2. Attach latch-type burs to the contra-angle attachment on the low-speed handpiece, ensuring that the bur is locked in place.

3. Attach friction-grip burs to the high-speed handpiece, ensuring that the bur is locked in place.
4. Correctly attach abrasive discs to the mandrel by screwing to tighten or by positioning the metal opening onto the mandrel, ensuring that the disc is securely locked.

Chapter Exercises

Multiple Choice

Circle the letter next to the correct answer.

1. A discoid-cleoid is a double-ended variety of this type of instrument: _____
   a. Condenser
   b. Excavator
   c. Gingival margin trimmer
   d. Carver

2. The dental hygienist may select what type of handpiece as an addition to but not a substitute for manual scaling and instrumentation in the removal of calculus?
   a. High-speed
   b. Laser
   c. Ultrasonic
   d. Low-speed

3. What hand cutting instrument is primarily used for the removal of decay and soft dentin?
   a. Explorer
   b. Hatchet
   c. Hoe
   d. Spoon excavator

4. A prophy angle attaches to the _____ handpiece.
   a. Straight, slow-speed
   b. High-speed
   c. Laser
   d. Ultrasonic

5. The high-speed handpiece uses what type of mechanism when inserting and locking the bur?
   a. Friction-grip
   b. Latch-type
   c. Mandrel
   d. Snap-on

6. The most commonly used sizes of round burs are _____.
   a. 1/4 to 8
   b. 33 to 37
   c. 169 to 171
   d. 556 to 558

7. Inverted cone burs are designed to _____.
   a. open the pulp chamber during endodontic treatment
   b. place retention grooves
   c. remove tooth structure
   d. b and c

8. A mandrel is a device used for _____.
   a. attaching abrasive accessories to the handpiece
   b. carving the occlusal surface of a restoration
   c. etching the interproximal surface of a preparation
   d. b and c

9. What type of hand instrument is designed to contour the composite resin to its normal anatomy while the resin is still soft?
   a. Burnisher
   b. Carver
   c. Plastic instrument
   d. Condenser

10. A low-speed handpiece operates at speeds up to _____ rpm.
    a. 7000
    b. 30,000
    c. 200,000
    d. 450,000

Apply Your Knowledge

1. You are assisting in a restorative procedure, and Dr. Campbell has just completed the removal of the decay with the high-speed handpiece. She asks for the hand cutting instrument that would assist in the removal of the decay. What instrument will you have in the transfer zone for exchange of the handpiece?

2. Dr. Campbell has just completed the restorative procedure and is ready to adjust the patient's lower partial. What handpiece is used to adjust a partial outside of the mouth? How would you prepare the handpiece, and what type of bur would be inserted?

3. While setting up for your next procedure, you notice that the handpiece from the previous procedure is still attached to the dental unit. To save time, can you disinfect the handpiece and place a new sterile bur in the handpiece?

CHAPTER 13

The Dental Examination

http://evolve.elsevier.com/Robinson/essentials/

LEARNING OBJECTIVES	1. Pronounce, define, and spell the key terms.
	2. List and describe the components of a dental examination, including the examination techniques used in dentistry.
	3. Describe the procedure for a soft tissue examination.
	4. List and describe the two types of tooth diagrams used for charting.
	5. Describe Black classification of cavities.
	6. Identify charting symbols as related to dental needs and treatment.
	7. Identify charting abbreviations and describe the procedure for the charting of teeth.
	8. Describe the significance of a treatment plan.
	9. Provide a sample entry of dental treatment in a patient record.
KEY TERMS	cavity classifications diagnosis treatment plan

A thorough dental examination is necessary for the dentist to make a **diagnosis** (identification of disease) and to recommend to proceed with a **treatment plan** for a patient. A dental examination consists of the extraoral areas of the head and neck structures and the intraoral areas, which include soft tissue, periodontal tissue, and teeth. Your role in this data-gathering process is to prepare the setup, assist in the collection of information, and record the information in the patient's record as dictated by the operator.

Components of the Dental Examination

The dental examination begins after the patient has completed the medical and dental history form, and vital signs have been obtained and recorded by the dental assistant. Your role in assembling what is necessary for the dentist to diagnose a patient's dental status consists of gathering all completed forms that are necessary and then charting or recording the dentist's findings during the examination. The dental team (dentist, dental hygienist, and dental assistant) is responsible for gathering and recording specific components of this information:

- Head and neck examination
- Soft tissue examination
- Examination of the teeth
- Examination of the periodontal tissue

- Diagnostic radiographic and imaging
- Impressions to create a diagnostic cast or model
- Photographs

Examination Techniques

The dentist will use a variety of techniques to accomplish a thorough examination. A review of examination techniques is provided in Table 13.1.

Recording the Dental Examination

Dental recording, also referred to as *charting,* can be described as "shorthand" for the dentist. The dentist will dictate their findings, and the assistant will record these findings on the patient's clinical examination form or in the patient's electronic chart. Symbols, abbreviations, and color-coding are all used to indicate various conditions. To chart the information dictated by the dentist accurately and quickly, it is imperative that you learn the dentist's preferred system.

Elements That Make up a Charting System
- Tooth diagrams, numbering systems, and color coding
- Cavity classifications
- Charting symbols
- Abbreviations of tooth surfaces
- Abbreviations of treatments

TABLE 13.1
Examination Techniques

Technique	Description
Visual evaluation	The dentist will visually inspect the extraoral areas of the face: the lymph nodes, the temporomandibular joint (TMJ), the neck, and the lips. The intraoral areas include the tongue, gingiva, teeth, restorations, and missing teeth.
Palpation	The examiner's hands are used to examine texture, size, and consistency of hard and soft tissue in the mouth and facial areas.
Instrumentation	The examiner will use a mirror and explorer to examine imperfections in teeth, detect decay, and evaluate existing restorations.

Continued

TABLE 13.1

Examination Techniques—cont'd

Technique	Description
Radiographic Images	Intraoral and extraoral radiographic images provide a visual evaluation to identify decay, bone loss, and evaluation of impacted teeth.
Intraoral imaging 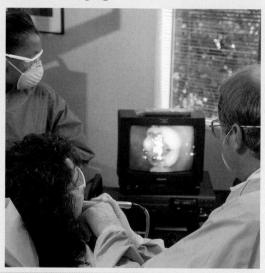	A broad scope of dental technology used to identify decay, defective restorations, periodontal conditions, pathology, developmental conditions, and other abnormalities. The camera projects an image on a screen. The magnification allows the dentist to better evaluate a specific tooth or area of the mouth, which makes it easier for the patient to understand what the dentist is examining.
Photography	Photographs are an excellent tool for identification, treatment planning, case presentations, and patient education.

Oral Examination

A thorough oral examination includes more than simply checking the teeth. It includes a careful examination of the neck, face, and lips and all soft tissue within the mouth.

Soft Tissue Examination

The soft tissue examination involves a complete examination of the lymph nodes, neck, cheeks, lips, mucosa, palate, tonsil area, tongue, and floor of the mouth. This examination requires the use of visual examination and palpation. The objective of this part of the examination is to detect any abnormalities in the extraoral and intraoral areas of a patient. See Procedure 13.1: Soft Tissue Examination (Expanded Function).

Examination of the Periodontal Tissue

A periodontal examination is a routine component of an adult patient dental examination. It is common practice for the dental hygienist to perform the periodontal examination for a patient at their scheduled recall appointment. After completing this appointment, the dental hygienist and dentist will confer to determine whether the patient should require a more thorough periodontal appointment. (For further discussion on the periodontal examination, see Chapter 24.)

Examination of the Teeth

A clinical examination of the teeth includes a thorough examination of each tooth. With the use of hand instruments and radiographic images, the dentist examines the surface of each tooth. The dentist dictates the findings to the dental assistant, who records them in the clinical examination form of the patient's record. Regardless of whether findings are manually recorded or entered in the patient's electronic record, it is essential that all entries are correctly entered and confirmed by the dentist.

Tooth Diagrams, Numbering Systems, and Color Coding

Tooth diagrams for recording dental conditions come in a variety of diagram styles; the most commonly used diagrams are the anatomic and geographic designs, which include the roots of the teeth as well.

In the **anatomic diagram**, the illustration resembles the shapes of actual teeth. (Fig. 13.1).

In the **geometric diagram**, a circle represents each tooth. The circle is divided to represent each tooth surface (Fig. 13.2).

Tooth Numbering

To ensure greater accuracy, the teeth on the diagram are numbered in the appropriate sequence. The dentist selects

FIGURE 13.1 Electronic charting showing an anatomic diagram. (Courtesy Patterson Office Supplies, Inc.)

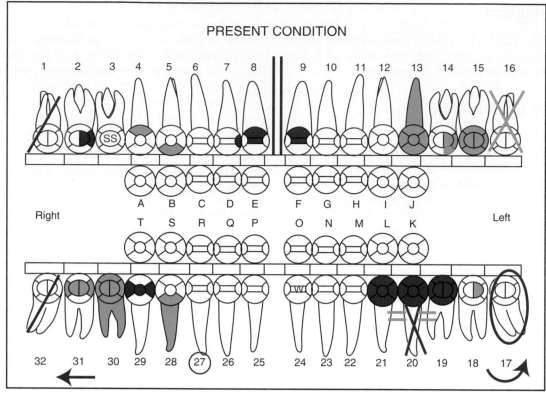

FIGURE 13.2 Geometric diagram. (From Gaylor LJ: The *administrative dental assistant,* ed 3, St. Louis, 2012, Saunders.)

the numbering system. (Numbering systems are discussed in Chapter 4.)

Tooth Arrangement

On the charting diagram, the teeth are arranged as if you are looking into the patient's mouth. Thus the right quadrants are on the left side of the page and the left quadrants are on the right side of the page.

Color Coding

Different colors are used to chart on the diagram to provide visual information about each entry. **Blue** or **black** represents dental treatment that has been completed. **Red** indicates dental needs detected and to be completed at future dental appointments.

Cavity Classifications

To better understand the types of restorations placed in teeth throughout the mouth, a standard cavity classification system was designed to describe the types and locations of decay requiring a restoration. G.V. Black (father of modern dentistry) developed the most commonly used system in the 1900s. Black's original classification included Classes I through V. Class VI was added later. **Cavity classifications** are described in Fig. 13.3.

Charting Symbols

A variety of symbols and abbreviations are used in dentistry. Unlike the Universal Tooth Designation System and the Black cavity classifications, which are standardized, there are many ways of using symbols and color in charting. Each dentist has their individual preferences and learning the dentist's preferred system is important.

The symbols shown in Table 13.2 commonly represent these conditions and materials either when charting by hand or when using a dental software program.

Charting Abbreviations
Treatment Abbreviations

When in doubt about the meaning or the use of an abbreviation, it is better to spell out the term or record what has taken place without using abbreviations. Abbreviations can be used to indicate the single surface or a combination of tooth surfaces. **Single Surface Abbreviations.** These and the other charting abbreviations involve the names of the tooth surfaces, such as **O** for occlusal (see Chapter 4 for names of all surfaces).

Combination of Surfaces. When two tooth surfaces are involved, such as distal and occlusal, the combined surfaces are referred to as **DO** for distal-occlusal. If three surfaces are combined, the same rule applies (e.g., **MOD** for mesial-occlusal-distal).

When referring to these combined surfaces, the letters are separately pronounced, for example, a **D-O cavity** or an **M-O-D restoration.**

See Procedure 13.2: Charting of Teeth.

Treatment Plan

Once the diagnostic information has been gathered, recorded, and reviewed, the dentist will conclude with a dental treatment plan of the patient's dental conditions and needs.

Black's Classification of Cavities

Classification	Location and Description
Class I	• Pits and fissures of the occlusal surfaces of molars and premolars. • Buccal or lingual pits of molars, and the lingual pits of maxillary incisors. Composite resins are the restorative material of choice. Selection will depend primarily on where the lesion is and what type of strength is required from the material.
Class II	• Proximal (mesial or distal) surfaces of premolars and molars. Because this surface area is difficult to detect visually, a radiograph is used to determine the location of decay. The design of the preparation/restoration will include the occlusal surface and involve proximal surfaces. The type of dental material used to restore this classification is composite (tooth-colored) resins designed for posterior teeth. If the tooth has extensive decay, the dentist may choose to restore the tooth with amalgam, gold or porcelain inlay, onlay, or crown.
Class III	• Proximal (mesial or distal) surfaces of incisors and canines. This decay is like a class II, except that it involves the anterior teeth. It is easier for the dentist to access these surfaces with less tooth structure affected. The type of dental material used to restore this classification consists of composite (tooth-colored) resins (for esthetic appearance).
Class IV	• Proximal (mesial or distal) surfaces of incisors and canines. The difference between class IV and class III decay is that class IV involves the incisal edge or angle of the tooth. The type of dental material used to restore this classification is composite (tooth-colored) resins. If the tooth has extensive decay, the dentist may choose to restore the tooth with a porcelain crown.
Class V	• Gingival third of the facial or lingual surface of any tooth. This is also referred to as *smooth-surface decay.* The type of dental material used to restore this classification depends on which teeth are affected. If decay occurs in posterior teeth, the dentist may choose silver amalgam; if anterior teeth are involved, composite (tooth-colored) resin will be used.
Class VI	• Incisal edges of the anterior teeth and the cusp tips of the posterior teeth. Class VI decay is caused by abrasion (wear) and defects. The dental material chosen is composite (tooth-colored) resins.

FIGURE 13.3 Black classification of cavities.

A dental treatment plan is presented and described to the patient by the dentist. It outlines exactly what dental services the dentist recommends, in what time frame, and how much it will cost after insurance. If the patient agrees and accepts the plan, then the patient is required to provide a signature and date, verifying their understanding of the process.

Types of Treatment Plans

Optional treatment plans can be presented to a patient based on consideration of their medical and financial stability. These plans can represent the following levels of care:

Level I—Emergency Care: Relieves immediate discomfort and provides relief to the patient.

Level II—Standard Care: Relieves immediate discomfort and restores the teeth to normal function, which can include permanent restorations, root canal therapy, periodontal therapy, or fixed and removable prosthetics.

Level III—Optimum Care: Relieves immediate discomfort and restores the teeth and surrounding tissue to maximum function and esthetic acceptability. This treatment level can include cosmetic dentistry, orthodontics, periodontics, implants, and reconstructive surgery.

TABLE 13.2
Commonly Used Charting Symbols

Conditions	Explanation	Charting Symbol	Procedure
Missing Tooth	Tooth or teeth that are not present or congenitally missing		Draw a black/blue "X" through the tooth. It does not matter whether the tooth was extracted or is congenitally missing. If a quadrant, or arch, is edentulous, make one "X" over all teeth missing.
Impacted or Unerupted Tooth	Tooth or teeth that have not erupted and are not exposed in the mouth		Draw a red circle around the whole tooth, including the root.
Tooth to Be Extracted	Tooth that has been diagnosed to be extracted		Draw a red diagonal line through the tooth. An alternative method is to draw two red parallel lines through the tooth.
Caries/Restore Class I	Decay affecting the pits and fissure of the occlusal surface		Outline the area involved if using composite filling material and color in the area if using amalgam filling material. Complete in red if needed, and black/blue for already restored.

TABLE 13.2

Commonly Used Charting Symbols—cont'd

Conditions	Explanation	Charting Symbol	Procedure
Caries/Restore Class II	Decay affecting the occlusal and interproximal surfaces of posterior teeth		Outline the area involved if using composite and, if using amalgam, color in the area in red to complete and black/blue for the area already restored.
Caries/Restore Class III	Decay affecting the occlusal and interproximal surfaces of anterior teeth		Outline the area to indicate composite in red to complete and black/blue for the area already restored.
Caries/Restore Class IV	Decay affecting the interproximal and incisal surface of an anterior tooth		Outline the area to indicate composite in red to complete and black/blue for the area already restored.
Caries/Restore Class V	Decay affecting the gingival third of a tooth		Outline the area involved if using composite and, if using amalgam, color in the area in red to complete and black/blue for the area already restored.

Continued

TABLE 13.2
Commonly Used Charting Symbols—cont'd

Conditions	Explanation	Charting Symbol	Procedure
Recurrent Decay	Decay is diagnosed from radiograph or from the margin of an existing restoration.		Outline the existing restoration in red to indicate decay in the area.
Sealant	Resin material placed in the pits and fissures of occlusal surface as a preventive means.		Place an "S" on the occlusal surface in red to complete and black/blue for already restored.
Periapical Abscess	Infection is within the pulp of a tooth.		Draw a red circle at the apex of the root to indicate infection.
Root Canal	Disease has affected the pulp of the tooth and requires pulp therapy.		Draw a line through the center of each root involved in red to be completed and black/blue for already restored.

TABLE 13.2
Commonly Used Charting Symbols—cont'd

Conditions	Explanation	Charting Symbol	Procedure
Veneer	Thin shell-like covering made from porcelain or composite to cover the facial aspect of a tooth surface.		Outline the facial portion only in red to be completed and black/blue for already restored.
Inlay	Cast restoration made from either porcelain or gold for a conservative Class II restoration.		Outline the shape of the restoration in red or black/blue if using porcelain and place diagonal lines if using gold.
Onlay	Cast restoration made from either porcelain or gold for more coverage of the occlusal surface.		Outline the shape of the restoration in red or black/blue if using porcelain and place diagonal lines if using gold.
Porcelain Fused to Metal (PFM) Crown	Full crown of a single tooth using two types of materials, porcelain for esthetics and metal for strength.		Outline the coronal portion of the tooth and add diagonal lines to indicate gold on the facial surface, in red to be completed and black/blue for already restored.
Gold Crown	Full crown of a single tooth using gold.		Outline the crown of the tooth and place diagonal lines in red to be completed and black/blue for already restored.

Continued

TABLE 13.2

Commonly Used Charting Symbols—cont'd

Conditions	Explanation	Charting Symbol	Procedure
Stainless Steel Crown	Full metal crown used for primary molars.		Outline the crown of the tooth and place "SS" on the occlusal surface in red to be completed and black/blue for already restored.
Post and Core	Used for additional strength in an endodontically treated tooth.		Draw a line through the root requiring the post; then continue the line into the gingival one third of the crown, making a triangle shape in red to be completed and black/blue for already restored.
Fixed Bridge	Cast unit to restore an area where one or more teeth are missing.		Draw an "X" through the root(s) of the missing tooth or teeth involved. Then draw a line to connect all teeth that make up the bridge. The type of material used to make the bridge will determine whether you outline the crowns for porcelain, use diagonal lines for gold, or use a combination of the two in red to be completed and black/blue for already restored.
Implant	Complete replacement of a tooth and root.		Draw horizontal lines through the root or roots of a tooth in red to be completed and black/blue for already placed.
Rotated Tooth	Tooth that has rotated from its normal position.		Indicate the direction the tooth has turned by placing a red arrow above the tooth.

TABLE 13.2
Commonly Used Charting Symbols—cont'd

Conditions	Explanation	Charting Symbol	Procedure
Drifting	Tooth or teeth that have shifted from their normal position.		Place a red arrow that points to the direction in which a tooth is drifting.
Diastema	Additional space existing between two teeth with no contact.		Draw two red vertical lines between the teeth.
Fractured Tooth or Root	Surface of a tooth that has fractured because of trauma or extensive caries.		If a tooth or a root is fractured, draw a red zigzag line where the fracture occurred.
Denture	Removal prosthetic to replace a full arch.	CLD PUD PUD	Draw a complete line beneath the roots of the teeth connecting the teeth in red if denture is to be fabricated, or in blue/black if already fabricated.

Recording Dental Treatment

At the completion of every procedure, a specific sequence regarding treatment is followed when recording what was provided for the patient at the visit. This information is located in the patient's clinical record under "Treatment Provided." The chart entry should be clear, complete, and concise.

Treatment Information to Be Included in a Patient's Record

- Date of treatment
- Medical history update, including vital signs
- The tooth treated and the surfaces involved
- Anesthetic used
- Types of moisture control
- Types of dental materials used
- How the patient tolerated the procedure
- Type of treatment to schedule patient's next appointment.
- Signature of dentist

See Procedure 13.3: Recording the Completed Dental Treatment.

About Fees

In most practices, a *super bill* is provided to the patient at the completion of a visit. This form is part of the bookkeeping system but is not part of the patient record. The information on this form is used to itemize what was completed during the appointment, providing the procedure(s), tooth number(s), and surfaces, as well as the fee charged for each procedure. This form also has an area to schedule the patient for their next appointment and the length of time required. The super bill can also be used to generate an insurance claim, if necessary.

■ Ethical Implications

Knowledge and skill in recording a patient's past and present dental conditions are especially important. Charting is a critical skill for the dental team. If the dentist's dictation or the recording is not correctly documented in the patient record, then legally it is *not completed*.

The dentist must always review the patient record and provide a signature for verification on any entry made in a patient record.

Procedure 13.1

Soft Tissue Examination (Expanded Function)

This procedure is legal for certified dental assistants to complete in many states.

Equipment and Supplies

- Gauze squares (2 × 2 and 4 × 4)
- Tongue depressor (optional)
- Mouth mirror
- Patient record to document findings

Procedural Steps

Patient Preparation

1. When escorting the patient to the treatment area, observe the patient's general appearance, speech, and behavior.
Purpose: Unusual behavior or appearance must be immediately noted or called to the dentist's attention.
2. Seat the patient in the dental chair in an upright position. Drape the patient with a patient napkin.
3. Explain the procedure to the patient.
Purpose: The patient who knows what to expect will be more comfortable and more willing to participate in the examination.

Extraoral Features

1. Examine the face, neck, and ears for asymmetry and/or abnormal swelling.
Purpose: The two sides of the face should be symmetric.

2. Look for abnormal tissue changes, skin abrasions, and discoloration.
Purpose: Unusual bruising, scratches, or cuts may require further evaluation of the area.
3. Evaluate the texture, color, and continuity of the vermilion border, the commissures of the lips, the philtrum, and the smile line.
Purpose: Lumps, dryness, and cracking of the tissue are deviations from normal and may indicate the need for further evaluation of the area.
4. Document all findings in the patient record.

Cervical Lymph Nodes

1. Position yourself behind the patient so that you can easily place your fingers just below the patient's ears.
2. To examine the right side of the neck, use your left hand to steady the patient's head. Using your fingers and thumb of your right hand, gently follow the chain of lymph nodes downward, starting in front of the right ear and continuing to the clavicle (collarbone).

Purpose: You are looking for swelling, abnormal formation, and tenderness of the area.

3. To examine the left side of the neck, use your right hand to steady the patient's head. Using your fingers and thumb of your left hand, gently follow the chain of lymph nodes downward, starting in front of the left ear and continuing to the clavicle (collarbone).
4. Document all findings in the patient record.

Temporomandibular Joint

1. To evaluate the temporomandibular joint (TMJ) movements in centric, lateral, protrusive, and retrusive movements, ask the patient to open and close the mouth normally and then to move the jaw from side to side.
2. To further evaluate the movement of the TMJ, gently place your fingers just in front of the external opening of the ear. Ask the patient to open and close the mouth normally.

3. To determine whether there is noise in the TMJ during movement, listen as the patient opens and closes the mouth. A stethoscope placed on the joint may be used.
4. Note in the patient record any abnormalities or patient comments on pain, tenderness, or other problems related to opening and closing of the mouth.

Indications of Oral Habits

1. Look for indications of oral habits, such as thumb sucking, tongue-thrust swallow, mouth breathing, and tobacco use.

Purpose: These habits can affect the patient's oral health.

2. Look for signs of other oral habits, such as bruxism, grinding, and clenching. Indications include abnormal wear on the teeth and problems in the TMJ.

Interior of the Lips

1. Ask the patient to open their mouth slightly.
2. Examine the mucosa and labial frenum of the upper lip by gently retracting the lip with your thumbs and index fingers.
3. Examine the mucosa and labial frenum of the lower lip by gently retracting the lip with your thumbs and index fingers.
4. Gently palpate the tissue to detect lumps or similar abnormalities.

Oral Mucosa and Tongue

1. Gently palpate the tissue of the buccal mucosa by placing the thumb of one hand inside the patient's mouth and the index and third fingers of your other hand on the exterior of the cheek.

Continued

2. Examine the tissue covering the hard palate.

3. Visually examine the buccal mucosa and the opening of the Stensen duct. A warm mouth mirror may be used to view the flow of saliva from the duct.
   Purpose: The mouth mirror is warmed to prevent fogging.
4. Ask the patient to extend their tongue and then to relax it. Using sterile gauze, gently grasp the tip of the tongue and pull it forward.
5. Observe the dorsum (top) of the tongue for color, papillae, presence or lack of a coating, and abnormalities.
6. Gently move the tongue from side to side to examine the lateral (side) and ventral (underneath) surfaces.

7. Use a warm mouth mirror to observe the posterior area.
   Caution: To avoid triggering the gag reflex, this mirror is very carefully placed and is moved very little.
8. Examine the uvula, base of the tongue, and posterior area of the mouth by placing a mouth mirror or tongue depressor firmly at the base of the tongue.
   Caution: Firm but gentle placement reduces the possibility of triggering the gag reflex.

9. With the mouth mirror firmly depressing the base of the tongue, ask the patient to say "ahh."
   Purpose: The oropharynx expands, allowing a better view of the upper portion of the throat.

Floor of the Mouth

1. With the patient's teeth closed, palpate the soft tissue of the face above and below the mandible.
   Purpose: Tori and other abnormalities can be detected.

Soft Tissue Examination (Expanded Function)—cont'd

2. Gently palpate the interior of the floor of the mouth by placing the index finger of one hand on the floor of the mouth and placing the fingers of the other hand on the outer surface under the chin.

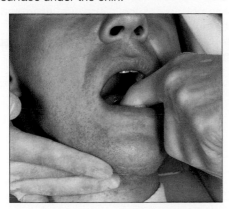

3. Instruct the patient to touch the tongue to the hard palate. **Purpose:** The floor of the mouth, lingual frenum, and salivary ducts can be visually examined.

4. Observe the quantity and consistency of the flow of saliva. Depending on the patient's general health, diet, and medications, the saliva may vary in consistency from watery to thick and ropy.
5. Accurately document all information in the patient record.

Date	Extraoral examination: no changes, schedule for a 6-month examination.	Signature

Procedure 13.2

Charting of Teeth

Equipment and Supplies
- Mouth mirror
- Explorer
- Cotton pliers
- Periodontal probe
- Gauze sponges (2 × 2)
- Dental floss
- Articulating paper
- Articulating paper holder
- Air-water syringe
- Pencil or pen (red and black)
- Paper/electronic clinical examination form

Procedural Steps

Patient Preparation

1. The patient is seated and draped with a patient napkin.
2. The patient is placed in a supine position.
   Purpose: The dentist has better intraoral vision and instrumentation with the patient in a supine position.

Examination of the Teeth and Occlusion

1. Ensure that colored pencils or pens, the clinical examination form, and a flat surface are readily available.
   Purpose: The more organized you are, the fewer errors and stops will be made.
2. Throughout the procedure, use the air syringe to clear the mouth mirror, and adjust the operating light, as necessary.

Continued

Purpose: Better visualization is provided for the dentist as the teeth are examined.

3. Transfer the mirror and the explorer to the dentist. The dentist will begin with tooth #1 and will continue to #32. The dentist will examine every surface of each tooth.
4. Record the specific notations as the dentist calls them out.
5. The dentist will examine the patient's occlusion (bite). Place the articulating paper within the holder and transfer the instrument with the paper correctly positioned for that side of the mouth.
   Note: The holder is positioned closest to the cheek with the paper between the teeth.

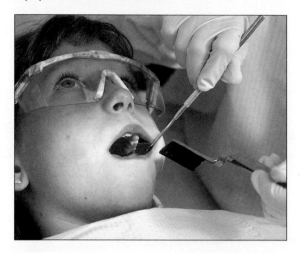

6. Any marks made by the paper will remain on the patient's occlusal and incisal surfaces.
   Purpose: The dentist will look for any abnormal markings to indicate improper occlusion.
7. At the completion of the procedure, rinse and dry the patient's mouth.
8. Accurately document all information in the patient record and sign.

Date	Intraoral examination. Patient has MO decay on tooth #4. Reschedule patient for a 2-unit appointment.	Signature

---

Equipment and Supplies

- Black ink pen
- Patient's record

Procedural Steps

1. In the Date column, record the date the treatment was provided, using numbers in a month/date/year format, such as 9/7/16.
2. In the Progress Notes column, record all areas of the dental procedure, such as the tooth, the surfaces of the tooth restored, the type and amount of anesthetic agent, the dental materials used, and the patient's tolerance of the appointment.
3. If appropriate, then describe the procedure that was performed with appropriate details, such as whether the tooth was prepared for a crown.

Purpose: The treatment is documented, which serves as a reference for future appointments.

4. After entering the complete treatment, sign the entry.
   Note: Always make sure to have the dentist sign the dental record, which verifies that the entry is accurate and was completed.
5. Return the completed dental record to the business office.
   Purpose: The patient returns to the business office area to make payment for services and to schedule any additional appointments.

DATE	PROGRESS NOTES
	New patient examination, reviewed health history. Vital signs: BP 117/76, temp 98.4° F, resp 21, pulse 76. Intraoral and extraoral examination, 4 bite-wing radiographs, preliminary impression. Schedule patient for cleaning and composite resin on #12.
	E. Campbell, DDS/L. Stewart, CDA

Chapter Exercises

Multiple Choice

Circle the letter next to the correct answer.

1. Charting a condition that requires treatment should be color coded in _____.
   a. green
   b. red
   c. black
   d. pencil

2. An intraoral imaging system is used to _____.
   a. view soft tissue in areas that are hard to reach
   b. magnify conditions in the mouth
   c. replace radiographs
   d. make a commercial for a dental product

3. The abbreviation PFM represents _____.
   a. patient faints momentarily
   b. porcelain filling on mesial
   c. porcelain fused to metal
   d. protrusive forward movement

4. During the soft tissue examination, the dentist may use _____ to pull the tongue forward gently.
   a. cotton pliers
   b. Howe pliers
   c. sterile gauze
   d. suture material

5. If using the Universal Numbering System when looking at a charting diagram, the patient's right quadrant will be located on the _____ side of the diagram.
   a. left
   b. right

6. During routine charting of a patient, the dentist dictates for the patient to receive a gold crown for tooth #4. This charting should show the crown outlined with _____.
   a. blue and blue diagonal lines
   b. red and red diagonal lines
   c. blue and colored in solid blue
   d. red and colored in solid red

7. Which of the following teeth would a class III cavity classification be charted on?
   a. #3
   b. #12

c. #24
d. #29

8. A small red circle at the root apex indicates _____.
   a. an abscess
   b. an impacted tooth
   c. completed endodontic treatment
   d. root caries

9. According to the Black classification, Class _____ cavities are also known as smooth surface cavities.
   a. I
   b. II
   c. V
   d. VI

10. Treatment entries in the patient's chart must be recorded _____.
    a. by a computer entry
    b. in ink to make it permanent
    c. in pencil in case it needs to be corrected
    d. a or b

Apply Your Knowledge

1. When charting a patient's findings, Dr. Campbell prefers to call out cavity classifications. If Dr. Campbell indicated a Class II on the "mesial / distal of tooth #4," a Class III on the "mesial of tooth #6," a Class IV on the "distal of tooth #7," and a Class I on the "lingual of tooth #8," how would these be charted?

2. Dr. Campbell is dictating her findings on a patient during a recall appointment and indicates that tooth #12 has recurrent decay. When you look at the chart, you notice that tooth #12 has a mesial occlusal (MO) amalgam. How would recurrent decay appear?

3. If a dental examination is more than simply "checking someone's teeth," then what else would it include?

CHAPTER 14

Moisture Control

http://evolve.elsevier.com/Robinson/essentials/

One of the key responsibilities of the clinical assistant is to maintain moisture control throughout the dental procedure. The tooth, surrounding tissue, and oral cavity can become a catch all for water, saliva, blood, and tooth fragments, which interferes with visibility of the area for the operator.

The type of procedure and access of the operative area will determine the best isolation method to use. This chapter describes several techniques and applications that will help you determine what works best for the situation.

Mouth Rinsing

The two basic types of rinsing procedures used in dentistry are limited-area rinsing and complete mouth rinsing.

Limited-area rinsing is frequently performed throughout a procedure because debris can accumulate during the preparation of a tooth. A limited-area rinse must be quickly and efficiently accomplished without causing any delay in the procedure and is routinely used when the dentist pauses for a closer inspection.

The **complete mouth rinse** is performed at the completion of a dental procedure and is always used to leave the patient with a comfortable and fresh feeling.

See Procedure 14.1: Performing a Mouth Rinse.

Oral Evacuation Methods

Throughout a dental procedure, the water from either the air-water syringe or from the high-speed handpiece is expressed to cool the tooth and remove debris. A specific type of oral evacuation method will be selected to remove the liquids and debris from the mouth.

Saliva Ejector

The saliva ejector is used to remove small amounts of saliva or water from the patient's mouth. This small straw-like tube has the flexibility to conform to many areas in the mouth (Fig. 14.1). Placement of the saliva ejector is simple and comfortable for the patient. To maintain its position in the mouth, it is bent in the shape of a candy cane and placed under the tongue on the opposite side from which you are working.

High-Volume Oral Evacuation

The **high-volume evacuator** (HVE) is a strong source of moisture control that is consistently used during a dental procedure when the handpiece is being used.

The HVE system, also referred to as the oral evacuator, works on a vacuum principle similar to that of a household vacuum cleaner.

The HVE is used to:

- Keep the mouth free from saliva, blood, water, and debris
- Retract the tongue or cheek away from the procedure site
- Reduce the bacterial aerosol caused by the high-speed handpiece

HVE Tips

The most commonly used HVE tips are made of a durable plastic and are disposed of after a single use. HVE tips are also made of stainless steel, which must be sterilized before reuse (Fig. 14.2).

HVE tips are available straight or with a slight angle in the middle. All types have two beveled working ends (**beveled** meaning slanted). The positioning of the bevel is determined by where it is placed in the mouth. It is slanted downward for use in the **anterior** portion of the mouth and slanted upward for use in the posterior portion of the mouth.

When the HVE tip is placed into the handle of the suction unit, the tip is pushed into place through a plastic protective barrier, which will cover the HVE handle. If the incorrect end of the tip has been placed in the suction, do not turn it around; the HVE tip is now contaminated and must be replaced with a new tip.

Holding the Oral Evacuator

The oral evacuator can be held in one of two ways: the thumb-to-nose grasp or the pen grasp (Fig. 14.3). Either method provides control of the tip, which is necessary for efficient use and patient comfort and safety. It is common to alternate between positions, depending on the area being treated or the resistance of the tissue to retract.

When assisting a right-handed dentist, hold the evacuator in the right hand. When assisting a left-handed dentist, hold the evacuator in the left hand. The other hand is then free to use the air-water syringe or to transfer instruments to the dentist as needed.

To be most efficient in HVE placement, position the HVE tip in the mouth first and then allow the dentist to position the handpiece and the mouth mirror (Fig. 14.4).

See Procedure 14.2: Positioning the High-Volume Evacuator During a Procedure

FIGURE 14.3 Methods of holding the oral evacuator tip. *Top,* Thumb-to-nose grasp. *Bottom,* Pen grasp.

FIGURE 14.1 Saliva ejector.

FIGURE 14.2 High-volume evacuator (HVE) tips. (From Boyd LRB: *Dental instruments: a pocket guide,* ed 5, St. Louis, 2015, Saunders.)

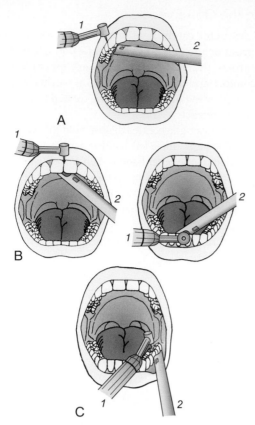

FIGURE 14.4 Placement of the high-volume evacuator (HVE) tip. A, Maxillary right buccal/occlusal surface. *1.* Operator's position with handpiece is buccal or occlusal. *2.* Assistant's position with suction tip is lingual. **B,** Maxillary/Mandibular central incisors. *1.* Operator's position with handpiece is facial. *2.* Assistant's position with suction tip is lingual. **C,** Mandibular left occlusal surface. *1.* Operator's position with handpiece is lingual/occlusal. *2.* Assistant's position with suction tip is buccal.

FIGURE 14.5 Isolite dental isolation system. (From Boyd LRB: *Dental instruments: a pocket guide*, ed 7, St. Louis, 2021, Elsevier.)

Dental Isolation System

This hand-free suction isolation system involves a mouthpiece that combines retraction and continuous suction, allowing the dental assistant to increase productivity (Fig. 14.5). The system easily integrates into the dental unit.

Oral Evacuation Caution

Improper or careless placement of the HVE can cause soft tissue to be accidentally *sucked* into the tip, resulting in the possibility of harming localized tissue. Keeping the tip at an angle with the

soft tissue helps prevent this from occurring. If the soft tissue is accidentally sucked into the tip, then rotate the angle of the tip to break the suction or quickly turn off the vacuum control to release the tissue.

Isolation Techniques

The common isolation techniques used in dentistry are cotton rolls, dental dam, and dry angles. **Isolation**, as used here, means to keep the area isolated and dry.

Cotton Rolls

One method of ensuring a dry environment is with the use of **cotton rolls**. When placing a permanent restorative material, cementing a crown, or applying sealants, a clean and dry environment is necessary. Cotton rolls are available in a variety of sizes and are flexible to be formed to fit in an available space. Some cotton rolls have a light coating on the surface to make them slightly stiff. A softer type of cotton roll is not coated but is wrapped with a cotton thread.

Advantages and Disadvantages of Cotton Rolls

Advantages
- Easy to apply.
- Comfortable for the patient.
- No additional equipment is needed for placement.

Disadvantages
- Does not prevent contamination of the area by saliva and moisture.
- Does not protect the patient from aspiration.
- If improperly removed, then dry cotton rolls may adhere to the oral mucosa, which can injure the tissue.
- Must be frequently replaced.
- Cotton rolls have limited retraction.

Cotton Roll Placement

To isolate a specific area of the maxillary arch, a cotton roll is placed on the cheek side of the teeth in the **mucobuccal fold**. This fold securely holds the cotton roll in place and is the area where the masticatory mucosa covering the alveolar ridge turns upward and becomes the lining mucosa of the cheek (Fig. 14.6).

Because of movement of the tongue and the tendency of saliva to pool in the floor of the mouth, cotton roll isolation is more difficult to achieve in the **mandibular arch**. Cotton rolls are placed in both the mucobuccal fold and the lingual side of the arch parallel to each other (Fig. 14.7).

When the anterior portion of the mandible is isolated, cotton rolls are positioned in the lingual area, instructing the patient to raise their tongue for secure placement. The other cotton roll is placed between the lip and teeth (Fig. 14.8).

Depending on the location, cotton rolls are placed and removed with cotton pliers or with gloved fingers. If the cotton roll becomes saturated before the procedure is completed, then it should be replaced, as necessary.

See Procedure 14.3: Placing and Removing Cotton Rolls.

FIGURE 14.6 Cotton roll placement for the posterior maxillary arch.

FIGURE 14.8 Cotton roll placement for the anterior section of the mandibular arch.

FIGURE 14.7 Cotton roll placement for the posterior mandibular arch.

FIGURE 14.9 Application of a dry angle.

Related Aids

Dry Angles

A dry angle is a triangle-shaped absorbent pad to help isolate posterior areas in both the maxillary and mandibular arches. The pad is placed on the buccal mucosa over the Stensen duct (Fig. 14.9). (This duct from the parotid gland is located opposite the maxillary second molar.)

These pads collect the flow of saliva and protect the tissue in this area. Follow the manufacturer's directions for placement and, if necessary, replace the pads if they become saturated before the procedure is completed. To remove, use water from the air-water syringe to wet the pad thoroughly before separating it from the soft tissue in the mucosa.

Dental Dam

The **dental dam** is a thin latex barrier used to isolate either a single tooth or several teeth during a dental procedure. These teeth are referred to as being isolated.

Indications for Using a Dental Dam

- An infection control protective barrier.
- Safeguards the patient's mouth against contact with debris, acid-etch materials, and other materials during treatment.
- Protects the patient from accidentally inhaling or swallowing debris, such as small fragments of a tooth or scraps of restorative material.
- Protects the tooth from contamination of saliva or debris if pulpal exposure accidentally occurs.
- Protects the oral cavity from exposure to infectious material when an infected tooth is opened during endodontic treatment.
- Provides moisture control that is essential for the placement of restorative materials.
- Improves access during treatment by retracting the lips, tongue, and gingiva.
- Provides better visibility because of the contrast of color of the dam and the tooth.
- Enhances dental team efficiency, discourages patient conversation, and may reduce the time required for some treatments.

Before placing the dental dam, review the patient's medical history for any indications of latex sensitivity or allergy. If this is an indication, then the dentist must be consulted before the application is continued.

The dental dam is applied after the local anesthetic has been administered and while the dentist is waiting for the anesthesia to take effect.

The teeth to be isolated should be clean and free of plaque or debris. When indicated, tooth brushing or selective coronal polishing is performed before placing the dental dam (see Chapter 21). If not removed, the plaque or debris can become dislodged and may irritate the gingival tissue.

Dental Dam Equipment

The equipment used for preparation, placement, and removal of the dental dam is described in Table 14.1.

TABLE 14.1
Dental Dam Equipment

Type of Equipment	Description of Equipment
Dam material (From Boyd LRB: *Dental instruments: a pocket guide,* ed 5, St. Louis, 2015, Saunders.)	Comes in latex or latex-free material. Available sizes are 6 × 6 and 5 × 5. Comes in a wide range of colors and in three gauges of thickness (thin, medium, and heavy).
Dental dam frame (From Boyd LRB: *Dental instruments: a pocket guide,* ed 5, St. Louis, 2015, Saunders.)	This U-shaped frame is made of plastic or metal that stretches the dam material away from the face and the worked area.

TABLE 14.1
Dental Dam Equipment—cont'd

Type of Equipment	Description of Equipment
Dental dam napkin	This cotton absorbent sheet is placed between the dental dam and the patient.

(From Heymann HO, Swift EJ Jr., Ritter AV: *Sturdevant's art and science of operative dentistry,* ed 6, St. Louis, 2013, Mosby.)

Type of Equipment	Description of Equipment
Lubricant	This water-soluble material can be placed on the underside of the dam around the punched area for easy placement between tight contacts.
Dental dam punch	This hole-punch device is used to create holes in the dam that expose the teeth to be isolated. Different sizes are used for specific teeth.

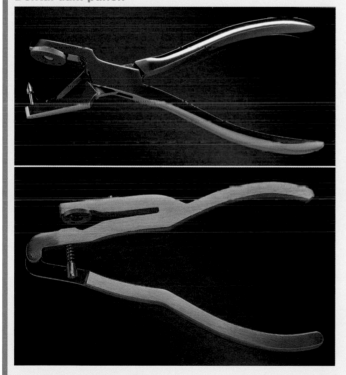

(From Boyd LRB: *Dental instruments: a pocket guide*, ed 5, St. Louis, 2015, Saunders.)

Continued

TABLE 14.1
Dental Dam Equipment—cont'd

Type of Equipment	Description of Equipment

5 Largest hole (clamped)
4 Large hole (molars)
3 Medium hole (premolars)
2 Small hole (maxillary anteriors)
1 Smallest hole (mandibular anteriors)

(From Bird DL, Robinson DS: *Modern dental assisting*, ed 11, St. Louis, 2015, Saunders.)

Dental dam stamp	Stamp designed in the shape of a dental arch and imprints teeth on the dental dam to be punched.

MAXILLARY

MANDIBULAR

(From Boyd LRB: *Dental instruments: a pocket guide*, ed 5, St. Louis, 2015, Saunders.)

Dental dam forceps	This type of forceps is used to place and remove the dental dam clamp.

TABLE 14.1
Dental Dam Equipment—cont'd

Type of Equipment	Description of Equipment
Dental dam clamps 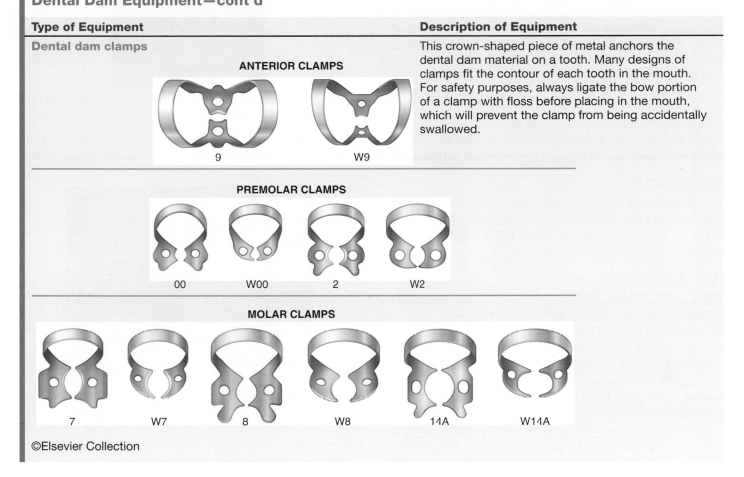	This crown-shaped piece of metal anchors the dental dam material on a tooth. Many designs of clamps fit the contour of each tooth in the mouth. For safety purposes, always ligate the bow portion of a clamp with floss before placing in the mouth, which will prevent the clamp from being accidentally swallowed.

©Elsevier Collection

Preparation of the Dental Dam Application

Each application of the dam is preplanned to accommodate the dentist's preferences, the tooth or teeth involved, and the procedure to be performed.

Several important factors are to be incorporated when planning for punching the dental dam:
- The arch, its shape, and any irregularities, such as missing teeth or a fixed prosthesis
- Number of teeth to be isolated
- Identification of the anchor tooth and location of the key-punch hole
- Size and spacing of the other holes to be punched (the **anchor tooth** holds the dental dam clamp, and the **key-punch hole** covers the anchor tooth)

Maxillary Arch Applications

In preparing for the maxillary application, the dam material is stamped or marked. This mark automatically designates the margin of the dam for these holes. If the patient has a mustache or a thick upper lip, then allowing extra space for the anterior teeth area may be necessary.

Mandibular Arch Applications

In preparing for the mandibular application, the dam is stamped or marked to accommodate the small size of the mandibular anterior teeth; the holes are punched closer together than those for posterior teeth.

Curve of the Arch

Adjusting the punched holes to accommodate an extremely narrow or wide arch is necessary. Failure to make such adjustments will increase the difficulty when inverting the edges of the punched holes of the dam into the gingival sulcus.

Bunching and stretching on the lingual aspect of the dental dam will occur if the curve of the arch is punched too narrow or too wide. Folds and stretching of the dam on the facial aspect occur if the arch is punched too curved or too narrow.

Maligned Teeth

If a single tooth or teeth are **maligned** within the dental arch, then special consideration is taken before the dental dam is punched. (Maligned and **malposed** mean that the individual tooth is not in its normal position within the dental arch.)

If a tooth is lingually positioned, then the hole-punch size remains the same, but the hole is placed approximately 1 mm lingually from the normal arch alignment. If the tooth is facially positioned, then the hole-punch size remains the same, but the hole is placed approximately 1 mm facially from the normal arch alignment.

Teeth to be Isolated

Single-tooth isolation is indicated to isolate selective teeth for restorative procedures, such as for Class I and Class V. It is also common to use single tooth isolation for endodontic treatment.

By applying **multiple-tooth isolation**, the dam provides more stability and better visibility for the operator. One concept is to have two teeth isolated so that the most posterior tooth acts as an anchor tooth to hold the clamp. For additional stability in the posterior area of the quadrant, however, isolating multiple teeth within the quadrant is the most effective (Fig. 14.10). When anterior teeth are being restored, maximum stability is achieved by isolating the six anterior teeth (canine to canine).

Key-Punch Hole

The **anchor tooth** holds the dental dam clamp. The **key-punch hole** is punched in the dental dam to cover the anchor tooth. A larger no. 5–size hole is necessary for the key punch because it must also accommodate the clamp.

Hole Size and Spacing

The size of each hole selected on the dental dam punch must be appropriate for the tooth to be isolated. A correctly sized hole allows the dam to slip easily over the tooth and snugly fit in the cervical area, which is important to prevent leakage around the dam.

In general, the holes are spaced from 3.0 to 3.5 mm between the edges, not the centers, of the holes, which allows adequate spacing between the holes to create a **septum** that slips between the teeth without tearing or injuring the gingiva.

The septum is the portion of the dental dam between the holes of the punched dam. During application, this portion of the dam is passed between the contacts. (*Septum* is singular, *septa* is plural.)

See Procedure 14.4: Preparation, Placement, and Removal of the Dental Dam (Expanded Function).

Preframed Dental Dam

A preframed dental dam is available that provides easy application for a single tooth or multiple teeth (Fig. 14.11). Its single-use design provides the flexibility for access with suction, handpiece, and radiographic films or sensors.

FIGURE 14.10 Application of dental dam isolating full quadrant for better visibility and stability. (From Boyd LRB: *Dental instruments: a pocket guide*, ed 7, St. Louis, 2021, Elsevier.)

FIGURE 14.11 Preframed dental dam isolating mandibular anterior teeth. (From Boyd LRB: *Dental instruments: a pocket guide,* ed 7, St. Louis, 2021, Elsevier.)

▪ Ethical Implications

During the application of the dental dam, you may be left alone to place the dam by yourself. If this is the case, then verify that applying a dental dam is a legal function in your state for dental assistants and that you have had special training in the application process.

Performing a Mouth Rinse

Equipment and Supplies

- HVE tip
- Saliva ejector
- Air-water syringe

Procedural Steps

1. Decide which oral evacuation system will be best for the rinsing procedure.
2. Grasp the air-water syringe in your left hand and the HVE or saliva ejector in your right hand.

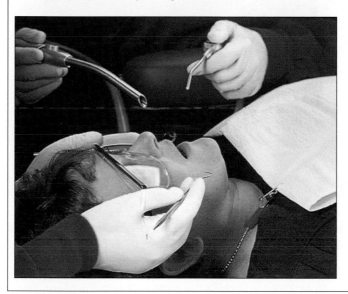

Limited-Mouth Rinse

1. Turn on the suction and position the tip toward the site for a limited-area rinse.
2. Spray the combination of air and water onto the site to be rinsed.
   Purpose: The combination of air and water provides more force to clean the area thoroughly.
3. Suction all fluid and debris from the area, being sure to remove all fluids.
4. Dry the area by pressing the air button only.

Full-Mouth Rinse

1. Have the patient turn toward you.
   Purpose: Turning the head allows the water to pool on one side, making it easier for you to suction all of the water.
2. Turn on the HVE or the saliva ejector and position the tip in the vestibule of the patient's left side.
   Note: Carefully position the tip so that it does not come into contact with soft tissue.
3. With the HVE or saliva ejector tip positioned, direct the air-water syringe from the patient's maxillary right across to the left side, spraying all surfaces.
4. Continue along the mandibular arch, following the same sequence from right to left.
   Purpose: This pattern of rinsing forces debris to the posterior mouth, where the suction tip is positioned for easier removal of fluids and debris.

HVE, High-volume evacuator.

Positioning the High-Volume Evacuator During a Procedure

Equipment and Supplies

- Sterile HVE tip
- Plastic barrier cover for the HVE handle and hose
- Cotton rolls

Procedural Steps

1. Place the HVE tip in the holder by pushing the end of the tip into the holder through the plastic barrier.
   Purpose: Leaves the opposite end exposed and ready for use.
2. If necessary, use the HVE tip or a mouth mirror to retract the cheek or tongue gently.

Posterior Placement

1. For a mandibular site, place a cotton roll under the suction tip.
   Purpose: Provides patient comfort, aids in stabilizing tip placement, and prevents injury to the tissue.
2. Place the bevel of the HVE tip as close as possible to the tooth being prepared.
   Purpose: Suction will draw the water into the tip immediately after it leaves the tooth being prepared.
3. Position the bevel of the HVE tip parallel to the buccal or lingual surface of the tooth being prepared.
4. Place the upper edge of the HVE tip so that it extends slightly beyond the occlusal surface.
   Purpose: Suction will catch the water spray from the handpiece as it leaves the tooth being prepared.

Anterior Placement

1. When the dentist is preparing the tooth from the lingual aspect, position the HVE tip so that it is parallel to the facial surface and slightly beyond the incisal edge.

2. When the dentist is preparing the tooth from the facial aspect, position the HVE tip parallel to the lingual surface and slightly beyond the incisal edge.

HVE, High-volume evacuator.

Procedure 14.3

Placing and Removing Cotton Rolls

 (icon at top right)

Equipment and Supplies

- Basic setup
- Cotton rolls
- Air-water syringe

Maxillary Placement

1. Have the patient turn toward you with their chin raised.
   Purpose: Provides better visualization and ease in the placement of the cotton roll.

2. Using cotton pliers, pick up a cotton roll so that it is evenly positioned within the beaks of the cotton pliers.

3. Transfer the cotton roll to the mouth, and securely position it in the mucobuccal fold closest to the working field.
   Note: Once you place the cotton roll with the pliers, you may want to use your gloved finger or the handle end of the cotton pliers to push the cotton roll into the mucobuccal fold.

4. Maxillary placement can be used for any location on the maxillary arch.

Mandibular Placement

1. Have the patient turn toward you with their chin lowered.

Placing and Removing Cotton Rolls—cont'd

Purpose: Provides better visualization and ease in the placement of the cotton roll.

2. Using the cotton pliers, pick up a cotton roll so that it is evenly positioned within the beaks of the cotton pliers.

3. Transfer the cotton roll to the mouth, and securely position it in the mucobuccal fold closest to the working field.
4. Carry the second cotton roll to the mouth, and position it in the floor of the mouth between the working field and the tongue.
   Note: Have the patient lift the tongue during placement and then relax the tongue to help secure the cotton roll in position.

5. If you are placing cotton rolls for the mandibular anterior region, bend the cotton roll before placing for a contoured fit.

6. If using a saliva ejector for the procedure, then place it after the cotton roll is in position in the lingual vestibule.

Cotton Roll Removal

1. At the completion of a procedure, remove the cotton roll before the full-mouth rinse. If the cotton roll is dry, then moisten it with water from the air-water syringe.
   Purpose: Dry cotton rolls will adhere to the lining of the oral mucosa, and tissue may become irritated when a dry cotton roll is pulled away from the area.
2. Using cotton pliers, retrieve the contaminated cotton roll from the site.
3. If appropriate for the procedure, then perform a limited rinse.

Equipment and Supplies

- Basic setup
- Precut 6 × 6 inch dental dam
- Dental dam stamp and inkpad or template and pen
- Dental dam punch
- Dental dam clamp or clamps with ligature attached
- Dental dam clamp forceps
- Young frame
- Dental dam napkin
- Dental tape or waxed floss
- Cotton rolls
- Lubricant for patient's lips
- Lubricant for dam
- Black spoon
- Crown and bridge scissors

Patient Preparation

1. Check the patient's record for any contraindications to latex or past use and identify the area to be isolated. Inform the patient of the need to place a dental dam, and explain the steps involved.
2. Assist the dentist in the administration of a local anesthetic. Ask the operator which teeth are to be isolated. Examine the area for any malposed teeth to be accommodated.
3. Apply lubricating ointment to the patient's lip with a cotton roll or a cotton-tip applicator.
   Note: The patient's comfort is a concern throughout the placement and removal of the dental dam.
4. Use the mouth mirror and explorer to examine the site where the dam is to be placed. This area should be free of plaque and debris.
   Purpose: If the dam is placed in an area with plaque and debris, then the dam could push the plaque and debris into the sulcus and irritate the gingival tissue.
   Note: If debris or plaque is present, selective tooth brushing or coronal polishing is performed on these teeth before applying the dental dam.
5. Floss all contacts involved in the placement of the dental dam.
   Purpose: Any tight contacts may tear the dam.

Punching the Dental Dam

1. Use a template or stamp to mark the teeth to be isolated on the dam.

2. Correctly punch the marked dam according to the teeth to be isolated. Be sure to use the correct size of punch hole for the specific tooth.
3. If teeth have tight contacts, then lightly lubricate the holes on the tooth surface (undersurface) of the dam.
   Purpose: Lubrication eases placement of the dam over the contact area of the teeth.

Placing the Clamp and Frame

1. Select the correct size of clamp.
   Note: The W7 clamp has been selected for this procedure.
2. Secure the clamp by tying a ligature of dental tape on the bow of the clamp.
3. Place the beaks of the rubber dam forceps into the holes of the clamp. Grasp the handles of the rubber dam forceps, and squeeze to open the clamp. Turn upward and allow the locking bar to slide down to keep the forceps open for placement.
4. Place yourself in the operator's position and adjust the patient for easy access.
5. Retrieve the rubber dam forceps. Position the lingual jaws of the clamp first, then the facial jaws. During placement, keep an index finger on the clamp to prevent the clamp from coming off before it has been stabilized on the tooth. Check the clamp for fit.
   Purpose: Lingual jaw placement serves as a fulcrum for placement of the facial jaws.

6. Transfer the dental dam to the site; stretch the punched hole for the anchor tooth over the clamp.

Preparation, Placement, and Removal of the Dental Dam (Expanded Function)—cont'd

7. Using cotton pliers, retrieve the ligature and pull it through so that it is exposed and easy to grasp, if necessary.
8. Position the Young frame over the dam and slightly pull the dam, allowing it to hook onto the projections of the frame.
   Purpose: This position ensures a smooth and stable fit.
9. Fit the last hole of the dam over the last tooth to be exposed at the opposite end of the anchor tooth.
   Purpose: This position stabilizes the dam and aids in locating the remaining punch holes for the teeth to be isolated.
10. Using the index fingers of both hands, stretch the dam on the lingual and facial surfaces of the teeth so that the dam slides through each contact area.
11. With a piece of dental tape or waxed floss, floss through the contacts, pushing the dam below the proximal contacts of each tooth to be isolated.
    Note: Slide the floss through the contact rather than pulling it back through the contact. This process will keep the dam in place.

12. If the contacts are extremely tight, then use floss or a wedge placed into the interproximal area to separate the teeth slightly.
13. A ligature is placed to stabilize the dam at the opposite end of the anchor tooth.

Inverting the Dam

1. Invert, or reverse, the dam by gently stretching it near the cervix of the tooth.
   Purpose: Inverting the dam creates a seal to prevent the leakage of saliva.
2. Apply air from the air-water syringe to the tooth being inverted to help in turning the dam material under.
   Purpose: When the tooth surface is dry, the margin of the stretched dam usually inverts into the gingival sulcus as the dam is released.
3. A black spoon or burnisher can be used to invert the edges of the dam.
4. When all punched holes are properly inverted, the dental dam application is complete.

5. If necessary, for patient comfort, a saliva ejector may be placed under the dam and positioned on the floor of the patient's mouth on the side opposite the area being treated.
6. If the patient is uncomfortable and has trouble breathing only through the nose, then cut a small hole in the palatal area of the dam by pinching a piece of the dam with cotton pliers and cutting a small hole near the palatal area.

Removing the Dam

1. If a ligature was used to stabilize the dam, then remove it first. If a saliva ejector was used, then remove it.
2. Slide your finger under the dam parallel to the arch and pull outward so that you are stretching the holes away from the isolated teeth. Working from posterior to anterior, use the crown and bridge scissors to cut from hole to hole, creating one long cut.
3. When all septa are cut, the dam is lingually pulled to free the dam from the interproximal space.
4. Using the dental dam forceps, position the beaks into the holes of the clamp, and open the clamp by squeezing the handle. Gently slide the clamp from the tooth.

5. Remove both the dam and the Young frame at one time.
6. Use a tissue or the dam napkin to wipe the patient's mouth, lips, and chin free of moisture.
7. Inspect the dam to ensure that the entire pattern of the torn septa of the dental dam has been removed.
8. If a fragment of the dental dam is missing, use dental floss to check the corresponding interproximal area of the oral cavity.
   Purpose: Fragments of the dental dam left under the free gingiva can cause gingival irritation.

Chapter Exercises

Multiple Choice

Circle the letter next to the correct answer.

1. You are assisting in the restoration of tooth #10 with a Class V on the facial surface; the HVE tip should be placed on the _____.
   a. facial surface
   b. lingual surface
   c. opposite side of where the dentist is working
   d. b and c

2. Hole size no. _____ is used for the anchor tooth, which holds the rubber dam clamp.
   a. 1
   b. 3
   c. 4
   d. 5

3. While placing the dental dam, you notice the contacts are extremely tight. A(n) _____ may be used to help push the material interproximal.
   a. explorer
   b. tape or floss
   c. wooden wedge
   d. separating disc

4. The HVE handle should be held in a _____ grasp.
   a. palm
   b. pen
   c. thumb-to-nose
   d. b or c

5. The purpose of inverting the dental dam is to _____.
   a. prevent saliva leakage
   b. prevent the clamp from coming off
   c. stabilize the dam
   d. a, b, and c

6. If a patient's cheek or tongue is accidentally sucked into the HVE tip, then you should _____.
   a. inform the dentist
   b. quickly turn off the vacuum control
   c. rotate the angle of the tip to break the suction
   d. b or c

7. During oral evacuation for tooth #19, the bevel of the HVE tip should be positioned _____ the occlusal surface of the tooth being prepared.
   a. even with
   b. slightly below
   c. slightly above

8. Cotton roll isolation is not the best selection for a _____ procedure.
   a. restorative
   b. cementation
   c. sealant
   d. a and b

9. A limited rinse is one that _____.
   a. is completed at the beginning of the procedure
   b. is completed at the end of the procedure
   c. rinses the whole mouth
   d. rinses a specific area in the mouth

10. When using a saliva ejector, position the tip _____ on which you are working.
    a. in the buccal mucosa area
    b. under the tongue on the same side
    c. under the tongue on the opposite side
    d. in the palatal area

Apply Your Knowledge

1. You are assisting in an amalgam procedure and notice the cotton rolls that were placed have become saturated with saliva and debris. After removing the cotton rolls, you notice that the patient's mucosa is red and irritated. What caused this, and what could have prevented this?

2. Dr. Stewart is restoring tooth #25 on the facial surface. Where is the best position for you to place the HVE tip during the tooth preparation?

3. How would you prepare the dental dam for placement for tooth #25?

CHAPTER 15

Pain and Anxiety Management

http://evolve.elsevier.com/Robinson/essentials/

The dental profession has access to a wide range of pain and anxiety control procedures to provide oral health care to individuals who would otherwise remain untreated because of their fear of pain. Pain and anxiety control are defined as the exposure of chemical, physiologic, and psychological approaches to prevent and treat preoperative, operative, and postoperative pain and anxiety.

For most dental procedures, pain control is accomplished with the application of a topical and local anesthetic agent. There are some patients, however, that are apprehensive about receiving dental treatment. This type of patient may require additional methods to help control their anxiety. The administration of nitrous oxide–oxygen and antianxiety drugs may be prescribed to provide comfort to the patient when receiving dental care.

A new direction for confronting anxiety with a patient is introducing relaxation techniques. Relaxation techniques can help reduce levels of stress hormones, as well as pain and anxiety.

Use of intravenous (IV) sedation or **general anesthesia** is recommended for a patient with the need for invasive or extensive dental treatment or for one who is medically or physically compromised.

The dental assistant must be familiar with the procedures, types of equipment, and the range of anesthetics used in all areas of dentistry.

Topical Anesthesia

Topical anesthesia is a procedure where a concentrated anesthetic agent, such as benzocaine, is topically applied to the area where the local anesthetic injection is to take place. It provides a temporary numbing effect on the nerve endings on the surface of the oral mucosa. These agents are available in the form of ointments, liquids, sprays, and patches (Fig. 15.1).

FIGURE 15.1 Topical anesthetics. (Courtesy Premier Dental Products Company, Plymouth Meeting, Pennsylvania.)

Local Anesthetic Solution	Color of Cartridge Band
Articaine HCl 4% with epinephrine 1:100,000	Gold
Bupivacaine 0.5% with epinephrine 1:200,000	Blue
Lidocaine HCl 2%	Light blue
Lidocaine HCl 2% with epinephrine 1:50,000	Green
Lidocaine HCl 2% with epinephrine 1:100,000	Red
Mepivacaine HCl 3%	Tan
Mepivacaine HCl 2% with levonordefrin 1:20,000	Brown
Prilocaine HCl 4%	Black
Prilocaine HCl 4% with epinephrine 1:200,000	Yellow

FIGURE 15.2 Color-coding system for anesthetic cartridges. (Anesthetic syringe and color-coding illustrations from Malamed SF: *Handbook of local anesthesia,* ed 6, St. Louis, 2013, Mosby.)

Topical Anesthetic Ointment

Topical anesthetic ointment can lessen or even eliminate that initial "pinch" from an injection. For maximum effectiveness, the ointment is applied to the dried mucosal surface at the site of the injection with a cotton-tip applicator for 2 to 5 minutes.

See Procedure 15.1: Applying a Topical Anesthetic Ointment.

Local Anesthesia

Local anesthesia is a procedure that was first introduced in the 1800s. A local anesthetic agent is the most frequently used form of pain control in dentistry and is the drug of choice to reduce or relieve associated pain that may take place during and immediately after a dental procedure. This type of anesthesia provides a safe, effective, and dependable method for a suitable duration in virtually all forms of dental treatment.

Local Anesthetic Agents

The chemical makeup of local anesthetic agents blocks the ability of the nerve membrane to generate an impulse. Because of this block, the impulse does not transmit the feeling of pain to the brain. To receive local anesthesia, the agent is injected near the nerve specifically affecting the tooth or teeth receiving dental treatment.

Composition of Local Anesthetic Solution
- Local anesthetic drug—blocks nerve conduction
- Sodium chloride—allows solution to be isotonic with body tissues
- Sterile water—gives volume to the concentration
- Sodium—acts as an antioxidant to prevent damage to cells

Local anesthetic agents are broadly classified under two chemical groups: amides and esters. The difference between the two is in how they are metabolized by the body: amides by the liver and esters primarily in the plasma. The amides were first introduced to clinical practice in the 1940s and provide the standards by which all other local anesthetic agents are measured. Ester-type anesthetics are used primarily as topical anesthetics.

A color-coding system designed by the American Dental Association created an easily recognizable standardization for all injectable local anesthetics (Fig. 15.2).

Induction and Duration of an Anesthetic

Induction is the time frame from when the injection is given until the complete effective numbing sensation. **Duration** is the time frame from when the injection is given until the numbing sensation is gone. Duration varies among anesthetic agents, between pulp and soft tissues, and between maxillary infiltration and mandibular blocks. Duration will also vary from patient to patient. In general, local anesthetic agents follow this time frame:
- Short-acting duration local anesthetic agents can last approximately 30 minutes.
- Intermediate-acting duration local anesthetic agents will last approximately 60 minutes (most local anesthetic agents are in this group and are used for general dental procedures).
- Long-acting duration local anesthetic agents will last approximately 90 minutes.

Vasoconstrictors

A **vasoconstrictor** is an added drug to the local anesthetic agent to slow down the intake of the anesthetic agent and increase the duration of action. The action of a vasoconstrictor can:
- Prolong the effect of the anesthetic agent by decreasing blood flow in the immediate area of the injection
- Decrease bleeding in the area, which is beneficial during surgical procedures

The most common vasoconstrictors used are epinephrine, levonordefrin, and Neo-Cobefrin. The ratio of vasoconstrictor to anesthetic solution is supplied as 1:50,000, 1:100,000, or 1:200,000. A concentration of 1:100,000 indicates that one part of the vasoconstrictor is diluted in 100,000 parts of anesthetic solution. The lower the second number, the larger the amount of epinephrine in the solution.

Health Status of the Patient

Local anesthetic agents and vasoconstrictors are considered safe drugs when properly administered. Certain health conditions may affect the dentist's choice in the type of anesthetic solution and whether or not that solution contains a vasoconstrictor. Health conditions are noted in the patient's medical history, and the dentist must be alerted to the health conditions when selecting a local anesthetic agent.

Health Conditions Affecting the Selection of a Local Anesthetic Agent

- Hypertension
- Cardiovascular disease
- Hyperthyroidism
- Liver disease
- Kidney disease
- Pregnancy

Local Anesthesia Techniques

The location and the nerves of the tooth or teeth to be anesthetized determine the type of injection method to be used.

By knowing the location and teeth affected, the assistant is better prepared with the setup and transfer of the procedure.

Maxillary Anesthesia

Because of the **porous** nature of the alveolar cancellous bone in the maxilla, local anesthesia diffuses through the bone and reaches the nerve at the apices of the tooth. There are three major types of local anesthetic injections applied for the maxillary arch (Fig. 15.3).

- *Infiltration anesthesia* involves injecting the anesthetic solution into the tissue near the apices of the tooth being treated.
- *Field block* refers to injecting the anesthetic near a larger terminal nerve branch, thus numbing a larger surface area.
- *Nerve block* occurs when local anesthetic is deposited close to a main nerve trunk, thus numbing an even larger area.

Palatal Anesthesia

Local anesthesia in the palatal area may be necessary for procedures that involve the soft tissue or the palate (Fig. 15.4).

- *Greater palatine nerve block* numbs the posterior portion of the hard palate
- *Nasopalatine nerve block* numbs the anterior hard palate.

FIGURE 15.3 Maxillary injections. (From Malamed SF: *Handbook of local anesthesia*, ed 6, St Louis, 2013, Mosby.)

FIGURE 15.4 Palatal injections. (Courtesy Margaret J. Fehrenbach, RDH, MS.)

FIGURE 15.5 Mandibular injections. (From Malamed SF: *Handbook of local anesthesia*, ed 6, St Louis, 2013, Mosby.)

Mandibular Anesthesia

Because of the dense, compact nature of the mandibular bone, anesthetic solution does not diffuse easily through it. Therefore block anesthesia is the type of injection for mandibular teeth (Fig. 15.5).

- *Inferior alveolar nerve block,* also referred to as *mandibular block,* is injected into the inferior alveolar nerve, which numbs half of the lower jaw, including the teeth, tongue, and lip.
- *Buccal nerve block* numbs the mandibular molars within the quadrant.
- *Incisive nerve block* numbs the mandibular premolar and anterior teeth.

FIGURE 15.6 Periodontal ligament injection. (From Logothetis DD: *Local anesthesia for the dental hygienist*, ed 2, St Louis, 2017, Elsevier.)

Periodontal Ligament Injection

An alternative infiltration technique involves directly injecting the anesthetic solution into the periodontal ligament and surrounding gingival tissue. This type of injection can be completed with the use of a conventional syringe or a specialized periodontal ligament injection syringe (Fig. 15.6).

Local Anesthesia Setup

When preparing the local anesthetic setup, the dental assistant will review the treatment plan in the patients record to gather specific information about the procedure before assembling the setup (Table 15.1).

Specifics include (1) reviewing the patients' medical history for contraindications to anesthesia, (2) confirming with the dentist the type of local anesthetic to set out, and (3) knowing which tooth or teeth to be anesthetized to determine the needle length and gauge.

See Procedure 15.2: Assembling the Local Anesthetic Syringe.

Transferring the Anesthetic Syringe

The transfer of an anesthetic syringe takes place in the transfer zone just below the patient's chin. If the patient is apprehensive or if the dentist is anesthetizing a child, then behind the patient's head may be a more suitable zone for transferring the syringe.

Always be alert to infection control and protocol. The transfer of a sterile syringe is appropriate, but once the syringe has been used, it becomes contaminated, and the dentist will need to recap and retrieve the syringe for additional injections.

Patients should never be left alone after the anesthesia has been given. Continually observe the patient to ensure that they are not in distress or developing an allergic reaction.

See Procedure 15.3: Assisting in the Administration of Local Anesthesia.

Local Anesthetic Cautions

Needlestick injuries are serious, and care must be taken to prevent such accidents when handling a contaminated syringe.

TABLE 15.1
Local Anesthetic Setup

Part	Description
Anesthetic syringe Thumb ring Finger grip Finger bar Barrel of syringe Piston rod Harpoon Threaded tip	• The *thumb ring, finger grip*, and *finger bar* make it possible for the dentist to hold the syringe firmly when giving the injection. • The *harpoon* is pushed into the rubber stopper of the anesthetic cartridge; by pulling back, the piston rod retracts the rubber stopper. This action makes aspiration possible. An aspirating syringe is used to administer the local anesthetic agent to enable the dentist to aspirate (aspirate means to draw back) after insertion of the needle. • The *barrel* of the syringe holds the anesthetic cartridge in the syringe. The cartridge is loaded into the syringe through the large open area on the side of the barrel. The other side has a large window, enabling the dentist to watch for blood in the cartridge as he or she aspirates. • The *piston rod* pushes down on the rubber stopper of the anesthetic cartridge and pushes the anesthetic solution out through the needle. • The *threaded tip* where the needle is screwed onto the syringe.
Disposable needle **Short Needle** From Boyd LRB: *Dental instruments: a pocket guide*, ed 5, St. Louis, 2015, Elsevier. **Long Needle** From Boyd LRB: *Dental instruments: a pocket guide*, ed 7, St. Louis, 2021, Elsevier.	1. Cartridge end of needle that is screwed into the anesthetic cartridge. 2. Needle hub rests on the syringe 3. Needle (short – maxillary / long – mandibular and infiltration) 4. Lumen of the needle is the opening (in different sizes 25, 27, and 30 gauge). The larger the gauge, the thinner the needle 5. Bevel is the slanted end of needle 6. Protective cap for cartridge end 7. Seal of cap 8. Needle guard removed before injection

Continued

TABLE 15.1
Local Anesthetic Setup—cont'd

Part	Description
Anesthetic cartridge *[image of anesthetic cartridge with labeled parts 1–6 and close-up of rubber diaphragm]*	1. Rubber diaphragm where the cartridge end of needle syringe needle is inserted 2. Aluminum cap that holds the diaphragm in place 3. Glass cartridge (carpule) of anesthetic solution 4. Marking of type of anesthetic 5. Color coded band of type of anesthetic 6. Rubber plunger where harpoon is inserted for injection of anesthetic

From Boyd LRB: *Dental instruments: a pocket guide*, ed 7, St. Louis, 2021, Elsevier

A needlestick injury can occur during usage, after usage, in recapping, and in the disposal. It is imperative for the dental office to have a written exposure control plan that incorporates universal precautions, work practice controls, and hepatitis B vaccinations.

A directive from the Centers for Disease Control and Prevention (CDC) states that contaminated needles used in dental procedures should be recapped by a recapping device or by a single-handed scoop technique (Fig. 15.7).

A **recapping device** allows the dentist to slide the needle into the guard without touching it. With a **single-handed scoop technique**, the needle guard is placed on the tray, and the end of the needle is slid into its cover. Once the end of the needle is covered, the other hand may safely be used to complete bringing the cap into position.

Pain and Anxiety Control Methods

Many people have some form of pain or anxiety when it comes to receiving dental care. Several methods described in this section are used to reduce the pain and anxiety during preoperative, operative, and postoperative care.

Relaxation Techniques

Fear can be minimized during a dental procedure when the staff is empathetic (understanding) toward patients. Several techniques can be used to help alleviate the fear before and during dental treatment.

- Asking the patient to imagine a pleasant memory or a soothing place can help reduce the fear.
- Devices such as headsets with music or having a video available to watch can distract and calm the patient before the injection and throughout the procedure.

FIGURE 15.7 Needle recapping devices. (Left photo from Boyd LRB: *Dental instruments: a pocket guide,* ed 5, St Louis, 2015, Saunders. Right photo courtesy Hu-Friedy Mfg. Co., LLC, Chicago, Illnois.)

- Having the patient take slow and deep breaths supplies the body with oxygen and other chemicals that relax the central nervous system and help reduce discomfort.

Nitrous Oxide Analgesia

Nitrous oxide analgesia is one of the most common forms of in-office pain and anxiety control. The gas is inhaled through the nose and primarily acts as a sedative to help eliminate fear and to relax the patient. The terms *inhalation sedation, nitrous oxide–oxygen analgesia,* and *psychosedation* are interchangeable when describing nitrous oxide. In this discussion, the term *nitrous oxide analgesia* will be used.

The combination of nitrous oxide and oxygen gases produces nitrous oxide analgesia (Fig. 15.8). The patient inhales a combination of nitrous oxide gas and oxygen through a nosepiece, feeling the effect almost immediately. The mix produces a pleasant, relaxing experience for the patient with easy onset, minimal side effects, and rapid recovery.

FIGURE 15.8 Nitrous oxide gas–oxygen (N₂O) system unit. (From Boyd LRB: *Dental instruments: a pocket guide,* ed 5, St. Louis, 2015, Saunders.)

When used alone, nitrous oxide analgesia dulls the perception of pain, such as during the injection of a local anesthetic agent or for a simple procedure, but it must be used in conjunction with an effective local anesthetic solution to achieve total pain control for most dental procedures.

After the completion of treatment, the flow of nitrous oxide is discontinued, and complete oxygen is delivered through the nosepiece for approximately 5 minutes. Some patients may require more time on 100% oxygen to oxygenate (clear) or completely recover from the effects of the nitrous oxide analgesia. Indications and contraindications for the use of nitrous oxide should be considered before use.

Indications for Using Nitrous Oxide Analgesia

- Administration is relatively simple and is easily managed by the dentist.
- Special training is required for the dentist and dental team; the services of anesthetist or other special personnel is not necessary.
- Nitrous oxide–oxygen sedation has an excellent safety record with minimal side effects.
- The patient is awake and able to communicate at all times.
- Recovery is rapid and complete within a matter of minutes.
- Nitrous oxide–oxygen sedation may be used with patients of all ages.

Contraindications for Using Nitrous Oxide Analgesia

- Pregnancy: Although no evidence indicates that enough nitrous oxide crosses the placenta to damage the fetus, nitrous oxide analgesia is administered to a pregnant patient only with the permission of her obstetrician.
- Nasal obstruction: Cold or allergy symptoms can prevent the patient from obtaining the benefit of the drug.
- Emphysema or other pulmonary diseases: These diseases cause breathing difficulties. Increased oxygen during the administration of nitrous oxide analgesia may lower the stimulus to breathe as often as necessary.
- Emotional instability: This reaction can be intensified because of the altered perception of reality produced by the nitrous oxide analgesia. It is important to consult with the patient's physician first.

Equipment for Administering Nitrous Oxide

The dental office may be equipped with either built-in N_2O/O_2 equipment in the dental unit or use a portable unit that can be moved from operatory to operatory. Table 15.2 review the components that would be included for the setup for administering nitrous oxide/oxygen.

Safety Precautions with Nitrous Oxide

Nitrous oxide is used only during patient treatment. It is never unnecessarily administered or used for recreational purposes. For staff and patient safety, the maximum allowable amount of nitrous oxide in the dental environment is 50 parts per million (ppm).

Masks are designed to have a **scavenger system** attached for the protection of the dental team. A scavenger system should always be used to reduce the amount of nitrous oxide exhaled into the air by the patient and thus breathed by members of the dental team (Fig. 15.9). The use of a scavenger system is recommended to reduce the amount of nitrous oxide released into the treatment area.

Patient Assessment and Monitoring

In specific states, credentialed dental assistants are certified to assess and monitor nitrous oxide–oxygen analgesia under the direct supervision of the dentist. Before the administration of nitrous oxide analgesia begins, the patient must be informed about what to expect. This includes:

- Explaining the process of administering the gases
- Describing how to use the mask and explaining the importance of nasal breathing
- Describing the sensations of warmth and tingling that the patient may experience
- Reassuring the patient that they will remain conscious, aware, and in control of their actions

The baseline is the ratio of nitrous oxide to oxygen that is most effective for each patient. At the baseline, the patient is conscious and cooperative but pleasantly relaxed. The dentist determines the volumes of nitrous oxide and oxygen and the time necessary for the patient to reach baseline. The least amount of nitrous oxide should always be used. For most patients, 30% nitrous oxide or less is effective. Small children typically require less. Once the baseline has been determined, this information is recorded on the patient's record at each appointment.

TABLE 15.2
Nitrous Oxide Analgesia Equipment

Equipment	Description
Cylinders From Boyd LRB: *Dental instruments: a pocket guide*, ed 7, St. Louis, 2021, Elsevier	Nitrous oxide and oxygen are dispensed in steel cylinders, which are color coded. Cylinders should be stored in an upright position, away from a heat source, and secured to the wall (or a portable unit) to prevent them from falling on the valve stem, which could cause the cylinder to explode. 1. Blue for nitrous oxide 2. Green for oxygen
Gas machines	Nitrous oxide gas machines are available as a portable or a central system. Components of gas machines include the following: • Yokes, which hold the cylinder in the machine • Control valves, which are used to control the flow of each gas • Flow meter, which indicates the rate of flow of the gas The greater the flow of gas, the higher the ball rises. Separate color coded flow meters are used for nitrous oxide and for oxygen: • Pressure gauge, which indicates the pressure of cylinder contents • Reservoir bag, which is where the two gases are combined and from which the patient draws for breathing
Nitrous Oxide Nasal Mask 	Masks, which are the nasal inhalers through which the patient breathes the gases. They are available in a disposable variety, which is discarded after a single use, and in rubber, which can be sterilized or disinfected for reuse. 1. Gas hose, which carries the gases from the reservoir bag to the mask or nosepiece 2. Scavenger hose to evacuate excess gas 3. Nasal mask in different sizes for adults and children

FIGURE 15.9 Scavenger system attached to the mask and evacuation unit to redirect unused nitrous oxide gas.

See Procedure 15.4: Assisting in the Administration and Monitoring of Nitrous Oxide–Oxygen Sedation (Expanded Function).

Antianxiety Agents

Antianxiety drugs can be prescribed for the relief of anxiety. These medications can produce sleep, sedation, and anesthesia. Antianxiety agents can be orally or intravenously administered. Before administering any form of an antianxiety drug, the dentist is required to have specialized training in the prescribing of agents and the method of delivery.

Antianxiety agents commonly prescribed include secobarbital (Seconal), chlordiazepoxide (Librium), and diazepam (Valium), which can suppress mild to moderate anxiety. Chloral hydrate (Noctec) is a sedative that is often used for sedating children.

When these drugs are prescribed, the patient will be asked to take the drug orally 30 to 60 minutes before the appointment. Patients must be informed that these drugs induce drowsiness and that they should not drive themselves to and from the appointment.

Indications for the Use of Antianxiety Drugs
- The patient is apprehensive about a procedure.
- The procedure is long and/or difficult.
- The patient is mentally or physically compromised.
- The patient is a child in need of extensive treatment.

Intravenous Sedation

Dental specialists, such as the oral and maxillofacial surgeon or the periodontist, will provide IV sedation for patients undergoing extensive procedures. The process of starting, monitoring, and removing IV sedation is completed only by an individual trained and certified.

IV conscious sedation results in a minimally depressed level of consciousness. The patient maintains the ability to keep an open airway and respond appropriately to physical or verbal stimulation. Specific antianxiety drugs are administered intravenously throughout the procedure at a slower rate, providing state I analgesia.

LEONARD S. TAYLOR, D.D.S.
2100 WEST PARK AVENUE
CHAMPAIGN, ILLINOIS 61820

Telephone: 367-6671   DEA NO. 0000000

Name _John Doe_   Age _45_

Address _789 Broad Street, Urbana, IL_   Date _4/15/XX_

Rx

Drug name   Form   Dosage

Drug ABC   tabs   350 mg.
#50 ←— Dispense

Sig: 1 tab   QID   prn   pain

1 tablet, 4 times daily as needed for pain

☐ Label

Refill _O_ Times   _Leonard S. Taylor_ , D.D.S.

FIGURE 15.10 Sample prescription blank. (Courtesy Patterson Office Supplies, Champaign, Illinois.)

Analgesic Agents

Analgesic agents are drugs that dull the perception of pain without producing unconsciousness. They may be prescribed to relieve a toothache or to relieve postoperative pain. Patients may be less anxious if they are assured of adequate pain control after their procedure.

Mild analgesic drugs, such as aspirin, ibuprofen, or acetaminophen, are used for the relief of low-intensity pain. These analgesic agents provide adequate pain relief for many types of dental pain, including a toothache or the discomfort that may follow the extraction of a tooth.

Strong analgesic drugs can include a narcotic drug and are only to be prescribed for patients with severe pain, such as that which follows extensive surgical procedures. Examples of narcotic drugs include codeine, oxycodone (Percodan), meperidine (Demerol), morphine, and hydromorphone (Dilaudid). Narcotic drugs are capable of producing physical and psychologic dependence, and their extended use should be avoided.

Prescriptions

A prescription is a written order authorizing the pharmacist to supply a certain drug to a patient. The prescription itself is made up of the components shown in Fig. 15.10. When the dentist prescribes medication, a record of the prescription is recorded in the patient's record.

Under no circumstance may a dental assistant prescribe medication. Medicine is dispensed only with explicit instructions and under the direct supervision of the dentist.

Brand names or **trade names** of a drug are controlled by the business firm as a registered trademark; for example, Tylenol is a brand name of acetaminophen. Brand names are always capitalized.

Generic names are those drug names that any business firm may use. All common and unprotected names fall into this second group. Generic names are not capitalized.

For example, Valium is the brand name of a drug used to treat anxiety. The generic name for Valium is diazepam.

Documentation of Anesthesia and Pain Control

Keeping accurate records is an essential aspect of pain and anxiety analgesia. The following information is documented in the progress notes section of the patient record:
- Preoperative and postoperative vital signs
- Tidal volume if inhalation sedation is provided
- Time anesthesia began and ended
- Peak concentration administered
- Postoperative time (in minutes) for patient recovery
- Adverse events or patient complaints

Ethical Implications

Prescribed drugs come in many forms and are supplied in many applications. The drugs used in dentistry provide a great range in help for patients to feel at ease from anxiety or relief from pain. Drugs can also pose great potential for harming patients. Caution must always be taken when preparing and assisting in the administration of drugs.

A patient of the practice may have a substance abuse problem and may come to your office "under the influence" or may even try to solicit prescriptions from the dentist. Pay special attention to managing the prescription pads, controlled substances, and nitrous oxide in your office.

Procedure 15.1

Applying a Topical Anesthetic Ointment

Equipment and Supplies
- 2 × 2-inch gauze squares
- Topical anesthetic ointment
- Sterile cotton-tip applicator

Procedural Steps

Preparation

1. Place a small amount of topical ointment on the end of the cotton-tip applicator. Replace the cover of the ointment.
   Note: Never insert the same applicator into the ointment after it has been used and contaminated.
2. Explain the procedure to the patient.
   Purpose: Patients are more comfortable and less anxious when they are well informed and know what to expect.
3. Determine the injection site, and gently dry the site with a 2 × 2 gauze square.

Purpose: Drying the site allows the ointment to penetrate the surface area better and not become diluted by saliva, which would decrease its effectiveness.

Placement

1. Place the ointment directly on the injection site.

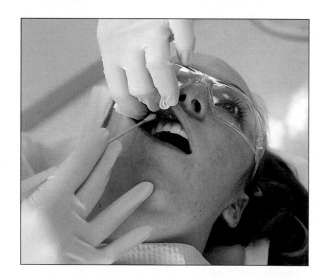

2. Allow the applicator to remain on the site for 3 to 5 minutes.
3. Remove the applicator just before the dentist gives the injection.
   Purpose: The site should not be wet with saliva, which would decrease the effect of the ointment.

Assembling the Local Anesthetic Syringe

Equipment and Supplies

- Sterile syringe
- Sealed disposable needle or needles
- Sterile local anesthetic cartridges
- Needle guard

From Boyd LRB: *Dental instruments: a pocket guide*, ed 7, St. Louis, 2021, Elsevier

Procedural Steps

Selecting the Anesthetic Setup

1. The location of the injection will determine the needle length. The dentist determines the type of anesthetic solution.
   Purpose: The choices of anesthetic solution and needle length depend on the patient's medical and dental history and the procedure.
2. Organize supplies and position the items at chairside out of the patient's view.
3. Wash hands before preparing the syringe.

Loading the Anesthetic Cartridge

1. Hold the syringe in one hand and use the thumb ring to pull back the plunger.

2. With the other hand, load the anesthetic cartridge into the syringe. The stopper end goes in first, toward the plunger.

3. Release the thumb ring and allow the harpoon to engage into the stopper.
4. Use gentle finger pressure to engage the piston forward until the harpoon is engaged into the stopper.

Note: Do not hit the piston with the palm of your hand in an effort to engage the harpoon. This could lead to fracturing of the glass cartridge.

5. To ensure that the harpoon is securely in place, gently pull back on the plunger.
   Purpose: The harpoon must be securely engaged so that the dentist can aspirate during the injection.

Placing the Needle on the Syringe

1. Break the seal on the needle and remove the protective cap from the needle. The protective guard (clear plastic) is removed at this time. The needle guard is not yet removed.

Continued

Assembling the Local Anesthetic Syringe—cont'd

2. Screw the needle into position on the syringe. Take care to position the needle so that it is straight and attached.
Purpose: If the needle is not correctly positioned, then the anesthetic solution may leak or may not flow properly.

3. Place the prepared syringe on the tray ready for use and out of the patient's sight.
Note: Previous teaching suggested that the needle be attached to the syringe before placing the anesthetic cartridge. Stanley Malamed recommends the aforementioned sequence of steps because it virtually eliminates the possibility of a broken cartridge or leakage of anesthetic solution during the procedure.

Photos from Malamed SF: *Handbook of local anesthesia,* ed 6, St. Louis, 2013, Mosby.

Procedure 15.3

Assisting in the Administration of Local Anesthesia

Equipment and Supplies

- Topical anesthetic ointment
- Sterile cotton-tip applicators
- Sterile gauze sponges
- Sterile assembled local anesthetic syringe

Note: This exchange takes place just below the patient's chin and out of the patient's line of vision.

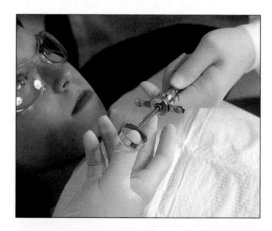

Procedural Steps

1. Apply a topical anesthetic solution to the appropriate area of injection (see Procedure 15.1).
2. Loosen the needle guard.
3. Transfer the syringe to the operator by placing the thumb ring over the dentist's thumb.

4. While the dentist is giving the injection, monitor the patient for any adverse reactions and project a calming and relaxed manner.
5. The dentist will return the contaminated syringe to the tray and will replace the needle guard by using a one-handed scoop technique or a recapping device.
Purpose: This step prevents the possibility of a needle stick injury.

Procedure 15.3

Assisting in the Administration of Local Anesthesia—cont'd

6. After the injection is completed, have the patient turn toward you. Rinse the patient's mouth using the air-water syringe and the high-volume evacuator or saliva ejector.
7. Continue monitoring the patient throughout the procedure for any adverse effects.
8. At the completion of the procedure, instruct the patient about the numbness and not to bite their lip or cheek.
9. Before leaving the dental treatment area, remove the used needle with the needle guard still in place and dispose of it in the sharp's container.
10. Remove the anesthetic cartridge and dispose of it with the medical waste. Place the syringe on the tray to be returned to the sterilization center.
11. Record the type and amount of anesthesia used for the procedure.

(From Boyd LRB: *Dental instruments: a pocket guide,* ed 5, St. Louis, 2015, Saunders.)

■ Procedure 15.4

Assisting in the Administration and Monitoring of Nitrous Oxide–Oxygen Sedation (Expanded Function)

Equipment and Supplies

- Nitrous oxide–oxygen sedation system
- Scavenger-type masks (adult and child sizes)
- Equipment for measuring vital signs

Procedural Steps

1. Check the tanks for an adequate supply of gases. Select and place the appropriate size of mask on the tubing.
2. Seat the patient, update the medical history, and take and record vital signs.
3. Review the use of nitrous oxide with the patient.
   Purpose: Informing the patient before administration helps eliminate fear of the unknown.
4. Place the patient in a supine position.
5. Have the patient position the mask over their nose and adjust the fit.
6. Tighten the tubing once it is comfortable for the patient.

Purpose: Tightening the tubing eliminates the need for the patient to hold the mask in place and to prevent leakage from around the mask.

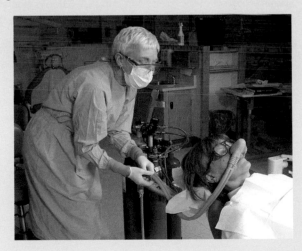

Continued

Assisting in the Administration and Monitoring of Nitrous Oxide–Oxygen Sedation (Expanded Function)—cont'd

7. If the mask pinches or causes discomfort, then place a gauze square under the edge.

Administration

1. At the dentist's instructions, begin adjusting the flow meter for oxygen flow only. The patient is given 100% oxygen for at least 1 minute.
2. At the dentist's direction, adjust the flow of nitrous oxide in increments of 0.5 to 1 liter per minute and reduce the oxygen flow by a corresponding amount.
   Note: Most machines automatically perform this function.
3. At 1-minute intervals, the previous step is repeated until the dentist determines that the patient has reached the baseline reading.
   Purpose: This slow process minimizes the risk for administering too much nitrous oxide.
4. Note the patient's baseline level.
5. Closely monitor the patient throughout the procedure.

Oxygenation

1. Toward the end of the procedure, nitrous oxide is depleted and 100% oxygen is administered, as directed by the dentist.
   Purpose: Oxygenation of patients for a minimum of 5 minutes helps prevent diffusion hypoxia, which creates a feeling of lightheadedness.

2. After the oxygenation is complete, remove the mask. Slowly position the patient upright.
   Purpose: Bringing the patient upright too quickly may cause postural hypotension (fainting).

3. Record the patient's baseline levels of nitrous oxide and oxygen and his or her response during analgesia.
   Purpose: This documentation provides a legal record of care and serves as a reference for future care and the administration of nitrous oxide–oxygen sedation (analgesia).

Photos from Malamed SF: *Sedation: a guide to patient management,* ed 5, St Louis, 2009, Mosby.

Chapter Exercises

Multiple Choice

Circle the letter next to the correct answer.

1. _____ is a medical condition in which the dentist should be alerted when selecting an anesthetic with a vasoconstrictor.
   a. Arthritis
   b. Paralysis
   c. Liver disease
   d. Migraine headaches

2. Oxygen and nitrous oxide gases are supplied in steel cylinders. The color coding for the nitrous oxide tanks is _____.
   a. yellow
   b. blue
   c. green
   d. red

3. Anesthetic cartridges should be _____.
   a. maintained in the refrigerator until their use
   b. sterilized before use
   c. maintained in their packaging
   d. disinfected before use

4. A vasoconstrictor is a drug that has been added to local anesthetic agents to cause the blood vessels to _____.
   a. expand
   b. constrict
   c. bleed
   d. dissolve

5. _____ anesthesia is achieved by the dentist injecting the anesthetic solution into the nerve trunk.
   a. Block
   b. Infiltration
   c. Topical
   d. Analgesia

6. A _____-inch needle is selected when administering infiltration injection of a local anesthetic.
   a. 1
   b. 1 5/8
   c. 2
   d. 2 5/8

7. Topical anesthetics should remain on the oral mucosa for _____.
   a. 30 seconds
   b. 1 minute
   c. 2 to 5 minutes
   d. 7 to 10 minutes

8. _____ is the most commonly used form of topical anesthetic for a local anesthesia procedure.
   a. Patch
   b. Liquid
   c. Ointment
   d. Spray

9. After a procedure, the contaminated needle is discarded in the _____.
   a. sharps container
   b. sterilization center
   c. treatment room
   d. garbage

10. Before applying topical anesthetic ointment, _____.
    a. gently dry the tissue
    b. thoroughly rinse the area
    c. blow air on the site from the air-water syringe
    d. tightly pull the mucosa

Apply Your Knowledge

1. You are assisting in a restorative procedure for teeth #2, #3, and #5. As you prepare the local anesthetic setup, what should be retrieved for the setup? Remember the type of injection and how many teeth will be involved.

2. The dentist has just completed administering the injection, and he transfers a contaminated uncapped syringe back to you over the patient's chest. Will you receive the syringe? If not, what will you do?

3. A patient is receiving nitrous oxide–oxygen sedation analgesia during a procedure. The patient has no indication in the record about any adverse effects, but your patient seems anxious and fidgety. What is your sense of the situation, and how do you handle this situation?

CHAPTER 16

Principles and Concepts of Radiation

http://evolve.elsevier.com/Robinson/essentials/

LEARNING OBJECTIVES

1. Pronounce, define, and spell the key terms.
2. Explain the benefits of dental radiography and its uses in dentistry.
3. Define x-rays and the anatomic structure of matter, and describe ionization.
4. Describe the properties of x-ray beams.
5. Differentiate among the types of radiation.
6. Identify the components of the dental x-ray machine.
7. Explain how x-rays are produced
8. Define radiopaque and radiolucent.
9. List and describe the four factors that affect the quality of a radiograph.
10. Complete the following related to radiation hazards and protection:
    • Define maximum permissible dose.
    • Explain the ALARA principle.
11. Discuss the biologic effects of radiation, including the differences between somatic and genetic effects of x-rays.
12. Discuss the methods used to protect patients from radiation.
13. Discuss the methods used to protect the operator from radiation.

KEY TERMS

absorbed dose
acute radiation exposure
ALARA principle
anode
background radiation
cathode
cervical collar
chronic radiation exposure
collimation
collimator
contrast
control panel
cumulative effects

density
digital imaging
dose equivalence
filter
filtration
focusing cup
F-speed film
genetic changes
ionization
latent period
leakage radiation
maximum permissible dose (MPD)

object-film distance (OFD)
photon
position indicator device (PID)
primary radiation
radiation monitoring
radiolucent
radiopaque
scatter radiation
secondary radiation
somatic changes
source-film distance
tubehead

Dental images, commonly known as *x-ray images*, are essential in the practice of dentistry and are produced using either a conventional x-ray film or with digital imaging. Regardless of the method used, a quality image is necessary to identify and diagnose dental conditions that otherwise may go undetected.

The benefits of using x-ray images in dentistry certainly outweigh the risks when proper safety procedures are followed. Nevertheless, as essential as radiology is to dentistry, it is imperative that operators and patients be informed that exposure to radiation has the ability to cause damage to living tissue.

This chapter discusses the production of x-ray images, and the methods used to protect the patient and operator from the harmful effects of exposure to radiation.

Radiation Physics

All things in the world are composed of energy and matter. Energy is defined as the ability to do work. Although energy cannot be created or destroyed, it can change form. Atoms are the basic form of *matter,* and they contain energy. Matter is anything that occupies space and has form or shape.

Atomic Structure

Understanding the basic anatomic structure of matter is important because it relates to the ways in which x-ray beams are produced, emitted (given off) from the machine, and absorbed by the body tissue of both patient and the operator.

All matter is made of atoms. Atoms are extremely minute and consist of (1) an inner core, or *nucleus,* that consists of positively charged particles called *protons* and particles called *neutrons* that have no charge and (2) negatively charged particles called *electrons* that orbit around the nucleus (Fig. 16.1). In the neutral or stable atom, the number of orbiting electrons (–) equals the number of protons (+) in the nucleus; therefore the atom is electrically neutral.

Ionization

Ionization is one of the principal ways that radiation transfers its energy to matter. Ionization occurs when an x-ray beam strikes the patient's tissue. It is the process that changes the electrical balance within an atom by either gaining or losing an electron to form a charged ion. Ions are atoms that gain or lose an electron and become electrically unbalanced. X-rays have enough energy to produce ions.

During the process of ionization, electrons remain stable in their orbit around the nucleus until radiograph photons collide with them. A **photon** is a minute bundle of pure energy that has no weight or mass.

Properties of X-Ray Beams

An x-ray is a type of radiation that has a shorter wavelength with a high frequency capable of penetrating bone and soft tissue within the body, creating an image on a film. X-ray beams are a form of energy that can penetrate matter and have unique characteristics.

Similar to visible light, radar, radio, and television waves, x-ray beams belong to a group called *electromagnetic radiation* (Fig. 16.2). Electromagnetic radiation is made of photons that travel through space at the speed of light in a straight line with a wavelike motion.

The shorter the wavelength of radiation, the greater its energy (Fig. 16.3). Because of the high energy of short wavelengths, they

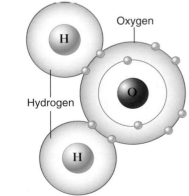

FIGURE 16.1 Diagrammatic representation of an oxygen atom. (**B**, From Patton KT, Thibodeau GA: *Anatomy and physiology,* ed 9, St Louis, 2016, Mosby.)

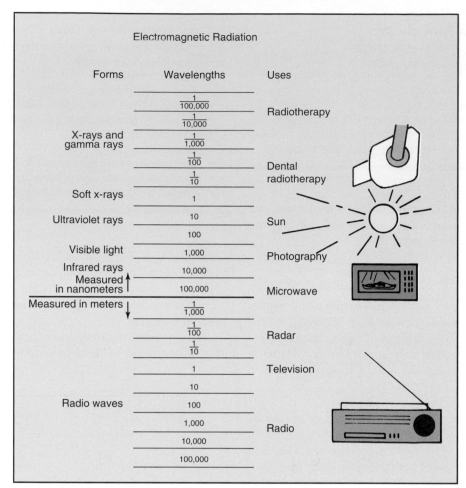

FIGURE 16.2 Electromagnetic spectrum, showing the various wavelengths of radiation typically used.

are able to penetrate matter more easily than longer wavelengths. The unique properties of x-ray beams make them especially valuable in dentistry.

Dental X-Ray Machine

Dental X-ray machines can vary in size and appearance, but all have three primary components: the tubehead, an extension arm, and the control panel.

Tubehead

The primary function of the tubehead is to house the dental x-ray tube (Fig. 16.4). The tubehead is made of metal and has a protective lead lining to prevent radiation from escaping.

The Dental X-Ray Tube

The dental x-ray tube is made of glass and is approximately 6 inches long and 1½ inches in diameter. The air has been removed from the tube to create a vacuum. This vacuum environment allows electrons to flow with minimal resistance between the electrodes (cathode and anode; Fig. 16.5).

Cathode

The **cathode** (−) is a tungsten filament. Tungsten is a metal capable of withstanding the intense heat given off during the

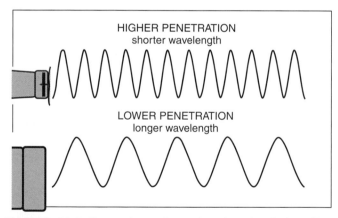

FIGURE 16.3 Comparison of wavelengths of radiation. (From Hagen-Ansert SL: *Textbook of diagnostic sonography*, ed 7, St Louis, 2012, Mosby.)

generation of x-ray beams. Electrons are generated in the x-ray tube at the cathode. The hotter the filament becomes, the more electrons are produced.

The **focusing cup**, which is a part of the cathode, keeps the electrons suspended in a cloud at the cathode. When the exposure button is pressed, the circuit within the tubehead is completed, and the electrons very rapidly cross from the cathode (−) to strike the anode (+). This process occurs because positive and negative attract each other.

FIGURE 16.4 Dental x-ray tubehead. (From White SC, Pharoah MJ: *Oral radiology: principles and interpretation*, ed 7, St Louis, 2014, Mosby.)

FIGURE 16.5 X-ray tube with the major components labeled. (From White SC, Pharoah MJ: *Oral radiology: principles and interpretation*, ed 7, St Louis, 2014, Mosby.)

Anode

The **anode** (+) acts as the target for the electrons. It consists of a **tungsten target** (a small block of tungsten) that is embedded in the larger copper stem. The copper around the target conducts the heat away from the target, thus reducing wear and tear on the target.

The oil in the x-ray tube absorbs approximately 99% of the energy generated by this process, and this energy is given off as heat. The remaining 1% exits the tubehead as x-ray beams through the window (opening) as a divergent beam toward the patient. The center portion of this x-ray beam is known as the *central ray* or *primary beam*.

Collimator

The collimator, similar to the filter, is a metal disc, usually lead; it has a small opening in the center to control the size and shape of the x-ray beam as it leaves the tubehead (Fig. 16.6A).

Filter

The filter is an aluminum disc located at the port of the tubehead where the position indicator device (PID) is connected (see Fig. 16.6B). The filter removes low-energy, long-wavelength x-ray beams, which may be absorbed by the patient but are not necessary for producing the radiograph.

Position Indicator Device

The PID is an open-ended, lead-lined cylinder that is placed against the patient's face during film exposure to aim the x-ray beam at the film in the patient's mouth (Fig. 16.7). The PID may be rectangular or cylindrical.

FIGURE 16.6 **A,** Collimator. **B,** Filter.

FIGURE 16.7 Rectangular position indicator device (PID). (Courtesy Margraf Dental Manufacturing, Inc. Jenkintown, PA, http://www.margafdental.com.)

Extension Arm

The extension arm encloses the wires between the tubehead and the control panel. It also plays an important role in positioning the tubehead.

The tubehead is attached to the extension arm by means of a yoke that can be horizontally turned 360 degrees. (**Horizontally** means to move in a side-to-side motion; **vertically** means to move in an up-and-down direction.) This design permits maximum flexibility in positioning the tubehead.

If the tubehead drifts, then the arm should be immediately repaired. The patient or the operator must never hold the tubehead in place during exposure.

Control Panel

The **control panel** of an x-ray unit is located on a wall outside the x-ray area to prevent radiation exposure to the operator while the film is exposed (Fig. 16.8). It contains the *master switch,* an *indicator light, selector buttons,* an *exposure timer,* and a selector button, which controls the exposure time, mA, and kV selector.

Master Switch and Indicator Lights

The master switch turns the machine on and off. An orange indicator light shows when the master switch is on. The x-ray machine may be safely left on all day; it does not produce radiation unless the electronic timer is being pushed.

The red emission indicator light comes on only when the electronic timer is being pushed and radiation is being emitted.

FIGURE 16.8 X-ray unit. (Courtesy Instrumentarium Dental Inc., Milwaukee, Wisconsin)

Exposure Button

The exposure button controls the flow of electricity to generate the x-rays. The button is electronically controlled to provide precise exposure time, and x-rays are generated *only* while the exposure timer is pressed. The exposure time is measured in fractions of a second called *impulses* (60 impulses = 1 second: 30 impulses = 0.5 second).

Milliamperage Selector

The mA selector controls the number of electrons produced. Increasing the mA increases the quantity of electrons available for the production of x-ray beams.

Kilovoltage Selector

The kilovoltage peak (kVp) selector is used to control the penetrating power or the beam. Dental x-ray machines generally operate at 70 or 90 kVp.

X-Ray Production

When the x-ray machine is turned on, the electrical current enters the control panel, and the following events occur in an instant (Fig. 16.9):

- Pushing the exposure button activates the high-voltage circuit. The electrons in the cloud are shot across the x-ray tube to the anode. The molybdenum cup in the cathode directs the electrons to the tungsten target in the anode.
- The electrons speed from the cathode to the anode. When the electrons strike the tungsten target, their energy of motion *(kinetic energy)* creates x-rays and heat. Less than 1% of the energy is converted to x-rays, with 99% lost as heat.
- The heat is carried away from the copper stem and is absorbed by the insulating oil in the tubehead.

FIGURE 16.9 The production of dental images. (From Langlais RP, Miller CS: *Exercises in oral radiology and interpretation*, ed 5, St Louis, 2017, Elsevier.)

- The x-rays travel through the unleaded glass window of the tube, the tubehead seal, and the aluminum filter. The aluminum filter removes the longer-wavelength x-rays from the beam.
- The x-ray beam then travels through the collimator, where its size is restricted; it travels down the PID and exits at the opening.

Types of Radiation

Primary radiation, also known as the central ray or primary beam, is the stream of radiation emitted from the x-ray unit. The primary beam travels in a straight line, producing diagnostically useful radiographs (Fig. 16.10A).

Secondary radiation in dentistry is given off after the primary beam comes into contact with matter, such as the soft tissue of the head, the bones of the skull, and the teeth. Secondary radiation is less penetrating than primary radiation because the rays become weaker after they contact the tissue; however, the patient still may absorb these rays (see Fig. 16.10B).

Scatter radiation is a form of secondary radiation that occurs when an x-ray beam is deflected from its path during impact with the patient. (*Deflected* means turned aside.) Scatter radiation travels in all directions and is impossible to confine. Without adequate protective barriers, the operator and others nearby may be affected by exposure to scatter radiation (see Fig. 16.10C).

Characteristics of X-Ray Beam

There are three characteristics of the x-ray beam. They are described as the *quality, quantity,* and *intensity* of the x-ray beam. These characteristics determine the *contrast, density,* and *image detail*—the qualities necessary for a good image (Table 16.1).

Quality

In dental radiography, the term *quality* is used to describe the energy or penetrating ability of the x-ray beam. The quality or

FIGURE 16.10 Types of radiation interaction. **A**, Primary. **B**, Secondary. **C**. Scatter.

—	A. Primary beam
- - -	B. Secondary
– –	C. Scatter

TABLE 16.1
Visual Characteristics and Influencing Factors

Visual Characteristics	Influencing Factors	Effect of Influencing Factors
Density	mA	↑ mA = ↑ density &↓ mA = ↓ density
	kVp	↑ kVp = ↑ density &↓ kVp = ↓ density
	Time	↑ time = ↑ density &↓ time = ↓ density
	Subject thickness	↑ thickness = ↓ density &↓ thickness = ↑ density
Contrast	kVp	↑ kVp = long-scale contrast; low contrast &↓ kVp = short-scale contrast; high contrast

mA, Milliamperage; *kVp*, kilovoltage peak.

wavelength and energy of the x-ray beam is controlled by kV. A higher kV is used when the area to be exposed is dense or thick. Density is the overall blackness or darkness of a radiograph. A radiograph with the correct density helps the dentist to view black areas (air space), white areas (enamel, dentin, and bone), and gray areas (soft tissue).

Quantity

Quantity of the x-ray beam refers to the number of x-rays produced in the dental x-ray unit. The A is the unit of measurement used to describe the number of electrons or current flowing through the cathode filament. Because the number of amperes needed to operate a dental x-ray unit is small, amperage is measured in milliamperes (mA). One mA is equal to 1/1000 of an A. In dental radiography, the use of 7 to 15 mA is required.

FIGURE 16.11 Bite-wing radiograph shows radiopaque (white *a*) area of amalgam restoration and radiolucent (black *b*) areas of air and cheek tissue.

Intensity

Intensity is the combination of the number of x-ray photons (quantity) and the energy of each photon (quality). The intensity of the x-ray beam is affected by a number of factors, including the kVp, mA, exposure time, and distance.

Characteristics of Images

There are specific characteristics that affect the image detail.

Contrast

The image on a radiograph appears in a range of shades from black to white with multiple shades of gray. This range is referred to as the *gray scale*. The range of shades of gray to black to white is called *contrast*.

Images that appear on radiographs are referred to as being **radiolucent** or **radiopaque** (Fig. 16.11). Radiolucent structures appear dark or black on the radiograph. Air spaces, soft tissues of the body, and dental pulp appear as radiolucent images. Radiopaque structures appear white or light gray on the radiograph. Metal, enamel, and dense areas of bone appear as radiopaque images.

The ideal contrast of a film clearly shows the radiopaque white of a metal restoration, the radiolucent black of air, and the many shades of gray between these extremes. *Higher* kV produces more penetrating radiographs and *lower* radiographic contrast, as follows:

- A 90-kVp setting requires less exposure time and produces an image that has low contrast (more shades of gray).
- A 70-kVp setting requires a slightly longer exposure time and produces an image with high contrast (fewer shades of gray).

Density

Density is the overall blackness or darkness of a film. An image with the correct density enables the dentist to view black areas (air spaces), white areas (enamel, dentin, and bone), and gray areas (soft tissues). The degree of density is controlled by the *milliampere seconds (mAs)*.

Other factors that influence the density of an image include the following:

- Amount of radiation reaching the film
- Distance from the x-ray tube to the patient (length of PID)
- Processing of dental film if using conventional film
- Patient's body size

Image Detail

Three characteristics that affect the detail of the image include: sharpness, magnification, and distortion.

Sharpness refers to how well an image reproduces the fine details or distinct outlines of an object. Sharpness is sometimes referred to as *detail, resolution,* or *definition,* as is seen on a high-definition television. The sharpness of an image is influenced by the following factors: focal spot size, film composition, and movement. *Magnification* refers to the proportionate enlargement of a dental image. *Distortion* refers to the disproportionate change in the size of image. Elongation and foreshortening of images can produce distortion. For more information, see Chapter 17.

Radiation Effects

All ionizing radiation is harmful and produces biologic changes in living tissues. Although the amount of x-radiation used in dental imaging is small, biologic changes do occur. Thus the dental assistant must know how the harmful effects of radiation occur and how to discuss radiation risks with patients. The entire x-ray area is considered a radiation hazard area, and a radiation hazard area sign must be posted in sight of all personnel and patients (Fig. 16.12).

Tissue Damage

In dental radiography, not all x-rays pass through the patient and reach the dental film; the patient's tissues absorb some x-rays. When the energy from the x-ray photon is absorbed, chemical changes result in biologic damage.

Biologic Effects

Exposure to radiation can bring about changes in body chemicals, cells, tissues, and organs (Table 16.2). The effects of radiation may not become evident for many years after the time the x-rays were absorbed. This lag time is called the **latent period.**

Ionization

Ionization results in the harmful effects of x-rays in humans. Ionization can cause disruption of cellular metabolism and permanent damage to living cells and tissues. The atoms that lose

FIGURE 16.12 Comparison of somatic and genetic effects of radiation. (Courtesy Elsevier Collection.)

electrons become positive ions; as such, they are unstable structures capable of interacting with and damaging other atoms, tissues, or chemicals.

Cumulative Effects

Exposure to radiation has a cumulative effect over a lifetime. This means that when tissues are exposed to x-rays, some damage occurs. Although tissues can repair some damage, the tissues do not return to their original state.

Acute and Chronic Radiation Exposure

Acute radiation exposure occurs when a large dose of radiation is absorbed in a short period, such as in a nuclear accident. *Chronic radiation exposure* occurs when small amounts of radiation are absorbed repeatedly over a long period.

TABLE 16.2
Equivalent Traditional and SI Units of Radiation Measurement

Quantity	SI Units	Traditional Units	Conversion
Exposure	Coulombs per kilogram (C/kg)	Roentgen (R)	1 C/kg = 3380 R
Dose	Gray (Gy)	Rad	1 Gy = 100 rad
Dose equivalence	Sievert (Sv)	Rem	1 Sv = 100 rem

SI, Système Internationale d'Unités.

From Miles DA, Van Dis ML, Williamson GF, et al: *Radiographic imaging for the dental team,* ed 4, St Louis, 2009, Saunders.

Genetic and Somatic Effects

X-rays affect both genetic and somatic cells. *Genetic* cells are the reproductive cells (sperm and ova). Damage to genetic cells is passed on to succeeding generations. These changes from **genetic effects** are referred to as *genetic mutations*. All other cells in the body belong to the group of *somatic* tissues (*somatic* refers to the body) and are not passed on to future generations.

Critical Organs

Although the risk associated with dental x-rays is minimal, some tissues and organs are exposed to more radiation. The following organs are more sensitive to radiation and thus are called *critical organs*: skin, thyroid glands, lens of the eye, and bone marrow.

Radiation Measurement

Radiation can be measured in a manner similar to time, distance, and weight. Just as distance can be measured in miles or kilometers and time can be measured in hours or minutes, two sets of systems are used to define the ways in which radiation is measured. The older system is referred to as the *traditional,* or *standard* system. The newer system is the metric equivalent known as the Système Internationale d'Unités (SI).

The traditional units of radiation measurement include (1) the *roentgen* (R), (2) the *radiation absorbed dose* (rad), and (3) the *roentgen equivalent in* [hu]*man* (rem). SI units include (1) *coulombs* per kilogram (C/kg), (2) the *gray* (Gy), and (3) the *sievert* (Sv). Both systems are presented in Table 16.3.

TABLE 16.3
Relative Radiation Sensitivity of Cells and Tissues

Sensitivity to Radiation	Cell Type or Tissue
High	Small lymphocyte
	Bone marrow
	Reproductive cells
	Intestinal mucosa
Fairly high	Skin
	Lens of the eye
	Oral mucosa
Medium	Connective tissue
	Small blood vessels
	Growing bone and cartilage
Fairly low	Mature bone and cartilage
	Salivary gland
	Thyroid gland
	Kidney
	Liver
Low	Muscle
	Nerve

Modified from Miles DA, Van Dis ML, Williamson GF, Jensen CW: *Radiographic imaging for the dental team,* ed 4, St. Louis, 2009, Saunders.

Two important concepts are basic to radiation protection. The first is the concept of maximum permissible dose (MPD), and the second is the ALARA principle.

Maximum Permissible Dose

The **MPD** is defined by the National Council on Radiation Protection and Measurements (NCRP) as the maximum dose equivalent that a body is permitted to receive in a specified period of time. The MPD is the dose of radiation that the body can endure with little or no injury.

The NCRP publishes recommendations specifying dose limits for exposure to ionizing radiation. The most recent report states that the current MPD for persons occupationally exposed to radiation is 5000 millirem (mrem), or 5.0 rems/year (0.05 Sv/year). For non–occupationally exposed persons, the current MPD is 0.1 rem/year (0.001 Sv/year).

Dental personnel should strive for an occupational dose of *zero* by adhering to strict radiation protection practices. Zero exposure is not difficult to achieve when radiation safety precautions are taken.

The ALARA principle or concept states that all exposure to radiation must be kept As Low As Reasonably Achievable. Every possible method of reducing exposure to radiation should be used. The radiation protection measures can be used to minimize exposure to both the patient and the operator.

Radiation Safety

We are exposed to radiation every day of our lives. **Background radiation** comes from natural sources, such as radioactive materials in the ground and cosmic radiation from space. Exposure from medical or dental sources is an additional risk. Because of their concern, patients frequently ask, "I've heard x-rays are bad for me. Do you really have to take them?" The dental assistant must anticipate this patient reaction and be able to explain to the patient the risks and diagnostic benefits of dental radiation, the safety precautions used during radiographic exposure, and the benefits of detecting disease that might not otherwise be detected, all of which far outweigh the risks from receiving small doses of radiation.

Protective Devices

Measures that provide protection include the use of properly operating radiographic equipment. The x-ray tubehead must be equipped with appropriate aluminum filters, lead collimators, and PIDs. Equipment should be checked on a regular basis by state or federal regulations.

Proper Equipment

Another factor limiting the amount of radiation the patient receives is the use of proper equipment. The dental x-ray **tubehead** must be equipped with the appropriate aluminum **filter**, lead collimator, and position indicator device. The other components of the dental x-ray unit and tubehead are discussed in detail in Chapter 17.

Aluminum Filtration

The purpose of the aluminum filter is to filter out longer-wavelength, low-energy x-rays from the x-ray beam (Fig. 16.13).

FIGURE 16.13 Aluminum discs are placed in the path of the x-ray beam to filter out low-energy long wavelengths, which are harmful to the patient. (From Iannucci JM, Jansen Howerton L: *Dental radiography: principles and techniques*, ed 4, St. Louis, 2012, Saunders.)

Low-energy, longer-wavelength x-rays are harmful to the patient and are not useful in producing a diagnostic image. **Filtration** of the x-ray beam results in higher energy and a more penetrating, useful beam.

Collimation

The **collimation** is used to restrict the size and shape of the x-ray beam and to reduce patient exposure. The **collimator** is a lead plate with a hole in the center. It is placed directly over the opening in the machine housing where the x-ray beam exits the tubehead. The collimator may have a round or a rectangular opening. The rectangular collimator restricts the size of the x-ray beam to slightly larger than No. 2 intraoral film. (Film size is discussed in Chapter 17.) The round collimator produces a beam that is 2¾ inches in diameter—considerably larger than No. 2 intraoral film. When the shape and size of the beam are changed to a rectangle, the amount of tissue exposed can be reduced by more than one half (Fig. 16.14).

Position Indicator Device

The **PID** is used to aim the x-ray beam at the film in the patient's mouth, thereby minimizing the amount of radiation to the patient's face. PIDs used in dentistry are usually 8, 12, or 16 inches long. The radiographic technique being used determines the length selected (see Chapter 17). To minimize patient exposure, the long PID is preferred because less divergence (spread) of the x-ray beam occurs. Faulty or malfunctioning equipment should be repaired immediately.

☐ Area exposed to radiation using a circular collimator

■ Area exposed to radiation using a rectangular collimator

FIGURE 16.14 Collimation of tubehead to film size.

Patient Protection

Lead Aprons and Thyroid Collars

The thyroid gland is susceptible to radiation during dental x-ray procedures. The function of lead aprons and thyroid collars is to reduce radiation exposure to the gonads and thyroid gland. A lead apron and thyroid collar must be used on all patients for all exposures (Fig. 16.15). This rule applies to all patients, regardless of the patient's age or sex or the number of films to be taken. The lead apron should cover the patient from the thyroid and extend over the lap area.

The thyroid collar, also known as a **cervical collar**, covers the thyroid gland during the exposure and reduces radiation exposure to the gland. Most thyroid collars are part of the lead apron; however, they are also available as separate items.

The lead apron and the thyroid collar should be hung up or laid over a rounded bar rather than folded when not in use. (Folding eventually cracks the lead and allows radiation leakage.)

Prescribing Radiographs

The dentist is responsible for prescribing dental radiographs for every patient based on their individual needs. To limit the amount of radiation a patient receives, the dentist must use professional judgment about the number, type, and frequency of dental radiographs. Table 16.4 provides examples for prescribing radiographs.

Pregnancy

The manual *Guidelines for Prescribing Dental Radiographs,* issued by the American Dental Association (ADA) and the

FIGURE 16.15 *1.* Lead apron. *2.* Lead apron with thyroid collar, *3.* Lead apron poncho for front and back protection. (From Boyd LR: *Dental instruments: a pocket guide*, ed 7, St Louis, 2021, Elsevier.)

TABLE 16.4

Examples of Selection Criteria for Prescribing Radiographs

Type of Patient	Child (Mixed Dentition)	Adult
New patient	Individualized examination consisting of panoramic examination with posterior bitewings or posterior bitewings with selected periapical views	Individualized examination consisting of posterior bitewings and selected periapicals; a full mouth survey is appropriate when patient presents with clinical evidence of generalized dental disease or a history of extensive dental treatment
Recall patient with no clinical caries and low risk factors for caries	Posterior bitewing examination at 12- to 24-month intervals	Posterior bitewing examination at 24- to 36-month intervals
Recall patient with clinical caries and high risk factors for caries	Posterior bitewing examination at 6-month intervals until no carious lesions are evident	Posterior bitewing examination at 12- to 18-month intervals

From Miles DA, Van Dis ML, Williamson GF, et al: *Radiographic imaging for the dental team,* ed 4, St Louis, 2009, Saunders.

U.S. Food and Drug Administration (FDA), states that dental radiographic procedures "do not need to be altered because of pregnancy." When a lead apron is used during dental imaging procedures, the amount of radiation received in the pelvic region is nearly zero. The embryo or fetus receives no detectable exposure with the use of a lead apron.

Although scientific evidence indicates that dental x-ray procedures can be performed during pregnancy, many dentists and pregnant patients prefer to postpone such x-ray procedures because of patient concerns, especially within the first trimester of pregnancy.

Pediatric Patients

If the patient is a child who is unable to cooperate, the child is seated on the parent's lap in the dental chair. Both the parent and child are covered with the lead apron, and the parent holds the film in place. If the patient is an adult with disabilities, ask the caregiver to hold the film in place, and give the caretaker a lead apron to wear. Having the parent or caregiver hold the film is acceptable because this is a single exposure for that individual. If a dental assistant were to hold the film in this manner, they would have repeated exposures and would suffer the **cumulative effects** of radiation.

Fast-Speed Film

When using the conventional film-based technique, fast-speed film is the single most effective method of reducing a patient's exposure to x-ray beams. The faster the film speed, the less radiation is necessary for each exposure.

The film speed is determined by the amount of x-radiation needed to produce a high-quality radiograph. Film speed is rated in a range from A to F. Currently, **F-speed film**, or InSight, is the fastest intraoral film available. The film speed is determined by the size of the crystals in the emulsion that coats the film. Larger crystals (F speed) are more sensitive to radiation and need less radiation. Film sizes and types of radiographs are discussed further in Chapter 17.

Digital Imaging

Digital imaging requires **significantly less x-radiation** than conventional film-based radiography because the sensor used to capture the image is more sensitive to x-ray beams than in conventional film. Exposure times for digital images are 70% to 80% less than those required with conventional film. It is no longer a matter of *if* but rather *when* most dental practices will transition to digital imaging. Digital radiography is discussed in greater detail in Chapter 17.

Proper Film Exposure Technique

Unnecessary radiation exposure to patients is caused by the need for retakes. Every time a film must be retaken because of an error in operator exposure technique or a processing error, the patient is exposed to double the amount of radiation. (Exposure techniques are discussed in Chapter 17.)

Film-Holding Instruments

Patients are sometimes asked to use their finger to hold the film in their mouth. This technique is not acceptable because the patient's hands and fingers are exposed to radiation.

A variety of film-holding instruments can be used to keep the patient's hand and fingers from being exposed to the x-ray beams. Film holders also hold the film in a stable position and aid the operator in properly positioning the film in the PID. (The technique for using film holders is discussed in Chapter 17.)

Operator Protection and Monitoring

The dental assistant must use proper operator protection measures to avoid occupational exposure to radiation, including primary radiation, leakage radiation, and scatter radiation. The assistant must carefully follow the safety guidelines and use radiation monitoring devices.

Radiation Monitoring

Radiation monitors can be worn by the operator or placed on x-ray equipment or on walls. **Radiation monitoring** protects the operator by identifying occupational exposure to radiation.

Personnel Monitoring

A film badge (pocket dosimeter) is used to measure the amount of occupational exposure. The badge contains a film packet, similar to dental film, embossed with the wearer's name and identification number (Fig. 16.16).

Employees are provided their own individual badge to be worn at all times while at work. Film badges should not be worn outside of the office, especially in bright sunlight. Film badges must be removed when the person being monitored is having medical or dental x-ray images taken because the badge is intended to measure only occupational exposure.

Equipment Monitoring

Dental x-ray machines should be monitored for leakage radiation. (Leakage radiation is any radiation, with the exception of the primary beam, that is emitted from the dental tubehead.) Dental x-ray equipment can be monitored through the use of a film device that can be obtained from the manufacturer or from the state health department.

FIGURE 16.16 A film badge is used to monitor the amount of radiation that reaches the dental radiographer. (Courtesy Global Dosimetry Solutions, Irvine, California.)

Rules of Operator Protection

An assistant who fails to follow the rules of radiation protection may suffer the results of chronic radiation exposure. By following the rules of radiation protection, dental personnel can keep their radiation exposure at zero.

> **Rules of Radiation Protection**
> - Never stand in the direct line of the primary beam.
> - Always stand behind a lead barrier or a proper thickness of drywall. If a lead barrier is not available, stand at right angles to the beam.
> - Never stand closer than 6 feet from the x-ray unit during an exposure unless you are behind a barrier.

Documentation

Exposure of dental radiographs must always be documented in the patient's dental record, which should include the following information:

- Informed consent
- Number and type of radiographs exposed
- Rationale for exposing such radiographs
- Diagnostic information obtained from the radiograph

> **Ethical Implications**
>
> Following all radiation safety procedures and being aware of the legal implications involved in taking dental radiographs are the ethical and legal responsibilities of the dental assistant. Federal and state regulations control the use of dental x-ray equipment. For example, the Consumer-Patient Radiation Health and Safety Act is a federal law that establishes guidelines for the proper maintenance of x-ray equipment and requires persons taking dental radiographs to be professionally trained and certified. Some state regulations require dental offices, clinics, and dental schools to be inspected every 1 to 3 years to check the safety of the x-ray equipment.
>
> As a dental assistant, being informed about the specific radiation safety requirements in your state is your responsibility.

Chapter Exercises

Multiple Choice

Circle the letter next to the correct answer.

1. The ALARA goal can be achieved by _____.
   a. well-trained and competent operators
   b. using fast-speed film
   c. placing lead aprons on all patients
   d. all of the above

2. The fastest film speed used in dentistry is _____.
   a. C   c. E
   b. D   d. F

3. Dental film badges are used to record _____.
   a. the radiation received by the operator
   b. the radiation received by the patient
   c. the number of films taken
   d. all of the above

4. Dental personnel should strive for _____ exposure to radiation.
   a. zero
   b. the maximum possible dose
   c. 0.05 rem
   d. 0.01 Sv

5. The process in which cells are altered by exposure to radiation is _____.
   a. electromagnetic force
   b. ionization
   c. matter
   d. photon

6. Which of the following has an influence on radiation safety?
   a. Safe equipment
   b. Skilled operator
   c. Lead apron and thyroid collars
   d. All of the above

7. Dental radiographs are used to _____.
   a. detect dental decay in the early stages
   b. detect bone loss in the early stages
   c. evaluate growth and development
   d. accomplish all of the above

8. Which of the following are characteristics of x-ray beams? They are _____.
   a. invisible
   b. weightless
   c. travel in straight lines
   d. all of the above

9. Which of the following affects the density of a radiograph?
   a. Amount of radiation reaching the film
   b. Distance from the x-ray tube to the patient
   c. Size of the patient's body
   d. All of the above

10. The results of radiation that are passed on to future generations are called _____ effects.
    a. somatic
    b. genetic
    c. acute
    d. cumulative

11. The term for images that appear dark or black on radiographs is _____.
    a. radiopaque
    b. radiolucent

12. Filters in dental x-ray units are made from _____.
    a. lead
    b. aluminum
    c. steel
    d. tungsten

13. The purpose of a collimator is to _____.
    a. remove long wavelengths of radiation
    b. remove short wavelengths of radiation
    c. restrict the diameter of the beam
    d. enlarge the diameter of the beam

14. The purpose of the filters in dental x-ray machines is to _____.
    a. remove long wavelengths of radiation
    b. remove short wavelengths of radiation
    c. restrict the diameter of the beam
    d. enlarge the diameter of the beam

15. The purpose of the PID is to _____.
    a. aim the x-ray beam at the film
    b. generate x-rays
    c. minimize the amount of radiation
    d. accomplish all of the above

Apply Your Knowledge

1. Mr. Lopez indicates a reluctance to have the prescribed dental radiographs be taken. On careful questioning, you determine that his reluctance is because of his lack of understanding about the effects of radiation. How would you manage this situation?

2. Your dentist employer has given you the responsibility of selecting a new dental x-ray unit for your office. One of the choices you must make is the type of collimator in the new machine. What things would you consider? Why?

3. Mrs. Collins brings her 3-year-old son, Dennis, into your dental office to be seen on an emergency basis. He fell and cracked his front tooth, and the dentist asks you to take an x-ray image. Dennis is too small to sit in the chair himself and is unable to hold the film holder in his mouth. How would you take the prescribed radiograph?

4. Your mother has stated that she is concerned about your safety because you work around x-ray machines on a daily basis. What would you tell her?

5. As a child, you probably played "shadow casting" using sunlight or a flashlight. Try this experiment using a flashlight and a wall. Shine the light on the wall, and place one hand between the light beam and the wall. If you move your hand closer to the wall and away from the light source, the shadow is close to the actual size of your hand. If you move your hand away from the wall and nearer to the light source, the image of your hand is magnified (larger) but is distorted in shape. How does this experiment on shadow casting relate to dental radiography?

CHAPTER 17

Oral Radiography

http://evolve.elsevier.com/Robinson/essentials/

LEARNING OBJECTIVES

1. Pronounce, define, and spell the key terms.
2. Discuss the components of film-based radiography, including the film packet and x-ray film.
3. Describe the advantages and disadvantages of digital radiography and describe the two main technologies used in digital dental imaging.
4. Identify the three types of intraoral views.
5. Describe the care of dental films, including storage and film care during exposure.
6. Describe infection control techniques in dental radiography and demonstrate how to practice infection control during film exposure.
7. Complete the following related to intraoral radiography techniques:
   • Compare and contrast the paralleling technique and the bisecting angle technique.
   • Assemble the XCP (extension-cone paralleling) instruments.
   • Describe vertical and horizontal angulation.
8. Complete the following related to the full-mouth radiographic survey:
   • Produce a full-mouth radiographic survey using the paralleling technique.
   • Produce a four-film radiographic survey using the bite-wing technique.
9. Describe the basic principles of the occlusal technique and produce maxillary and mandibular radiographs using the occlusal technique.
10. Identify errors in exposure and processing technique and describe the steps for prevention.
11. Demonstrate the infection control techniques necessary during film processing, both in the darkroom and with use of a daylight loader.
12. List the steps in manual processing and in automatic processing of dental radiographs, as well as the steps in duplicating radiographs.
13. Mount a full series of periapical and bite-wing dental radiographs.
14. Complete the following related to panoramic imaging:
   • Describe the purposes, uses, advantages, and disadvantages of panoramic imaging.
   • Describe the equipment used in panoramic imaging.
   • Demonstrate the procedure for exposing a panoramic image
   • Discuss common errors and infection control in panoramic imaging.
15. Describe additional types of extraoral images used in dentistry.
16. Discuss informed consent, documentation, and ownership of dental radiographs when it comes to dental radiography.

KEY TERMS

automatic processing techniques
bisecting angle technique
bite-wing image
cassette
charge-coupled device (CCD)
diagnostic quality image
digital image
digitizes

film duplicating
horizontal angulation
latent image
manual processing
occlusal technique
panoramic radiography
paralleling technique
periapical views

phosphor storage plates (PSPs)
point of entry
radiograph
scanning
sensor-holding device
vertical angulation

X-rays have been an essential part of dentistry for decades. Traditional dental x-rays were exposed with film much like the cameras we used. The film is placed in the mouth, the "image" is taken, and then the film is developed in a darkroom.

Since the 1980s, digital imaging has revolutionized dental radiology and has largely replaced traditional film-based techniques. Because some dental offices still use traditional x-rays, it is important to be skilled with all forms of dental radiography, which include film-based techniques and digital technology. Developing the clinical skills to effectively use the dental x-ray equipment, x-ray film and processing, and infection control techniques. to avoid technique errors, recognize them when they do occur, and prevent errors in the future is critical.

When discussing digital radiography, the term digital image is used instead of radiograph, film, or x-ray. A radiograph is an image on conventional dental film.

Digital Radiography

Digital radiography is a type of x-ray imaging that uses digital x-ray sensors to replace traditional photographic x-ray film. It produces enhanced computer images of the teeth and other oral structures and conditions. Digital dental images can be taken inside (intraoral) or outside (extraoral) the mouth (Fig. 17.1).

Although digital imaging systems are high tech, a conventional x-ray machine is still used to expose the image, and the position of the image receptor (sensor or phosphor storage plate [PSP]) in the mouth is identical to positioning the traditional dental film. There are many reasons for the steady increase in the use of digital technologies. Table 17.1 provides the advantages and disadvantages of digital radiography.

Types of Digital Imaging Systems

There are two basic systems used to acquire a digital image: **direct imaging** and **indirect imaging.**

FIGURE 17.1 Radiographic image display. (Courtesy Dentsply Sirona, York, Pennsylvania.)

Table 17.1
Advantages and Disadvantages of Digital Radiography

Advantages	
Gray-scale resolution	Gray-scale resolution is excellent, which is important because an accurate diagnosis is often based on contrast.
	The dentist may manipulate the contrast on the computer.
Reduced radiation exposure to the patient	Digital radiographic systems require 50%–80% less radiation exposure than conventional x-ray units.
Faster viewing of images	Images are almost immediately ready for viewing.
Lower equipment and film costs	Costs for x-ray film and processing solutions are eliminated.
	No environmental concerns related to disposal of processing chemicals are present.
Patient education	Patients can see and understand conditions within the teeth.
	Can increase the patient's willingness to accept treatment plans.
Disadvantages	
Initial setup costs	Digital radiography systems require an initial investment estimated at $10,000, depending on the type of computer and other auxiliary features.
Quality of images	Not everyone agrees, but the images appear to be satisfactory to diagnose dental disease.
Sensor size	Some patients find the sensors bulky and complain about the thickness.
	Some patients tend to gag more frequently than when traditional film is used.
Infection control	The sensor must be protected with disposable control barriers because the digital sensor cannot be heat sterilized.

TrueComfort™ Design [1]

To maximize both patient comfort and ease of use, DEXIS has enhanced its own great sensor housing design by refining the curvatures, redesigning the cable exit, upgrading the materials, and giving it a slimmer profile.

Four beveled corners and a smooth, rounded casing ensure there are no sharp edges against the palate or soft tissue. The smaller, angled dome makes precise placement in posterior regions easy.

Integrated Electronics [2]

A smart design places the electronics on the sensor's back to maximize the active imaging area. The on-board electronics provide the USB functionality, allowing direct connection to the computer.

ScatterGuard™ [3]

A protective shield affixed to the interior wall of the rear housing protects the patient by preventing X-ray back scattering.

PureImage™ Technology

The ability to see subtleties in x-ray images is crucial to diagnosis, collaboration, and patient communication. Through a combination of advanced hardware and software technologies, the DEXIS Platinum sensor is able to deliver clinically meaningful images that are extremely clear and highly detailed.

A premium quality **Caesium Iodide scintillator** [4] converts the x-ray beam into visible light and guides it through its micro-columnar structures.

Fiber optics [5] then transmit the light precisely to the CMOS sensor surface. This efficient design allows for a high signal-to-noise ratio, resulting in clean images with virtually no visual noise.

Our **high-resolution CMOS sensor** [6] features an exclusive architecture that maximizes active area at the pixel level to bring out the smallest details.

FIGURE 17.2 Dexis platinum sensor. (Courtesy KaVo Kerr, Brea, California.)

Direct Digital Imaging

In direct imaging, a solid-state sensor is the image receptor (Fig. 17.2). It contains an x-ray–sensitive silicon chip with an electronic circuit embedded in the silicon. The sensor, available in a variety of sizes, is positioned in the patient's mouth instead of film (Fig. 17.3).

The sensor, or **charge-coupled device (CCD)**, is the most commonly used digital receptor. The technology is used in a variety of other imaging devices, such as telescopes, fax machines, personal data assistants (PDAs), video cameras, and even some panoramic machines and other extraoral imaging systems, such as cone beam volumetric imaging.

Like telephones, some CCDs are wireless, and other types have a cable connected directly from the sensor to the computer. The wireless type of sensor uses radio frequency transmission to instantly transmit the image to the computer via radio waves.

Indirect Digital Imaging
Phosphor Storage Imaging

In **PSP** imaging systems, the image receptor is a thin, flexible plate, the size of a conventional x-ray film, that has been coated with phosphor crystals (Fig. 17.4). The phosphor layer is able to store the energy of the x-ray photons for a period of time. The PSP is placed in a barrier envelope to be ready for use on a patient. After exposure, the plate is scanned to "read" the information stored on the plate by using a laser beam that releases

FIGURE 17.3 Various sizes of digital sensors. (Courtesy Dentsply Sirona, York, Pennsylvania.)

the energy from the plate and converts it into a digital image. The latent image will remain on the phosphor plate before the scanning phase for minutes to hours, depending on the environment in which the plates are stored. They should not be exposed to bright light or warmth because this will release the energy before it is read by the scanner. After the plates are scanned, they are exposed to bright light that erases all remaining energy, and the plates are ready to be used again. For infection control,

FIGURE 17.4 A, Barrier envelope. **B,** Front and back sides of a phosphor plate.

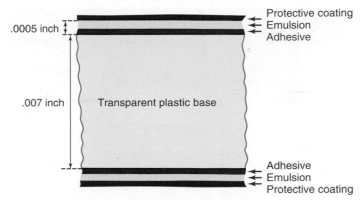

FIGURE 17.5 A cross-sectional diagram of film base and emulsion. (From Frommer H, Stabulas-Savage JJ: *Radiology for the dental professional*, ed 9, St Louis, 2011, Mosby.)

the imaging plate is inserted into a specially designed barrier envelope. The barrier envelope is sealed by removing the adhesive strip and pressing the envelope closed. The imaging plate is protected and then can be used intraorally. The imaging plate is positioned in the patient's mouth using the same positioning techniques as are used with conventional dental x-ray film. After exposure, the imaging plate is carefully removed from the barrier envelope and then is placed in a scanner that uses a laser to display the image on the computer.

The imaging plates cannot be autoclaved, and extreme care must be taken when handling to avoid scratches or dust.

Digital Imaging Software Programs

Most computer software programs that are used in digital imaging are capable of performing electronic image enhancement. This means that the operator can change the following image variables together or separately:

- Contrast
- Brightness
- Image size (zoom)
- Sharpness
- Inversion (white to black and black to white)
- Pseudocolor alteration

Film-Based Radiography

Film-based dental radiography uses photographic film that has been adapted for dental use. Place a film in the patient's mouth and then expose it to an x-ray beam to capture the image on film. The latent image (invisible) on the film becomes visible only after the film is processed in a darkroom (a light-tight room) or in an automatic film-processing machine. Once the film is processed and dried, it becomes a radiograph; it is placed into a film mount and is ready to be viewed and interpreted by the dentist.

Intraoral Dental X-Ray Film

Intraoral dental film consists of a semiflexible plastic film base coated on both sides with an emulsion containing x-ray–sensitive crystals of silver bromide, silver halide, and silver iodine embedded in gelatin (Fig. 17.5). The size of the crystals determines the film speed. (Film speed is discussed in Chapter 16.)

- The film base is made of clear cellulose acetate.
- The thin adhesive layer attaches the emulsion to the film base.
- The gelatin suspends the emulsion of microscopic silver crystals over the film base. During film processing, the gelatin absorbs the processing solutions and allows the chemicals to react with the silver halide crystals.
- The silver halide crystals absorb radiation during x-ray exposure and store energy emitted from the radiation.
- The protective layer is a thin transparent coating that protects the emulsion surface.

Film Packet

The film is supplied in a sealed packet to protect it from light and moisture. The film packet will contain either one film or two films. By having two films, you are able to have a duplicate to be used for insurance or referrals.

The film packet includes the following layers (Fig. 17.6):

- Outer vinyl packet, with one corner of the film having a small raised bump. This bump differentiates the left or right size when film is placed for mounting purposes.
- Black paper wrapper protects the film from light.
- A lead foil sheet is positioned behind the film to shield it from secondary scattered radiation.

Intraoral film packets are provided in five sizes: (#0) for children younger than 3 years, (#1) anterior views on adults and children, (#2) adult size – universal, (#3) preformed bite-wing, (#4) infrequently used, and (#5) occlusal (Fig. 17.7).

Care of Dental Films

Film Storage

All dental films should be stored according to the manufacturer's instructions to protect them from light, heat, moisture,

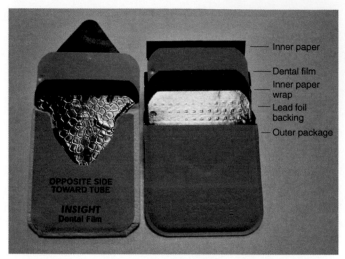

FIGURE 17.6 Contents of a moisture-proof dental film packet. (Courtesy Carestream Health, Inc., Rochester, New York.)

FIGURE 17.7 The white side of the film packet faces the tube. **A,** Size 4 occlusal film. **B,** Size 2 film. **C,** Size 1 film.

chemicals, and scatter radiation. The box of radiographic film is marked with an expiration date.

Film Care During Exposure

Films to be exposed are dispensed before the radiographic procedure begins. They are placed on a clean towel just outside the room where the films are to be exposed.

Never leave films, whether exposed or unexposed, in the room where additional films are being exposed. By doing this, it could result in the new films being exposed to scatter radiation, which results in film fog and reduces their diagnostic value.

Infection Control in Dental Radiography

Dental radiographic procedures present special infection control challenges. The operator contacts the patient's saliva while placing and removing the sensors or film packets and touches many things while exposing and processing film. Protective measures and barriers used while producing radiographs are illustrated in Fig. 17.8.

FIGURE 17.8 A, x-ray equipment with barriers in place. **B,** Radiography operatory with barriers in place. **C,** Protective barrier on x-ray film.

Surfaces Likely to Be Contaminated During X-Ray Procedure

- X-ray tubehead
- Position indicator device (PID)
- X-ray control panel
- Exposure button
- Computer keyboard
- Digital sensors and cables
- Phosphor storage plates (PSPs)
- Lead apron
- Dental chair controls
- Operatory counter surfaces
- Darkroom equipment
- Sleeves on automatic processors

Dental film is now available with plastic barriers over the packet. The film is exposed as usual, and then the plastic barrier cover is removed. The infection control protocol is more efficient and effective when the dental assistant plans for the procedure before the patient is seated.

The sensor or phosphor plate must be carefully covered with a barrier because, at this time, they cannot be heat sterilized. Care must be taken when removing the barrier to avoid contamination of the sensor under the barrier. Follow the manufacturer's recommendations regarding surface disinfection of the sensor.

See Procedure 17.1: Practicing Infection Control With Digital Sensors; Procedure 17.2: Practicing Infection Control with Phosphor Storage Plates; and Procedure 17.3: Practicing Infection Control During Film Exposure.

CDC Guidelines for Digital Radiology

1. Wear gloves when exposing radiographs and handling contaminated film packets. Use other PPE (e.g., protective eyewear, mask, gown) as appropriate if spattering of blood or other bodily fluids is likely.
2. Use heat-tolerant or disposable intraoral devices whenever possible (e.g., film-holding and positioning devices). Clean and heat sterilize heat-tolerant devices between patients.

3. Transport and handle exposed film in an aseptic manner to prevent contaminating the developing equipment.
4. The following apply for digital radiography sensors:
   a. Use FDA-cleared barriers.
   b. Clean and heat sterilize, or high-level disinfect, between patients; barrier protect semi-critical items. If an item cannot tolerate these procedures, then, at a minimum, protect it between patients with an FDA-cleared barrier, and clean and disinfect with an EPA-registered hospital disinfectant with intermediate-level (i.e., tuberculocidal claim) activity. Consult the manufacturer for methods of disinfecting and sterilizing digital radiography sensors and for protecting associated computer hardware.

CDC, Centers for Disease Control and Prevention; *EPA,* U.S. Environmental Protection Agency; *FDA,* U.S. Food and Drug Administration; *PPE,* personal protection equipment.

Intraoral Views

Types of Intraoral Views

Whether you are using a digital or a film-based technique, there are three types of intraoral views: (1) periapical, (2) bite-wing, and (3) occlusal. Each type of intraoral view presents specific information (Table 17.2).

TABLE 17.2
Types of Dental Images

Type	Primary Uses	Example
Periapical	Shows images of the entire length of the tooth, plus 3–4 mm beyond the apices. Is used to diagnose abscesses and other pathologic conditions around the root area of the teeth. Is also used to identify unerupted teeth.	
Bite-wing	Shows images of the crowns of the teeth on both arches on one film. A bite-wing survey (BWX) can consist of two or four films and is used to diagnose interproximal caries, recurrent caries, pulpal pathologic conditions, and conditions of the crestal bone.	
Occlusal	Is used to locate impactions, supernumerary teeth, pathologic conditions, and fractures of the maxilla or mandible. #4 film is used.	

Occlusal radiograph from Miles DA, Van Dis ML, Williamson GF, et al: *Radiographic imaging for the dental team,* ed 4, Philadelphia, 2009, Saunders.

Intraoral Imaging Techniques

There are two basic techniques used to obtain periapical images: the **paralleling technique** and the **bisecting (bisection of the angle) technique** (Figs. 17.9A and B). The American Academy of Oral and Maxillofacial Radiology and the American Dental Education Association (ADEA) recommend use of the paralleling technique because it provides the most accurate image with the least amount of radiation exposure to the patient.

Paralleling Technique

The paralleling technique is also known as the *extension-cone paralleling (XCP)*, *right-angle*, or *long-cone* technique. To use the paralleling technique competently, you must understand the terminology, which include: *parallel*, *intersecting*, *perpendicular*, *right angle*, *long axis* of the tooth, and *central ray (CR)*, along with the following five basic rules:

1. Image receptor/film *placement* so that it will cover the correct teeth to be examined.
2. Image receptor/film *positions* so that it is parallel to the long axis of the tooth. The image receptor in the appropriate holder (positioning instrument) must be placed away from the teeth and toward the middle of the mouth (Fig. 17.10).
3. *Vertical angulation* for the CR of the x-ray beam directed perpendicular (at a right angle) to the image receptor/film and the long axis of the tooth (Fig. 17.11).

A. Longitudinal axis of tooth
B. Imaginary bisecting line
C. Plane of film
CR. Central ray

FIGURE 17.9 Intraoral x-ray techniques. **A,** Paralleling, **B,** Bisecting technique.

FIGURE 17.10 Position of the film sensor, teeth, position indicator device, and central ray of the x-ray beam. (From Iannucci J, Jansen Howerton L: *Dental radiography: principles and techniques*, ed 5, St Louis, 2017, Elsevier.)

FIGURE 17.11 Vertical angulation of the position indicator device (PID) refers to PID placement in an up-and-down (head-to-toe) direction.

X-ray beam

Receptor

FIGURE 17.12 Correct horizontal angulation. (From Iannucci J, Jansen Howerton L: *Dental radiography: principles and techniques*, ed 5, St Louis, 2017, Elsevier.)

4. *Horizontal angulation* for the CR of the x-ray beam directed through the contact area between the teeth (Fig. 17.12).
5. *Central ray* for the x-ray beam centered on the image receptor/film to ensure that all areas are exposed. Failure to center the x-ray beam results in a partial image, or *cone cut* (Fig. 17.13).

Sensor or Film Holding Instruments

To place and keep the sensor/film in its proper position in rela tion to the tooth, the paralleling technique requires the use of holding instruments. A commonly used type of sensor/film device is the Rinn XCP instrument (Fig. 17.14). In addition to film or sensor positioning, these instruments include a localizing ring, also known as an *aiming ring,* which facilitates aligning the position indicator device (PID) with the film or sensor in both horizontal and vertical planes. This alignment increases the accuracy and reduces the need for unnecessary

FIGURE 17.13 This radiograph demonstrates that the position indicator device (PID) was not centered on the film, causing an unexposed area of film. (From Frommer HH, Stabulus JJ: *Radiology for the dental professional,* ed 9, St Louis, 2011, Mosby.)

retakes. The procedures that use the XCP film- and sensor-holding instruments follow the basic principles of placement and paralleling. See Procedure 17.4: Assembling Extension-Cone Paralleling (XCP) Instruments.

Bisecting Angle Technique

The bisecting angle technique is applied in special circumstances, such as in difficult or unusual anatomy (e.g., in patients with a very shallow palate or a very short lingual frenum or when palatal or mandibular tori [bone growths] are present). In addition, small children and some endodontic views may require the use of this technique. Using the proper technique, diagnostic images can be obtained with this method.

Basic Principles

The bisecting angle technique is based on the geometric principle of bisecting a triangle (bisecting means dividing into two equal parts: Fig. 17.15).

FIGURE 17.14 Rinn extension-cone paralleling (XCP) instruments are color-coded for easy assembly. **A,** The red instruments are for bite-wing placement, the yellow are for posterior placement, and the blue are for anterior placement. **B,** Rinn sensor suitable for Gendex, VisualiX, USB/GX Cygnus, and Visiodent.

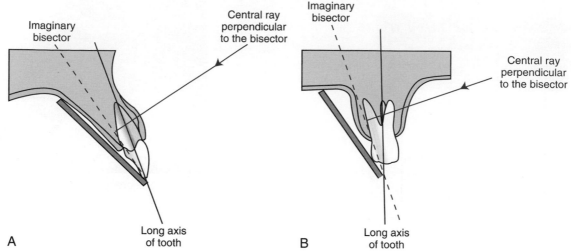

FIGURE 17.15 A, Anterior tooth with the central ray perpendicular to the *imaginary* bisector of the angle between the long axis of the tooth and the film plane. **B,** A posterior tooth using the bisecting angle concept. (From Miles D, Van Dis ML, Williamson GF, et al: *Radiographic imaging for the dental team,* ed 4, Philadelphia, 2009, Saunders.)

The angle formed by the long axis of the teeth and the sensor/film is bisected, and the x-ray beam is directed at a right angle (perpendicular) to the bisecting line.

In this technique, the sensor/film is placed close to the crowns of the teeth to be radiographed and extends at an angle into the palate or floor of the mouth. Sensor/film holders for the bisecting angle technique, including some with alignment indicators, are commercially available.

Available types of image receptor holders for the bisecting technique include the following:

- The bisecting-angle instrument (BAI; Dentsply Rinn) includes plastic bite-blocks, plastic aiming rings, and metal indicator arms.
- The Stabe bite-block (Dentsply Rinn) is a disposable bite-block that can be used with the paralleling technique or the bisecting technique. With the bisecting technique, the scored front section is removed, and the image receptor is placed *as close as possible* to the teeth.
- The EeZee-Grip holder (Dentsply Rinn) is a sensor-holding device that is used in the bisecting technique (Fig. 17.16).

Patient Positioning

The patient's midsagittal plane should be perpendicular to the floor, which means that the patient's head is upright for maxillary film and is slightly tipped back for the mandibular arch.

A #2 sensor/film is used in both the anterior (in a vertical position) and posterior (in a horizontal position) region. Only three films are needed in the maxillary anterior region because all four maxillary incisors can be imaged on the #2 sensor/film.

Beam Alignment

The x-ray beam is directed to pass between the contacts of the teeth being radiographed in the horizontal dimension, just as it does in the paralleling technique. The vertical angle, however, must be directed at 90 degrees to the imaginary bisecting line. Too much vertical angulation will produce images that are too short (foreshortened), and too little vertical angulation will result in images that are too long (elongated). The beam must be centered to prevent cone cutting. A short or a long PID can be used (Table 17.3).

FIGURE 17.16 A, Snap a Ray Xtra Film and phosphor plate holder for the bisecting technique. **B,** The EeZee-Grip Digital Sensor Holder for the bisecting technique.

TABLE 17.3
Vertical Angulations for the Bisecting Angle Technique

Teeth Being Imaged	Vertical Angulations (in degrees)
Maxillary incisors	−40 to −50
Maxillary cuspids	−45 to −55
Maxillary premolars	−30 to −40
Maxillary molars	−20 to −30
Mandibular incisors	−15 to −25
Mandibular cuspids	−20 to −30
Mandibular premolars	−10 to −15
Mandibular molars	−5 to 0

If the patient positioning is correct, then these vertical angulations will produce reasonable film images for most patients.

Full-Mouth Radiographic Survey

An intraoral *full-mouth survey (FMX)* contains both *periapical* and *bite-wing* images. The periapical image shows the entire tooth from occlusal surface or incisal edge to about 2 to 3 mm beyond the apex to show the periapical bone. This view is used to diagnose decay; pathology of the tooth, root, and bone; and tooth formation and eruption (Fig. 17.17). Periapical exposures are essential in endodontics and in oral surgical procedures.

For the average adult, a full-mouth series consists of 18 to 20 images—generally, 14 periapical views and 4 to 6 bite-wing views. The number may vary, however, depending on the dentist's preference and the number of teeth present. For example, for the patient without teeth, 14 periapical views are enough to cover the edentulous arches; bite-wings are not necessary. For the patient with a full dentition, the number of periapical views varies depending on whether the paralleling or the bisecting technique is used.

A

B

FIGURE 17.17 **A,** Full-mouth survey using digital sensor. **B,** Mounted full-mouth series with eight anterior films using the paralleling technique. (Courtesy KaVo Kerr, Brea, California.)

A
- Entire crown and tooth of canine, including apex and surrounding structures.
- Interproximal alveolar bone and mesial contact of canine.
- Lingual cusp of first premolar usually obscures distal contact of canine.

B
- Entire crown and roots of one lateral and one central incisor, including apices of teeth and surrounding structures.
- Interproximal alveolar bone between central and lateral contact areas, mesial and distal contact areas, and surrounding regions of bone.
- Mesial contacts of adjacent central incisor and adjacent canine.

C
- Entire crown and root of canine, including apex and surrounding structures.
- Interproximal alveolar bone and mesial and distal contacts.

D
- Entire crown and roots of four mandibular incisors, including apices of teeth and surrounding structures.
- Contacts between central incisors and between central and lateral incisors.
- In most cases, not necessary to see distal contacts of lateral incisors.

FIGURE 17.18 Anterior periapical film placement shows structures visible on the radiograph. (From Iannucci J, Jansen Howerton L: *Dental radiography: principles and techniques*, ed 5, St Louis, 2017, Elsevier.)

The *anterior* area is the region in which the number of images varies. Variables include the size of the sensor, if you are using digital, and the technique used (Fig. 17.18). When using dental film and the bisecting technique, three anterior views are taken on each arch (maxillary and mandibular) with size #2 film. For the paralleling technique, three or four size #1 films would be used on each arch (Fig. 17.19).

Film Placement

There are specific teeth and structures that must be clearly visible on each image for every projection.

Guidelines for Film Placement
- Anterior films are always vertically placed.
- Posterior films are always horizontally placed.
- The film holder is always positioned away from the teeth and toward the middle of the mouth.
- The film is always centered over the areas to be examined.
- The film is always placed parallel to the long axis of the teeth.
- If using traditional film:
  - The white side of the film always faces the teeth.
  - The identification dot on the film is always placed in the slot of the film holder (dot in the slot).

See Procedure 17.5: Producing a Full-Mouth Radiographic Survey Using the Paralleling Technique.

Producing Bite-Wing Views

The bite-wing image shows the upper and lower teeth in occlusion. Only the crowns and a small portion of the root are seen. This view is used for detecting interproximal decay, early periodontal disease, recurrent decay under restorations, and the fit of metallic fillings or crowns (Fig. 17.20).

A
- All crowns and roots of first and second premolars and first molar, including apices, alveolar crests, contact areas, and surrounding bone

B
- All crowns and roots of first, second, and third molars, including apices, alveolar crests, contact areas, surrounding bone, and tuberosity region

C
- All crowns and roots of first and second premolars and first molar, including apices and surrounding bone
- Distal contact of mandibular canine

D
- All crowns and roots of first, second, and third molars, including apices and surrounding bone

FIGURE 17.19 Posterior periapical film placement showing structures visible on the radiograph. (From Iannucci J, Jansen Howerton L: *Dental radiography: principles and techniques,* ed 5, St Louis, 2017, Elsevier.)

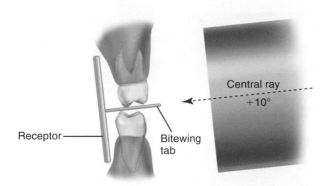

Central ray
+10°

Receptor

Bitewing
tab

FIGURE 17.20 Positions of the receptor, bite-wing tab, and central ray in the bite-wing technique. (From Iannucci J, Jansen Howerton L: *Dental radiography: principles and techniques*, ed 5, St Louis, 2017, Elsevier.)

The film or sensor is positioned (by a bite tab or a holding device) parallel to the crowns of both the upper and the lower teeth, and the CR is directed perpendicular to the film or sensor.

The premolar **bite-wing image** should include the distal halves of the crowns of the cuspids, both premolars, and often the first molars on both the maxillary and the mandibular arches. The molar film should be centered over the second molars.

Correct horizontal angulation is crucial to the diagnostic value of a bite-wing view. Even a slight amount of overlapping of the proximal (contact) surfaces on the image may lead to a misdiagnosis.

See Procedure 17.6: Producing a Four-Film Radiographic Survey Using the Bite-Wing Technique.

Occlusal Technique

The occlusal technique is used to examine large areas of the upper or lower jaw. The occlusal technique is so named because the patient bites or *occludes* the entire film.

Uses for Occlusal Radiographs

- To locate retained roots of extracted teeth
- To locate supernumerary (extra) unerupted or impacted teeth
- To locate salivary stones in ducts of the submandibular gland
- To locate fractures of the maxilla and mandible
- To examine the area of a cleft palate
- To measure changes in the size and shape of the maxilla or mandible

---

This technique requires the use of conventional dental film. In adults, #4 intraoral film is used, but #2 film is used in children. The occlusal technique is used when large areas of the maxilla or mandible must be radiographed.

Basic Principles

The basic principles of the occlusal technique are as follows:

1. Film is positioned with the white side facing the arch being exposed.

2. Film is placed in the mouth between the occlusal surfaces of the maxillary and mandibular teeth.
3. Film is stabilized when the patient gently bites on the surface of the film.
4. Vertical angulation between 35 and 65 degrees is used.

See Procedure 17.7: Producing Maxillary and Mandibular Radiographs Using the Occlusal Technique.

Exposure and Technique Errors

A **diagnostic quality image** is one that has been properly placed, exposed, and processed. Only diagnostic quality images are of benefit to the dentist, and retakes require the patient to be subjected to additional radiation. It is important for the dental assistant to recognize errors, identify their causes, and know how to correct the problem (Fig. 17.21).

Processing Radiographs

Processing dental film consists of a series of steps that change the latent (invisible) image into a visible image on the radiograph. Most practices now use an automatic processor on their films. In some dental offices, however, knowing how to process the film manually is necessary. This section discusses both methods.

Infection Control During Film Processing

After completing the exposures, remove your gloves and wash your hands. Carefully carry the paper cup or plastic bag containing the contaminated films to the processing area. Be careful not to touch the contaminated films with your bare hands. Regardless of whether you use a manual or an automatic processor with a daylight loader, you must remember that the used film packets are considered contaminated and should be appropriately handled.

See Procedure 17.8: Practicing Infection Control in the Darkroom and Procedure 17.9: Practicing Infection Control with the Use of the Daylight Loader.

Processing Solutions

Processing solutions are considered to be hazardous chemicals and are subject to special chemical labeling and disposal requirements. Always wear your personal protective equipment when handling these chemicals, and check disposal requirements specific to your state (see Chapter 6).

Care and Maintenance of Processing Solutions

You must always follow the manufacturer's instructions for storing, mixing, and using the processing solution (developer, fixer, and replenisher). These solutions deteriorate with exposure to air, continued use, and chemical contamination. Overused and old solutions cause radiographs to be too light and nondiagnostic (Table 17.4).

Developer Solution

The first step in processing begins with the developer solution. The developer solution softens the emulsion. After developing,

FIGURE 17.21 Radiographic exposure errors. **A,** Clear. **B,** Black. **C,** Dark. **D,** Light. **E,** No apices. **F,** Overlapped contacts. **G,** Foreshortened image. **H,** Elongated image. **I,** Cone cut. **J,** Distorted image with dark lines on corners. **K,** Double image. **L,** Blurred image. **M,** Light image with herringbone pattern. *PID,* Position indicator device; *XCP,* extension-cone paralleling. (Radiographs from Iannucci J, Jansen Howerton L: *Dental radiography: principles and techniques,* ed 4, St. Louis, 2012, Saunders.)

TABLE 17.4
Maintenance of Processing Solutions

Type of Processing Chemicals	Schedule of Maintenance
Manual chemicals	Solutions should be changed every 3–4 weeks.
Automatic chemicals	Solutions should be changed every 2–6 weeks.
Replenisher chemicals	Developer and fixer solutions should be replenished daily in both manual and automatic processing. Follow the manufacturer's instructions for the amount to remove and replace.

partially processed films are rinsed in water to remove any remaining chemical.

Note: There must be no exposure to light at this point in the processing or the film will turn black.

Fixer Solution

The fixer solution removes the unexposed silver halide crystals and creates white-to-clear areas on the radiograph.

After the films have been fixed, they are thoroughly washed in water to remove any remaining chemicals.

Replenisher Solution

Replenishers are solutions of developer and fixer that are added to compensate for the loss of volume and the strength of the solutions that results from use.

Manual Processing

Manual processing depends on a combination of:
1. Solution temperature
2. Time in the solution
   Note: Both are critical for the successful processing of film.
   See Procedure 17.10: Manual Processing of Dental Radiographs.

Darkroom

Manual film processing requires that the darkroom be light-tight and have adequate working space and good ventilation and be clean and dry at all times. It should be equipped with the following:

- Items required for infection control (e.g., gloves, disinfectant spray, paper towels)
- Disposal container for contaminated film packets or barriers
- Recycle container for lead foil pieces (*Caution:* Lead should not be thrown in the trash.)
- Separate processing tanks for the developer solution, the rinse water, and the fixer solution
- Hot and cold running water supply, with mixing valves to adjust the temperature
- Safelight and a source of white (normal) light. (A safelight is a device that provides enough illumination in the darkroom to work without the danger of fogging the film. Red light bulbs are not safelights.)

- Timer accurate to minutes and seconds
- Accurate thermometer that floats in the tanks to indicate the temperature of solutions
- Stirring rod or paddle to mix the chemicals and to equalize the temperature of solutions
- Safe storage space for chemicals
- Film hangers
- Film-drying rack and film dryer

Processing Tanks

In most darkrooms, the developer solution is in the tank on the left, the water bath (rinse) is the center tank, and the fixer solution is in the tank on the right. Always check the location of each chemical before processing (Fig. 17.22).

Keep the tank covered except when placing and removing films to prevent evaporation of the solutions.

Automatic Film Processing

Automatic film processing is a simple method used to process dental x-ray films (Fig. 17.23).

Advantages of Automatic Film Processor
- Less processing time is required.
- Time and temperature are automatically controlled.
- Less equipment is required.
- Less space is needed.

An automatic film processor consists of a series of rollers that transport the films through the steps and solutions necessary for complete processing (Fig. 17.24).

The temperature of the developer in automatic processors ranges from 85°F to 105°F (29.4°C to 40.5°C), which significantly reduces the developing and overall processing time. Automatic film processing requires 4 to 6 minutes to develop, fix, wash, and dry a film, whereas manual processing and drying techniques require approximately 1 hour.

Units with a daylight loading capability do not require a darkroom because they have light-tight baffles into which the hands

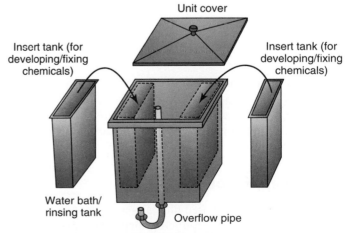

FIGURE 17.22 Processing tanks showing developing and fixing tank inserts in a bath of running water.

FIGURE 17.23 Automatic film processors. **A,** Without the daylight loader. **B,** With the daylight loader. (**B,** Courtesy Air Techniques, Inc., Melville, New York.)

FIGURE 17.24 Workings of an automatic film processor. The operator opens the film packet in the darkroom and inserts the film into the opening. The film is carried on rollers through the processing solutions. The finished film is returned in 4 to 5 minutes. A series of rollers transports the film through developing, fixing, and washing stations. (From White SC, Pharoah MJ: *Oral radiology: principles and interpretation,* ed 7, St. Louis, 2014, Mosby.)

are placed while the film is opened and inserted into the rollers. In a daylight loading unit, the exposed film is unwrapped and processed within the machine.

An automatic processor without daylight loading capability requires the use of a darkroom while unwrapping and placing films into the processor.

Care of the Automatic Processor

The automatic processor must be routinely cleaned and disinfected according to the manufacturer's directions. In addition, automatic processors must have routine preventive maintenance.

The two most common causes of automatic processor breakdown are (1) failure to keep the rollers clean and (2) inadequate replenishing of chemicals. The manufacturer's recommendations for daily and monthly cleaning of the automatic processor must be carefully followed.

Processing Errors

Proper processing of exposed film is as important as the exposure technique used in producing diagnostic quality radiographs. Dental assistants should readily recognize errors and understand how to avoid them (Fig. 17.25). See Procedure 17.11:

Automatic Processing of Dental Radiographs Using the Daylight Loader.

Duplicating Radiographs

Duplicate radiographs are identical copies of an intraoral or an extraoral radiograph; they may be necessary when:

- Referring a patient to a specialist
- Filing insurance claims
- A patient changes their dentist

Equipment and Film Requirements

To duplicate radiographs, you will need a special duplicating type of film and a duplicating machine (Fig. 17.26).

Duplicating film is only used for duplication and is never exposed to x-ray beams. Duplicating film is available in periapical sizes and in 5 × 12-inch and 8 × 10-inch sheets.

The duplicating machine uses white light to expose the film. Because the film is light sensitive, the duplication process is performed in the darkroom with the safelight.

Note: The longer the duplicating film is exposed to light, the lighter the duplicate films will become. This is the opposite of x-ray films, which will become darker when exposed to light.

Steps in Duplicating Radiographs

- Turn on the safelight and turn off the white light.
- Place the radiographs on the duplicator machine glass.
- Place the duplicating film on top of the radiographs with the emulsion side (darker side) against the radiographs.
- Turn on the light in the duplicating machine for the manufacturer's recommended time. Purpose: The light passes through the radiographs and strikes the duplicating film.
- Remove the duplicating film from the machine, and process it normally, using manual or automatic processing techniques.

Mounting Radiographs

Processed radiographs are arranged in anatomic order in holders, called *mounts,* to make it easy for the dentist to study and review the film. The mount is always labeled with the patient's name and the date that the radiographs were exposed. The dentist's name and address should also be on the mount.

FIGURE 17.25 Radiograph processing errors. **A,** Overdeveloped. **B,** Developer splash. **C,** Scratched film. **D,** Water spots. **E,** Solution too low. **F,** Roller marks. **G,** Fingerprints. **H,** Overlapped films. **I,** Underdeveloped. **J,** Reticulation. **K,** Fixer spots. **L,** Developer cutoff. **M,** Number of errors. **N,** Fixer cutoff. **O,** Air bubbles. **P,** Black fingerprint. **Q,** Static electricity. **R,** Exposure to light. **S,** Fogged film. (From Iannucci J, Jansen Howerton L: *Dental radiography: principles and techniques,* ed 4, St. Louis, 2012, Saunders.)

Selecting the Mount

Mounts are available in many sizes with different numbers and sizes of windows (openings) to accommodate the number and sizes of exposures in the patient's radiographic survey. The mounts most commonly used for radiographic surveys are available in black, gray, and clear plastic.

Methods of Mounting Films

Two methods can be used when mounting radiographs. Knowing how the dentist prefers to have radiographs mounted is important. Mistakes in mounting radiographs can result in errors in the dental treatment. Both methods rely on the identification of the raised (embossed) dot found on the film:

FIGURE 17.26 Film duplicator. (Courtesy DENTSPLY Rinn, Elgin, Illinois.)

In the first method, the films are placed in the mount with the raised dots facing up (convex). The American Dental Association (ADA) recommends this method of mounting radiographs. Radiographs are viewed as if the viewer is looking directly at the patient; the patient's left side is on the viewer's right, and the patient's right side is on the viewer's left.

In the second method, the radiographs are placed in the mount with the raised dots facing down (concave). Radiographs are viewed as if the viewer is inside the patient's mouth and is looking out; the patient's left side is on the viewer's left, and the patient's right side is on the viewer's right.

Tips for Mounting Radiographs

Images of normal anatomy can help you correctly place the films in the mount (Fig. 17.27). Using dental restorations and missing teeth as aids is also helpful in mounting films. To mount the films with the raised dot facing up, remember that it should look like a pimple, not a dimple (see Procedure 17.12: Mounting Dental Radiographs).

Extraoral Images

Extraoral images are useful when large areas of the jaw or skull must be examined. Almost all extraoral images are becoming digital to provide better resolution than traditional film-based images.

Panoramic Imaging

Panoramic radiographs allow the dentist to view the entire dentition and related structures on a single large film (Fig. 17.28).

Uses for this type of projection:
- Locate impacted teeth
- Observe tooth eruption patterns
- Detect lesions in the jaw
- Detect features in the bone
- Provide an overall view of the mandible and maxilla

Panoramic units can use panoramic film or be digital. In panoramic radiography, both the film and the tubehead rotate around the patient, producing a series of individual images. When these images are combined to present a single image, an overall view of the maxilla and mandible is created (Fig. 17.29).

Advantages and Disadvantages

As with all radiographic techniques, panoramic radiography has both advantages and disadvantages (Table 17.5).

Equipment

Many styles of panoramic x-ray units are available. Although each manufacturer's panoramic unit is slightly different, all machines have similar components. The primary components of the panoramic unit include the panoramic x-ray tubehead, head positioner, and exposure controls (Fig. 17.30).

Tubehead. The panoramic x-ray tubehead is similar to an intraoral tubehead in that it has a filament to produce electrons and a target to produce radiographs. Unlike the intraoral tubehead, the vertical angulation of the panoramic tubehead is not adjustable.

Head Positioner. Each panoramic unit has a head positioner that is used to align the patient's teeth as accurately as possible. Each head positioner consists of a chin rest, a notched bite-block, a forehead rest, and lateral head supports or guides (Fig. 17.31). Each panoramic unit is unique, and the operator must follow the manufacturer's instructions to position the patient correctly.

Exposure Controls. Exposure controls allow the milliamperage and kilovoltage settings to be adjusted to accommodate patients of different sizes. Step-by-step procedures for exposure of a panoramic film include equipment preparation.

Guidelines for Exposing Panoramic Image

To produce a diagnostic panoramic image and minimize patient exposure, you must follow the guidelines for exposing panoramic image.

See Procedure 17.13: Preparing the Equipment for Panoramic Radiography; Procedure 17.14: Preparing the Patient for Panoramic Radiography; and Procedure 17.15: Positioning the Patient for Panoramic Radiography.

Additional Extraoral Projections Used in Dentistry

Specialized areas of dentistry are using state-of-the-art equipment to assess the maxillofacial areas of the head and neck. The following technology include:

Lateral cephalometric projection, which is used to evaluate facial growth and development, trauma, disease, and developmental abnormalities. This projection shows the bones of the face and skull and soft tissue.

Cone beam computed tomography (CBCT), which is a technology that provides three-dimensional (3D) information. The views provide the mouth, face, and jaw from any direction, which is beneficial to the dental specialist in varying areas, such as impacted teeth, temporomandibular joint (TMJ) disorder, dental implants, tumors of the jaw, pathology, orthodontics, and reconstructive surgery.

Informed Consent

Informed consent includes explaining to the patient the purpose for taking radiographs and helping the patient understand the risks and benefits of dental images. An example would be informing the patient of the conditions and diseases that might go undetected without the image and what the consequences might be. If the patient is a minor or a legally incompetent adult, then the parent or guardian must give consent.

FIGURE 17.27 Radiographic landmarks of normal anatomy. **A,** Structures of the tooth. **B–D,** Maxillary structures. Radiographic landmarks of normal anatomy. **E–G,** Maxillary structures. **H–L,** Mandibular structures.

1. Pterygomaxillary fissure
2. Posterior border of maxilla
3. Maxillary tuberosity
4. Maxillary sinus
5. Floor of the maxillary sinus
6. Medial border of maxillary sinus/ lateral border of the nasal cavity
7. Floor of the orbit
8. Infraorbital canal
9. Nasal cavity
10. Nasal septum
11. Floor of the nasal cavity
12. Anterior nasal spine
13. Incisive foramen
14. Hard palate/floor of the nasal cavity
15. Zygomatic process of the maxilla
16. Zygomatic arch
17. Articular eminence
18. External auditory meatus
19. Styloid process
20. Mandibular condyle
21. Sigmoid notch
22. Coronoid process
23. Posterior border of ramus
24. Angle of mandible
25. Hyoid bone
26. Inferior border of mandible
27. Mental foramen
28. Mandibular canal
29. Cervical vertebrae
30. Epiglottis

FIGURE 17.28 **A,** Panoramic image of an adult patient. **B,** The diagram outlines some of the structures that can be visualized on a panoramic image. (From White SC, Pharoah MJ: *Oral radiology: principles and interpretation,* ed 7, St Louis, 2014, Mosby.)

FIGURE 17.29 The film and tubehead move around the patient in opposite directions. (Courtesy Dr. Robert M. Jaynes, Assistant Professor, Oral Radiology Group, The Ohio State University College of Dentistry.)

TABLE 17.5
Advantages and Disadvantages of Panoramic Radiography

Advantages	
Field size	The entire maxilla and mandible can be visualized on one panoramic film.
Ease of use	Learning how to expose a panoramic radiograph is relatively quick and easy.
Patient acceptance	Most patients prefer the panoramic radiograph because they do not have to hold uncomfortable film in their mouths.
Less radiation exposure	The patient receives less radiation exposure compared with the full-mouth radiographic survey (FMX).
Disadvantages	
Image sharpness	The images seen on a panoramic radiograph are not as sharp as those visualized on an intraoral film.
Focal trough limitations	Structures must be within the focal trough or they will appear out of focus.
Distortion	Even when the proper technique is used, some overlapping of the teeth and distortion of the images will always be noted.
Cost of equipment	Compared with the cost of an intraoral radiograph unit, a panoramic unit is more expensive.

FIGURE 17.30 Primary components of a panoramic unit.

FIGURE 17.31 Head positioner, consisting of a notched bite-block, forehead rest, and lateral head supports, is used to position the patient's head.

Documentation

Exposure of dental images must always be documented in the patient dental record and should include the following information:

- Informed consent
- Number and type of images exposed
- Rationale for exposing such images
- Diagnostic information obtained from the images

Ownership of Dental Images

Although the patient or the insurance company paid the fee for the radiographic images, the dentist owns the images. Radiographic images are diagnostic aids and are considered a part of the patient's permanent record.

Patients have a right to reasonable access to their records, including a copy of the images. If a patient moves or transfers to another dentist, then the patient can request in writing that their radiographs or digital images be forwarded to that dentist. Duplicate images should be made and forwarded to the new dentist, and the original radiographs and digital images should be retained in the patient's record.

☐ Ethical Implications

You must be aware of the laws in your state regarding the use of ionizing radiation in dentistry and must comply with all licensing or certification requirements.

Exposing patients to radiation has health and safety considerations and implications for the proper diagnosis of dental disease and treatment planning. In addition, legal action is a possibility if an improper diagnosis is made or if a lack of treatment results from dental radiographs that are not properly exposed or processed.

Practicing Infection Control with Digital Sensors

Goal

To perform all infection control practices using digital sensor exposure

Equipment and Supplies

- Barriers for the operatory, including the sensor, computer keyboard, and mouse
- Paper towels or gauze squares
- Digital sensor (sizes as necessary)
- Packaged positioning device
- Wraps or cushions for sensor (optional)
- Sensor and cable barriers
- Lead apron with thyroid collar
- Surface cleaner or disinfectant

(From Bird DL, Robinson DS: *Modern dental assisting,* ed 11, St. Louis, 2015, Saunders.)

Procedural Steps

1. Wash and dry your hands.
2. Place surface barriers on equipment, computer keyboard and mouse, and work area.
3. Set out the packaged positioning device, barriers for the sensor and cable, a paper towel or gauze squares, and miscellaneous items you might choose.
   Purpose: Once gloved, you should not have to leave the operatory area for additional materials.
4. Secure the barrier around the digital sensor.

(Courtesy Crosstex, Hauppauge, New York.)

Purpose: Sensors are reused on patients and cannot be heat sterilized. Therefore protecting them with FDA-cleared barriers is essential.

1. Seat the patient and place the lead apron.
2. Wash and dry your hands, and don gloves.
3. After all exposures are complete, remove the lead apron and dismiss the patient.
   Note: To remove the lead apron and still maintain the aseptic technique, you can wear over gloves to remove the apron or you can take off your gloves and remove the apron bare handed.
4. Put on utility gloves, and remove barriers from the x-ray equipment, taking care not to touch the surfaces underneath.
   Purpose: Chemical-resistant utility gloves are necessary when performing surface disinfection. If you touch a surface underneath the barrier while you are removing it, then that surface will be contaminated and must be disinfected.
5. Dispose of barriers and paper towels.
6. Place the positioning device on a tray to be returned to the instrument-processing area.
7. Disinfect the lead apron and any surfaces that may have become contaminated during the removal of surface barriers.
8. Carefully disinfect the sensor according to the manufacturer's recommendations.
   Purpose: Sensors are very expensive and can be damaged if improperly handled. Several leading brands of digital sensors are available. Cleaning and disinfecting protocols may vary according to the individual manufacturer.
9. Wash and dry your hands.

FDA, U.S. Food and Drug Administration.

Practicing Infection Control with Phosphor Storage Plates

Goal

To perform all infection control practices when using phosphor storage plates (PSPs)

Equipment and Supplies

- Barriers for the operatory
- Barriers for the computer and mouse
- Paper towels or gauze
- Cotton rolls
- PSPs (sizes as necessary)
- Barrier PSP envelopes
- Packaged positioning device
- Lead apron with thyroid collar
- Black transfer box
- Paper cup
- Image scanner
- Surface cleaner or disinfectant

Procedural Steps

1. Turn on the computer.
2. Log on to link the patient's images to their chart.
3. Choose the image layout you wish to use.

4. Wash and dry your hands.
5. Place surface barriers on equipment and work area.

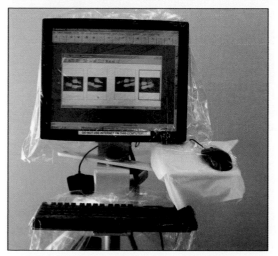

6. Slide the PSPs into barrier envelopes. Seal the barrier envelope by removing the protective strip and by gently pressing to seal the edge.

7. Set out the packaged positioning device, paper cup, transfer box, paper towel, and other miscellaneous items you might need.
   Purpose: Once gloved, you should not have to leave the operatory area for additional materials.

Exposures

1. Seat the patient and place the lead apron.
2. Wash and dry your hands, and don gloves.
3. Place the PSP into the film holder for each exposure.

Continued

Practicing Infection Control with Phosphor Storage Plates—cont'd

4. After each exposure, wipe excess saliva from the PSP envelope using a paper towel.
5. Place each exposed PSP into the paper cup labeled with the patient's name or directly into the black transfer box.

6. After the exposures are complete, remove the lead apron and dismiss the patient.
7. While still gloved, remove barriers, taking care not to touch the surfaces underneath.
   Purpose: You must wear gloves while removing barriers because they are contaminated. If you touch a surface underneath the barrier while you are removing it, then that surface will be contaminated and must be disinfected.
8. Dispose of barriers and paper towels.
9. Place the used positioning device on a tray to be returned to the instrument-processing area.

Preparing PSPs for Scanning

Note: If **scanning** is immediately performed after exposure, the black transfer box step is not necessary, and the PSPs can be immediately scanned. The black transfer box is necessary because PSPs should not be exposed very long to bright light or warmth because this exposure will release the energy before it is read by the scanner.

1. While gloved, remove each PSP from the paper cup, carefully open the sealed envelope, and allow the PSP to drop into the black transfer box. Use care not to touch the outside of the transfer box to avoid contamination.
   Purpose: Gloves must be worn because the PSP envelopes are contaminated.
2. Dispose of the contaminated envelopes.
3. Remove your gloves, and wash and dry your hands.

Scanning the PSP

1. Scanning machines vary greatly, depending on the manufacturer; therefore reading the specific instructions for the specific machine being used is critical.

2. Insert the PSP into the scanner according to the manufacturer's instructions.
   Purpose: The scanning machine will convert the fluorescent signal into a digital image that will appear on the monitor.

3. When the imaging is complete, log off the system.
4. Document the procedure in the patient's record.

Photos from Bird DL, Robinson DS: *Modern dental assisting,* ed 11, St. Louis, 2015, Saunders.

Goal

To perform all infection control practices during film exposure

Equipment and Supplies

- Barriers for the operatory
- Paper towels
- X-ray film or digital sensors (sizes as necessary)
- Packaged film- or sensor-holding device
- Sensor or phosphor storage plate (PSP) barriers (optional)
- Lead apron with thyroid collar
- Disposable container for exposed films (labeled with the patient's name)
- Surface cleaner or disinfectant

Procedural Steps

1. Wash and dry your hands.
2. Place surface barriers on equipment and work area.

3. Set out the packaged film- or sensor-holding device, film, labeled container for exposed film, paper towel, and other miscellaneous items you might need.
   Purpose: Once gloved, you should not have to leave the operatory area for additional materials.

4. Seat the patient and place the lead apron.
5. Wash and dry your hands, and don gloves.
6. After each exposure, wipe the excess saliva from the film or sensor using a paper towel.
   Note: If you are using a digital sensor, then be careful not to damage or dislodge the barrier between exposures.
7. Place each exposed film or PSP into the container, being careful not to touch the external surface.
   Purpose: Your contaminated gloves will contaminate the outer surface of the container.

8. After the exposures are complete, remove the lead apron and dismiss the patient.
   Note: To remove the lead apron and still maintain aseptic technique, you can wear over gloves to remove the apron, or you can take off your gloves and remove the apron barehanded. If you remove the lead apron while gloved, then you must disinfect the lead apron.
9. While still gloved, remove barriers, taking care not to touch the surfaces underneath.
   Purpose: You must wear gloves while removing barriers because they are contaminated. If you touch a surface underneath the barrier while you are removing it, then that surface will become contaminated and must be disinfected.
10. Dispose of barriers and paper towels.
11. Place the film- or sensor-holding device on a tray to be returned to the instrument-processing area.
12. Wash and dry your hands.
13. Take the exposed films to the processing area.

Goal

To assemble Rinn XCP instruments for all areas of the mouth in preparation for radiographic surveys.

Equipment and Supplies

- Rinn XCP instruments (for film or digital sensors)

Procedural Steps

Anterior Assembly

1. Lay out the blue parts for the anterior XCP instrument.

2. Assemble the anterior XCP instrument by inserting the two prongs of the blue anterior indicator arm into the openings in the blue anterior bite-block.

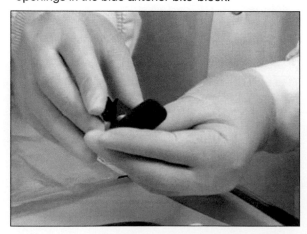

3. Insert the anterior indicator arm into the opening on the blue anterior aiming ring.

4. Flex the plastic backing of the blue bite-block to open the film slot for easy insertion of the anterior film packet.

5. The blue anterior XCP instrument is correctly assembled when the film is seen centered in the middle of the aiming ring.

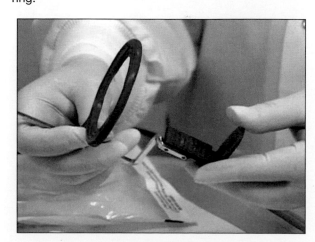

Assembling Extension-Cone Paralleling (XCP) Instruments—cont'd

Posterior Assembly

1. Lay out the yellow parts for the posterior XCP instrument.

2. Assemble the yellow posterior XCP instrument by inserting the two prongs of the yellow posterior indicator arm into the openings in the yellow posterior bite-block.

3. Insert the yellow posterior indicator arm into the opening on the yellow posterior aiming ring.

4. Flex the plastic backing of the yellow bite-block to open the film slot for easy insertion of the posterior film packet.

5. The posterior XCP instrument is correctly assembled when the film is seen centered in the middle of the aiming ring.

Producing a Full-Mouth Radiographic Survey Using the Paralleling Technique

Goal

To follow the proper steps to produce a full-mouth radiographic survey (FMX) using the paralleling technique.

Equipment and Supplies

- Appropriate number and size of x-ray films or sensors
- Appropriate infection control materials (paper cup, barriers, paper towel, and impervious surface cover)
- Lead apron and thyroid collar
- Sterile packaged extension-cone paralleling (XCP) instruments
- Cotton rolls
- Patient chart

Procedural Steps

Preparation Before Seating Patient

1. Prepare the operatory with all infection control barriers.
   Purpose: Any object that is touched and was not covered with a barrier must be disinfected after the patient is dismissed.
2. Determine the number and type of views to be exposed through a review of the patient's chart, directions from the dentist, or both.
3. If you are using film or phosphor storage plates (PSPs), then label a paper cup with the patient's name and the date. Place it outside the room where the x-ray machine will be used.
   Purpose: This is the transfer cup for storing and moving exposed films or PSPs.

4. Turn on the x-ray machine, and check the basic settings (kilovoltage, milliamperage, and exposure time).
5. Wash and dry your hands.
6. Dispense the desired number of films and store them outside the room where the x-ray machine is being used.
   Purpose: This step prevents fogging caused by scatter radiation.

Positioning the Patient

1. Comfortably seat the patient in the dental chair with their back in an upright position and the head supported.
2. Ask the patient to remove eyeglasses and bulky earrings.
   Purpose: These objects may cause radiopaque images to be superimposed on the radiographs.

3. Ask the patient to remove prosthetic appliances or objects from the mouth.
   Note: Always wear gloves when handling a prosthetic appliance.
4. Position the patient so that the occlusal plane of the jaw being x-rayed is parallel to the floor when the mouth is open.
5. Drape the patient with a lead apron and a thyroid collar.
6. Wash and dry your hands and put on clean examination gloves.
7. Open the package and assemble the sterile film- or sensor-holding instruments.
   Purpose: Allowing the patient to observe you washing your hands, putting on clean gloves, and opening the sterile package of instruments assures the patient that appropriate infection control measures are being taken.

Maxillary Canine Region

1. Vertically insert the #1 film packet or sensor into the anterior bite-block.
   Note: Not all digital sensors are available in the #1 size.
2. Position the film packet or sensor with the canine and first premolar centered. Position the film as far posterior as possible.
3. With the film- or sensor-holding instrument and film in place, instruct the patient to close the mouth slowly but firmly.
4. Position the localizing ring and position indicator device (PID); then make the exposure.

Producing a Full-Mouth Radiographic Survey Using the Paralleling Technique—cont'd

Note: The image of the lingual cusp of the first premolar is usually superimposed on the distal surface of the canine because of the curvature of the maxillary arch. This contact area must be opened on the view of the premolar region.

Continued

Producing a Full-Mouth Radiographic Survey Using the Paralleling Technique—cont'd

Maxillary Central or Lateral Incisor Region

1. Vertically insert the #1 film packet or sensor into the anterior block.
   Note: Not all digital sensors are available in the #1 size.
2. Center the film packet or sensor between the central and lateral incisors. Position the film or sensor as posterior in the mouth as possible.

3. With the instrument and film in place, instruct the patient to close the mouth slowly but firmly.
4. Position the localizing ring and PID, then make the exposure.

Producing a Full-Mouth Radiographic Survey Using the Paralleling Technique—cont'd

Mandibular Canine Region

1. Vertically insert the #1 film packet or sensor into the anterior block.

   Note: Not all digital sensors are available in the #1 size.

2. Center the film or sensor on the canine. Position the film or sensor as far in the lingual direction as the patient's anatomy will allow.

Note: A cotton roll may be placed between the maxillary teeth and the bite-block to prevent rocking of the bite-block on the canine tip and to increase patient comfort.

3. With the instrument and film in place, instruct the patient to close the mouth slowly but firmly.

4. Position the localizing ring and PID, then make the exposure.

Continued

Producing a Full-Mouth Radiographic Survey Using the Paralleling Technique—cont'd

Mandibular Incisor Region

1. Vertically insert the #1 film packet or sensor into the anterior bite-block.
   Note: Not all digital sensors are available in the #1 size.
2. Center the film or sensor packet between the central incisors. Position the packet as far in the lingual direction as the patient's anatomy will allow.
   Note: A cotton roll may be placed between the maxillary teeth and the bite-block to prevent rocking of the bite-block on the canine tip and to increase patient comfort.

3. With the instrument and film in place, instruct the patient to close the mouth slowly but firmly.
4. Slide the localizing ring down the indicator rod to the patient's skin surface.
5. Position the localizing ring and PID, then make the exposure.

Producing a Full-Mouth Radiographic Survey Using the Paralleling Technique—cont'd

Maxillary Premolar Region

1. Horizontally insert the film or sensor into the posterior bite-block, pushing the film or sensor all the way into the slot.
2. Center the film or sensor on the second premolar. Position the film in the midpalatal area.

3. With the instrument and film in place, instruct the patient to close the mouth slowly but firmly.
4. Position the localizing ring and PID, then make the exposure.

Continued

Producing a Full-Mouth Radiographic Survey Using the Paralleling Technique—cont'd

Maxillary Molar Region

1. Horizontally insert the film or sensor into the posterior bite-block.
2. Center the film or sensor on the second molar. Position the film or sensor in the midpalatal area.

3. With the instrument and film in place, instruct the patient to close the mouth slowly but firmly.
4. Position the localizing ring and PID, then make the exposure.

Producing a Full-Mouth Radiographic Survey Using the Paralleling Technique—cont'd

Mandibular Premolar Region

1. Horizontally insert the #2 film or sensor into the posterior bite-block.
2. Center the film or sensor on the contact point between the second premolar and the first molar. Position the film or sensor as far lingual as the patient's anatomy will allow.

3. With the instrument and film in place, instruct the patient to close the mouth slowly but firmly.
4. Slide the localizing ring down the indicator rod to the patient's skin surface.
5. Position the localizing ring and PID, then make the exposure.

Continued

Producing a Full-Mouth Radiographic Survey Using the Paralleling Technique—cont'd

Mandibular Molar Region

1. Horizontally insert the #2 film or sensor into the posterior bite-block.
2. Center the film or sensor on the second molar. Position the film or sensor as far lingual as the tongue will allow.
   Note: This position will be closer to the teeth than the position for the premolar and anterior views.

3. With the instrument and film in place, instruct the patient to close the mouth slowly but firmly.
4. Slide the localizing ring down the indicator rod to the patient's skin surface.
5. Position the localizing ring and PID, then make the exposure.

Producing a Four-Film Radiographic Survey Using the Bite-Wing Technique

Goal

To produce a four-view series of radiographs using the bite-wing technique.

Equipment and Supplies

- Four #2 films, digital sensors, or phosphor storage plates (PSPs)
- Paper cup
- Lead apron and thyroid collar
- Bite-wing tab or film- or sensor-holding device

Procedural Steps

Premolar Bite-Wing Exposure

1. Set vertical angulation at −10 degrees.

   Purpose: A positive angulation means that the position indicator device (PID) points downward, which places the beam so that it is nearly perpendicular to both the upper and the lower halves of the film or sensor.

2. Position the patient so that the occlusal plane is parallel to the floor. If necessary, ask the patient to lower or raise the chin.

3. Position the film or sensor in the patient's mouth by placing the lower half between the tongue and the mandibular teeth. Position the film or sensor with the anterior border at the middle of the canine.

4. Hold the film or sensor in place by pressing the tab over the occlusal aspect of the mandibular teeth.

   Purpose: This step prevents the film or sensor from slipping out of position.

5. Ask the patient to close the mouth slowly. Take care not to allow the patient to close on the fingertip of your glove.

6. Do not pull the film or sensor too tightly against the lower teeth as the patient closes the mouth.

   Purpose: Doing so can cause the film or sensor to push against the lingual aspect of the maxillary alveolar ridge and force the film down into the floor of the mouth.

7. Stand in front of the patient to set the horizontal angulation. To better visualize the curvature of the arch, place your index finger along the premolar area. Align the open end of the PID parallel with your index finger and the curvature of the arch in the premolar area.

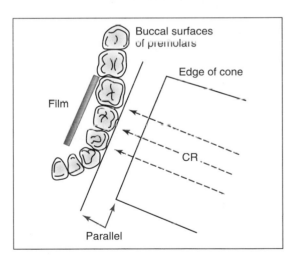

Molar Bite-Wing Exposure

1. Set vertical angulation at −10 degrees.

   Purpose: A positive angulation means that the PID points downward. This angulation places the beam so that it is nearly perpendicular to both upper and lower halves of the film.

2. Position the patient so that the occlusal plane is parallel with the floor. If necessary, ask the patient to lower or raise the chin.

Continued

3. Position the film in the patient's mouth by placing the lower half between the tongue and the mandibular teeth. Center the film or sensor on the second molar; the front edge of the film or sensor should be aligned with the middle of the mandibular second premolar.

4. Hold the film or sensor in place by pressing the tab over the occlusal aspect of the mandibular teeth.
   Purpose: This step prevents the film or sensor from slipping out of position.

5. Ask the patient to close the mouth slowly. Take care not to allow the patient to close on the fingertip of your glove.

6. Do not pull the film too tightly against the lower teeth as the patient closes the mouth.
   Purpose: Doing so can cause the film or sensor to push against the lingual aspect of the maxillary alveolar ridge and force the film down into the floor of the mouth.

7. Stand in front of the patient to set the horizontal angulation. To better visualize the curvature of the arch, place your index finger along the premolar area. Align the open end of the PID parallel with your index finger and the curvature of the arch in the molar area.
   Purpose: Different film placement and horizontal angulations are needed to open the proximal contact areas.

8. Make certain that the PID is positioned far enough forward to cover both the maxillary and the mandibular canines to prevent a cone cut.
   Purpose: To check for a cone cut, stand directly behind the tubehead and look along the side of the PID. No portion of the film or sensor should be visible; the film or sensor should be covered by the PID.

9. Direct the central ray through the contact areas.

10. Make the exposure.

Producing Maxillary and Mandibular Radiographs Using the Occlusal Technique

Goal

To follow the steps of the occlusal technique in producing diagnostic quality maxillary and mandibular radiographs.

Equipment and Supplies

- Two #4 films
- Paper cup
- Lead apron and thyroid collar

Procedural Steps

Maxillary Occlusal Technique

1. Ask the patient to remove prosthetic appliances or objects from the mouth.
2. Place the lead apron and thyroid collar.
3. Position the patient's head so the film plane is parallel to the floor and the midsagittal plane is perpendicular to the floor.
4. Place the film packet in the patient's mouth with the white side of the film on the occlusal surfaces of the maxillary teeth. The long edge of the film is placed in a side-to-side direction.
5. Place the film as far posterior as possible.
6. Position the PID so that the central ray (CR) is directed at −65 degrees through the center of the film. The top edge of the PID is placed between the eyebrows on the bridge of the nose.

7. Press the activating button on the x-ray machine for the exposure.

8. Document the procedure.

Mandibular Occlusal Technique

1. Recline the patient and position the head with the midsagittal plane perpendicular to the floor.
2. Place the film packet in the patient's mouth with the white side of the film on the occlusal surfaces of the mandibular teeth. The long edge of the film is placed in a side-to-side direction.
3. Position the film as far posterior on the mandible as possible.
4. Position the PID so that the CR is directed at a 90-degree angle to the center of the film packet. The PID should be centered approximately 1 inch below the chin.

Continued

Producing Maxillary and Mandibular Radiographs Using the Occlusal Technique—cont'd

5. Press the exposure button and make the exposure.

6. Document the procedure.

Procedure 17.8

Practicing Infection Control in the Darkroom

Goal
To practice infection control measures when in the darkroom.

Equipment and Supplies
- Paper towels
- Clean gloves
- Clean paper cup
- Container for lead foil

Procedural Steps
1. Place a paper towel and a clean cup on the counter near the processor.
   Purpose: The paper towel provides a barrier for the work surface, and the cup is used to discard the opened film packets.
2. Wash your hands, and put on a new pair of gloves, preferably the type that does not contain powder.
   Purpose: Powder remaining on the hands can cause artifacts on the exposed film.
3. Turn on the safety light, and then turn off the white light. Open the film packets and allow each exposed film to drop onto the paper towel. Be careful that the unwrapped films do not come into contact with the gloves.
   Purpose: The film must remain free from contamination. A contaminated film may remain contaminated even after processing.

7. Place the films into the processor or on developing racks with your bare hands.

4. Remove the lead foil from the packet, and place it in the foil-recycling container.
   Purpose: Lead foil is considered an environmental hazard and should not be discarded with the general waste.
5. Place the empty film packets into the clean cup.
6. Discard the cup. Remove your gloves by turning them inside out, then discard them.

Note: If you used films with plastic barriers, then you would have already removed the protective barrier in the operatory with gloved hands. You would then open the packets with your bare hands and feed the films into the processor.

Procedure 17.9

Practicing Infection Control with the Use of the Daylight Loader

Goal

To practice infection control measures when using the daylight loader in processing dental radiographic films

Equipment and Supplies

- Paper towels
- Clean gloves
- Clean cup
- Container for lead foil

Procedural Steps

1. Wash and dry your hands, and then place a paper towel or a piece of plastic as a barrier to cover the bottom of the daylight loader.

2. Place the following into the bottom of the daylight loader.
   a. Cup containing the contaminated film
   b. Clean pair of gloves
   c. Second empty paper cup

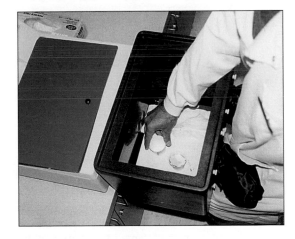

3. Close the top of the daylight loader.
4. Put your clean hands through the sleeves of the daylight loader, then put on the gloves.
   Purpose: Clean hands prevent contamination of the sleeves. Contaminated gloves should never be placed through the sleeves of the daylight loader.

Continued

Practicing Infection Control with the Use of the Daylight Loader—cont'd

5. Open the packets and allow the films to drop onto the clean barrier.
   Purpose: The clean barrier keeps dust or powder from the film.
6. Place the contaminated packets into the second cup and place the lead foil into the foil-recycling container.
   Purpose: The cup confines the contaminated film packets and makes disposal easier.
7. After you open the last packet, remove your gloves by turning them inside out. Insert the films into the developing slots.
   Purpose: The film remains uncontaminated and eliminates the question of whether organisms can survive in the solutions.

8. After you insert the last film, pull your ungloved hands through the sleeves.
9. Open the top of the loader, and then carefully pull the ends of the barrier over the paper cup and used gloves and discard.

Note: Be careful not to touch the contaminated parts of the barrier with your bare hands.

Procedure 17.10

Manual Processing of Dental Radiographs

Goal
To process dental radiograph films using a manual tank.

Equipment and Supplies

- Fully equipped darkroom
- Surface barriers or disinfecting solution for counters
- Exposed films
- Film rack

- Timer
- Pencil
- Film dryer (optional)

Procedural Steps

Preparation

1. Follow all the infection control steps discussed in this chapter.

2. Stir solutions with the corresponding paddle.
   Purpose: The chemicals are heavy and tend to settle to the bottom of the tank. Do not interchange mixing paddles, or cross-contamination will occur.
3. Check the temperature of the solutions and refer to the processing chart to determine the times.
   Purpose: The temperature of the solution determines the processing time.
4. Label the film rack with the patient's name and date of exposure.
5. Turn on the safelight, and then turn off the white light.
6. Wash your hands and put on gloves.
7. Open the film packets and allow the films to drop onto the clean paper towel. Take care not to touch the films.
   Purpose: The films have not been contaminated. Films that have been touched become contaminated and may remain contaminated even after processing.

Processing

1. Attach each film to the film rack so that the films are parallel and not touching each other.

2. As you immerse the film rack in the developer solution, slightly agitate (jiggle) the rack.
   Purpose: Agitating the film rack prevents air bubbles from forming on the film.
3. Start the timer. The timer is set according to the recommendations stated on the processing chart (e.g., 5 minutes if the solution is 68°F).
4. When the timer goes off, remove the rack of films and rinse the rack in the circulating water in the center tank for 20 to 30 seconds. Allow the excess water to drip off the films.
   Purpose: Water dripping from the racks into the fixer will dilute it.
5. Insert the rack of films into the fixer tank and set the timer for 10 minutes.
   Purpose: For permanent fixation, the film is kept in the fixer for a minimum of 10 minutes. For a wet reading, however, films may be removed from the fixing solution after 3 minutes for viewing. Films must be returned to the fixer to complete the process.
6. Return the rack of films to the center tank of circulating water for at least 20 minutes.
   Purpose: Incomplete washing will cause the films to turn brown eventually.
7. Remove the rack of films from the water and place it in the film dryer. If a film dryer is not available, then hanging the films to air-dry is recommended.
   Purpose: Films may be air-dried at room temperature in a dust-free area or placed in a heated drying cabinet. Films must be completely dried before they can be handled for mounting and viewing.
8. When the films are completely dry, remove them from the rack and mount and label.

Procedure 17.11

Automatic Processing of Dental Radiographs Using the Daylight Loader

Equipment and Supplies
- Automatic x-ray processor with the daylight loader
- Exposed dental films
- Chemical disinfection spray
- Two disposable cups or containers for lead foil and film packets
- Paper towel

Procedural Steps
1. At the beginning of the day, turn on the machine and allow the chemicals to warm up according to the manufacturer's recommendations.
   Purpose: The heating unit must warm the chemicals to the correct temperature to ensure that the films will be of diagnostic quality.

2. Follow the infection control steps discussed in the section earlier in this chapter.
   Purpose: Film packets are contaminated because they have been in the patient's mouth.
3. Wash and dry your hands.
4. Open the lid on the daylight loader and place a paper towel over the bottom. Then place two disposable cups on the towel.
   Purpose: The paper towel will act as a surface barrier on the bottom of the daylight loader. One disposable cup is for the lead foil in the film packet; the other is used to dispose of the paper towel, film packets, and gloves.
5. Put on gloves and slide your gloved hands through the sleeves of the daylight loader.

Continued

Automatic Processing of Dental Radiographs Using the Daylight Loader—cont'd

6. Remove the film from its packet, and check to ensure that the black paper has not stuck to the film. If the black paper is left on the film or if double film packets have not been separated, then the films will be damaged, and the automatic processor could jam.
7. Feed the film into the machine.
   Note: Open the film packets, and feed films in one at a time to prevent having films overlap during loading.
8. While the film is feeding into the machine, remove the lead foil from the packet and place it in one of the disposable cups. Then drop the empty packet onto the paper towel.
9. Keep the films straight as they are slowly fed into the machine. Allow at least 10 seconds between insertion of each film into the processor and the insertion of the next film. Place films in alternate film slots when possible.
10. After the last film is inserted into the machine, carefully remove your gloves and drop them into the center of the paper towel. While touching only the corners and underside of the paper towel, wrap the paper towel over the contaminated film packets and gloves. Place the wrapped paper towel into the second cup.
    Purpose: Handling the paper towel only by the corners and underside will help eliminate cross-contamination during film-processing procedures.
11. Remove the cup containing the lead foil and take it to the foil-recycling container.
12. Remove the processed radiographs from the film recovery slot on the outside of the automatic processor. Allow 4 to 6 minutes for the automated process to be completed.
    Note: When processing extraoral films, carefully remove the film from the **cassette**. Handle all films only by the edges to prevent fingerprints and scratches on the films.

Mounting Dental Radiographs

Goal
To mount a full-mouth series of dental radiographs.

Equipment and Supplies
- Appropriate size of film mount
- Pencil
- View box
- Paper towel
- Processing for full-mouth series of radiographs

Procedural Steps
1. Place a clean paper towel over the work surface in front of the view box.
   Purpose: To keep the films clean.
2. Turn on the view box.
3. Label and date the film mount.

4. Wash and dry your hands.
   Purpose: Washing and drying the hands prevents finger marks on the radiographs.
5. Identify the embossed dot on each radiograph; place the film on the work surface with the dot facing up.
   Purpose: The American Dental Association (ADA) recommends mounting with the dot up.
6. Sort the radiographs into three groups: bite-wing, anterior periapical, and posterior periapical views.
7. Arrange the radiographs on the work surface in anatomic order. Use your knowledge of normal anatomic landmarks to distinguish maxillary from mandibular radiographs.
8. Arrange all maxillary radiographs with the roots pointing upward and all mandibular radiographs with the roots pointing downward.
9. Place each film in the corresponding window of the film mount. The following order is suggested for film mounting:
   a. Maxillary anterior periapical films
   b. Mandibular anterior periapical films
   c. Bite-wing films
   d. Maxillary posterior periapical films
   e. Mandibular posterior periapical films

Procedure 17.12

Mounting Dental Radiographs—cont'd

10. Check the mounted radiographs to ensure that (1) the dots are all properly oriented, (2) the films are properly arranged in anatomic order, and (3) the films are secure in the mount.

Procedure 17.13

Preparing the Equipment for Panoramic Radiography

Goal

To prepare the equipment necessary for a panoramic radiograph.

Equipment and Supplies

- Extraoral film
- Cassette
- Infection control barriers

Procedural Steps

1. Load the panoramic cassette in the darkroom under safelight conditions. Handle the film only by its edges to prevent fingerprints.
   Purpose: The panoramic film is sensitive to light, and the remainder of the film in the box will be ruined if exposed to light.
2. Place all infection control barriers and containers.
3. Cover the bite-block with a disposable plastic barrier. If the bite-block is not covered, it must be sterilized before it is used on the next patient.
   Purpose: The bite-block is considered a semi-critical item and must be disposable or sterilized.
4. Cover or disinfect (or both) any part of the machine that comes in contact with the patient.

Purpose: Parts of the machine touching the patient but not intraorally used are considered noncritical items and must be disinfected with a high-level disinfectant.

5. Set the exposure factors (kilovoltage, milliamperage) according to the manufacturer's recommendations.
6. Adjust the machine to accommodate the height of the patient, and properly align all movable parts.
7. Load the cassette into the carrier of the panoramic unit.

Preparing the Patient for Panoramic Radiography

Goal
To prepare a patient for a panoramic x-ray image.

Equipment and Supplies
- Double-sided lead apron (or style recommended by the manufacturer)
- Plastic container

Procedural Steps
1. Explain the procedure to the patient. Give the patient the opportunity to ask questions.
   Purpose: The patient has the right to be informed and give consent to the procedure.
2. Ask the patient to remove all objects from the head and neck area, including eyeglasses, earrings, lip-piercing and tongue-piercing objects, necklaces, napkin chains, hearing aids, hairpins, and complete and partial dentures. Place the objects in a container.
   Purpose: If not removed, these objects will appear on the radiograph and could superimpose diagnostic information.
3. Place a double-sided (for protecting the front and back of the patient) lead apron on the patient, or use the style of lead apron recommended by the manufacturer.

Note: A thyroid collar is not recommended for all panoramic units because it blocks part of the beam and obscures important anatomic structures. Refer to the manufacturer's instructions for the unit you use.

Goal
To position the patient for a panoramic radiograph

Procedural Steps

1. Instruct the patient to sit or stand "as tall as possible" with the back straight and erect.
   Purpose: The spinal column is very dense; if the spine is not straight, then a white shadow will appear over the middle of the radiograph and obscure diagnostic information.
2. Instruct the patient to bite on the plastic bite-block and then slide the upper and lower teeth into the notch (groove) on the end of the bite-block.
   Purpose: The groove aligns the teeth in the focal trough.

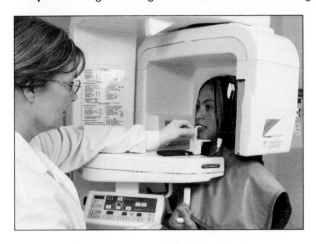

3. Position the midsagittal plane (the imaginary line that divides the patient's face into right and left sides) perpendicular to the floor.
   Purpose: If the patient's head is tipped or tilted to one side, then a distorted image will result.
4. Position the Frankfort plane (the imaginary plane that passes through the top of the ear canal and the bottom of the eye socket) parallel with the floor.

Purpose: The occlusal plane will be positioned at the correct angle.

5. Instruct the patient to position the tongue on the roof of the mouth and then close the lips around the bite-block.
   Purpose: If the tongue is not placed on the roof of the mouth, a radiolucent shadow will be superimposed over the apices of the maxillary teeth.
6. After the patient has been positioned, instruct them to remain still while the machine rotates during exposure.
   Purpose: Any movement of the patient will result in a blurred image on the radiograph.
7. Expose the film and proceed with film processing.
8. Document the procedure.

DATE	PROCEDURE	OPERATOR
1/25/21	Exposed panoramic radiograph	DLB

Chapter Exercises

Multiple Choice

Circle the letter next to the correct answer.

1. Images on radiographs that appear black are called _____.
   a. radiopaque
   b. radiolucent
2. The overall darkness of a radiographic image is called the _____.
   a. density
   b. contrast
   c. sharpness
   d. gray tones
3. The colored side of the film packet is always placed _____ the position indicator device.
   a. away from
   b. toward
   c. does not matter
4. If the dentist suspects an abscess at the apex of a tooth, then what type of radiograph would most likely be prescribed?
   a. bite-wing
   b. periapical
   c. occlusal
5. The image that exists on the film after exposure and before processing is called the _____ image.
   a. ghost
   b. latent
   c. hidden
   d. radiation
6. The type of radiograph that shows the crowns of the teeth on both arches at one time is called a _____ view.
   a. bite-wing
   b. occlusal
   c. periapical
7. The film size that is usually used for children younger than 3 years is _____.
   a. 0
   b. 1
   c. 2
   d. 3
8. The radiographic technique that requires the film to be placed at a right angle to the teeth is the _____ technique.
   a. paralleling
   b. bisection angle
9. Bite-blocks for holding the film in the patient's mouth should be _____.
   a. sterilized
   b. disposable
   c. either of the above
10. What processing error would cause the film to be too dark?
    a. Insufficient processing time
    b. Insufficient fixing time
    c. Developer temperature too warm
    d. Developer temperature too cold
11. What technique error would cause the image of the teeth on the radiograph to look too long?
    a. Foreshortening
    b. Closed contacts
    c. Elongation
    d. Incorrect vertical angulation
12. What technique error would cause closed contacts on a bite-wing?
    a. Excessive vertical angulation
    b. Insufficient vertical angulation
    c. Incorrect horizontal angulation
13. Which type of radiograph shows the maxillary and mandibular teeth on one film?
    a. Periapical view
    b. Bite-wing view
    c. Panoramic view
14. Digital radiography requires _____ radiation than traditional machines.
    a. more
    b. less
15. An advantage of panoramic radiographs is the excellent detail of the images.
    a. True
    b. False

Apply Your Knowledge

1. After exposing and processing a maxillary premolar radiograph, you notice that the teeth appear unusually short on the film, and the dentist asks you to retake the image. What change will you make when you retake the image?
2. You are preparing to take an FMX on an adult patient. What materials would you set out, and where would you place surface barriers?
3. An 18-year-old patient is scheduled for a prophy and bite-wing films. How many films would is normally prescribed?
4. Recently you noticed that the radiographs have streaks on them when they come out of the automatic processor. What could be the problem?
5. Mrs. Li has been a patient in your office for almost 5 years and is now moving out of the area. Mrs. Li comes into the office and wants her radiographs to take with her. She said she paid for the radiographs and that they belong to her. How would you handle this situation?

CHAPTER 18

Restorative and Esthetic Dental Materials

http://evolve.elsevier.com/Robinson/essentials/

LEARNING OBJECTIVES

1. Pronounce, define, and spell the key terms.
2. Discuss the criteria that must be met before a dental material is brought onto the market.
3. Describe the basic properties required of dental materials to be used within the environment of the oral cavity.
4. Describe amalgam and its importance in dentistry and demonstrate how to mix and transfer dental amalgam.
5. Describe composite resins and their importance in dentistry and demonstrate how to prepare composite resin materials.
6. Complete the following as related to dental liners:
   - Describe dental liners and their importance in dentistry.
   - List the three most commonly placed types of liners.
   - Demonstrate the application of calcium hydroxide and cavity varnish.
7. Discuss etching systems and demonstrate how to apply an etchant material.
8. Discuss bonding systems and demonstrate how to apply a bonding system.
9. Discuss intermediate restorative material and demonstrate the mixing process.
10. Complete the following as related to cements used for restorative dentistry.
    - List the types of dental cements.
    - Discuss the three methods that are used for preparation of a cement product.
    - Demonstrate how to mix zinc oxide-eugenol (ZOE) for a base, temporary cementation, and permanent cementation.
    - Demonstrate how to mix glass ionomer for permanent cementation.
    - Demonstrate how to mix zinc phosphate for a base and permanent cementation.
    - Demonstrate how to mix polycarboxylate for a base and permanent cementation.
11. Describe the use of tooth-whitening products in the esthetic aspect of restorative dentistry.

KEY TERMS

alloy	curing	polymerization
amalgam	etching	retention
amalgamator	exothermic	strain
bonding	force	stress
cements	galvanic	tooth whitening
composite resins	pestle	trituration

Restorative is a term used in dentistry to describe the ability to remove decay or disease from the tooth structure and restore it back to health and its proper function. This can be accomplished by a *direct restoration*, which is a dental restoration completed within the mouth, or by the cementation of an *indirect restoration* (which is further discussed in Chapter 23). **Esthetic** is a term that refers to restoring the tooth or teeth to deliver an artistically attractive appearance.

The types of dental materials used by the general dentist for direct restorative procedures include:

- Amalgam is one of the most affordable and durable restorative materials. Its common name "silver filling" was first introduced in 1826 and was perfected by G.V. Black in 1895.
- Composite resins are the most widely accepted material of choice by dentists and patients because of their natural and esthetic appearance and new advances in their strength.
- Tooth-whitening products provide one of the fastest and most cost-effective ways of restoring the esthetic appearance of teeth.

Supplemental materials that are integrated in restorative procedures to contribute to the health and wellbeing of the tooth include: (1) **cavity liners, cavity sealers, desensitizers, bases, etchants**, and **bonding agents**—which are a variety of materials applied based on the design and need in the restoration process; (2) **temporary restorative materials**— which are selected for a provisional restoration; and (3) cements—which are dental materials that provide a temporary or permanent adhesion for indirect restorations such as inlays, onlays, and crowns and bridges directly to tooth structure.

Characteristics of Dental Materials

When a dental material is introduced to the profession, the product must meet strict guidelines before it can be marketed for use. The Council of Dental Materials, Instruments, and Equipment, a subcommittee of and formed by the American Dental Association (ADA), provides these standards and specifications.

Criteria That Must Be Met Before a Dental Material Is Brought onto the Market

A dental material must:

- *Not* be poisonous or harmful to the body.
- *Not* be harmful or irritating to the tissue of the oral cavity.
- Protect the tooth and oral tissue of the oral cavity.
- Resemble the natural dentition as closely as possible so as to be esthetically pleasing.
- Be easily formed and placed in the mouth to restore natural contours.
- Conform and function, despite limited access, wet conditions, and poor visibility.

Properties Affecting a Dental Material

The oral cavity presents every possible challenge to the dentist when selecting a dental material suitable for the mouth. Table 18.1 provides the basic properties required of dental materials, considering their limitations within the environment of the oral cavity.

TABLE 18.1
Properties of Dental Materials

Property	Description
Mechanical	Involves biting and chewing in the posterior area of the mouth. Mechanical properties include force, which is the biting and chewing, especially in posterior teeth; stress, which is the internal resistance or force that can cause distortion; and strain, which is the change or deformation of a material as the result of stress.
	Types of Stress and Stain
	Tensile stress and strain pull and stretches the material.
	Compressed stress and strain results from two forces pushing toward each other.
	Shear stress and strain occurs when two forces parallel slide in opposite directions.
Ductility and malleability	Involves the measure of a metal's capability to withstand permanent deformation by either tensile or compressive forces.
Thermal change	Involves the temperature changes in the mouth. Thermal changes can cause a dental material to contract and expand, resulting in microleakage of fluid, debris, and microorganisms when the dental material pulls away from the tooth structure.
Electrical	Involves the galvanic current, which can take place with the condition of metals interacting with s aliva.
Corrosive	Involves the corrosive reaction within a metal when it comes into contact with corrosive products. Certain foods and beverages can corrode or discolor metals.
Hardness	Involves the resistance or wearability of an alloy or metal to scratching or abrasion.
Solubility	Involves the degree to which a substance will dissolve in a wet environment.
Application	Involves the four specific steps in the application process: (1) flow of material, (2) adhesion of the material to the tooth, (3) retention to the tooth, and (4) curing of the material.

FIGURE 18.1 Example of class II amalgam restoration. (From Heymann HO, Swift EJ, Ritter AV: *Sterdevant's art and science of operative dentistry,* ed 6, St Louis, 2013, Mosby.)

FIGURE 18.2 The mercury and alloy powder are in their purest forms before trituration. (From Hatrick CD, Eakle WS: *Dental materials: clinical applications for dental assistants and dental hygienists,* ed 3, St. Louis, 2016, Saunders.)

Amalgam

Dental amalgam is a safe, affordable, and durable material predominantly used to restore premolars and molars (Fig. 18.1). The name "amalgam" refers to the end result of mixing approximately equal parts of mercury (43% to 54%) and an amalgam alloy powder (57% to 46%) together (Fig. 18.2).

Composition of Amalgam Alloy Powder

Silver—gives it strength
Tin—gives it workability and strength
Copper—gives it strength and low corrosion
Zinc—suppresses oxidation

Application of Dental Amalgam

Amalgam is supplied by the manufacturer in sealed single-use capsules with the proper ratio of alloy powder in one side of the capsule and mercury in the other side and separated by a thin membrane. The single-use capsule ensures an accurate ratio of alloy powder and mercury and reduces the possibility of exposure to any of the materials. Immediately after use, the capsule is reassembled and discarded with nonregulated waste.

Capsules are available in 600 mg of alloy, which is the appropriate amount of material for a small or single-surface restoration, or 800 mg of alloy, which is used for a larger restoration (Fig. 18.3). If more amalgam is required, then additional capsules are placed with the setup and triturated as needed.

Trituration is the process by which mercury and alloy powders are mixed together to form the mass of amalgam needed to restore the tooth. The preloaded capsule of amalgam alloy and mercury contains a pestle, which aids in the mixing process. Before the capsule is placed into the amalgamator, many types of capsules require the use of an activator, which breaks the separating membrane. The activated capsule is placed in the amalgamator, and the cover is closed to prevent mercury vapors from escaping during trituration. The amalgamator is set to operate for the length of time specified in the manufacturer's directions. Amalgam should appear soft, pliable, and easily shaped when first triturated.

FIGURE 18.3 Precapsulated amalgam.

The amalgam is carried to the tooth by the amalgam carrier and is placed in increments into the prepared tooth, with each increment immediately condensed with the use of an amalgam condenser. The purpose of condensation is to pack the amalgam tightly into all areas of the prepared cavity and to aid in removing any excess mercury from the amalgam mix.

With the use of hand-carving instruments, the dentist is able to carve back the amalgam material to the tooth's normal anatomy, which was removed during cavity preparation.

See Procedure 18.1: Mixing and Transferring Dental Amalgam.

Amalgam Disposal

Dentistry is committed to recycling dental amalgam. To help in that endeavor, the ADA developed "Best Management Practices for Amalgam Waste," a series of amalgam waste handling and disposal practices. The protocol includes the following practices:
- Use amalgam capsules.
- Have disposable chair-side traps.
- Install amalgam separators that are compliant.
- Use vacuum pump filters.

- Inspect and clean traps.
- Collect and recycle amalgam.

Composite Resins

Composite resin is a tooth-colored dental material that is the most widely used material by dentists and the most requested by patients (Fig. 18.4). Early in its use, this material had a composition that made it esthetically pleasing, but it was not able to withstand some of the properties discussed earlier in this chapter. The advantages of this tooth-colored material are that it can (1) withstand the environments of the oral cavity; (2) be easily shaped to the anatomy of a tooth; (3) match the natural tooth color; and (4) be directly bonded to tooth surfaces for strength. The composition of composite resins includes the resin matrix, inorganic fillers, and a coupling agent.

FIGURE 18.4 Class III composite restoration on the mesial surface of tooth #10. (Courtesy Premier Dental Products, Plymouth Meeting, Pennsylvania.)

Composition of Composite Resins
- **Resin matrix** (bisphenol A–glycidyl methacrylate [BIS-GMA])—fluidlike material used to make synthetic resins
- **Inorganic fillers**—quartz, glass, silica, and colorants to add the strength and characteristics necessary for a restorative material
- **Coupling agent**—to strengthen and chemically bond the filler to the resin matrix
- **Pigments**—to give it color

The inorganic fillers within composite materials are classified by particle size as *megafill, macrofill, midfill, minifill, microfill,* and *nanofill*. Some of the newer composites today include a combination of particle sizes, which are termed *hybrid* (Fig. 18.5).

Shade Selection

Color matching is one of the most critical aspects when working with composite resins. If the correct shade is not selected, then the difference will be apparent to the patient after the restoration is in place. The composite kit may include its own shade guide; most manufacturers cross-reference their shades with those of the VITA Shade Guide, which is a universally adopted guide (Fig. 18.6).

Application of Composite Resins

Composite resins are supplied in lightproof syringes, as a paste, or in capsules (Fig. 18.7). The material is supplied in a kit that includes varying shades of the composite resin, along with an etching and bonding system that specifically works for the application process of that material.

Polymerization is the process by which resin material is changed from a pliable state (in which it can be molded or

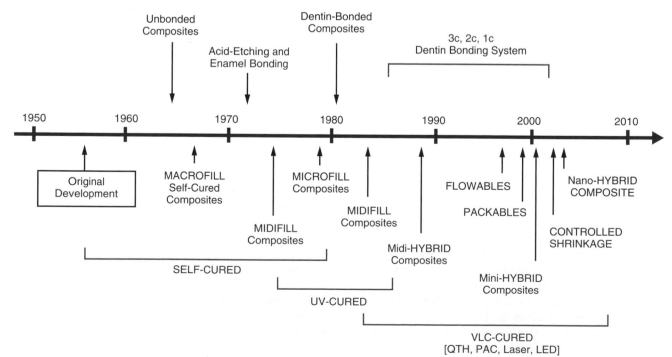

FIGURE 18.5 Summary of the historical evolution of dental composites, curing methods, and accompanying bonding systems. (Courtesy SC Bayne. From Heymann HO, Swift EJ, Ritter AV: *Sturdevant's art and science of operative dentistry,* ed 6, St. Louis, 2013, Mosby.)

FIGURE 18.6 Types of shade guides. (From Boyd LRB: *Dental instruments: a pocket guide,* ed 5, St. Louis, 2015, Saunders.)

FIGURE 18.7 Composite resin kit. Z100 Restorative 3m ESPE. (From Dastin KG: *Dental material pocket guide.* Saunders. 2014. St Louis.)

FIGURE 18.8 Placement of a liner.

shaped) into a hardened restoration. Polymerization occurs through an auto-curing or a light-curing process. Light cured resins do not require mixing and are directly applied from the syringe with the addition of a syringe tip. The paste contains both the photo initiator and the amine activator and will not polymerize until it is exposed to the curing light.

The **light-curing process** uses a high-intensity blue light source that provides an effective curing of resins. The blue light source is a combination of tungsten and a halogen lighting system. The exact curing time depends on the following:

- Composite manufacturer's instructions (most often 20 to 60 seconds)
- Thickness and size of the restoration (When larger quantities of the material are being placed, each increment is cured before the next is placed.)
- Shade of the restorative material used (The darker the shade, the longer the required curing time.)

Finishing and Polishing

The finishing and polishing of composite resins are significantly different from the completion steps in an amalgam procedure.

Because composite materials go from a soft pliable state to being completely hardened by polymerization, the dentist is not able to carve or adjust with hand instruments. Finishing burs and abrasive materials are used to contour and polish a finished composite resin.

See Procedure 18.2: Preparing Composite Resin Materials.

Cavity Liners

As their name implies, a cavity liner is a material that is placed to line the deepest portion of the cavity preparation. Their function is to provide pulpal protection or dentinal regeneration. The health of the tooth and the type of restorative material selected will determine what type of liner should be placed. The most common types of liner are calcium hydroxide and glass ionomer.

Calcium Hydroxide

Calcium hydroxide is a frequently selected cavity liner because of its unique characteristics. Calcium hydroxide (1) helps protect the pulp from chemical irritation, (2) has the ability to stimulate reparative dentin, and (3) is compatible with all types of restorative materials. Calcium hydroxide is supplied as a two-paste and is light cured (Fig. 18.8). Common brands used are Dycal, Hydrox TM, and Life.

See Procedure 18.3: Application of Calcium Hydroxide (Expanded Function).

Glass Ionomer

A resin-modified glass ionomer liner is indicated to form a strong bond to dentin, sealing the restoration to reduce microleakage and help reduce postoperative sensitivity. Examples include vitrebond, Ketac Bond, and Fuji Lining.

Cavity Sealers

Cavity sealers, such as **Varnish**, are materials that consist of one or more natural resins in an organic solvent. Examples include Copalite, Plasodent, and Barrier. Application of a varnish accomplishes the following (Fig. 18.9):
- It seals the dentinal tubules.
- It reduces microleakage around a restoration.
- It protects the tooth from highly acidic cements such as zinc phosphate.

Cavity varnish is contraindicated with composite resins and glass ionomer restorations because of interference with the materials.

Fluoride varnish is a highly effective cavity varnish and desensitizer. This gel-like material is designed to release fluoride on enamel, root structure, and dentin structure.

See Procedure 18.4: Application of Cavity Varnish (Expanded Function).

Desensitizers

A **desensitizer** is a type of sealer used to protect the tooth from hypersensitivity. This material works like a varnish, but the makeup of the product is GLUMA, which acts as a barrier and seals the dentin tubules with hydroxyethyl methacrylate (HEMA) and glutaraldehyde.

Because of the makeup and the toxic element, this material is used sparingly and should not come into contact with soft tissue

Dental Bases

When a tooth preparation becomes moderately deep to deep, placement of a base is necessary before placing the final restoration (Fig. 18.10). This additional layer helps protect the pulp. A base can provide pulpal protection in three ways: as a protective base, as an insulating base, or as a sedative base.

Many of the dental cements that are discussed later in the chapter (zinc oxide-eugenol [ZOE], polycarboxylate, zinc phosphate, and glass ionomer) are used as a base by altering the measurements to the proper consistency.

Dental Etching

Etching, also referred to as a tooth conditioner, is a technique applied to a prepared tooth surface to create a microscopic etched layer (Fig. 18.11). This system was first designed for the preparation of the enamel structure for composite materials and sealants, but research has found that etching a surface of enamel or dentin allows the dental material to have better retention to the tooth surface.

The primary ingredient in an etchant material is a phosphoric or maleic acid. This liquid or gel substance is applied to the enamel or dentin surface for a specified period to form a better chemical bond between the tooth and the permanent restorative material.

See Procedure 18.5: Applying an Etchant Material (Expanded Function).

Dental Bonding

Bonding systems involve a liquid material that flows into the etched surface of a tooth, creating a **micromechanical retention** (Fig. 18.12). This self-cured or light-cured material improves the adherence between the tooth and the permanent restoration.

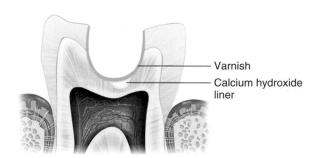

FIGURE 18.9 Placement of a cavity varnish. (Copyright Elsevier Collection.)

— Varnish
— Calcium hydroxide liner

FIGURE 18.10 Placement of a base. (Copyright Elsevier Collection.)

— Cement base
— Calcium hydroxide liner

FIGURE 18.11 Microscopic view of dentin after etching. (From Heymann HO, Swift EJ, Ritter AV: *Sturdevant's art and science of operative dentistry,* ed 6, St Louis, 2013, Mosby.)

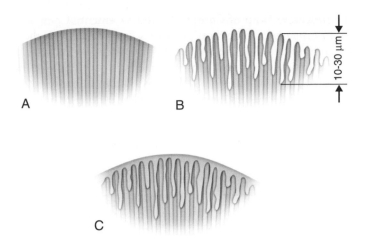

FIGURE 18.12 Process of Bonding. (Copyright Elsevier Collection.)

FIGURE 18.14 Placement of intermediate restorative material into a class II prepared molar.

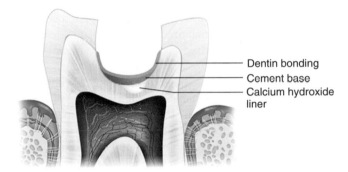

- Dentin bonding
- Cement base
- Calcium hydroxide liner

FIGURE 18.13 Placement of dentin bonding. (Copyright Elsevier Collection.)

Enamel bonding allows for the placement of sealants, orthodontic brackets, resin-bonded bridges, and bonded veneers. **Dentin bonding** allows for the adhesion of another permanent material to the etched tooth structure. A major factor in the success of bonding a material to dentin is the removal of the smear layer. The smear layer is a thin layer of debris that consists of fluids and tooth components that have remained on the dentin after cavity preparation (Fig. 18.13).

See Procedure 18.6: Applying a Bonding System (Expanded Function).

Intermediate Restorative Materials

An intermediate restoration is recommended as a short-term restoration. The dental material most often used is **intermediate restorative material**, also referred to as **IRM**. IRM is a reinforced ZOE material. The eugenol in this material has a sedative effect on the pulp, and fillers are added to improve the strength and durability of the material (Fig. 18.14). Common uses include:

- Temporary restoration
- Restoration of primary teeth
- Caries management
- Placement as a base

See Procedure 18.7: Mixing and Placing Intermediate Restorative Material (Expanded Function).

Dental Cements

Dental cements represent a category of dental materials that are versatile in their use. The ADA has classified dental cements according to their properties and their intended use.

- *Type I cements* are classified as a **luting agent.** This type of cement is designed to act as an adhesive to cement an indirect restoration to the tooth structure or to adhere brackets to the tooth surface during orthodontic treatment. This group includes permanent and temporary cements.
- *Type II cements* involve materials that can be used as a restorative material, such as intermediate restorative material and dental sealants (see Chapter 21).
- *Type III cements* include the liners and bases that are placed within the cavity preparation. These were discussed earlier in the chapter.

Mixing Dental Cements

Dental cements are supplied in various forms: liquid-powder mixes, capsules, and syringes. If using a liquid-powder method, then each type is mixed in a methodical manner. The differences include how the liquid and powder are dispensed and the ratios of liquid to powder.

> **Guidelines for Mixing Dental Cements**
> - Follow the manufacturer's instructions.
> - Measure the powder and liquid according to the manufacturer's instructions.
> - Place the powder toward one end of the glass slab or paper pad and the liquid toward the opposite end. (The space in the middle is for mixing.)
> - Divide the powder into increments. Each manufacturer uses a slightly different system for sectioning the powder. Some divide it into equal parts; others divide the powder into progressively smaller increments. When increment sizes vary, the smaller increments are brought into the liquid first.
> - Incorporate each powder increment into the liquid, and then thoroughly mix. (The mixing time per increment varies.)

Automix Systems

Many types of cements today are supplied in a cartridge where they are automatically mixed as they are expressed onto the pad or directly onto the tooth surface you are working on. The advantages of using an automix system are that it provides an exact measurement of material, easy mix and application, and easy cleanup.

Types of Cements

Glass Ionomer Cements

Glass ionomer cements are one of the most versatile types of cements used in dentistry. It can bond to enamel, dentin, and metallic materials.

Advantages of Glass Ionomer Cement

- Is an acid-soluble calcium fluoroaluminosilicate glass; the slow release of fluoride from this powder inhibits recurrent decay.
- Causes less trauma to the pulp than many other types of cement.
- Has low solubility in the mouth.
- Slightly adheres to moist tooth surfaces.
- Has a very thin film thickness for excellent ease of seating.

Types of Glass Ionomer Cements

Type I cement is used for cementation of indirect restorations

Type II is designed for restoring areas of erosion near the gingival.

Type III is used as a liner and dentin bonding agent.

Type IV is used for pit and fissure sealants.

Type V is used in the cementation of orthodontic bands and brackets.

Type VI is used for the core buildup of a restoration.

During preparation for glass ionomer cementation, the tooth should never be overdried, which can increase postoperative sensitivity. Glass ionomers are available in self-curing and light-cured formulas. They are supplied in powder and liquid, which are manually mixed, or in premeasured capsules, which are triturated. The capsules have the advantages of (1) being more convenient to use, (2) requiring less mixing time, and (3) producing consistent mixes because of the controlled powder-to-liquid ratio.

See Procedure 18.8: Mixing Glass Ionomer for Permanent Cementation.

Composite Resin Cements

A newer classification of cement material is the **composite resin cement,** which has been designed especially for the following indications:

- Ceramic or porcelain inlays, onlays, crowns, and bridges
- Ceramic veneers
- Orthodontic bands
- Direct bonding of orthodontic brackets
- Metal-based crowns and bridges

Chemical Makeup of Composite Resin Cement. Composite resin cements have physical properties comparable with those of composite resins, including thin film thickness and virtual insolubility in the mouth. An important aspect of the selection of composite resin cements is that the tooth must be free of all plaque and debris and must be prepared by etching or by treating the tooth surface with a bonding system before cementation.

Application. Composite resin cements are supplied (1) as a powder and liquid mix, (2) in a syringe-type applicator as a base and catalyst, and (3) in a versatile light-cured/dual-cured system.

See Procedure 18.9: Mixing Composite Resin for Permanent Cementation.

Zinc Oxide–Eugenol Cement

ZOE cement is one of the most versatile cements available. There are four classifications for ZOE based on the makeup of the material and its use.

Type I ZOE (TempBond) is supplied as a two-paste system and is a temporary cement. The material is supplied either in a syringe or as two pastes that are dispensed in equal lengths on a paper pad and then mixed according to the manufacturer's directions.

Type II ZOE is used as a base for permanent cementation of cast restorations or appliances. With a pH level of approximately 7.0, which is less acidic than most other cements, this is one of the least irritating of all dental cements.

Type III ZOE is indicated as a thermal base and for the placement of a temporary restoration (IRM is the brand name) and is prepared and placed in the cavity preparation.

Type IV ZOE is for use as a cavity liner.

See Procedure 18.10: Mixing Zinc Oxide–Eugenol for Temporary Cementation, as a Base, and for Permanent Cementation.

Polycarboxylate Cement

Polycarboxylate cement, also known as *polyacrylic cement,* is used as a luting agent for cast restorations and cementation of orthodontic bands. The material is supplied as a powder and a liquid. Polycarboxylate maintains its versatility as a nonirritating base under composite and amalgam restorations and as an intermediate or temporary restoration.

The liquid is made up of polyacrylic acid and water. The liquid has a limited shelf life because it thickens over time when the water evaporates. If evaporation occurs, then the liquid should be discarded.

See Procedure 18.11: Mixing Polycarboxylate for a Base and Permanent Cementation.

Zinc Phosphate Cement

Zinc phosphate, one of the oldest dental cements in use, can be classified as follows:

Type I (fine grain) zinc phosphate cement is used for the permanent cementation of cast restorations.

Type II (medium grain) zinc phosphate cement is recommended for use as an insulating base for deep cavity preparations.

Zinc phosphate cement is exothermic in action. (**Exothermic** means giving off heat.) To dissipate heat before placing in the casting or in the cavity preparation, the cement must be spatulated over a wide area of a cool, dry, thick glass slab.

The temperature of the glass slab is an important variable in the mixing of zinc phosphate cement. The ideal temperature for the slab is 68°F (20°C). A warmer slab will shorten the setting time of the cement, and a colder slab will increase the setting time. Colder temperatures can cause condensation on the slab, and the moisture can weaken the material.

See Procedure 18.12 Mixing Zinc Phosphate for a Base and Permanent Cementation.

Tooth-Whitening Materials

Tooth whitening has become one of the most popular esthetic dental treatments. Tooth-whitening products are available in everyday items, such as toothpaste, floss, mouth rinses, and even chewing gum. Most tooth-whitening products are made from a peroxide-based ingredient and are supplied in different concentrations (10%, 16%, and 22%). The peroxide-based whitening product works deep within the enamel to remove staining and discoloration that have come from years of accumulated stain and aging. When the peroxide-based product contacts the teeth, it allows oxygen to enter the enamel and then whitens the colored substances. See Chapter 22 for methods of tooth whitening.

Ethical Implications

Preparing and mixing restorative materials must be precise and exact. The dentist expects the clinical assistant to be knowledgeable and experienced with the materials used in the dental office. The dental team is responsible for educating patients about what to expect with a newly placed restoration and how they should feel and care for that restoration.

Procedure 18.1

Mixing and Transferring Dental Amalgam

Equipment and Supplies

- Amalgam capsule
- Capsule activator
- Amalgamator
- Amalgam well or cloth
- Amalgam carrier

2. Place the capsule in the amalgamator.

Procedural Steps

1. Activate the capsule using the activator, if required, for the type of amalgam.
   Purpose: The activator breaks the separating membrane to allow the mercury and alloy powder to mix.

Continued

Mixing and Transferring Dental Amalgam—cont'd

3. Adjust the settings on the amalgamator.
4. Close the cover on the amalgamator and begin trituration.
5. Remove the capsule, twist it open, and dispense amalgam in the well or amalgam cloth.

6. Fill the small end of the carrier first; then transfer the carrier, making sure that the end of the carrier is directed toward the preparation.

7. Transfer the carrier to the operator with the small end facing toward the tooth to be filled.

8. Continue this process until the preparation is overfilled.

Preparing Composite Resin Materials

Equipment and Supplies

- Shade guide
- Composite resin material
- Treated paper pad or material dispenser
- Composite instrument
- 2 × 2-inch alcohol gauze pads
- Curing light

(Courtesy 3M ESPE, St. Paul, Minnesota.)

Preparing Composite Resin Materials—cont'd

Procedural Steps

1. Select the shade of the tooth.
   Purpose: Composites are supplied in varying shades. With the use of a shade guide, select the shade that most closely resembles the patient's natural tooth color.
   Note: Use natural lighting for making this decision. Fluorescent lighting can alter the natural tooth color.
2. Once the shade is selected, prepare the composite syringe or express the amount for the restoration onto the treated pad or in the light-protected well.
   Note: Most often, you will need a very small amount; therefore do not waste the material.
3. Transfer the composite instrument and material to the transfer zone for the dentist.
4. The dentist may ask for the liquid bonding resin or alcohol gauze to be available during the placement of material increments.
   Purpose: These will aid in the flow of material.

5. Have the curing light ready during the placement of the material. The best time to light-cure the material is as the increments are placed.
   Purpose: This step completes the final setting of the material.

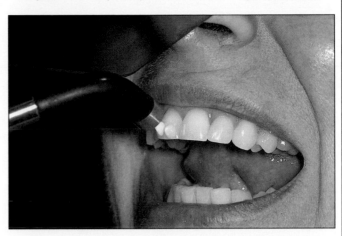

■ ### Procedure 18.3

Application of Calcium Hydroxide (Expanded Function)

Equipment and Supplies

- Small paper mixing pad
- Small spatula
- Calcium hydroxide applicator
- Calcium hydroxide base and catalyst paste (from the same manufacturer)
- 2 × 2-inch gauze pads

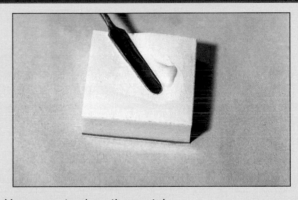

3. Use gauze to clean the spatula.
4. With the tip of the applicator, pick up a small amount of the material, and apply a thin layer at the deepest area of the preparation.
5. Use an explorer to remove any material from the enamel before drying.
6. Clean and disinfect the equipment.

Procedural Steps

1. Dispense small, equal amounts of the catalyst and base pastes onto the paper mixing pad.
   Purpose: The area to be covered will be 0.5 to 1 mm, depending on the size of the cavity preparation.
2. Using a circular motion, quickly mix (10 to 15 seconds) the material over a small area of the paper pad with the spatula.

Application of Dental Varnish (Expanded Function)

Equipment and Supplies

- Microbrush applicators (2)
- Cotton pliers and cotton pellets (2)
- Dental varnish

Procedural Steps

1. Retrieve a new applicator or cotton pellets in cotton pliers.
2. Open the bottle of varnish and place the tip of the applicator or cotton pellet into the liquid.

3. Immediately replace the cap on the bottle.
   Purpose: When varnish is exposed to the air, evaporation causes this liquid to thicken. If it becomes too thick, then a thinning agent must be added.
4. Place a thin coating of varnish on the walls, floor, and margin of the cavity preparation. Allow it to air-dry.
5. Apply a second coat, and repeat steps 1 through 4.

(From Heymann HO, Swift EJ, Ritter AV: *Sturdevant's art and science of operative dentistry,* ed 6, St. Louis, 2013, Mosby.)

Applying an Etchant Material (Expanded Function)

Equipment and Supplies

- Basic setup
- Cotton rolls and/or dental dam for isolation
- Applicator (cotton pellets for liquid etchant and syringe tip for gel)
- Etchant material
- High-velocity evacuator
- Air-water syringe
- Timer

(Courtesy 3M ESPE, St. Paul, Minnesota.)

Procedural Steps

1. The prepared tooth must be isolated from contamination. A dental dam or cotton rolls are placed before the etching process begins.
   Purpose: Saliva must not contaminate the preparation.
2. The surface of the tooth structure must be clean and free of any debris, plaque, or calculus before etching.
   Purpose: Debris on the surface may interfere with the etching process.
3. After cleaning, the surface is carefully dried but is not desiccated.
   Purpose: Too much drying of the tooth structure will harm the tooth.

Applying an Etchant Material (Expanded Function)—cont'd

4. The etchant material is selected. Most manufacturers supply a gel etchant in a syringe that can be applied to enamel or dentin.
   Purpose: The gel allows the etchant to be carefully placed only where needed.

(Courtesy Dr. William Libenberg. From Hatrick CD, Eakle WS, Bird WF: *Dental materials: clinical applications for dental assistants and dental hygienists,* ed 2, St. Louis, 2011, Saunders.)

5. The tooth structure is etched for the time recommended by the manufacturer, usually ranging from 15 to 30 seconds.
   Purpose: The exact time depends on the material and its use. For example, etching time for placing sealants is not the same as etching time for bonding orthodontic brackets.
6. After etching, the surface is thoroughly rinsed and dried for 15 to 30 seconds.
7. An etched surface has a frosty-white appearance. If the surface does not have this appearance or has been contaminated with moisture, then repeat the etching process.

■ **Procedure 18.6**

Applying a Bonding System (Expanded Function)

Equipment and Supplies

- Bonding agent
- Applicator device or brush
- Air-water syringe
- Oral evacuation system
- 2 × 2-inch gauze pads

Procedural Steps

1. If a metal matrix band is used, then the band is prepared with cavity varnish or wax before placing it around the tooth.
   Purpose: This step prevents the bonding resin and amalgam from adhering to the surface (see Chapter 21 for the application of a matrix).

2. The cavity preparation and the enamel margins should be etched according to the manufacturer's directions.
3. A primer is applied to the entire preparation in one or multiple coats, depending on the manufacturer's directions.
4. The dual-cured adhesive resin is placed in the entire cavity preparation and is lightly air-thinned. The resin should appear unset or partially set.

5. The restorative material is mixed and then readied for placement into the cavity preparation.
   Purpose: This step integrates the restorative material and bonding material at the preparation walls before the resin has had time to polymerize (set).

Equipment and Supplies

- Treated paper pad
- Spatula (flexible stainless steel)
- Intermediate restorative materials (IRMs)—powder and dispenser
- IRM liquid and dropper
- 2 × 2-inch alcohol gauze

- Basic setup
- Tofflemire matrix retainer/Matrix band/Wedge (for class II)
- Plastic instrument
- Condenser
- Discoid/cleoid carvers
- Hollenback carver
- Cotton pellet
- Articulating paper

Mixing Material Steps

1. Shake the powder before dispensing, and then measure the powder onto the mixing pad.
   Purpose: When the powder is fluffed, it will not be as packed, thus creating a drier mix.
2. IRM is dispensed in equal ratios, meaning one scoop of powder to one drop of liquid. Make a well in one half of the powder, and then dispense the liquid into the mix. Recap the containers.
3. Incorporate the remaining powder into the mixture in two or three increments, and thoroughly mix with the spatula. The mix will be quite stiff at this stage.
4. Wipe the mix back and forth on the mixing pad for 5 to 10 seconds. The resulting mix should be smooth and adaptable. The mix must be completed within 1 minute.
5. Immediately clean and disinfect the equipment.

Procedural Steps

1. Clean, dry, and isolate the site with cotton rolls or a dental dam.
2. Examine the tooth and preparation, making sure to keep a mental note of the outline of the preparation.
   Purpose: When you begin carving, you need to know how far to carve back to the tooth structure.

3. If the preparation includes a proximal wall, you will need to place the appropriate matrix and wedge for the preparation. (See Chapter 21 for matrix selection and application.)
4. Mix the IRM to the appropriate consistency.
5. Using your plastic instrument (FP-1), take increments of the material to the preparation. If an interproximal box is present, begin filling this area first.
   Purpose: This area is more difficult to see, and material must be packed against the tooth for proper contour.
6. After each increment, condense the material while first using the small end of the condenser.
7. Continue filling the preparation until it becomes overfilled.
   Purpose: You want enough material to be able to carve back to the tooth structure.

Carving Stage

8. If a matrix system was used, use an explorer to run around the matrix band to remove any excess material from the marginal ridge and the proximal box. Remove the matrix at this time, leaving the wedge in place.
9. Remove any excess material from the occlusal surface, using the discoid/cleoid carver.
   Purpose: To keep the interproximal space open for easier carving.
10. Complete the final carving of the occlusal surface with the discoid/cleoid carver, making sure to carve back to the normal anatomy of the tooth.
    Note: Look at the same tooth on the opposite side of the arch for anatomic landmarks.

11. If an interproximal surface was involved, use the Hollenback carver to remove any excess material from the interproximal area, making sure not to create an overhang or indentation in the material.
12. Once carving has been completed, remove the wedge.
13. To check the occlusion, instruct the patient to bite down gently on articulating paper.
14. After the final carving, take a wet cotton pellet and wipe over the restoration.
15. Inform the patient that this restoration is "short term," and instruct them to not chew sticky foods on that side.

Procedure 18.8

Mixing Glass Ionomer for Permanent Cementation

Equipment and Supplies

- Paper mixing pad
- Spatula (flexible stainless steel)
- Glass ionomer powder and dispenser
- Glass ionomer liquid and dropper
- 2 × 2-inch gauze pads

Procedural Steps

1. Dispense the manufacturer's recommended proportion of the liquid on one half of the paper pad.
2. Dispense the manufacturer's recommended proportion of the powder on the other half of the pad; the powder is usually divided into two or three increments.
3. Incorporate the powder and the liquid, following the recommended mixing time. The material should have a glossy appearance.
4. Immediately clean and disinfect the equipment.

Mixing Composite Resin for Permanent Cementation

Equipment and Supplies

- Basic setup
- Etching system
- Cotton pellets
- Applicators
- Bonding system
- Resin cement (supplied in powder/liquid or syringe type)
- Mixing pad
- Spatula
- 2 × 2–inch gauze pads

Procedural Steps

1. Apply etchant to enamel and dentin for 15 seconds, then rinse. Blot excess water with a moist cotton pellet, leaving the tooth moist.
   Purpose: During this procedure, you do not want the tooth completely dry.
2. Apply a bond adhesive to enamel and dentin, then dry gently. Avoid excess adhesive on all prepared surfaces.
3. Light cure each surface for 10 seconds.
4. Apply primer to etched porcelain or roughened metal surfaces. Dry for 5 seconds.
5. Dispense a 1:1 ratio onto a mixing pad; then mix for 10 seconds. Apply a thin layer of cement to the bonding surface of the restoration.

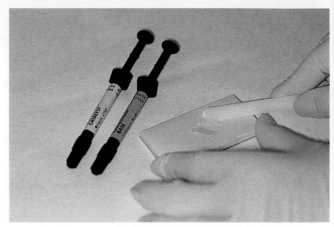

(From Hatrick CD, Eakle WS: *Dental materials: clinical applications for dental assistants and dental hygienists*, ed 3, St Louis, 2016, Elsevier.)

6. Once the crown is seated, margins may be light-cured for 40 seconds or allowed to self-cure for 10 minutes from the start of the mixing.
   Note: For porcelain and precured composite crowns, margins must be light-cured for 40 seconds.

Mixing Zinc Oxide-Eugenol for Temporary Cementation as a Base and for Permanent Cementation

Procedural Steps for Temporary Cementation

1. Measure the pastes onto the mixing pad at equal lengths, approximately ½ inch per unit of restoration.
2. Replace the caps immediately.
3. Incorporate the two pastes together.
4. Mix while wiping the material over an area of the mixing pad.

5. The material should be smooth and creamy and prepared within 20 to 30 seconds.

6. Immediately fill the temporary restoration with the cement.
   Purpose: Because the material has weaker properties than are seen in the permanent cement, fill the provisional rather than line it.
7. Clean and disinfect the equipment immediately.

Procedure Steps for a Base

(From Bird DL, Robinson DS: *Modern dental assisting,* ed 11, St. Louis, 2015, Saunders.)

Mixing Zinc Oxide-Eugenol for Temporary Cementation as a Base and for Permanent Cementation—cont'd

Procedural Steps for Base

1. Measure the powder onto the mixing pad. Immediately replace the cap.
2. Dispense the liquid near the powder on the mixing pad. Immediately replace the cap.
3. Incorporate half of the powder into the liquid and mix with the spatula for 20 to 30 seconds.
4. Incorporate the remaining portion into the mixture. Continue mixing for an additional 20 to 30 seconds. The material should be thick and have a puttylike appearance.

Procedural Steps for Permanent Cementation

1. Measure the powder and place it onto the mixing pad or glass slab. Immediately replace the cap on the powder.
2. Dispense the liquid near the powder. Immediately replace the cap on the liquid container.
3. Incorporate the powder and liquid all at once, and then mix with the spatula for 30 seconds.
4. Initially, the mix is puttylike; with additional mixing for 30 seconds; however, the mix will become more fluid for loading into the casting.
5. Immediately clean and disinfect the equipment.

(From Baum L, Phillips RW, Lund MR: *Textbook of operative dentistry,* ed 3, Philadelphia, 1995, Saunders.)

Mixing Polycarboxylate for a Base and Permanent Cementation

Equipment and Supplies

- Treated paper pad or glass slab
- Spatula (flexible stainless steel)
- Polycarboxylate powder and dispenser
- Polycarboxylate liquid (in plastic squeeze bottle or calibrated syringe)
- 2 × 2-inch gauze pads

Continued

Mixing Polycarboxylate for a Base and Permanent Cementation—cont'd

Polycarboxylate for a Base

Procedural Steps

1. Dispense the powder and liquid onto the pad.
   Note: When used for a base, the liquid portion is decreased to make a thicker consistency.
2. Incorporate all the powder into the liquid; the total mixing time should not exceed 45 seconds.
3. Form the completed mix into a small ball.

Polycarboxylate for Permanent Cement

Procedural Steps

1. Gently shake the powder to fluff the ingredients. Measure the powder onto the mixing pad, and immediately recap the container.
2. Dispense the liquid, and then recap the container.
3. Use the flat side of the spatula to incorporate all the powder quickly into the liquid at one time. The mix must be completed within 30 seconds.
4. A correct mix should be somewhat thick and have a shiny, glossy surface.

5. Immediately clean and disinfect the equipment.

Mixing Zinc Phosphate for a Base and Permanent Cementation

Equipment and Supplies

- Glass slab (cool)
- Spatula (flexible stainless steel)
- Zinc phosphate powder and dispenser
- Zinc phosphate liquid and dropper
- 2 × 2-inch gauze pads

Zinc Phosphate for a Base

Procedural Steps

Dispense the powder and liquid onto the pad.
Note: When used for a base, the liquid portion is decreased to make a thicker consistency.
Incorporate all the powder into the liquid; the total mixing time should not exceed 45 seconds.
Form the completed mix into a small ball.
Ready material for placement

Zinc Phosphate for Permanent Cementation

Procedural Steps

Preparing the Mix

1. Dispense the powder toward one end of the slab and the liquid at the opposite end.
2. Recap the containers.
   Purpose: These materials are damaged by prolonged exposure to air and humidity.
3. Divide the powder into small increments as directed by the manufacturer.

4. Incorporate each powder increment into the liquid.
   Note: When increment sizes vary, the smaller increments are used first. Mixing time per increment also varies; the time is approximately 15 to 20 seconds.
5. Thoroughly spatulate the mix, using broad strokes or a figure-eight movement over a large area of the slab.

Purpose: This step helps dissipate the heat that is generated during mixing.

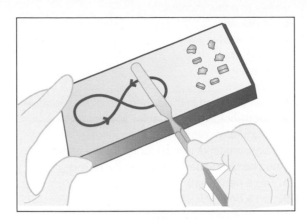

6. Test the material for appropriate cementation consistency. The cement should string up and break approximately 1 inch from the slab. Total mixing time is approximately 1 to 2 minutes.

Placing Cement in the Casting

In addition to preparing and mixing the material, the assistant will have the important responsibility of placing the cement in the casting.

7. Hold the casting with the inner portion facing upward.
8. Retrieve the cement onto the spatula. Scrape the edge of the spatula along the margin to cause the cement to flow from the spatula into the casting.

9. Place the tip of the spatula or a black spoon into the bulk of the cement; move the material so that it covers all internal walls with a thin lining of cement.
10. Turn the casting over in your palm and transfer it to the dentist.

    Purpose: By having the outer portion of the casting facing up, the dentist can safely rotate it to obtain a better grasp for seating it.
11. Transfer a cotton roll so that the patient can bite down on it to help seat the crown and displace the excess cement.
12. Immediately clean and disinfect the equipment.

Multiple Choice

Circle the letter next to the correct answer.

1. Dental cements are versatile in their use. Which method of dental cement can be applied in a restorative procedure?
   a. As a liner
   b. As an insulating base
   c. For permanent cementation
   d. b and c

2. When two metals touch in the mouth, a small shock is created. This shock is known as a _____.
   a. deformation
   b. galvanic action
   c. microleakage
   d. thermal conduction

3. Glass ionomer cement is unique because it can be used as a _____.
   a. base
   b. luting agent
   c. restorative material
   d. a, b, and c

4. Before dentin bonding, the smear layer is removed from the prepared tooth surface by the process of _____.
   a. drying
   b. etching
   c. sealing
   d. varnish

5. The completed mix of polycarboxylate cement should appear _____.
   a. dull
   b. glossy
   c. puttylike
   d. stringy

6. The slow release of fluoride in _____ cements is capable of inhibiting recurrent decay.
   a. zinc oxide–eugenol
   b. IRM
   c. zinc phosphate
   d. glass ionomer

7. When working with light-cured composite resins, the darker the shade of the material, the _____ curing time required.
   a. longer
   b. shorter

8. A(n) _____ restoration is expected to last from a few weeks to a few months.
   a. amalgam
   b. composite resin
   c. temporary
   d. sealant

9. An alloy is a _____.
   a. cement used in the adherence of a restoration
   b. tooth-colored material for anterior teeth
   c. mixture of metals
   d. base material placed for insulating effects

10. Zinc phosphate cement should be mixed _____.
    a. on a paper pad
    b. on a cool, thick glass slab
    c. on a treated paper pad
    d. in an amalgamator

Apply Your Knowledge

1. You are preparing to mix zinc phosphate material for a permanent cementation of a crown. You notice after you have incorporated half of the powder that the cement is starting to thicken. What could have happened? Should you (1) stop mixing and use the mix at this point, (2) keep incorporating all of the powder, or (3) start over?

2. A patient comes in for an emergency appointment because of losing a "filling" and describes discomfort in the tooth. The tooth involved is tooth #4. What treatment could be indicated for this patient until they can be scheduled for a restorative procedure?

3. The patient from the emergency appointment comes back to have a new amalgam restoration placed in tooth #4. Dr. Smith explains that the decay is close to the pulp and that some sensitivity may be felt in the area. What material could the dentist use to decrease the sensitivity for the patient?

CHAPTER 19

Impression Materials and Laboratory Procedures

http://evolve.elsevier.com/Robinson/essentials/

LEARNING OBJECTIVES

1. Pronounce, define, and spell the key terms.
2. Complete the following related to impressions and impression trays:
   - List the three types of impressions obtained.
   - Describe the types of impression trays and their characteristics of use.
3. Discuss various impression materials and their properties, uses, mixing techniques, and applications, and perform the following associated procedures:
   - Alginate impression material.
   - Prepare a mandibular and maxillary preliminary impression.
   - Mix a two-paste final impression material.
   - Prepare an automix final impression material.
4. Describe the importance of a bite registration and its uses in a procedure.
5. List the types of equipment in the dental laboratory
6. List the uses of a diagnostic cast and perform the following procedures:
   - Mix dental plaster.
   - Pour dental models using the inverted-pour method.
   - Trim and finish dental models.

KEY TERMS

alginate	impression	polysulfide
automix	irreversible hydrocolloid	registration
centric	model trimmer	silicone
diagnostic cast	plaster	stone
extrude	polyether	viscosity

There are a variety of dental procedures that will require an impression to be taken of the patient's teeth and surrounding oral tissues. Three types of impressions obtained include:

1. **Preliminary impressions,** which are taken by the dentist or by the expanded function dental assistant (EFDA) or registered dental assistant (RDA). It is indicated for (a) diagnostic models, (b) custom trays, (c) provisional coverage, (d) dental and orthodontic appliances, and (e) pretreatment and posttreatment records (Fig. 19.1).
2. **Final impressions** are taken by the dentist and used to produce the most accurate replication of the tissue and tooth structure for the laboratory technician to make a cast restoration (inlay, onlay, veneer, crown, or bridge; Fig. 19.2).
3. **Occlusal (bite) registrations,** which are taken by the dentist or by the EFDA/RDA to reproduce the occlusal relationship of the maxillary and mandibular teeth when occluded (Fig. 19.3).

Because of the many uses of an impression, there are several types of impression trays and impression materials available. The dental assistant is responsible for knowing the different types of trays and impression materials to set up for the procedure, how the tray is prepared, and how the material is mixed. The dental assistant's role will be to either assist in the procedure or be delegated to take the impression.

Impression Trays

Impression trays are designed for obtaining an accurate impression of the area required. The type of tray selected for a procedure will depend on (1) the dentist's preference and (2) the type of tray that will provide the most accurate result for the type of impression material being used.

FIGURE 19.1 Example of a preliminary impression.

FIGURE 19.3 Example of a bite registration. (Courtesy 3M Dental Products, St Paul, Minnesota.)

FIGURE 19.4 Examples of quadrant, sectional and full arch impression trays.

Impression trays are supplied as **quadrant trays**, which cover one half of the arch; **section trays**, which are suited for the anterior teeth; and **full-arch trays**, which cover the complete arch (Fig. 19.4). Table 19.1 reviews the different types of trays.

Impression Materials

Impression materials are selected because of their unique qualities that allow the dentist to obtain the most accurate reproduction. An impression material is classified according to specific properties:

- **Mechanical property**—Indicates the flexibility of a material. The two types of material are inelastic and elastic. *Inelastic* material is rigid and will fracture when deformed. This type includes impression compounds, impression plaster, and zinc oxide–eugenol (ZOE) impression paste. *Elastic* materials can be deformed and returned to their natural appearance. This type includes alginate, elastomers, and agar.
- **Setting property**—*Irreversible* material indicates that a chemical reaction has occurred and that the material cannot go back to its original state. This type includes alginate, elastomeric impression materials, ZOE impression paste, and impression plaster. A *reversible* material can be altered by temperature and includes agar and impression compounds.

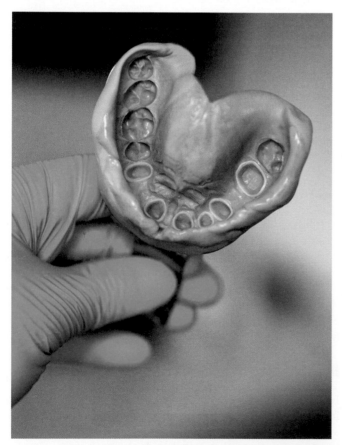

FIGURE 19.2 Example of a final impression. (©iStock.com/ deteetarkan.)

TABLE 19.1
Types of Impression Trays

Type		Characteristics	Use
Perforated tray		A preformed tray made from metal or hard plastic and is supplied in standard sizes for children through adult. The holes allow the impression material to form a mechanical lock with the tray.	Preliminary impressions
Custom tray		The tray is fabricated in the lab from a diagnostic model. Because of the smooth surface, it requires an adhesive to be applied to hold the impression material securely in the tray.	Final impression
Bite registration tray		Is a thin mesh like material that allows the patient to bite normally into the material that is added on both sides.	Bite registration

Continued

TABLE 19.1

Types of Impression Trays—cont'd

Type	Characteristics	Use
Triple tray	Is designed to eliminate steps by taking the final impression and bite registration at the same time.	Final impression and bite registration
 (From Boyd LRB: *Dental instruments: A pocket guide,* ed 5, St. Louis, 2015, Saunders.)		
Vacuum formed tray	Is customized to fit a patient's mouth and made from light-cured resin, acrylic resin, or thermoplastic resin.	Final impression, custom provisional, tooth whitening tray
Water-coolant tray	A metal tray that is attached to a coolant tubing used with reversible hydrocolloid impression material	Final impression
 (Courtesy Dux Dental, Oxnard, California.)		

Types of Impression Materials

Alginate

Alginate is an **irreversible hydrocolloid** (*hydro* meaning *water,* and *colloid* meaning a *gelatinous* substance) and is the material of choice when taking preliminary impressions. The make-up consists of potassium alginate, which is derived from seaweed, calcium sulfate, trisodium phosphate, diatomaceous earth, zinc oxide, and potassium titanium fluoride. Alginate goes through two physical phases during the setting process: a **sol** (solution) phase, during which the material is in a liquid or semiliquid form, and a **gel** (solid) phase, during which the material becomes semisolid.

There are two settings of alginate: **normal set**, which has a working time of 2 minutes and a setting time of up to 4½ minutes, and **fast set**, which has a working time of 1¼ minutes and a setting time of 1 to 2 minutes, which is important when you have a patient that easily gags.

Alginate is supplied as a powder and is packaged in either premeasured packages or in bulk canisters. A plastic scoop is provided for dispensing the powder, and a plastic cylinder is supplied for measuring the water (Fig. 19.5). The water-to-powder ratio for mixing alginate is 1 scoop of powder to 1 *measure line* of water. When mixing the material for a mandibular impression, generally 2 scoops of powder and 2 measure lines of water are required

FIGURE 19.5 Packaging of alginate material.

FIGURE 19.6 A plastic scoop and cylinder are supplied with alginate

(Fig. 19.6). For a maxillary impression, 3 scoops of powder and 3 measure lines of water are necessary.

Most alginate impression materials must be *poured up* within 1 hour of taking the impression—a requirement dictated by the environment. Because much of the material is derived from water, a slight change in its environment can distort the impression and cause **dimensional** change.

An alginate impression is sensitive to its environment; an example would be if you wrapped the impression in a wet paper towel, too much water is introduced, and it could cause the alginate to absorb and expand, causing a condition called **imbibition**. If an alginate impression were to remain in the open air, then moisture would evaporate from the material, causing it to shrink and distort, which is a condition called **syneresis**. The best step to take after taking an impression is to store the disinfected impression in a plastic biohazard bag and cover it with a slightly moistened towel, which will provide an atmosphere close to 100% relative humidity, causing the least amount of distortion.

See Procedure 19.1: Mixing Alginate Impression Material.
Taking alginate impressions. Preliminary impressions are used to create a negative reproduction of the teeth and their surrounding tissues and structures. When an impression is "poured up" in **stone** or **plaster** to make a model, also referred to as a **cast**, you are then creating a positive reproduction of the teeth and their surrounding structures.

It is important for the clinical assistant to be prepared to mix the alginate, load the tray, and help maintain comfort for the patient while taking the impression. If this procedure is a legal function in the state in which you are practicing, then you would proceed to take the impression. Before taking the impression, the procedure should be explained to the patient to ensure their comfort. The patient should be informed that:

- The material will feel cold, have no unpleasant taste, and will quickly set.
- They should breathe deeply through the nose, which will help them to relax and be more comfortable.
- They should not talk after the tray has been placed; if the need to communicate arises, then should do so through hand gestures.

See Procedure 19.2: Taking a Mandibular Preliminary Impression (Expanded Function) and Procedure 19.3: Taking a Maxillary Preliminary Impression (Expanded Function).

Reversible Hydrocolloid

Reversible hydrocolloid materials have the unique physical state that can go from a sol to a gel and then back to a sol. The change in temperature transforms from one physical state to another. A special bath is used to change the consistency of the material for use.

Elastomeric Impression Materials

Elastomeric impression materials are used when an accurate impression is essential. The term elastomeric indicates they have an elastic or rubberlike quality after setting. These materials are supplied as a **base** and **catalyst** and are self-curing.

The types of elastomeric materials commonly used in dental practice are **polysulfide**, **polyether**, **condensation silicone**, and **addition silicone**. Each type of material has different properties and characteristics. Table 19.2 provides a summary of the comparative properties of these materials.

Final impression materials are supplied in three forms or viscosities (**viscosity** is the ability of the material to flow):

1. **Light body** is the easiest-flowing material of the three forms. This material is expressed from a syringe around the tooth and into the sulcus of the prepared tooth or teeth, which provides the detail of the margin that was created by the dentist.
2. **Regular body** and **heavy body**, also referred to as tray-type, is used as a tray material and has the ability to force the light-bodied material into close contact with the prepared tooth and surrounding tissue to ensure a more accurate impression.

TABLE 19.2

Properties of Final Impression Materials

Type	Characteristics	Working Abilities
Polysulfide	A paste material is supplied in two tubes.	Harder material to mix
	A strong odor and taste are associated with the material.	Longer mixing time of 60 seconds
	The stiffness and stability of the material are poor.	Longer setting time of 10–20 minutes
Polyether	A paste material is supplied in tubes or cartridges.	An easy material to mix
	Has an acceptable odor and taste.	Short mixing time of 30–45 seconds
		Fast setting time of 6–7 minutes
Condensation silicone	The material is supplied as a paste and a liquid.	Easy material to mix
	Has an acceptable odor and taste.	Average mixing time of 30–60 seconds
	The stiffness and stability are average.	Average setting time of 6–10 minutes
Addition silicone (also referred to as vinyl polysiloxane)	A paste material is supplied as a two-paste system, as a putty material or cartridges.	Easy material to mix
	Has an acceptable odor and taste.	Short mixing time of 30–45 seconds
	The stiffness and stability are excellent.	Average setting time of 6–8 minutes

Mixing Impression Materials

Impression materials are packaged several ways to accommodate preference of use:

- **Paste system**. The material is supplied in tubes and involves the use of a spatula and paper pad. The catalyst is picked up and spatulated into the base until the material is uniform in appearance. The material is then gathered onto the spatula and loaded into the tray (Fig. 19.7).
- **Automix system**. Provides a homogeneous mix with the appropriate amount of material without waste. The extruder is used to mix and dispense elastomeric impression materials automatically (Fig. 19.8).
- **Table-top or wall-mounted mixing unit**. This unit saves time and mechanically mixes the material and expresses it into the tray (Fig. 19.9).
- **Putty impression material**. Provides the benefits of true putty, including a dense consistency and insertion force than observed with heavy-bodied materials. Because the material

is kneaded in the palms, the material is already warm when it is seated in the mouth.

FIGURE 19.8 Automix impression paste system. (Courtesy Kerr Corporation, Orange, California.)

FIGURE 19.7 Final impression paste system.

FIGURE 19.9 Tabletop impression system. (Courtesy Y-W Chen, University of Washington Department of Restorative Dentistry, Seattle, Washington.)

Sequence of use is an important process to understand when assisting in a final impression procedure. The most common steps include light- and heavy-bodied materials in this sequence:

1. The material is selected by the dentist as determined by the type of procedure.
2. The tooth is isolated using a retraction system (refer to Chapter 23), and the teeth are rinsed and carefully dried.
3. The light-bodied material (most commonly used in a cartridge system with a syringe tip) is placed in the sulcus, and the material is displaced around and over the prepared tooth and onto the surrounding tissue.
4. The impression tray is loaded with the heavy-bodied material and then is seated over the light-bodied material.
5. When the impression materials have reached final set, the impression is removed and inspected for accuracy.
6. The impression is disinfected, placed in a biohazard container or bag, and taken to the laboratory.

See Procedure 19.4: Mixing a Two-Paste Final Impression Material and Procedure 19.5: Preparing an Automix Final Impression Material.

Bite Registration

In addition to having an accurate impression of the prepared teeth, the dentist and the laboratory technician will require an accurate bite registration of the normal centric relationship of the maxillary and mandibular arches. (Centric is when the jaws are closed in a position that produces maximal stable contact between the occluding surfaces of the maxillary and mandibular teeth.)

This relationship is recorded as the **occlusal registration** or **bite registration**. When the casts of the upper and lower jaws are mounted on the articulator, this bite registration is used to establish the proper centric relationship. (An articulator is a device that simulates the movements of the jaws and the temporomandibular joint.)

Bite Registration Materials

Materials used for bite registration have a low flow ability, which allows the material to remain where it is placed. A wax bite or a bite gauze tray with registration material can be used, or the material can be directly extruded on the occlusal surface of the teeth.

Wax Bite Registration

A wax bite registration is used to show the occlusal relationship of the maxillary and mandibular teeth (Fig. 19.10). A baseplate wax is softened for this procedure. When taking a wax bite registration, you should:

- Instruct the patient to practice opening and closing their mouth normally.
- Use a heat source to soften the wax.
- Place the softened wax against the biting surfaces of the teeth.
- Instruct the patient to bite gently and naturally into the wax.
- Allow the wax to cool.
- Carefully remove the wax bite registration to prevent distortion.
- Store with impressions or casts.

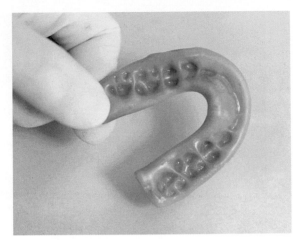

FIGURE 19.10 Wax bite registration.

Bite Registration Paste

Bite registration materials have gained popularity in taking a bite registration because the material:

- Is fast setting.
- Is convenient to use.
- Is supplied as a two-paste system or in cartridges.
- Can be directly applied to the arch or to a gauze tray into which the patient is instructed to bite.
  In addition, the paste has:
- No resistance to biting forces.
- No odor or taste.

Laboratory Procedures

The dental laboratory is a separate area of the dental office (away from the patient treatment area) where the dentist and the clinical staff perform specific procedures away from the patient. When working in the laboratory, safety is the first concern. Following safety precautions and infection control procedures is essential.

The major equipment found in the dental lab include the following:

- Model trimmer
- Specialized spatulas and bowls
- Vacuum former
- Dental vibrator
- Laboratory handpiece with specialized burs
- Articulator
- Dental lathe

Diagnostic Casts

A **diagnostic cast** is the model made from the impression. The material most commonly used to create diagnostic casts are derived from a **gypsum product**. The ADA has classified gypsum into different products because of their chemical property and strength. The two materials most commonly used to create diagnostic casts are model plaster and dental stone.

Model plaster, derived from plaster of Paris, is used when strength is not essential and dimensional accuracy is not critical.

FIGURE 19.11 Dental casts made from plaster.

FIGURE 19.13 Examples of pouring methods. Boxed *(upper left)*; inverted *(upper right)*; double pour *(lower)*.

FIGURE 19.12 Dental cast made from stone. (©iStock/Digender.)

Model plaster is easy to trim and is excellent for diagnostic casts because of its clean appearance (Fig. 19.11).

Dental stone is a form of gypsum and is stronger than model plaster and used when a more durable diagnostic cast is required, such as when used as a working model to make a retainer, a custom tray, or a casting by the laboratory technician (Fig. 19.12).

Water-to-Powder Ratios

Although plaster and dental stone have the same chemical formulas, their physical structures are different, and using specific water-to-powder ratios for each is necessary. The water-to-powder ratio has a dramatic effect on the setting time and strength of any gypsum product. Water is measured by **volume (mL)**, and powder is measured by **weight (g)**.

Each type of cast has an optimal water-to-powder ratio, which is specified by the manufacturer. These ratios should be carefully followed. The following are the recommended water-to-powder ratios for one impression, including the base:

- **Model plaster:** 45 to 50 mL of water to 100 g of powder
- **Dental stone:** 28 to 30 mL of water to 100 g of powder
- **High-strength stone:** 19 to 24 mL of water to 100 g of powder

Influences on Setting Time

Having adequate working time to mix the material and to place it into the impression is important. The setting time is the length of time it takes for the mixture of stone or plaster to turn into a rigid solid. See Procedure 19.6: Mixing Dental Plaster.

Factors Influencing the Setting of Gypsum

Factors	Action and Reaction
Type of gypsum	Model plaster sets faster than dental stone.
Water-to-powder ratio	The less water that is used, the faster the set.
Mixing	The longer and faster the mixing, the faster the set.
Temperature of water	For best results, water should be at room temperature and no warmer than 70°F (21.1°C). The warmer the water, the faster the set.
Humidity	On a humid day, the gypsum can absorb the moisture in the air, which will slow the set.

Pouring Diagnostic Casts

The three methods used for pouring diagnostic casts are: (1) the **double-pour** method, (2) the **box-and-pour** method, and (3) the **inverted-pour** method. These methods differ only in the way the base portion is formed (Fig. 19.13).

See Procedure 19.7: Pouring Dental Models Using the Inverted-Pour Method.

Trimming and Finishing Diagnostic Casts

When diagnostic casts are to be used for a case presentation or as part of the patient's permanent record, they should have an esthetic appearance. This is accomplished by trimming the casts to a geometric standard.

Casts are trimmed using a **model trimmer** (Fig. 19.14). A model trimmer is a device that is set up in the laboratory. The

FIGURE 19.14 Model trimmer.

FIGURE 19.15 Anatomic and art portions of a dental cast.

trimmer has a circular abrasive wheel that is set at 90 degrees to the cast. The wax bite **registration** is used to articulate the casts during the trimming process.

The cast consists of anatomic and art portions (Fig. 19.15).

The **anatomic portion** includes the teeth, oral mucosa, and muscle attachments. This portion should make up two thirds of the overall cast.

The **art portion** forms the base. This section should be no more than ½ inch thick and should make up one third of the overall cast.

See Procedure 19.8: Trimming and Finishing Dental Models.

Procedure 19.1

Mixing Alginate Impression Material

Equipment and Supplies

- Alginate
- Powder measure
- Water measure
- Medium-size rubber bowl
- Beavertail-shaped, wide-blade spatula

Procedural Steps

1. Place the appropriate amount of water in the bowl.
2. Shake the can of alginate to *fluff* the contents. After fluffing, carefully lift off the lid to prevent the particles from flying into the air.

   Purpose: Alginate is fluffed because the material tends to settle and pack down in the can, making the measurement inaccurate. When using preweighed packages, fluffing is not necessary.
3. Sift the powder into the water and use the spatula to mix with a stirring action to wet the powder until it has all been moistened.
4. Firmly spread the alginate between the spatula and the side of the rubber bowl.

Continued

Mixing Alginate Impression Material—cont'd

5. Mix with the spatula for the appropriate time. The mixture should appear smooth and creamy.
   Purpose: Inadequate mixing of alginate causes the mixture to contain air bubbles and a grainy texture, which may produce an unsatisfactory impression.

6. Wipe the alginate mix into one mass on the inside edge of the bowl.

Procedure 19.2

Taking a Mandibular Preliminary Impression (Expanded Function)

Equipment and Supplies

- Alginate powder
- Alginate measure scoop (provided by the manufacturer)
- Water measure (provided by the manufacturer)
- Room-temperature water (Cold water can increase the setting, and warm water can decrease the setting time.)
- Rubber bowl
- Wide-blade spatula
- Sterile impression trays
- Tray adhesive (used on nonperforated trays)
- Utility wax (if the tray needs to be extended)
- Saliva ejector
- Precaution (biohazard) bag

Preparation

1. Gather all necessary supplies.
2. Seat and prepare the patient.
3. Explain the procedure to the patient.
4. Select and prepare the mandibular impression tray.
5. Take 2 measures of room-temperature water with 2 scoops of alginate. Mix as specified in Procedure 19.1.

Loading the Mandibular Impression Tray

1. Gather half of the alginate in the bowl onto the spatula, then wipe alginate into one side of the tray from the lingual side. Quickly press the material down to the base of the tray.
   Purpose: This step removes any air bubbles trapped in the tray.

2. Gather the remaining half of the alginate in the bowl onto the spatula, then load the other side of the tray in the same way.
3. Smooth the surface of the alginate by wiping a moistened finger along the surface.

Seating the Mandibular Impression Tray

1. Place additional material over the occlusal surfaces of the mandibular teeth.
   Purpose: This step places any extra material in the fissures and interproximal surfaces to create less discrepancy in the anatomy of the impression.
2. Retract the patient's cheek with the index finger.
3. Slightly turn the tray sideways when placing it into the mouth.
4. Center the tray over the teeth.

5. First, gently press down the posterior border of the tray.
   Purpose: This step forms a seal.
6. Push down the anterior portion of the tray, and ask the patient to lift the tongue to the roof of the mouth and then to relax it.
   Purpose: This step allows the alginate to form an impression of the lingual aspect of the alveolar process.
7. Instruct the patient to breathe normally while the tray is in place.
8. Observe the alginate around the tray to determine when the material has set.
   Note: When set, the material should not register a dent when pressed with a finger.

Removing the Mandibular Impression

1. First, place your fingers on the top of the impression tray.
   Purpose: This step protects the maxillary teeth from damage during the removal of the mandibular tray.
2. Gently break the seal between the impression and the peripheral tissue by moving the inside of the patient's cheeks or lips with your finger.
3. Grasping the handle of the tray with your thumb and index finger, use a firm lifting motion to break the seal.
4. Snap up the tray and impression from the dentition.
5. Instruct the patient to rinse with water to remove any excess alginate material.
6. Evaluate the impression for accuracy.
7. Rinse, disinfect, wrap the impression in a slightly moistened towel, and place it in the appropriate precaution bag before pouring up.

Equipment and Supplies

- Maxillary tray
- Other equipment and supplies are the same as assembled for a mandibular impression (see Procedure 19.2). If the same bowl and spatula are reused, then make certain they are clean and dry before beginning the next mix. For a maxillary impression, 3 measures of water are mixed with 3 scoops of powder.

Preparation

1. The preparation of the material is the same as performed in Procedure 19.2.

Loading the Maxillary Impression Tray

1. Load the maxillary tray in one large increment, using a wiping motion to fill the tray from the posterior end.
   Purpose: This step helps prevent the formation of air bubbles in the material.

2. Place the bulk of the material toward the anterior palatal area of the tray.
   Purpose: This step prevents the alginate from flowing beyond the tray and into the patient's throat during tray placement.
3. Moisten your fingertips with tap water and smooth the surface of the alginate.

Seating the Maxillary Impression Tray

1. Use your index finger to retract the patient's cheek.
2. Slightly turn the tray sideways to position the tray into the mouth.

3. Center the tray over the patient's teeth.
4. Seat the posterior border (back) of the tray up against the posterior border of the hard palate to form a seal.
   Purpose: This step prevents the excess material from going toward the back of the mouth.
5. Direct the anterior portion of the tray upward over the teeth.
6. Gently lift the patient's lips out of the way as the tray is seated.
   Purpose: Retraction of the lips allows the material to flow into the vestibular areas.
7. Check the posterior border of the tray to ensure that no material is flowing into the patient's throat. If necessary, wipe excess material away with a cotton-tip applicator.
   Purpose: This technique helps prevent triggering the gag reflex when the material touches the soft palate area.
8. Firmly hold the tray in place while the alginate sets.

Removing the Maxillary Impression

1. To avoid injury to the impression and to the patient's teeth, place a finger along the lateral borders of the tray to push down and break the palatal seal.
2. Use a straight, downward snapping motion to remove the tray from the teeth.
3. Instruct the patient to rinse with water to remove any excess alginate impression material.

Caring for Alginate Impressions

1. Gently rinse the impressions under cold tap water to remove any blood or saliva.
   Purpose: Bioburden will interfere with the setting of gypsum products.
2. Spray the impression with an approved disinfectant.
3. If the impression must be stored before pouring, then wrap it in a damp paper towel and store the impression in a covered container or plastic bag labeled with the patient's name.

Before Dismissing the Patient

1. Examine the patient's mouth for any remaining fragments of alginate and remove them using an explorer and dental floss.
2. Use a moist facial tissue to remove any alginate from the patient's face and lips.

Equipment and Supplies

- Stock custom tray with appropriate adhesive
- Large, stiff, tapered spatulas (2)
- Large paper pads (2)
- Light-bodied base and catalyst
- Heavy-bodied base and catalyst
- Impression syringe with sterile tip
- 2 × 2-inch gauze pads

Procedural Steps

Preparing Light-Bodied Syringe Material

1. Dispense approximately 1½ to 2 inches of equal lengths of the base and catalyst of the light-bodied material onto the top one-third of the pad, making sure that the materials are not too close to each other.
   Purpose: Some paste materials tend to start spreading on the pad, and preventing a premature reaction is important.
2. Wipe the tube openings clean with gauze, and immediately recap.
   Purpose: Cleaning the top of the tube and the threads prevents the cap from becoming messy and sticking.
3. Place the tip of the spatula blade into the catalyst and base. Mix in a swirling direction for approximately 5 seconds.
4. Gather the material onto the flat portion of the spatula. Place it on a clean area of the pad, preferably in the center.
   Purpose: By beginning the mix on a clean area of the pad, a more homogeneous mix will be obtained.
5. Smoothly spatulate, wiping back and forth and trying to use only one side of the spatula during the mixing process.
   Purpose: Material is lost by using both sides of the blade.
6. To obtain a more homogeneous mix, pick the material up by the spatula blade and wipe it onto the pad.
   Purpose: The material is pulled from the bottom to the top of the mix.

7. Gather the material together and take the syringe tube and begin *cookie cutting* the material into the syringe. Insert the plunger and express a small amount of the material to make sure it is in working order.

8. Transfer the syringe to the dentist, making sure the tip of the syringe is directed toward the tooth.

Preparing Heavy-Bodied Tray Material

1. Dispense approximately 3 to 4 inches of equal lengths of the base and catalyst of the heavy-bodied material on the top third of the pad for a quadrant tray.
   Note: The amount of material placed depends on whether you are using a quadrant tray or a full-arch tray.
2. Place the tip of the spatula blade into the catalyst and base. Mix in a swirling direction for approximately 5 seconds.
3. Gather the material onto the flat portion of the spatula and place it on a clean area of the pad, preferably in the center.
   Purpose: Starting the mix on a clean area of the pad results in a more homogeneous mix.
4. Smoothly spatulate, wiping back and forth and trying to use only one side of the spatula during the mixing process.
   Purpose: Material is lost by using both sides of the blade.
5. To obtain a more homogeneous mix, pick up the material by the spatula blade and wipe it on the pad.

Continued

Mixing a Two-Paste Final Impression Material—cont'd

Purpose: The material is pulled from the bottom to the top of the mix.

6. Gather the bulk of the material with the spatula and load it into the tray. The best way to complete this step without incorporating air is to use the flat side of the spatula and to follow around the outside rim of the tray, *wiping* the material into the tray.

7. Using the tip of the spatula, evenly spread the material from one end of the tray to the other without picking up the material.

   Purpose: When the material is pulled in an upward direction, air is incorporated into the mixture.

8. Retrieve the syringe from the dentist and transfer the tray, making sure the dentist is able to grasp the handle of the tray properly.

Procedure 19.5

Preparing an Automix Final Impression Material

Equipment and Supplies

- Stock or custom tray with appropriate adhesive
- Extruder units (2)
- Extruder mixing tips (2)
- Light-bodied mixing tip
- Cartridge of light-bodied material
- Cartridge of heavy-bodied material
- 2 × 2-inch gauze pads

(From Hatrick CD, Eakle WS: *Dental materials: clinical applications for dental assistants and dental hygienists,* ed 3, St Louis, 2016, Saunders.)

Procedural Steps

1. Load the extruder with dual cartridges of the base and the catalyst of light-bodied material.
2. Remove the caps from the tube and extrude (force or push out) a small amount of unmixed material onto the gauze pad.

   Purpose: This step ensures that no air bubbles are in the mix and removes any hardened material that might remain.

3. Attach a mixing tip on the extruder along with a syringe tip for the light-bodied application by the dentist.

(Courtesy 3M ESPE, St Paul, Minnesota.)

4. When the dentist signals readiness, begin squeezing the trigger until the material has reached the tip.
5. Transfer the extruder to the dentist, ensuring that the tip is directed toward the area of the impression.
6. The dentist places the light-bodied material over and around the prepared teeth and onto the surrounding tissue.

(Courtesy 3M ESPE, St Paul, Minnesota.)

Preparing an Automix Final Impression Material—cont'd

7. Place the heavy-bodied cartridges in the extruder, making sure to express a small amount (the same as with the light-bodied material). Attach the mixing tip to the cartridge.
8. When the dentist signals readiness, begin squeezing the trigger, mixing the heavy-bodied material.
9. Load the impression tray with the heavy-bodied material, making sure not to trap air in the material.
   Note: Begin expressing the material at one end of the tray, and follow through to the other end without taking the tip out of the material.
10. Transfer the tray, making sure the dentist is able to grasp the handle of the tray.
11. When the impression materials have reached final set, the impression is removed and is inspected for accuracy by the dentist.
12. The impression is disinfected, placed in a precaution bag, labeled with the patient's name, and taken to the laboratory.

(Courtesy 3M ESPE, St Paul, Minnesota.)

Procedure 19.6

Mixing Dental Plaster

Equipment and Supplies

- Flexible rubber mixing bowl (clean and dry)
- Metal spatula (stiff blade with a rounded end)
- Scale
- Plaster (100 g)
- Water-measuring device
- Room-temperature water (70°F)
- Vibrator with a disposable cover

4. Add the powder to the water in steady increments. Allow the powder to settle into the water for approximately 30 seconds.
   Purpose: This step prevents the trapping of air bubbles.
5. Use the spatula to incorporate the powder slowly into the water. A smooth and creamy mix should be achieved in approximately 20 seconds.
   Purpose: This step helps avoid spilling the powder.

Procedural Steps

1. Measure 45 mL of room-temperature water into a clean rubber mixing bowl.
2. Place the paper towel on the scale and make necessary adjustments.
3. Weigh out 100 g of dental plaster.

6. Turn the vibrator to low or medium speed and place the bowl of plaster mix on the vibrator platform.
   Purpose: This step helps reduce the air in the mix.
7. Lightly press and rotate the bowl on the vibrator. Air bubbles will rise to the surface.
8. Complete mixing and vibration of the plaster for no longer than 2 minutes.

Equipment and Supplies

- Maxillary and mandibular impressions
- Glass slab or tile
- Laboratory spatula
- Laboratory knife and cutters
- 150 g of plaster (additional plaster is needed for the base)
- 60 mL of water (additional water needed for the base)
- Flexible rubber bowl
- Vibrator

Procedural Steps

Preparing the Impression

1. Use a gentle stream of air to remove excess moisture from the impression. Be careful not to dry out the impression.
   Purpose: Overdrying can cause distortion of the material.
2. Use your laboratory knife or laboratory cutters to remove any excess impression material that will interfere with the pouring of the model.

Pouring the Mandibular Model and Base

1. Mix the plaster and then set the vibrator at low to medium speed.
   Note: A separate mix is made for each impression.
2. Hold the impression tray by the handle and place the edge of the base of the handle on the vibrator.
3. Dip the spatula into the plaster mix, picking up a small increment (approximately ½ teaspoon).
4. Place the small increment in the impression near the most posterior tooth. Guide the material as it flows lingually.
   Purpose: The flowing action pushes out the air ahead of it and eliminates air bubbles.

5. Continue to place small increments in the same area as the first increment and allow the plaster to flow toward the anterior teeth.
6. Turn the tray on its side to provide the continuous flow of material forward into each tooth impression.
7. Once all of the teeth in the impression are covered, begin to add larger increments until the entire impression is filled.

8. Place the additional material onto a glass slab (or tile); shape the base to approximately 2 × 2 inches by 1 inch thick.
   Note: Commercial rubber molds are available for making bases. These molds provide symmetry to the cast and reduce the need for trimming.

Pouring Dental Models Using the Inverted-Pour Method—cont'd

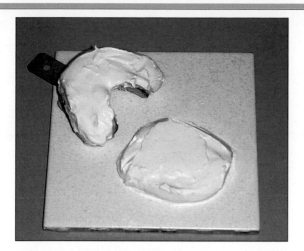

9. Invert the impression onto the new mix. Do not push the impression into the base.
   Purpose: When the poured impression is inverted onto the new mix, the fresh material tends to flow excessively, which can result in a base that is too large and too thin.
10. Holding the tray steady, use a spatula to smooth the plaster base mix up onto the margins of the initial pour. Be careful not to cover the impression tray with material; otherwise, removing the cast from the impression will be difficult.

Pouring the Maxillary Cast

1. Repeat steps 3 through 5, using clean equipment for the fresh mix of stone.

2. Place the small increment of plaster in the posterior area of the impression. Guide the material as it flows down into the impression of the most posterior tooth.
3. Continue to place small increments in the same area as the first increment and allow the plaster to flow toward the anterior teeth.
4. Rotate the tray on its side to provide the continuous flow of material into each tooth impression.
5. Once all the teeth in the impression are covered, begin to add larger increments until the entire impression is filled.
6. Place the mix onto a glass slab (or tile) and shape the base to approximately 2 × 2 inches by 1 inch thick.
   Note: Commercial rubber molds are available for making bases. These molds provide symmetry to the cast and reduce the need for trimming.
7. Invert the impression onto the new mix. Do not push the impression into the base.
   Purpose: When the poured impression is inverted onto the new mix, the fresh material tends to flow excessively, which can result in a base that is too large and too thin.
8. Holding the tray steady, use a spatula to smooth the stone base mix onto the margins of the initial pour. Be careful not to cover the impression tray with plaster; otherwise, removing the cast from the impression will be difficult.
9. Place the impression tray on the base so that the handle and the occlusal plane of the teeth on the cast are parallel with the surface of the glass slab (or tile).
   Purpose: This step helps form a base with uniform thickness.

Separating the Cast from the Impression

1. Wait 45 to 60 minutes after the base has been poured before separating the impression from the model.
   Purpose: The material needs to complete its initial setting stage, or teeth could fracture while removing the impression.
2. Use the laboratory knife to separate the margins of the tray gently.
3. Apply firm, straight, and upward pressure on the handle of the tray to remove the impression.
4. If the tray does not easily separate, then check to see where the tray is still attached to the impression. Again, use the laboratory knife to free the tray from the model.
5. Pull the tray handle straight up from the model.
   Note: Never wiggle the impression tray from side to side while it is on the cast. This movement can cause the teeth on the cast to fracture.
6. The models are ready for trimming and polishing.

Equipment and Supplies

- Poured stone maxillary and mandibular dental model
- Wax bite registration
- Pencil
- Ruler
- Laboratory knife
- Model trimmer

Procedural Steps

Preparing the Model

1. Soak the art portion of the model in a bowl of water for at least 5 minutes.
   Purpose: Soaking the art portion makes the trimming easier.

Trimming the Maxillary Model

1. Place the maxillary model on a flat countertop with the teeth setting on the table. Use your pencil to measure up 1¼ inches from the counter and draw a line around the model.

2. Turn on the trimmer. Firmly hold the model against the trimmer and trim the bottom of the base to the drawn line.
3. Draw a line ¼ inch behind the maxillary tuberosities. With the base flat on the trimmer, remove excess plaster in the posterior area of the model to the marked line.
4. To trim the sides of the model, draw a line through the center of the occlusal ridges on one side of the model. Measure out ¼ inch from this line and draw a line parallel to the previous drawn line.
   Note: If you need to measure beyond ¼ inch to ensure that the mucobuccal fold is not trimmed away, do so.
5. Repeat these measurements on the other side of the model.
6. Trim the sides of the cast to the lines drawn.

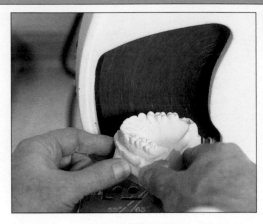

7. Draw a line behind the tuberosity that is perpendicular to the opposite canine, and trim to the drawn line. This step completes the maxillary heel cuts.
8. The final cut is made by drawing a line from the canine to the midline at an angle. Complete this on both sides, and trim to the drawn line.

Trimming the Mandibular Model

1. Occlude the mandibular model with the maxillary model using the wax bite.
2. With the mandibular base on the trimmer, trim the posterior portion of the mandibular model until it is even with the maxillary model.
3. Place the model's upside down (maxillary base on the table), measure 3 inches from the surface up, and mark a line around the base of the mandibular model.
4. Trim the mandibular model base to the drawn line.

5. With the models in occlusion with the wax bite, place the mandibular model on the trimmer and trim the lateral cuts to match the maxillary lateral cuts.
6. Trim the back and heel cuts to match the maxillary heel cuts.
7. Check that the mandibular anterior cut is rounded from the mandibular right canine to the mandibular left canine.
8. The models are now ready to be finished.

Finishing the Model

1. Mix a slurry of gypsum and water and fill in any voids.
2. Using a laboratory knife, remove any extra gypsum that occurs as beads on the occlusion or model.

Multiple Choice

Circle the letter next to the correct answer.

1. A maxillary alginate impression routinely requires _____ scoops of powder.
   a. 1
   b. 2
   c. 3
   d. 4

2. Diagnostic casts can be used by the dentist and the laboratory technician for _____ cases.
   a. orthodontic
   b. endodontic
   c. prosthodontic
   d. a and c

3. The light-bodied final impression material is most commonly applied to the prepared tooth using a _____.
   a. tray
   b. syringe
   c. crown form
   d. spatula

4. The dentist is taking a final impression specifically for tooth #24. The _____ tray design would be selected for this procedure.
   a. quadrant
   b. section
   c. full arch
   d. b or c

5. When an extruder unit is used, the impression material is actually mixed _____.
   a. on a paper pad first
   b. within the cartridges
   c. in the mixing tip
   d. in the tray

6. An acceptable diagnostic cast should be trimmed for a case presentation. The best way to trim the cast is to use _____.
   a. a slow-speed handpiece with a laboratory bur
   b. hand instruments
   c. sandpaper discs
   d. a laboratory model trimmer

7. The water-to-powder ratio for model plaster for a single cast and its base is 100 g of powder to _____ mL of water.
   a. 45 to 50
   b. 55 to 65
   c. 65 to 75
   d. 75 to 80

8. Before diagnostic casts are trimmed, the casts should be _____.
   a. set in a warm environment
   b. soaked in water
   c. placed in the refrigerator
   d. blown dry

9. A procedure that is used to replicate a patient's occlusion is a(n) _____.
   a. wax bite
   b. alginate
   c. bite registration
   d. a and c

10. When mixing a final impression paste material on a pad, incorporate the _____ into the _____.
    a. base; catalyst
    b. catalyst; base
    c. paste, liquid
    d. alginate; water

Apply Your Knowledge

1. You are assisting the dentist in taking a final impression of the upper-right quadrant for a single crown. You are using an automix system of impression material. While loading the tray, you notice that the cartridge has run out of material. What should you do?

2. The dentist has asked you to take an impression on the patient in the next room and to pour the models for an orthodontic consultation. Which type of impression can you legally take, and what material will you use to pour the impression?

3. The dentist is running behind schedule and has to get to the next patient. He asks you to go ahead and take the final impression on tooth #5. Is this your role in the procedure? If so, what steps do you take? If not, how do you handle this situation?

CHAPTER 20

Preventive Care

http://evolve.elsevier.com/Robinson/essentials/

KEY TERMS

active learning
biofilm
calculus
demineralization
dental decay
disclosing agents
fluoride

fluoride varnish
fluorosis
interdental aids
MyPlate
oral biofilm
plaque
preventive dentistry

remineralization
sodium fluoride
stannous fluoride
systemic fluorides
topical fluorides
white spot

The goal of **preventive dentistry** is to achieve and maintain optimal oral health for a lifetime. Through a comprehensive oral health program and a partnership between the patient and dental team, optimal oral health can become a reality for everyone.

Table 20.1 provides the five components of a comprehensive preventive dentistry program.

Process of Dental Disease

The interrelationship between the removal of biofilm, calculus, and good oral health is important for the patient to understand to maintain a healthy mouth. To educate patients effectively, you must first understand how dental diseases occur and how preventive dentistry is effective in reducing these occurrences.

TABLE 20.1

Comprehensive Preventive Dentistry Program

Preventive Measure	Description
Patient education	Education motivates patients, provides them with information, and assists them in developing the skills necessary to practice good oral hygiene.
Biofilm control	Daily removal of bacterial biofilm (plaque) from the teeth and adjacent oral tissue is the goal.
Fluoride therapy	Includes professionally applied fluorides, at-home fluoride therapy, and consumption of fluoridated community water.
Nutrition	Dietary counseling extends beyond limiting sugar consumption and includes a discussion of nutrition from the standpoint of oral health and general health.
Sealants	Resin-based material applied to occlusal surfaces of the primary and permanent teeth to prevent decay-causing bacteria from reaching into occlusal pits and fissures. (Chapter 21 discusses sealants.)

Bacterial Dental Biofilm

Bacterial dental **biofilm** (also known as **plaque** or **oral biofilm**) is a sticky, soft deposit of bacterial colonies that adhere to the teeth. Plaque biofilm naturally forms as soon as 1 hour after brushing. Biofilm forms on both supragingival and subgingival surfaces of a tooth. **Supragingival** biofilm is above the gingival margin, and **subgingival** biofilm is below the gingival margin. Plaque that remains on the teeth can harden and become *calculus* or *tartar*. The bacteria found in biofilm are the primary cause of **dental caries** and **periodontal disease**.

Stages in the Formation of Biofilm

I. *Pellicle formation*—The pellicle is a thin layer of glycoproteins from the saliva that forms on tooth surfaces and restorations. It reforms on the teeth within minutes after brushing and/or polishing. It serves to keep the tooth surfaces moist and may even provide a barrier against acids in biofilm.

II. *Bacteria attaches to the pellicle*—Bacteria colonize within the pellicle and begin to grow and multiply and produce acids. Organisms in the first few hours are gram-positive cocci and rods (see Chapter 5).

III. *Bacteria multiply and mature*—The longer the biofilm remains on the teeth, the greater the numbers and types of bacteria. Eventually *Streptococcus mutans* and *S. sanguinis* dominate the colonies. These bacteria are primarily responsible for dental caries and periodontal disease.

Dental Caries

Dental caries, also known as **dental decay**, occurs when the bacteria in the biofilm convert sugar from the foods we eat into acid. As the biofilm continues to attack the tooth, the area can turn into areas of caries (decay; Fig. 20.1).

FIGURE 20.1 A, Early carious lesion or white spot of demineralization. **B**, Overt carious lesions. **C**, Rampant caries. (**A**, Courtesy Dr. John D. **B**. Featherstone, School of Dentistry, University of San Francisco; **B** and **C**, Courtesy Dr. Frank Hodges, Santa Rosa, California.)

Demineralization and Remineralization

Demineralization is the loss of minerals (calcium, phosphorus, and fluoride), causing a breakdown of the enamel. The earliest sign of demineralization appears as a **white spot** on the tooth, which is actually the early lesion (Fig. 20.2).

When biofilm is present, the teeth are exposed to tooth acid formed by bacteria within the biofilm. These acid attacks cause demineralization.

Remineralization is the reverse process. Minerals are restored to the tooth surface that has been demineralized. When early remineralization occurs, the white spot hardens and may even be harder than the enamel around it. If the carious lesion has progressed too far, however, then remineralization cannot halt the process, and the tooth must be restored by a dentist. Fluoride itself cannot remineralize tooth structure, but it acts as a catalyst to repair damaged enamel by using calcium, phosphorus, and fluoride from the saliva.

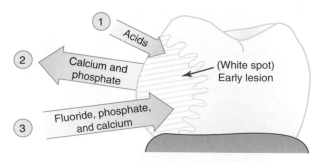

1. The tooth is attacked by acids in plaque and saliva.
2. Calcium and phosphate dissolve from the enamel in the process of demineralization.
3. Fluoride, phosphate, and calcium reenter the enamel in a process called remineralization.

FIGURE 20.2 Process of caries development.

Dental Calculus

Dental **calculus** is mineralized bacterial biofilm that forms a hard mass on the surface of natural teeth and on dentures and other dental prostheses. Calculus occurs at every age and on both primary and permanent teeth. Calculus plays an important role in periodontal disease. The rough surface of the subgingival calculus holds the disease-causing bacterial biofilm close to the gingival tissue, continuing the inflamed state of the tissue (Fig. 20.3).

Periodontal Disease

Periodontal disease can range from **gingivitis** (inflammation of the gingivae) to **periodontitis** (inflammation of the supporting tissues of the teeth). Dental biofilm is the primary cause of periodontal diseases. Periodontal diseases are discussed further in Chapter 24.

Home Care Techniques

Once the patient is motivated to want to learn and use skills to remove **biofilm** correctly, the dental professional will work with the patient to develop a program of oral hygiene that the patient will routinely follow at home. The goal of the program is to thoroughly remove biofilm at least once daily. After it has been thoroughly removed, it takes approximately 24 hours for biofilm to form again. Many home care techniques are used for biofilm removal; the technique selected must be based on the needs and abilities of the individual patient.

Patients can keep plaque under control by brushing, flossing, and using interdental cleaning aids. The dental hygienist and dental assistant can work with the patient to develop a program of oral hygiene strategies to be followed routinely at home.

Brushing

Toothbrush Selection

Choosing the size and style of a toothbrush depends on age and personal preference. The two basic types of toothbrushes are manual and powered (Fig. 20.4). The dental professional will assess the patient's needs and recommend the toothbrush and brushing method best suited to the individual patient.

Many styles of head size, tuft shape, and handle angle and shape are available (Fig. 20.5). Soft-bristled brushes are recommended for use because they are less likely to cause damage to the soft tissue or any exposed cementum or dentin. Soft bristles also adapt to the contours of the tooth better. Toothbrushes should be replaced as soon as the bristles show signs of wear, which is generally every 8 to 12 weeks.

Many people find using a powered toothbrush is easier than using a manual toothbrush. Powered toothbrushes today offer oscillating, pulsating, and cupping power for plaque removal. Powered toothbrushes are also beneficial for physically challenged individuals who are unable to manage a manual brush.

FIGURE 20.3 Heavy calculus deposits on the lingual surfaces of the lower anterior teeth. (Courtesy Dr. Edward J. Taggart, San Francisco, California.)

FIGURE 20.4 Example of a manual toothbrush and powered toothbrush. (From Newman M. Takei T, Klokkevold P, et al., eds: *Carranza's clinical periodontology,* ed 12, St Louis, 2015, Saunders.)

FIGURE 20.5 Examples of manual toothbrush designs. (Copyright iStock.com/undefinedundefined.)

FIGURE 20.6 Improper brushing techniques can result in abrasion *(arrows)* of the tooth surface, causing gingival recession. (Courtesy Dr. Robert Meckstroth.)

How Often to Brush

There is no single answer when patients ask, "How often should I brush?" The answer is based on complete biofilm removal rather than on the number of brushings.

To control bacterial biofilm and to prevent halitosis (bad breath), at least two brushings and flossing are recommended each day. Bacteria thrive in warm, moist, dark environments; therefore the mouth should be cleaned before going to bed at night. The longer the bacteria remain undisturbed, the more damaging the biofilm becomes. It is suggested that children use a timer to ensure that adequate time is spent brushing.

Tooth Brushing Precaution

The patient should be cautioned about the damage that can be caused by vigorously scrubbing the teeth. Over time, hard scrubbing can cause abnormal abrasion (wear) of the tooth structure, gingival recession, and exposure of the root surface (Fig. 20.6).

Oral Hygiene for 0 to 5 Years

Good oral health begins at birth. Even before the baby teeth have erupted, the parent should wipe the gums with a clean wet cloth after each feeding. As soon as the first teeth erupt, the parent can begin brushing in morning and before bedtime. A pea size of toothpaste can be used but then wiped off after. The first dental visit should occur by their first birthday.

Toothbrushing Techniques

Several brushing techniques are commonly used, but the **Bass method** (named after Dr. C. Bass, a pioneer in preventive dentistry) is the most commonly recommended technique (Table 20.2). This method is highly effective in removing biofilm directly beneath the gingival margin. The gingival margin is most important in controlling gingival inflammation. *Note:* Adding a rolling stroke after sulcular brushing modifies the Bass technique.

TABLE 20.2
Bass Method of Sulcular Brushing

Positioning the toothbrush	Place the toothbrush with the bristles directed straight into the gingival sulcus. The brush should be placed at a 45-degree angle to the long axis of the tooth.
Strokes	Press lightly so that the tips of the bristles go into the sulcus and embrasures. Vibrate the brush back and forth with very short strokes. Count at least 10 vibrations. Then reposition the brush over the next two or three teeth.

Continued

TABLE 20.2

Bass Method of Sulcular Brushing—cont'd

Cleaning the occlusal surfaces	Place the bristles on the occlusal surface and move the brush in back-and-forth or small circular motions.
Cleaning the lingual surfaces	Hold the brush in a vertical position and use gentle back-and-forth strokes.

Figure of positioning the toothbrush from Newman MG, Carranza FA: *Carranza's clinical periodontology,* ed 12, St. Louis, 2015, Saunders. Figures of cleaning occlusal and lingual surfaces from Carranza FA Jr: *Glickman's clinical periodontology,* ed 8, Philadelphia, 1996, WB Saunders.

Disclosing Agents

Because biofilm can be difficult to see, some people find it easier to learn tooth brushing and other biofilm removal techniques with the aid of a disclosing agent. **Disclosing agents** temporarily color the biofilm (usually red) to make it visible and therefore easier to remove (Fig. 20.7).

Disclosing agents are artificially sweetened and come as tablets or are formulated in a solution that is wiped over the teeth using a cotton-tip applicator. All ingredients in the tablet or solution are nontoxic and harmless if swallowed. Nevertheless, they stain clothing, so be careful with their use.

Instructions for Use of Disclosing Tablets

- A disclosing agent will temporarily color the tongue and gingivae along with the biofilm. In addition, the acquired pellicle will appear as a pale-stained surface sheen.
- Instruct patient to chew the tablet and swish the resulting solution around in the mouth for at least 30 seconds.
- Spit the excess liquid into a bowl of running water.
- Rinse the mouth with plain, cool water. Red remaining on the teeth indicates biofilm, which must be removed.
- After the biofilm has been removed, any remaining stain on the tissue will soon be rinsed away by the saliva.

Brushing the Tongue

Bacteria on the tongue must also be removed by brushing. The easiest method is to place the toothbrush at the back of the tongue and sweep forward several times across the dorsum (top) of the tongue.

Care of the Toothbrush

When brushing is completed, the toothbrush should be thoroughly rinsed to remove excess water. The toothbrush should then be placed in a position with good air circulation to permit air-drying.

Flossing

Removing biofilm from between the teeth is a critical part of good oral health. Dental floss is the most effective tool to use to remove biofilm from between the proximal surfaces of the teeth and reduce interproximal bleeding.

Dental floss comes in several different types: waxed or unwaxed, thick or extra fine, or even in a tufted texture that changes shape when tightened. Research has shown no difference in the effectiveness of waxed or unwaxed floss for removing biofilm. It depends on how well the dental floss is used.

Dental floss is also available in various colors and flavors. Even though colored and flavored dental flosses are no more

FIGURE 20.7 Dental biofilm made visible with a disclosing agent.

FIGURE 20.8 The dental assistant helps the patient with flossing.

FIGURE 20.9 Types of interdental aids. Interproximal cleaning devices include (**A** and **B**) wooden tips, (**C–F**) interproximal brushes, and (**G**) rubber-tip stimulator. (From Newman M, Takei T, Klokkevold P, et al., eds: *Carranza's clinical periodontology,* ed 12, St. Louis, 2015, Saunders.)

effective in removing biofilm, they may motivate patients, especially children, to floss more routinely (Fig. 20.8). The choice of dental floss is based on the patient's manual skills, needs, and preferences.

See Procedure 20.1: Assisting the Patient with Dental Floss (Expanded Function).

Toothpaste

Toothpaste contains ingredients designed to remove food residue with additional abrasives to remove stain. Most brands of toothpaste contain fluoride along with flavoring agents to give the mouth a fresh and clean feeling.

Today you can find toothpastes that are formulated as tartar control to help prevent calculus and stain, for sensitive teeth, and with chemical ingredients to help teeth look whiter.

Mouth Rinses

A mouth rinse does not replace tooth brushing and flossing, but it can be helpful as an addition to a person's daily oral hygiene. There are two types of mouth rinses that a patient would use: one provides a freshness from bad breath and the other is a therapeutic agent that can help reduce or control plaque, gingivitis, and tooth decay.

Mouth rinses are not recommended for children younger than 6 years of age because gargling reflexes are not developed and because the alcohol content in some rinses could cause an adverse event.

Oral Irrigation Devices

Oral irrigators, also known as "water picks," deliver a pulsating stream of water or a chemical agent through a nozzle to the teeth and gingiva to reduce plaque, control gingivitis, prevent gum bleeding, and improve bad breath. Using an oral irrigator can benefit patients with gum disease, implants, orthodontic appliances, and patients who are unable to floss.

Interdental Aids

Special **interdental aids** are recommended for cleaning between teeth with large or open interdental spaces (Fig. 20.9). These devices may be used in addition to dental floss but are not a substitute.

Interdental Aids

- **Interproximal brushes** are small brushes inserted between the teeth from the facial side and are moved with short back-and-forth strokes. This process is repeated from the lingual side.
- **Rubber and wooden-tip stimulators** are used to remove interproximal biofilm and to provide gingival stimulation.
- **Floss holder** makes flossing easier for individuals who have arthritis or poor manual dexterity or for those patients who believe their hands are too large.
- **Floss threader** is used to remove biofilm and debris from under fixed bridges and orthodontic appliances.

Fluoride

Fluoride is the primary defense used to combat dental caries. It is a naturally occurring mineral found in many forms. It may be present in our water, in the food we eat (which has absorbed fluoride from the soil), and as additives in many different products we use. Fluorides are effective in strengthening enamel, and when present in the outer layers of the enamel, the tooth is more resistant to demineralization and is resistant to dental decay.

Benefits of Fluoride

- Prevents demineralization
- Helps early lesions to remineralize
- Hardens tooth structure
- Increases enamel resistance

To achieve the maximum benefits of fluoride, an ongoing supply of both systemic and topical fluoride must be available throughout life.

Systemic fluorides, also known as dietary fluorides, are those consumed in water, foods, beverages, or supplements.

Topical fluorides are directly applied to the teeth in the form of fluoridated toothpaste, fluoride mouth rinses, and topical applications.

Safe Use of Fluoride

Fluorides added to the public water supply and present in dental products carry little or no risk when used as directed. Fluoride is beneficial in small amounts, but it can be harmful if instructions for use are not followed.

Long-term overexposure to fluoride, even at low concentrations, can result in dental fluorosis in children younger than 6 years of age who have developing teeth. (Fluorosis appears as white spots on the teeth. These spots do not weaken the teeth and are primarily a cosmetic problem.)

Children should always be supervised when brushing or using fluoride rinses and should not be allowed to swallow fluoride toothpaste or fluoride rinses.

It is important for any dental professional responsible for the application of fluoride to know how much fluoride they are giving to patients.

Sources of Systemic Fluoride

Fluoridated Water

Since 1945, hundreds of cities have started community water fluoridation; in 2016 nearly 73% of the United States had access to fluoridated water, with efforts to fluoridate additional communities ongoing.

In 2010 the US Department of Health and Human Services (DHHS) convened a panel of scientists from across the US government to review new information related to fluoride intake and to develop new recommendations for community water fluoridation.

These scientists reviewed the best available information on prevalence and trends in dental caries, water intake in children in relation to outdoor air temperature, changes in the percentages of US children and adults with dental fluorosis, and new assessments by the US Environmental Protection Agency (EPA) examining cumulative sources of fluoride exposure and the risks of children developing severe dental fluorosis. This new information led DHHS to propose changing the recommended level for community water systems to 0.7 milligrams per liter.

Levels of fluoride in controlled water fluoridation are so low that the danger of ingesting an acutely toxic quantity of fluoride from fluoridated water is nonexistent. Nevertheless, some communities have water that naturally contains more than twice the optimum level of fluoride. Prolonged exposure to these excessive amounts may cause dental fluorosis.

Other Dietary Sources

Foods and Beverages. Because many processed foods and beverages are prepared with fluoridated water, they must be considered as sources of dietary fluoride. In children who regularly drink them, processed juices and juice-flavored drinks can be a major source of dietary fluoride.

Prescribed Dietary Fluoride Supplements

Dietary fluoride supplements in the form of tablets, drops, or lozenges may be prescribed by the dentist for children ages 6 months to 16 years who live where no source of fluoridated water is available. Before prescribing, the dentist will take the following factors into consideration:
- Fluoride level of the child's drinking water
- Child's exposure to multiple water sources (e.g., a child whose home water source is not fluoridated but who attends a daycare center or a school in a fluoridated area)
- All potential sources of fluoride (e.g., many juices and prepared foods for young children)

The parents and patient must be willing to cooperate on an ongoing basis because supplementation is recommended until 16 years of age.

Topical Fluoride

Topical fluoride application is an essential part of a comprehensive dental preventive program. Stannous fluoride and sodium fluoride are effective in reducing dental decay. Topical fluorides are available in forms that are self-applied by the patient and in professionally applied formulations (Table 20.3).

TABLE 20.3
Types of Self-Applied Fluorides

Type	Form	Comments
Sodium fluoride (NaF) 0.24%	Dentifrices (gel or paste)	Approved by the American Dental Association (ADA).
Sodium monofluorophosphate (Na_2PO_3F) 0.76%	Dentifrices (gel or paste)	Is approved by the ADA.
Neutral NaF 0.025%	Mouth rinse	Is sold over the counter without a prescription.
Neutral NaF 0.20%	Mouth rinse	A prescription is required.
NaF 1.1%	Brush-on gel	Is not intended for use as a dentifrice; the teeth must be brushed first, then the gel is used.
Stannous fluoride (SnF_2) 0.4% in glycerin base	Brush-on gel	Is not intended for use as a dentifrice; the teeth must be brushed first, then the gel is used.

Types of Self-Applied Fluoride

Fluoride-Containing Toothpastes

Toothpastes containing fluoride are the primary source of topical fluoride. A major benefit of this fluoride is that the brushing action brings it into close contact with the surfaces of the teeth. Daily brushing with fluoride-containing toothpaste benefits patients of all age groups. Children younger than 6 or 7 years should be carefully supervised because ingestion of fluoride-containing toothpaste may cause dental fluorosis and nausea (Fig. 20.10).

Fluoride Mouth Rinses

Fluoride mouth rinses are most effective when used after brushing and flossing. Over-the-counter nonprescription rinses are designed to be used on a daily basis (Fig. 20.11). Prescription rinses are often used for their antibiofilm properties. Rinses containing stannous fluoride are effective in reducing dental hypersensitivity (sensitivity of the teeth).

Mouth rinses containing fluoride may be recommended as an additional source of topical fluoride for high-risk patients.

Brush-On Fluoride Gel

Brush-on gels are available with and without prescriptions. High-risk patients may use these at home by brushing them on the teeth or by applying them at home with a reusable custom tray.

FIGURE 20.10 Children younger than 8 years of age should be carefully supervised while they are brushing to ensure that all areas of their teeth have been thoroughly cleaned and that they do not swallow fluoride-containing toothpaste. (From Bird DL, Robinson DS: *Modern dental assisting,* ed 11, St. Louis, 2015, Saunders.)

The patient is instructed to use the tray at bedtime. A small amount of the brush-on gel is placed in the tray, and the tray is placed over the teeth for the amount of time recommended by the manufacturer.

If water in the area is fluoridated, then the patient is instructed to rinse and spit to prevent consuming excess fluoride. If the water in the area is not fluoridated, then the patient is told not to rinse after the application.

Professional Topical Fluoride Applications

Professional topical fluoride applications may be recommended for some children soon after the eruption of permanent teeth and for some patients at high risk for dental decay. Professionally applied topical fluoride may be performed by the dentist, the hygienist, or a qualified dental assistant.

1-Minute Versus 4-Minute Applications

Although the most benefit of fluoride occurs in the first minute, research shows that the full 4 minutes provides the best topical benefit.

The American Dental Association (ADA) states that "... *there are considerable data on caries reduction for professionally applied topical fluoride gel treatments of 4 minutes or more. In contrast, there is laboratory, but no clinical equivalency data on the effectiveness of 1-minute fluoride gel applications.*"

Upon examining current information on this topic, dental professionals need to determine whether professional topical fluoride applications are appropriate for all their patients, based on the caries risk factors.

See Procedure 20.2: Applying a Topical Fluoride Gel or Foam (Expanded Function).

Fluoride varnish is a concentrated topical fluoride within a resin or synthetic base that is painted on the teeth to prolong fluoride exposure (Fig. 20.12). Fluoride varnish is a complement to other fluoride treatments and can be applied instead of a fluoride gel at least twice a year for children up to age 18.

See Procedure 20.3: Applying Fluoride Varnish (Expanded Function).

FIGURE 20.11 Samples of over-the-counter 0.04% sodium fluoride rinses with the American Dental Association Seal of Acceptance. (**A**, Courtesy Chattem, Inc., Chattanooga, Tennessee. **B**, Courtesy Colgate Oral Pharmaceuticals, New York, New York.)

FIGURE 20.12 Fluoride varnish with tricalcium phosphate. (Photo Courtesy 3M, St. Paul, Minnesota.)

Nutrition

The study of nutrition is the science of how the body uses food for development, growth, repair, and maintenance. **Nutrients** are the components of food that are needed by the body. Good nutrition depends on an adequate supply of the nutrients that are effectively used by the body.

All nutrients are available through a well-balanced diet. Each nutrient has a specific role, and one nutrient cannot perform the functions of another. For optimal health, the foods we eat must meet our nutrient requirements and energy needs.

Every 10 years the US Department of Health and Human Services provides science-based *Health People* reports that describe goals and objectives for improving the health of all Americans.

Essential Nutrients

There are six essential nutrients the body cannot make on its own or in enough quantity for proper health and maintenance. These nutrients are vital for good health, growth, and disease prevention.

Carbohydrates

These foods provide energy, especially for your central nervous system and brain and protect you against disease. They should make up 45% to 65% of total daily calories. The type of carbohydrate you eat matters. Choose, grains, lentils, and fiber-rich vegetables and fruits over refined grains and products with added sugar.

Proteins

Proteins are essential for good health. These foods provide the building blocks of the body, which includes every cell, from bone to skin to hair. Meat, fish, and eggs are good sources, but you can also get protein from plant sources like lentils, soy, nuts, and some grains.

Fats

Healthy fats are an important part of a healthy diet. Fat supports many of the body's functions, such as vitamin and mineral absorption, blood clotting, building cells, and muscle movement. The most important types of fats for good health are unsaturated fats such as omega-3 and omega-6 fatty acids, which include nuts, seeds, fish, and vegetable oil.

Vitamins

Vitamins are vital for combating disease and staying healthy. Each vitamin plays an important role in the body and is essential for healthy vision, skin, and bones. There are 13 essential vitamins that the body needs to function properly (Table 20.4).

TABLE 20.4
Vitamins: Best Sources, Primary Functions, Deficiency Symptoms and Toxicity

Vitamin[a]	Sources	Functions	Deficiency Symptoms[b]	Toxicity
Vitamin A (carotene)	Yellow or orange fruits and vegetables, green leafy vegetables, oatmeal, liver, dairy products	Formation and maintenance of skin, hair, and mucous membranes; sight in dim light; bone and tooth growth	Night blindness, dry scaly skin, frequent fatigue	Toxic in high doses, although beta-carotene is nontoxic
Vitamin B1 (thiamine)	Cereal, oatmeal, meat, rice, pasta, whole grains, liver	Release of energy from carbohydrates, growth, and metabolism	Heart irregularities, fatigue, nerve disorders, mental confusion	Not toxic; high doses excreted by kidneys
Vitamin B2 (riboflavin)	Whole grains, green leafy vegetables, organ meats, milk, eggs	Release of energy from proteins, fats, and carbohydrates	Cracks in corners of mouth, rash, anemia	No toxic effects reported
Vitamin B6 (pyridoxine)	Fish, poultry, lean meats, bananas, prunes, dried beans, whole grains, avocados	Building of body tissue, metabolism of proteins	Convulsions, dermatitis, muscular weakness, skin cracks, anemia	Possible nerve damage in hands and feet from long-term mega doses

TABLE 20.4

Vitamins: Best Sources, Primary Functions, Deficiency Symptoms and Toxicity—cont'd

Vitamin[a]	Sources	Functions	Deficiency Symptoms[b]	Toxicity
Vitamin B12 (cobalamin)	Meats, milk products, seafood	Cell development, nervous system functioning, metabolism of proteins and fats	Anemia, nervousness, fatigue	No toxic effects reported
Biotin	Cereal/grain products, yeast, legumes, liver	Metabolism of proteins, fats, and carbohydrates	Nausea, vomiting, depression, hair loss, dry scaly skin	No toxic effects reported
Folate (folic acid, folacin)	Green leafy vegetables, organ meats, dried peas, beans, and lentils	Genetic material development, red blood cell production	Gastrointestinal disorders, anemia, cracks on lips	Some evidence of toxicity in large doses
Niacin	Meat, poultry, fish, cereal, peanuts, potatoes, dairy products, eggs	Metabolism of proteins, fats, and carbohydrates	Skin disorders, diarrhea, indigestion, general fatigue	Physician's care for nicotinic acid form
Pantothenic acid	Lean meats, whole grains, legumes, vegetables, fruits	Release of energy from fats and carbohydrates	Fatigue, vomiting, stomach distress, infection, muscle cramps	No toxic effects reported
Vitamin C (ascorbic acid)	Citrus fruits, berries, vegetables, peppers	Structure of bone, cartilage, muscle, and blood vessels; maintenance of capillaries and gums; absorption of iron	Swollen or bleeding gums, slow wound healing, fatigue, depression, poor digestion	Nausea, cramps, and diarrhea with 1 g or more
Vitamin D	Fortified milk/margarine, butter, eggs, fish, sunlight	Bone and tooth formation; maintenance of cardiac and nervous system function	*Children:* rickets and other bone deformities	Diarrhea and weight loss possible with high intake
			Adults: calcium loss from bones	
Vitamin E	Multigrain cereals, nuts, wheat germ, vegetable oils, green leafy vegetables	Protection of blood cells, body tissues, and essential fatty acids	Muscular wasting, nerve damage, anemia, reproductive failure	Relatively nontoxic
Vitamin K	Green leafy vegetables, fruit, dairy, and grain products	Blood clotting	Bleeding disorders in newborns and patients taking blood-thinning medications	Not toxic as found in food

[a]Specifics for each vitamin (recommended intakes and tolerable upper intake levels) vary by life-stage group and are available through the individual Dietary Reference Intake (DRIs) products developed by the Food and Nutrition Board of the Institute of Medicine and published by the National Academies Press. For more information, visit www.nap.edu.

[b]Many of these symptoms can also be attributed to problems other than vitamin deficiency. If you have these symptoms and they persist, see your physician.

Minerals

Much like vitamins, minerals help support the body. They are essential for building strong bones and teeth, maintaining a healthy blood pressure, regulating your metabolism, and remaining hydrated. Table 20.5 provides the sources, primary functions, and deficiency symptoms and toxicity.

Water

Approximately 62% of your body is water. Water is crucial for brain function; as a lubricant for your body; and to help carry nutrients to cells, hydrate the body, and flush out toxins. Besides just drinking water, a diet of fruits and vegetables can be a source.

Cariogenic Foods

Any food that contains sugars or carbohydrates that can be metabolized by bacteria in biofilm is described as being cariogenic. (*Cariogenic* means producing or promoting dental decay.)

A major factor in determining the carcinogenicity (ability to cause dental caries) of a carbohydrate is how long the food remains in the mouth. Refined carbohydrates such as candy and other sweets are cariogenic (caries producing) because their sugars are readily available.

Sugary liquids such as soft drinks quickly leave the mouth and are not as cariogenic as sticky foods that stay in the mouth longer. Foods such as crackers, although not sweet, are cariogenic

TABLE 20.5

Minerals: Best Sources, Primary Functions, Deficiency Symptoms, and Toxicity

Mineral[a]	Sources	Functions	Deficiency Symptoms[b]	Toxicity Symptoms
Calcium (Ca^{2+}, Ca^{++})	Milk and milk products, green leafy vegetables, soy products, sardines, salmon	Muscle and nervous system function, blood coagulation, bone and tooth formation	Poor bone growth and tooth development	Kidney stones
			Children: dental caries, rickets	
			Adults: soft and brittle bones	
Chloride (Cl^-)	Salt, fish, vegetables	Fluid and acid-base balance, activation of gastric enzymes	Growth retardation, psychomotor deficits, memory loss	Disturbances in acid-base balance
Magnesium (Mg^{2+}, Mg^{++})	Dark green vegetables, nuts, soybeans, whole grains, bananas, apricots, seafood	Bone and tooth formation, protein synthesis, lipid metabolism	Rare except in disease states: confusion, hallucinations, poor memory, muscle weakness, cramps	Drowsiness, weakness, lethargy Severe: skeletal paralysis, respiratory depression, coma, death
Phosphorus (PO_4)	Milk and milk products, eggs, meats, legumes, whole grains	Bone and tooth formation, energy metabolism, acid-base balance	*Malabsorption (rare):* anorexia, weakness, stiff joints, fragile bones	Muscle spasms
Potassium (K^+)	Milk and milk products, apricots, oranges, bananas, greens, meats, legumes	Fluid and acid-base balance, transmission of nerve impulses, enzyme reactions	Impaired growth, hypertension, bone fragility, central nervous system changes	Hyperkalemia (excess potassium in blood), cardiac disturbances
Sodium (Na^+)	*Major:* salt (sodium chloride) *Minor:* milk, vegetables	Acid-base balance, cell membrane permeability, impulse transmission	Weight loss, central nervous system abnormalities	Hypertension, leading to cardiovascular and kidney diseases
Chromium (Cr^{3+})	Liver, whole grains, cheese, legumes	Enzyme activation, glucose removal	Weight loss, central nervous system abnormalities	Inhibited insulin activity
Copper (Cu^{2+}, Cu^{++})	Shellfish, liver, nuts, whole grains, raisins	Red blood cell production, lipid metabolism	Anemia, bone fragility, impaired immune response	Neuron and liver cell damage from copper accumulation
Fluorine (F^-)	Foods cooked in fluoridated water, fish, gelatin	Bone and tooth formation	Increased susceptibility to caries	Fluorosis, mottling of teeth
Iodine (I^-)	*Major:* iodized salt *Minor:* fish, seaweed, vegetables	Energy metabolism, normal cell functioning	Goiter, cretinism (infants of iodine-deficient mothers)	Minimal toxic effect with normal thyroid functioning
Iron (Fe^{3+})	Organ meats, cereals, green leafy vegetables, whole grains	Hemoglobin formation, growth and development	Iron deficiency anemia, behavioral changes	Cirrhosis, diabetes, pigmentation, joint pain
Manganese (Mn^{2+})	Nuts, whole grains, vegetables and fruits, coffee, tea, cocoa, egg yolk	Normal bone structure, reproduction, normal functioning of cells and central nervous system	None observed in humans	Iron deficiency anemia through inhibiting effect on iron absorption; pulmonary changes, anorexia, apathy, impotence, headache, leg cramps, speech impairment; resembles Parkinson's disease at advanced stages of toxicity

TABLE 20.5

Minerals: Best Sources, Primary Functions, Deficiency Symptoms, and Toxicity—cont'd

Mineral[a]	Sources	Functions	Deficiency Symptoms[b]	Toxicity Symptoms
Selenium (Se)	Protein-rich foods (meat, eggs, milk), whole grains, seafood, liver and other meats, egg yolks, garlic	Part of an enzyme system; acts as an antioxidant with vitamin E to protect the cell from oxygen	Keshan disease (a human cardiomyopathy) and Kashin-Bek disease (an endemic human osteoarthropathy)	Physical defects of the fingernails and toenails, hair loss
Zinc (Zn^{2+})	Whole grains, wheat germ, crabmeat, oyster, liver and other meats, brewer's yeast	Involvement in protein synthesis; essential for normal growth and sexual development, wound healing, cell division and differentiation, smell acuity	Depressed immune function, poor growth, dwarfism, impaired skeletal growth, delayed sexual maturation, acrodermatitis	Severe anemia, nausea, vomiting, abdominal cramps, diarrhea, fever, hypocupremia (low blood serum copper), malaise, fatigue

[a]Specifics for each mineral (recommended intakes and tolerable upper intake levels) vary by life-stage group and are available through the individual Dietary Reference Intake (DRIs) products developed by the Food and Nutrition Board of the Institute of Medicine and published by the National Academies Press. For more information, visit www.nap.edu.

[b]Many of these symptoms can also be attributed to problems other than mineral deficiency. If you have these symptoms and they persist, see your physician.

because they stick to the teeth and remain in the mouth long enough to be broken down into sugars that can be used by the bacteria in biofilm.

Complex carbohydrates such as fruits and vegetables are less cariogenic because they leave the mouth before they are converted into simple sugars.

Dietary Guidelines

The dietary guidelines issued by the US Department of Agriculture (USDA) are important in helping find ways to reduce the rates of death and disease related to obesity, diabetes, cardiovascular disease, cancer, and other chronic illnesses.

Dietary Guidelines for Americans

Eat a variety of foods. Food contains combinations of nutrients and a varied diet, in the recommended proportions, will ensure an adequate supply of the key nutrients.

Maintain a healthy weight. Food intake should be balanced with exercise to maintain optimal health.

Choose a diet with plenty of grain products, vegetables, and fruits. These foods are important because they are a good energy source and provide a variety of nutrients and fiber.

Choose a diet low in fat, saturated fat, and cholesterol. Less than 30% of your daily caloric intake should come from fats. (Remember, fats have 9 calories per gram!)

Use sugars in moderation. Sugars primarily provide empty calories that can contribute to weight gain, and sugars are associated with dental disease. When calculating sugar intake, remembering that 4 grams equals a teaspoonful of sugar is helpful.

Use salt and sodium in moderation. In some people, salt is associated with hypertension (high blood pressure) and other health problems. Many processed foods have a high sodium content.

If you drink alcoholic beverages, do so in moderation. In addition to its intoxicating characteristics, alcohol contains 7 empty calories per gram.

MyPlate

In 2011 the USDA unveiled the most current government's new food icon, **MyPlate** (Fig. 20.13). "MyPlate" can be found on food packaging and is used in nutrition education in the United States. The MyPlate icon emphasizes the fruit, vegetable, grain, protein, and dairy food groups. Understanding these guidelines is important when planning your own dietary intake and in providing nutrition counseling to your patients. The MyPlate icon is simple and designed to help consumers think about building a healthy plate at mealtimes and to help them seek more information to plan their own dietary intake.

The MyPlate icon depicts a place setting with a plate and glass divided into five food groups. MyPlate is divided into sections of approximately 30% grains, 30% vegetables, 20% fruits,

FIGURE 20.13 MyPlate. United States Department of Agriculture, Choose MyPlate.

and 20% protein, accompanied by a smaller circle representing dairy, such as a glass of low-fat or nonfat milk or a yogurt cup.

MyPlate makes recommendations, such as "Make half your plate fruits and vegetables," "Switch to 1% or skim milk," "Make at least half your grains whole," and "Vary your protein food choices." The guidelines also recommend portion control while still enjoying food, as well as reducing sodium and sugar intakes.

Visit www.ChooseMyPlate.gov and browse from a special audience, such as children, students, adults, families, or professionals, and in 21 languages.

Preventive Dental Care

Patient Education

Patient education in oral health is the responsibility of all members of the dental health care team. Beginning with the initial examination, patient education is provided at every visit. An oral health program is based on motivation and education.

Motivation

The dental health professional should work with the patient to increase their motivational level so that the patient wants to learn and is willing to do the things necessary to achieve and maintain oral health. The lower the patient's level of motivation, the less their chance of success with an oral hygiene program.

The first step is to help the patient recognize a specific dental related need to be resolved. Then it is necessary for the patient to be willing to accept a role in solving the problem. As an example, the patient may not know that improper tooth brushing can damage the teeth and gums. Once the patient recognizes the problem and is willing to change their behavior, they will be more motivated to learn how to use proper techniques.

Education

Oral health education is not a lecture. It is listening more than talking and involves more problem solving than instruction. It is creating an awareness for the patient of the need to return regularly for professional prophylaxis, examination, and treatment. It is helping parents recognize the importance of preventive steps, such as the placement of sealants and the use of fluorides. It is counseling to increase the patient's awareness of the role of nutrition in achieving optimal dental and general health. In your role as a dental health educator, you must be enthusiastic about helping others achieve optimal oral health.

Acceptance

The patient can learn when they feel safe, accepted, and respected. Encouragement is freely given, and correction is structured in a positive manner. Most importantly, the patient is never scolded, embarrassed, or teased because of their ignorance or errors.

Active Learning

The most productive form of learning occurs when the patient is actively participating in the process, using as many of their senses as possible. Teaching biofilm control is an ideal situation for active learning.

Active Patient Education

- Establish open communication and a safe learning environment.
- Listen to the patient's concerns regarding their oral health.
- Jointly decide on an oral hygiene regimen.
- Present the skills to be learned one at a time and as simply as possible. When possible, use visual aids, such as disclosing tablets, to clarify the point.
- Give the patient an opportunity to practice new skills; for example, provide a toothbrush and guide the patient as they practice using a new brushing technique.
- Provide reinforcement and encouragement until the patient has mastered these skills; for example, use a disclosing tablet to demonstrate that all of the biofilm has been removed.
- Listen to the patient regarding their understanding of the information.
- Encourage the patient to continue these new actions at home until the desired habit pattern has been formed.

▪ Ethical Implications

Dental health professionals are concerned not only with treating oral diseases but also with preventing them. A comprehensive dental treatment plan must include a plan for disease prevention that consists of nutritional counseling, patient education, biofilm control, fluoride therapy, and dental sealants when indicated.

Prerequisites for Performing This Procedure

- Infection control protocol
- Patient communication skills
- Understanding of tooth morphologic form and structure
- Understanding of oral anatomy
- Manual dexterity

Equipment and Supplies

- Hand mirror for patient
- Dental floss

Procedural Steps

Preparing the Floss

1. Cut a piece of floss approximately 18 inches long. Wrap the excess floss around the middle fingers of both of your hands, leaving 2 to 3 inches of working space exposed.

2. Tightly stretch the floss between your fingers and use your thumb and index finger to guide the floss into place.
3. Tightly hold the floss between the thumb and forefinger of each hand. These fingers control the floss, and they should be no farther than 12 inches apart.

Flossing the Teeth

4. Gently pass the floss between the patient's teeth, using a sawing motion. Guide the floss to the gumline. Do not force or snap the floss past the contact area.
   Purpose: The floss may cut or injure the tissue.
5. Curve the floss into a C shape against one tooth. Gently slide it into the space between the gingiva and the tooth. Use both hands to move the floss up and down on one side of the tooth.
   Purpose: This step demonstrates how to remove biofilm from difficult-to-reach proximal areas.

6. Repeat these steps on each side of all the teeth in both arches, including the posterior surface of the last tooth in each quadrant.
7. As the floss becomes frayed or soiled, move a fresh area into the working position.
   Note: This procedure is described as it would be performed by the patient at home.

Documentation

DATE	PROCEDURE	OPERATOR
	Provided flossing demonstration and instruction. Patient practiced technique and did well.	DLB

Photos from Bird DL, Robinson DS: *Modern dental assisting*, ed 11, St. Louis, 2015, Saunders.

Prerequisites for Performing This Procedure

- Infection control protocol
- Patient communication skills
- Knowledge of oral anatomy
- Moisture control techniques

Equipment and Supplies

- Fluoride gel or foam
- Disposable trays of appropriate sizes
- Saliva ejector
- Cotton rolls
- Air-water syringe
- Timer

Procedural Steps

Selecting the Tray

1. Select a disposable tray that is the appropriate size for the patient's mouth. The tray must be long and sufficiently deep to cover all erupted teeth completely without extending beyond the distal surface of the most posterior tooth.

Purpose: Trays are available in sizes to fit primary, mixed, and adult dentition. If the patient's mouth can accommodate it, then you may use a double-arch tray, which saves time by simultaneously treating both arches. Remember, trays are discarded after a single use, and if you try a tray in the mouth but do not use it, then that tray must also be discarded.

Preparing the Teeth

2. Check to see whether calculus is present; if it is not, then no preparation is required.
   Purpose: Fluoride easily diffuses through the acquired pellicle and bacterial biofilm.
3. If calculus is present, then request that the dentist or dental hygienist remove it.
   Purpose: Calculus prevents fluoride from reaching the enamel of the tooth.
   Note: The presence of biofilm will not affect the uptake of fluoride.

Applying the Topical Fluoride

4. Seat the patient in an upright position and explain the procedure.
   Purpose: Having the patient upright prevents the gel from going into the throat.
5. Instruct the patient not to swallow the fluoride.
6. Select the appropriate tray and load it with a minimal amount of fluoride, following the guidelines according to the patient's age.
   Reminder: Containers that are handled with gloved hands during the appointment should be surface-disinfected during treatment room cleanup.

Applying a Topical Fluoride Gel or Foam (Expanded Function)—cont'd

7. Dry the teeth using air from the air-water syringe.
   Purpose: For fluoride to be maximally effective, the teeth must be dry when the fluoride is applied.

8. Insert the tray and place cotton rolls between the arches. Ask the patient to bite up and down gently on the cotton rolls.
   Purpose: This step allows the fluoride to be squeezed over all the tooth surfaces.
9. Promptly place the saliva ejector and tilt the patient's head forward.
   Purpose: This step prevents the patient from swallowing the fluoride.
10. Set the timer for the appropriate amount of time in accordance with the manufacturer's instructions. During this time, do not leave the patient unattended.

11. On completion, remove the tray but do not allow the patient to rinse or swallow. Promptly use the saliva ejector or the high-volume oral evacuator tip to remove excess saliva and solution. Do not allow the patient to close the lips tightly around the saliva ejector.
    Purpose: Removing excess saliva and fluoride solution will make the patient more comfortable and less likely to rinse with water.
12. Instruct the patient not to rinse, eat, drink, or brush the teeth for at least 30 minutes.
    Purpose: These activities could disturb the action of the fluoride.

Documentation

DATE	PROCEDURE	OPERATOR
	Applied APF fluoride gel. Instructed patient not to eat for 30 min.	DLB

Photos from Bird DL, Robinson DS: *Modern dental assisting*, ed 11, St. Louis, 2015, Saunders.

Prerequisites for Performing This Procedure

- Infection control protocol
- Patient communication skills
- Knowledge of oral anatomy

Equipment and Supplies

- 5% sodium fluoride varnish (unit dose)
- Cotton-tip applicator or syringe applicator
- 2 × 2 gauze squares or cotton rolls
- Saliva ejector

Procedural Steps

1. Gather supplies and single-unit dose for application.
   Purpose: Once you begin the procedure, you will not be able to stop in the middle to get something you forgot to set out.
2. Recline the patient to an ergonomically correct position.
   Purpose: You will have better access to the oral cavity and will be in a comfortable position.
3. Wipe the teeth to be varnished with the gauze or cotton roll, and insert the saliva ejector.
   Note: The varnish is not moisture sensitive and can be applied in the presence of saliva.
   Purpose: The saliva ejector is for patient comfort only.

4. Using a cotton-tip applicator, brush, or syringe-style applicator, apply 0.3 to 0.5 mL of varnish (unit dose) to the clinical crowns of teeth; application time is 1 to 3 minutes.

Note: Refer to the manufacturer's instructions for specific application time.

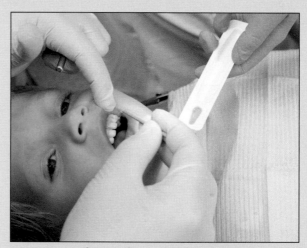

(Copyright iStock.com/BanksPhotos.)

5. Dental floss may be used to draw the varnish interproximally.
   Purpose: This step provides varnish protection for hard-to-reach surfaces.
6. Allow your patient to rinse after the procedure has been completed.
   Purpose: This step removes any residual taste.

Applying Fluoride Varnish (Expanded Function)—cont'd

7. Remind the patient to avoid eating hard foods, drinking hot or alcoholic beverages, brushing, and flossing for at least 4 to 6 hours, or preferably until the next day after the application. Drink through a straw for the first few hours after application.

Purpose: This step prolongs the contact of the varnish. Varnish can be removed the next day with tooth brushing and flossing.

Documentation

DATE	PROCEDURE	OPERATOR
	Applied 0.3 mL of 5% sodium fluoride varnish (insert brand name) on facial and lingual surfaces of teeth #6 to #14, and #19 to #30.	DLB

From Bird DL, Robinson DS: *Modern dental assisting*, ed 11, St. Louis, 2015, Saunders.

Multiple Choice

Circle the letter next to the correct answer.

1. What type of motion should be used when brushing the occlusal surfaces of the teeth?
   a. Back-and-forth
   b. Circular
   c. Sweeping stroke
   d. a and b

2. The patient learns most effectively when they _____.
   a. feel safe and accepted
   b. are actively involved
   c. recognize that they have a problem that needs to be solved
   d. all of the above

3. The most effective way to remove biofilm from the proximal tooth surfaces is by _____.
   a. flossing
   b. oral irrigation
   c. rinsing
   d. tooth brushing

4. When brushing the lingual surfaces of the anterior teeth, the head of the toothbrush is placed in a _____ position.
   a. horizontal
   b. vertical

5. A stiff-bristled toothbrush should not be used because it can _____.
   a. damage the soft tissue
   b. loosen a restoration
   c. affect exposed cementum
   d. a and c

6. Plaque biofilm can naturally form again within _____ hour(s) after brushing.
   a. 1
   b. 6
   c. 12
   d. 24

7. Fluoridated toothpaste is a source of _____ fluoride.
   a. systemic
   b. topical

8. In community water fluoridation, the recommended concentration of fluoride to water is _____ mg/L.
   a. 0.3
   b. 0.7
   c. 1
   d. 1.5

9. Prolonged exposure to excessive amounts of fluoride may cause _____.
   a. dental decay
   b. dental fluorosis
   c. periodontal disease
   d. all of the above

10. Only energy and no nutrients are provided by _____.
    a. carbohydrates
    b. empty calories
    c. fat
    d. protein

Apply Your Knowledge

1. Mrs. Barbara Lucas brings her three children—ages 9, 7, and 2 years old —into your office for a routine examination and dental prophylaxis. Eli, the youngest, is excited when his older sister, Carmen, receives tooth brushing instructions. Eli wants to use the same fluoride toothpaste as his sister and wants to brush his teeth by himself. What adaptations would you discuss with Eli and Mrs. Lucas regarding Eli's oral hygiene instructions?

2. Because dental biofilm is invisible, it can be difficult for patients to realize it is there. What can you use to make your home care demonstrations more effective?

3. Mrs. Slovin has telephoned your office with a concern that her child has been asked to participate in a school-based fluoride rinse program in her son's second-grade class. What questions would you ask the parent to help her move forward?

4. You and two of the other dental assistants in your office have decided to focus on healthy eating habits and physical exercise. Where could you find information about nutrition and personalized food plans?

CHAPTER 21

Coronal Polishing and Dental Sealants

http://evolve.elsevier.com/Robinson/essentials/

LEARNING OBJECTIVES

1. Pronounce, define, and spell the key terms.
2. Describe the difference between a prophylaxis and coronal polishing.
3. Give the indications and contraindications for a coronal polish procedure.
4. Name and describe the types of extrinsic and intrinsic stains.
5. Describe the difference between rubber cup polishing and air-powder polishing.
6. Discuss the following equipment and techniques used for coronal polishing:
   * Type of handpiece, grasp, and positioning for the prophy angle.
   * Fulcrum or finger rest per quadrant.
   * Use of prophy cup and bristle brushes on tooth surfaces.
   * Types of abrasive materials.
7. Describe the proper positioning for the operator and patient for the coronal polish procedure.
8. Give the rationale for the application of dental sealants.
9. Describe the two types of polymerization of dental sealants.
10. List the steps in the placement of dental sealants.

KEY TERMS

air-powder polishing
biofilm
calculus
clinical crown
dental sealants

endogenous
etching
exogenous
fulcrum
light-cured

oral prophylaxis
pits and fissures
rubber-cup polishing

Coronal Polishing

Coronal polishing (rubber-cup polish) is a dental procedure that removes **biofilm** (plaque) and stains from the coronal surfaces of the teeth to provide a polished feeling. Refer to Chapter 20 for a discussion of dental plaque. In some states, coronal polishing is delegated to the registered or expanded function dental assistant who has received additional instruction and credentialing for this procedure.

Coronal polishing is not a substitute for an oral prophylaxis. An **oral prophylaxis** is the complete removal of calculus, stains, and biofilm from the exposed and unexposed surfaces of the teeth by scaling and polishing as a preventive measure. The dentist and registered dental hygienist are the members of the dental team licensed to perform an oral prophylaxis.

Coronal polishing is a procedure strictly limited to the clinical crowns of the teeth and is performed with the use of a slow-speed dental handpiece, a rubber cup, a bristle brush, and an abrasive agent. (The **clinical crown** is that portion of the tooth that is visible in the oral cavity.)

Benefits of Coronal Polishing

* Patients like the feel of smooth, polished teeth.
* Fluoride is better received into polished enamel.
* There is better adherence of dental materials (etchants, sealants, bonding materials) to a polished tooth surface.
* A polished tooth surface is easier for patients to keep clean.
* The formation of new biofilm is slowed.

Selective Polishing

Selective polishing is a procedure in which only specific teeth or surfaces of a tooth are polished. The purpose of selective polishing is to avoid the unnecessary removal of even small amounts of surface enamel. There are specific indications and contraindications to performing a selective coronal polish.

Indications and Contraindications to Coronal Polishing

Indications
- For removal of extrinsic stain and plaque
- For preparation of occlusal surface for dental sealants
- For placement of dental dam
- For preparation of enamel surface for orthodontic bands and brackets
- For preparation of enamel for acid etching for a direct restoration
- For preparation of tooth surface for cementation of an indirect restoration

Contraindications
- When there is an absence of extrinsic stains
- Tooth sensitivity
- Teeth with dental caries, decalcification, hypoplasia, or exposed dentin or cementum
- Newly erupted teeth

Dental Stains

Stains are primarily an esthetic problem. Some stains can be removed, and others cannot. It is important to be able to identify stains to provide the patient with accurate information about the cause of the stain and possible options for removal.

Stains of the teeth occur in three basic ways:
- It directly adheres to the surface of the tooth.
- It is embedded in calculus and plaque deposits.
- It is integrated within the tooth structure.

Before coronal polishing is undertaken to remove stains, your role is to be able to distinguish between intrinsic and extrinsic stains (Fig. 21.1A and B).

Intrinsic stains are those that occur *within* the enamel and *cannot* be removed by polishing. Intrinsic stains may be **endogenous** (occurring during tooth development), or they may be **exogenous** (occurring after eruption; see Table 21.1 for types of intrinsic stains).

Extrinsic stains are those that occur on the *external* surfaces of the teeth and *can* be removed by scaling and/or coronal polishing (see Table 21.2 for types of extrinsic stains).

Methods of Removing Plaque and Stains

Two methods of stain removal are the **rubber-cup polishing** and the **air-powder polishing** techniques.

Remember to check the regulations in your state to see whether the coronal polishing procedure is delegated to a skilled dental assistant and, if so, which technique is permitted.

FIGURE 21.1 A, Intrinsic staining from dental fluorosis. **B,** Brown, and yellow extrinsic stains *(arrows)*. (Courtesy Dr. Frank Hodges.)

Rubber-Cup Polishing

Rubber-cup polishing is the most common technique for removing stains and plaque and for polishing teeth. An abrasive polishing agent is placed in a rubber polishing cup that is slowly and carefully rotated by a prophy angle attached to the slow-speed handpiece. (This form of coronal polishing is described in this chapter.)

Air-Powder Polishing

The air-powder polishing technique uses a specially designed handpiece with a nozzle that delivers a high-pressure stream of warm water and sodium bicarbonate. The powder and water, under high pressure, rapidly and efficiently remove stains; the flow rate is adjusted to control the rate of abrasion (Fig. 21.2).

Damaging Effects of Coronal Polishing

Coronal polishing has the potential to damage tooth surfaces, gingival tissue, and dental restorations. Table 21.3 provides information on the possible damaging effect of coronal polishing.

Equipment for Rubber-Cup Coronal Polishing

Polishing Cups

Soft, webbed polishing cups are used to clean and polish the smooth surfaces of the teeth (Fig. 21.3). The polishing cup is attached to the reusable prophy angle by a snap-on or screw-on attachment.

TABLE 21.1
Intrinsic Stains

Type of Stain	Appearance	Cause
Pulpless teeth	Not all pulpless teeth discolor. A wide range of colors exists—light yellow, gray, reddish brown, dark brown, or black; sometimes an orange or greenish color is seen.	Blood and pulpal tissue break down as a result of bleeding in the pulp chamber or death of the pulp tissue. Pigments from the blood and tissue penetrate the dentin and show through the enamel.
Tetracycline antibiotics	Is a light green to dark yellow or a gray-brown discoloration that depends on the dose, the length of time the drug was used, and the type of tetracycline.	Can occur in the child when the mother is given tetracycline during the third trimester of pregnancy or when given to the child in infancy and early childhood.
Dental fluorosis	Also termed *mottled enamel,* dental fluorosis is the result of ingestion of excessive fluoride during the mineralization period of tooth development.	Varying degrees of discoloration range from a few white spots to extensive white areas or distinct brown stains. (Fluorosis is discussed and illustrated in Chapter 17.)
Imperfect tooth development	Teeth are yellowish-brown or gray-brown and appear translucent or opalescent and vary in color.	May result from a genetic abnormality or environmental influences during development.
Silver amalgam	Appears as a gray or black discoloration around a restoration.	Metallic ions from the amalgam penetrate the dentin and enamel.
Other systemic causes	Appears as a yellowish or greenish discoloration in the teeth.	Causes include conditions of prolonged jaundice early in life and erythroblastosis fetalis (Rh incompatibility)

TABLE 21.2
Extrinsic Stains

Type of Stain	Appearance	Cause
Black stain	Is a thin black line on the teeth near the gingival margin; is more common in girls. Is frequently found in clean mouths. Is difficult to remove.	Is caused by natural tendencies.
Tobacco stain	Is a very tenacious dark brown or black stain.	Is caused by the products of coal tar in the tobacco and from the penetration of tobacco juices into pits and fissures, enamel, and dentin of the teeth. The use of any tobacco-containing products causes tobacco stains on the teeth and restorations.
Brown or yellow stain	Is most commonly found on the buccal surfaces of the maxillary molars and the lingual surfaces of the lower anterior incisors.	Is caused by poor oral hygiene or the use of a toothpaste with inadequate cleansing action.
Green stain	Appears as a green or green-yellow stain, usually occurring on the facial surfaces of the maxillary anterior teeth. Is the most common stain in children.	Is caused by poor oral hygiene when bacteria or fungi are retained in the bacterial plaque.
Antiplaque agents	Is a reddish-brown stain that appears on the interproximal and cervical areas of the teeth. Can also appear on restorations, in plaque, and on the surface of the tongue.	Is caused by the use of prescription mouth rinses that contain chlorhexidine. (Chlorhexidine is a disinfectant with broad antibacterial action.)
Food and drink	Is a light brownish stain and is lessened with good oral hygiene.	Is caused by tea, coffee, colas, soy sauce, berries, and other foodstuffs.

FIGURE 21.2 The air-powder polishing technique uses a specially designed handpiece with a nozzle that delivers a precise mixture of air, water, and sodium bicarbonate. The powder and water, under pressure, rapidly and efficiently remove stains and biofilm without contacting tooth enamel. The flow rate of the powder is adjusted to control the rate of abrasion. (Courtesy Dentsply Sirona, York, Pennsylvania.)

FIGURE 21.3 Various types of prophy angles.

Polishing cups are made from both natural and synthetic rubber. Natural rubber polishing cups are more resilient and do not stain the teeth. Synthetic rubber polishing cups are stiffer than natural polishing cups. If synthetic polishing cups are used, then white synthetic cups are preferable so as not to stain the teeth. Synthetic polishing cups should be used for patients with an allergy to latex products.

A disposable polishing cup or brush is also available, which is discarded after a single use. This disposable angle is manufactured with a polishing cup or a brush already attached.

Bristle Brushes

Bristle brushes are made from natural or synthetic materials and may be used to remove stains from the deep **pits and fissures** of the enamel surfaces. Bristle brushes can cause severe gingival lacerations and must be used with special care. Brushes are not recommended for use on exposed cementum or dentin because these surfaces are soft and easily abraded.

Use of Bristle Brush in Coronal Polishing

- Soak stiff brushes in hot water to soften them.
- Apply a mild abrasive polishing agent to the brush and spread the polishing agent over the occlusal surfaces to be polished using a light wiping stroke.
- Use your free hand and fingers to both retract and protect the cheek and tongue from the revolving brush.
- Establish a firm finger rest and bring the brush almost into contact with the tooth surface before activating the brush. Use the slowest speed, and then lightly apply the revolving brush to the occlusal surfaces. Use care to avoid contacting the gingivae.
- Use a short stroke brushing motion from the inclined planes to the cusps of the tooth.
- Frequently move from tooth to tooth to avoid generating frictional heat.
- Frequently replenish the supply of polishing agent to minimize frictional heat.

TABLE 21.3
Possible Damaging Effects of Coronal Polishing

Tooth Surfaces	• Newly erupted teeth are not completely mineralized, and excessive polishing with an abrasive could remove a small amount of surface enamel.
	• Avoid polishing exposed cementum in areas of recession because cementum is softer than enamel and is more easily removed.
	• Avoid polishing areas of demineralization because of the possibility of loss of surface enamel.
Gingival Tissue	• The potential to damage the gingival tissue exists if the cup is run at a high speed and is applied too long.
	• The potential to force particles of the polishing agent into the sulcus and to create a source of irritation exists with fast rotation.
Restorations	• Abrasive pastes can leave scratches or rough surfaces on gold, composite restorations, acrylic veneers, and porcelain-filled surfaces.

Prophylaxis Angle and Handpiece

The prophylaxis angle, commonly called a *prophy angle*, attaches to the slow-speed motor (see Chapter 12). The prophy angle must be thoroughly cleaned and sterilized after each use. (Handpiece maintenance is also discussed in Chapter 12.) When attaching the polishing cup or bristle brush to the prophy angle, be certain that the polishing cup or brush is securely fastened. If a polishing cup or brush falls off during the procedure, then the patient could swallow or inhale it.

> **Handpiece Operation**
> - The use of a low-speed handpiece is used for polishing to minimize frictional heat and gingival trauma from the rotation of the polishing cup.
> - The rheostat (foot pedal) controls the speed of the handpiece.
> - The toe of the foot is used to activate the rheostat and maintain a slow speed.
> - To produce a slow, even speed, apply steady pressure on the tooth to minimize frictional heat.
> - Use intermittent pressure on the tooth to allow the heat generated to dissipate between strokes.

Handpiece Grasp

The handpiece and prophylaxis angle are held in a pen grasp with the handle resting in the V-shaped area of the hand between the thumb and index finger (Fig. 21.4). A proper grasp is important because if the grasp is not secure and comfortable, then the weight and balance of the handpiece can cause hand and wrist fatigue.

Fulcrum and Finger Rest

The terms **fulcrum** and finger rest are interchangeable and are used to describe the placement of the third, or ring, finger of the hand that is holding the instrument or handpiece.

The fulcrum provides stability for the operator and must be placed in such a way as to allow movement of the wrist and forearm. You will reposition your fulcrum throughout the procedure

FIGURE 21.4 Close-up view of hand with handpiece and proper grasp.

as necessary and it can be intraoral or extraoral, depending on a variety of circumstances such as:
- Presence or absence of teeth
- Area of the mouth being polished
- How wide the patient can open their mouth.

Improper movement of the hand and fingers increases operator fatigue and, over time, can cause painful inflammation of the ligaments and nerves of the wrist.

Abrasives

Dental abrasives (polishing materials) are used to remove stains and to polish natural teeth, prosthetic appliances, restorations, and castings.

Abrasives are available in various grits. (Grit refers to the degree of coarseness of an abrasive agent.) Abrasives are available in extra coarse, coarse, medium, fine, and extra fine. The coarser the agent, the more abrasive the surface.

Even a fine-grit abrasive agent removes small amounts of the enamel surface. Therefore the goal is to always use the abrasive agent that produces the least amount of abrasion to the tooth surface.

> **Factors Influencing the Rate of Abrasion**
> - Amount of abrasive agent used (the more agent used, the greater the degree of abrasion)
> - Amount of pressure applied to the polishing cup (the lighter the pressure, the less abrasion)
> - Rotation speed of the polishing cup (the slower the rotation of the cup, the less abrasion)

Abrasives are available in commercial premixed pastes or in powders that are mixed with water or mouthwash to form slurry used in the polishing cup. Powder abrasives should be as wet as possible (but not runny) to minimize frictional heat. If the mixture is too wet, then splatter will occur and keeping the material in the cup will be difficult. The commercial type of premixed paste is packaged ready to use. Table 21.4 contains the most commonly used dental abrasives.

Coronal Polishing Technique

Proper positioning of both the operator and the patient is necessary so that the coronal polishing procedure may be performed with maximum comfort and efficiency for the patient and the operator.

Positioning the Patient
- The dental chair is adjusted so that the patient is approximately parallel to the floor with the back of the chair slightly raised.
- The movable headrest is adjusted for patient comfort and operator visibility.
- For access to the mandibular arch, position the patient's head with the chin down. (When the mouth is open, the lower jaw should be parallel to the floor.)
- For access to the maxillary arch, position the patient's head with the chin up.

TABLE 21.4
Commonly Used Abrasives

Agent	Action
Silex	Fairly abrasive and used for cleaning heavily stained tooth surfaces.
Superfine silex	Used to remove light stains on tooth enamel.
Fine pumice	A mild abrasive and used for more persistent stains, such as tobacco stains.
Zirconium silicate	For cleaning and polishing tooth surfaces. Zirconium silicate is highly effective and does not abrade tooth enamel.
Chalk	Also known as whiting and is precipitated by calcium carbonate. Chalk is frequently incorporated into toothpaste and polishing pastes to whiten the teeth.
Commercial premixed preparations	Premixed preparations contain an abrasive, water, a humectant to keep the preparation moist, a binder to prevent separation of the ingredients, flavoring agents, and color. Some commercial preparations are available in small plastic containers or individual packets that contribute to the cleanliness and sterility of the procedure.
Fluoride prophylaxis paste	Replaces some of the fluoride that is lost from the surface layer during the polishing process. A fluoride prophylaxis paste is not a substitute for the topical application of fluoride. Its use is contraindicated before acid etching of the enamel when followed by bonding of sealants or other bonded materials.

Positioning the Operator

- The operator positions described in this chapter are in reference to the face of a clock. (This concept is discussed in Chapter 11.)
- The operator should be comfortably seated at the patient's side and able to move around the patient to gain access to all areas of the oral cavity.
- The seated operator's feet should be flat on the floor with thighs parallel to the floor.
- The operator's arms should be at waist level and even with the patient's mouth.
- When performing a coronal polish procedure, the right-handed operator generally begins by being seated at the 8 o'clock to 9 o'clock position.
- When performing a coronal polish procedure, the left-handed operator generally begins by being seated at the 3 o'clock to 4 o'clock position.

Tip: For maximum support and safety, place the fulcrum as close as possible to the area you are polishing, preferably on the same dental arch.

Sequence of Polishing

If full-mouth coronal polishing is indicated, then it should be performed in a predetermined sequence to ensure that no area is missed. The best sequence is based on the operator's preference and the individual needs of the patient.

An affective sequence includes the positions and fulcrums described for a right-handed operator. (The concept of direct and indirect vision is discussed in Chapter 9).

To maintain patient comfort throughout the procedure, the patient's mouth is rinsed with water from the air-water syringe, as necessary. The assistant removes excess water and debris by using either the saliva ejector or the high-volume evacuator (HVE) tip.

Rubber-Cup Polishing Stroke

1. Fill the polishing cup with the polishing agent and spread it over several teeth in the areas to be polished.

2. Begin with the distal surface of the most posterior tooth in the quadrant and work forward toward the anterior.
3. Establish a finger rest and place the cup almost in contact with the tooth.
4. The stroke should be from the gingival third toward the incisal third of the tooth (Fig. 21.5).
5. Use the slowest speed, and then lightly apply the revolving cup to the tooth surface for 1 to 2 seconds.
6. Use light but enough pressure to make the edges of the polishing cup slightly flare (Fig. 21.6).
7. Move the cup to another area on the tooth, using a patting, wiping motion and an overlapping stroke to avoid creating frictional heat that could harm the tooth.
8. Frequently reapply the polishing agent, as needed.
9. Turn the handpiece to adapt the polishing cup to fit every area of the tooth to ensure that the cup covers all areas of the tooth.
10. If two polishing agents with different degrees of coarseness are being used, then always use a separate polishing cup for each abrasive. Use the coarsest abrasive agent first and finish with the finest (least abrasive). Always rinse between polishing agents. The finer abrasive agent will remove scratches left by the coarser abrasive agent.

See Procedure 21.1: Rubber Cup Coronal Polishing.

FIGURE 21.5 Use overlapping strokes to ensure complete coverage of the tooth.

FIGURE 21.6 Stroke from the gingival third to the incisal third with just enough pressure to make the cup flare.

Flossing After Coronal Polishing

Dental floss and tape have two purposes after coronal polishing. The first is to polish the interproximal tooth surface. The second is to remove any abrasive agent or debris that may be lodged in the contact area.

To polish these areas, an abrasive is placed on the contact area between the teeth, and the floss or tape is worked through the contact area with a back-and-forth motion. Because both operator and patient preferences vary, many kinds of floss and tape are available. After the interproximal surfaces are polished, a fresh piece of dental floss or tape is used to remove any remaining abrasive particles between the teeth.

If necessary, a floss threader can be used to pass the floss under any fixed bridgework to gain access to the abutment teeth. Flossing is discussed further in Chapter 20.

Evaluation of Polishing

When you have completed polishing and flossing, evaluate the effectiveness of your technique by reapplying the disclosing agent. Then use a mouth mirror to determine whether the following criteria have been met:

- No disclosing agent remains on any of the tooth surfaces.
- Teeth are uniformly glossy and reflect light from the mirror.
- No evidence of trauma to the gingival margins or any other soft tissue in the mouth is noted.

Pit and Fissure Sealants

Dental sealants are an effective procedure for preventing dental caries in the pit and fissure areas of primary and permanent teeth (See Chapter 4 for the location of pits and fissures throughout the dentition). In many states, the application of dental sealants is an expanded function procedure delegated to the credentialed dental assistant.

Although fluorides have the ability to increase the resistance of decay on the enamel surface of a tooth, the pits and fissures do not benefit from the effects of fluoride as much as smooth enamel surfaces do. Studies have shown 100% caries protection when dental sealants are properly placed and retained on the tooth surface (Fig. 21.7).

Oral bacteria and carbohydrates

FIGURE 21.7 Sealants act as a physical barrier to oral bacteria and carbohydrates. (From *Preventing pit and fissure caries: a guide to sealant use,* Boston, 1986, Massachusetts Department of Public Health and Massachusetts Health Research Institute.)

Questions Commonly Asked by Patients

Q. Do sealants hurt?
A. No. Sealants are easy and painless to apply.
Q. Does it take long to apply sealants?
A. It takes only a few minutes to seal each tooth.
Q. How long will sealants last?
A. Sealants can last 10 years, but need to be examined at regular dental visits and reapplied if necessary.

Dental sealants are applied as a fluid resin material to flow into the pits and fissures of teeth and then are allowed to chemically set or to be polymerized from a curing light. A dental sealant is successful only if it firmly adheres to the enamel surface and protects the pits and fissures from the oral environment.

The narrow width and uneven depth of pits and fissures make them ideal places for the accumulation of acid-producing bacteria (Fig. 21.8). Saliva, which helps remove food particles from other areas of the mouth, cannot clean deep pits and fissures in molars. The pits and grooves on the teeth are so small

FIGURE 21.8 Scanning electron micrograph (SEM) of occlusal pits and fissures. (From Daniel SJ, Harfst SA, Wilder RS: *Mosby's dental hygiene: concepts, cases, and competencies,* ed 2, St. Louis, 2008, Mosby.)

that even a single toothbrush bristle is too large to enter and clean pits and fissures (Fig. 21.9). The sealant acts as a physical barrier that prevents oral bacteria and dietary carbohydrates from creating the acidic conditions that cause demineralization and ultimately dental caries.

Placement of a dental sealant is a noninvasive technique that preserves the tooth structure and also prevents dental decay (Fig. 21.10).

Types of Sealant Materials

A wide variety of sealant materials is available, but most sealant materials fall into two main categories: resin-based sealants and glass ionomer sealants. The dental assistant should have a thorough understanding of the types and characteristics of the various sealant products and their use.

Method of Polymerization

One major difference among these materials is the method of polymerization (setting or curing). Some brands are self-cured,

FIGURE 21.9 Micrograph showing toothbrush bristle in a groove.

FIGURE 21.10 Molar with a properly placed sealant.

whereas others are light-cured. Both types are comparable in bond strength and rate of retention.

Self-cured materials are supplied as a two-part system (base and catalyst). When these pastes are mixed together, they quickly polymerize (harden), usually within 1 minute. The material must be in place before the initial setting occurs (Fig. 21.11).

Light-cured sealants do not require mixing. The material hardens when exposed to ultraviolet light. Currently, a one-step delivery system is available in which the material is provided in a light-protected preloaded syringe and is ready for direct application to the tooth. After the material is applied to the tooth, the curing light activates the setting of the material.

Color

Sealants may be clear, tinted, or opaque (white). Tinted or opaque sealants are more popular because they are easier to see during application and during checks for sealant retention on subsequent office visits. Some brands have a tint that is visible during the application but then turns clear after polymerization.

FIGURE 21.11 Dental Sealant kit with etchant, sealant, and tips.

Storage and Use

Because products and recommendations differ among manufacturers, it is important that you review the instructions specific to the brand being used.

Storage and Usage Tips for Sealant Materials

- Immediately replace caps on syringes and bottles after use.
- Do not expose materials to air or light.
- Do not store materials in proximity to eugenol-containing products.
- Most etchant and sealant materials are designed for use at room temperature. Check the manufacturer's recommendations.
- The shelf life of most sealant products at room temperature ranges from 18 to 36 months.
- Some brands of sealants must be stored in a refrigerator.

Sealant Placement Technique

Placement of dental sealants requires attention to detail. See Table 21.5 for guidelines to sealant placement.

Precautions for Dental Personnel and Patients

Etchant Precautions

Etching agents contain phosphoric acid. Patients and dental personnel should always wear protective eyewear when using etchants. Avoid contact with oral soft tissue, eyes, and skin. In case of accidental contact, immediately flush with large amounts of water. If eye contact is involved, immediately rinse with plenty of water and seek medical attention.

Sealant Precautions

Sealant material contains acrylate resins. Do not use sealants on patients with known acrylate allergies. To reduce the risk for an allergic response, minimize exposure to these materials. In particular, prevent exposure to uncured resin. Using protective gloves and a no-touch technique is recommended. If skin contact occurs, then wash the skin with soap and water. Acrylates may penetrate gloves. If the sealant contacts the gloves, then remove and discard the gloves, immediately wash the hands with soap and water, and put on new gloves. If accidental eye contact or prolonged contact with oral soft tissue should occur, then flush with large amounts of water. If irritation persists, contact a physician.

Protective glasses should be used by operators when ultraviolet or visible light-cured resins are used. Protective eyewear should also be provided for the patient during sealant procedures.

See Procedure 21.2: Application of Dental Sealants (Expanded Function).

Ethical Implications

The delegation of additional functions to dental assistants varies widely. In some states, the application of dental sealants and coronal polishing is an expanded function for dental assistants. In a few states, however, dental assistants will assist with the application of coronal polish and the placement of dental sealants. Check the regulations in your state and practicing according to your professional responsibilities. You play an important role in your patients' preventive care by educating them about routine visits and the importance of sealants.

TABLE 21.5
Guidelines for Sealant Placement

Steps	Principle
Maintenance of a dry tooth surface	Saliva contamination will interfere with retention of the sealant by the tooth. A dry field is maintained by using a dental dam, cotton roll holders, cotton rolls, and dry angles.
Preparation of the tooth	The tooth must be cleaned with a prophy brush (bristle) and a mixture of pumice and water. The pumice must not contain oil or fluoride because both would interfere with the conditioning of the tooth. After cleaning, the surfaces must be thoroughly rinsed and dried.
Conditioning/etching of the tooth	Conditioning the tooth is a critical step because retention of the sealant relies on proper conditioning. The tooth is etched or conditioned with a solution of phosphoric acid. After conditioning, the tooth is rinsed and dried.
	Once the tooth is conditioned, it must not be contaminated with water or saliva. If contamination occurs, then repeating the entire etching process will be necessary.
Sealant placement	Using a dispenser or brush applicator, adequate amount of sealant is placed to cover all fissures on the occlusal surface. A thin layer of sealant is carried into the buccal and lingual inclines of the occlusal surface to seal supplementary fissures. Follow the manufacturer's directions.

Rubber-Cup Coronal Polishing (Expanded Function)

Equipment and Supplies

- Sterile or disposable prophy angle
- Snap-on or screw-on polishing cup accessory
- Snap-on or screw-on bristle brush
- Prophy paste or other abrasive in slurry
- High-volume evacuator (HVE) tip or saliva ejector
- Basic setup
- Cotton-tip applicator (if disclosing solution is used)
- Dental tape
- Dental floss
- Bridge threader
- Air-water syringe and sterile tip

Procedural Steps

1. Check the patient's medical history for any contra-indications to the coronal polish procedure.
2. Seat and drape the patient with a waterproof napkin. Ask the patient to remove any dental prosthetic appliance that they may be wearing. Provide the patient with protective eyewear.
3. Explain the procedure to the patient and answer any questions.
4. Inspect the oral cavity for lesions, missing teeth, and tori.
5. Apply a disclosing agent to identify the areas of plaque.

Maxillary Right Posterior Quadrant, Buccal Aspect

1. Sit in the 8 o'clock to 9 o'clock position or move to the 11 o'clock to 12 o'clock position.
2. Ask the patient to tilt the head up and turn slightly away from you.
3. Hold the dental mirror in your left hand. Use it to retract the cheek or to gain indirect vision of more posterior teeth.

4. Establish a fulcrum on the maxillary right incisors.

Maxillary Right Posterior Quadrant, Lingual Aspect

1. Remain seated in the 8 o'clock to 9 o'clock position or move to the 11 o'clock to 12 o'clock position.
2. Ask the patient to turn theirs head up and toward you.
3. Hold the dental mirror in your left hand. Use direct vision in this position; the mirror provides a view of the distal surfaces.
4. Establish a fulcrum on the lower incisors and reach up to polish the lingual surfaces.

Maxillary Anterior Teeth, Facial Aspect

1. Remain in the 8 o'clock to 9 o'clock position.
2. Position the patient's head so that it is slightly tipped up and facing straight ahead. Make necessary adjustments by slightly turning the patient's head toward or away from you.
3. Use direct vision in this area.
4. Establish a fulcrum on the incisal edge of the teeth, adjacent to the ones being polished.

Maxillary Anterior Teeth, Lingual Aspect

1. Remain in the 8 o'clock to 9 o'clock position or move to the 11 o'clock to 12 o'clock position.
2. Position the patient's head so that it is slightly tipped upward.
3. Use the mouth mirror to gain indirect vision and to reflect light on the area.

4. Establish a fulcrum on the incisal edge of the teeth, adjacent to the ones being polished.

Maxillary Left Posterior Quadrant, Buccal Aspect

1. Sit in the 9 o'clock position.
2. Position the patient's head so that it is tipped upward and slightly turned toward you to improve visibility.
3. Use the mirror to retract the cheek and to gain indirect vision.
4. Rest your fulcrum finger on the buccal occlusal surface of the teeth toward the front of the sextant.

Alternative: Rest your fulcrum finger on the lower premolars and reach up to the maxillary posterior teeth.

Maxillary Left Posterior Quadrant, Lingual Aspect

1. Remain in the 8 o'clock to 9 o'clock position.
2. Ask the patient to turn the head away from you.
3. Use direct vision in this position. Hold the mirror in your left hand for a combination of retraction and reflecting light.
4. Establish a fulcrum on the buccal surfaces of the maxillary left posterior teeth or on the occlusal surfaces of the mandibular left teeth.

Maxillary Left Posterior Quadrant, Lingual Aspect

1. Remain in the 8 o'clock to 9 o'clock position.
2. Ask the patient to turn their head away from you.
3. Use direct vision in this position. Hold the mirror in your left hand for a combination of retraction and reflecting light.
4. Establish a fulcrum on the buccal surfaces of the maxillary left posterior teeth or on the occlusal surfaces of the mandibular left teeth.

Mandibular Left Posterior Quadrant, Buccal Aspect

1. Sit in the 8 o'clock to 9 o'clock position or move to the 11 o'clock to 12 o'clock position.
2. Ask the patient to turn the head slightly toward you.
3. Use the mirror to retract the cheek and for indirect vision of the distal and buccal surfaces.
4. Establish a fulcrum on the incisal surfaces of the mandibular left anterior teeth and reach back to the posterior teeth.

Mandibular Left Posterior Quadrant, Lingual Aspect

1. Remain in the 9 o'clock position.
2. Ask the patient to turn their head slightly away from you.
3. For direct vision, use the mirror to retract the tongue and to reflect more light to the working area.

Continued

4. Establish a fulcrum on the mandibular anterior teeth and reach back to the posterior teeth.

Mandibular Right Quadrant, Buccal Aspect

1. Sit in the 8 o'clock position.
2. Ask the patient to turn their head slightly away from you.
3. Use the mirror to retract tissue and to reflect light. The mirror may also be used to view the distal surfaces in this area.
4. Establish a fulcrum on the lower incisors.

Mandibular Anterior Teeth, Facial Aspect

1. Sit in the 8 o'clock to 9 o'clock position or move to the 11 o'clock to 12 o'clock position.
2. As necessary, instruct the patient to adjust their head position by turning toward or away from you or by tilting the head up or down.
3. Use your left index finger to retract the lower lip. Both direct and indirect vision can be used in this area.
4. Establish a fulcrum on the incisal edges of the teeth adjacent to the ones being polished.

Mandibular Anterior Teeth, Lingual Aspect

1. Sit in the 8 o'clock to 9 o'clock position or move to the 11 o'clock to 12 o'clock position.
2. As necessary, instruct the patient to adjust their head position by turning toward or away from you or by tilting the head up or down.
3. Use the mirror to gain indirect vision, to retract the tongue, and to reflect light onto the teeth. Direct vision is often used in this area when the operator is seated in the 12 o'clock position, but indirect vision can also be helpful.
4. Establish a fulcrum on the mandibular cuspid incisal area.

Mandibular Right Quadrant, Lingual Aspect

1. Remain in the 8 o'clock position.
2. Ask the patient to turn their head slightly toward you.
3. Retract the tongue with the mirror.
4. Establish a fulcrum on the lower incisors.

Mandibular Right Quadrant, Lingual Aspect

1. Sit in the 8 o'clock to 9 o'clock position or move to the 11 o'clock to 12 o'clock position.
2. Ask the patient to turn their head slightly toward you.
3. Retract the tongue with the mirror.
4. Establish a fulcrum on the lower incisors.

(From Boyd: *Dental instruments: a pocket guide*, ed 7, Elsevier, St Louis.)

Consider the following with this procedure: Confirm state guidelines before performing this procedure; personal protection equipment (PPE) is required for the health care team; ensure appropriate safety protocols are followed; and ensure the procedure is to be documented in the patient record.

Prerequisites for Performing this Procedure

- Mirror positioning
- Operator positioning
- Dental anatomy
- Fulcrum positioning
- Instrumentation

Equipment and Supplies

- Protective eyewear for patient and operator
- Basic setup
- Cotton rolls or rubber dam setup
- Etching agent (liquid or gel)
- Sealant material
- Applicator syringe or device
- Prophy brush
- Pumice and water
- High-volume oral evacuator (HVE)
- Curing light and appropriate shield
- Low-speed dental handpiece with contra-angle attachment
- Articulating paper and holder
- Round white stone (latch type)
- Dental floss
- Materials for occlusal adjustments (when a filled resin product is used)

Procedural Steps

1. Place dental dam or cotton rolls and saliva ejector to isolate teeth to be sealed.
   Note: Moisture contamination with saliva or water can cause a lost or leaking sealant.
2. Clean the surfaces of the teeth to be sealed with pumice or oil/fluoride-free paste.

3. Use a three-way syringe and HVE to rinse and dry teeth thoroughly. Remove any retained polishing paste.
   Note: Some dentists prefer to clean out the fissures with a small round or needle-shaped bur or diamond rotary instrument. This allows them to inspect the fissures for the presence of caries.

4. Place etchant on enamel to be sealed for 20 to 30 seconds.
   Note: Some teeth need longer etching times, such as primary teeth and teeth with fluorosis.

Continued

5. Rinse with water for 10 to 15 seconds.
6. If using cotton rolls, carefully replace them or dry them out with the HVE.
   Note: Be certain that saliva does not contaminate the freshly etched surfaces or the enamel will need to be re-etched for 15 seconds.
7. Dry the teeth thoroughly.
   Note: Properly etched enamel should appear frosty. If not adequately etched, re-etch for an additional 30 seconds. The fissures in this photo were opened minimally with a small bur before etching.

8. Apply sealant according to the manufacturer's instructions.
   Note: Sealant should be gently worked into the pits and fissures to displace trapped air. It should cover the entire fissure but should not overfill the groove pattern because that will probably interfere with the occlusion.
9. Cure appropriately for the required length of time (self-cure or light-cure).
   Note: If light-curing, each area under the light probe should be cured for at least 20 seconds. High-powered curing lights may require less time. Follow manufacturer's recommendations.

10. Check with explorer to ensure that all fissures and pits are covered, no holes in the material exist, and sealant is well retained. Apply more material, if needed.
11. Remove dental dam or cotton rolls and thoroughly rinse.
12. Check occlusion with articulating paper and adjust sealant where needed.
    Note: Follow state laws as to which health care practitioner is allowed to do adjustment.
13. Check contact areas with floss.
    Note: Excess material may have blocked these areas.
14. Check retention at each subsequent visit.
    Note: Sealants should be checked for partial or complete loss. Make sure fissures are still covered. With retained sealants, check periphery for staining that may indicate leakage. Extensive decay can occur under leaking sealants if not detected early. Replace lost or leaking sealants.
15. Document the procedure.

Date	Charting Notes	Signature
	Sealant applied to # 30	PJL

(All photos in this procedure were from Hatrick CD, Eakle WS, Bird WF: *Dental materials: clinical applications for dental assistants and dental hygienists,* ed 3, St Louis, 2016, Saunders.)

Chapter Exercises

Multiple Choice

Circle the letter next to the correct answer.

1. When is a coronal polishing procedure indicated?
   a. Before a prophylaxis
   b. Before dental dam placement
   c. To polish demineralized areas
   d. a, b, and c

2. Which of the following influence the rate of abrasion of a polishing agent?
   a. Amount of abrasive material used
   b. Amount of pressure applied during polishing
   c. Rotation speed of the polishing cup
   d. All of the above

3. The prophy angle is held in a _____ grasp.
   a. palm
   b. palm-thumb
   c. pen

4. Tetracycline is an example of an _____ stain.
   a. extrinsic
   b. intrinsic

5. A bristle brush should not be used on cementum or dentin because the surface is _____.
   a. stained by the abrasive
   b. soft and easily grooved
   c. a and b

6. For coronal polishing, the maximum recommended speed of the low-speed handpiece is _____ rpm.
   a. 10,000
   b. 20,000
   c. 100,000
   d. 200,000

7. Plaque and stain are removed from the interproximal areas with a(n) _____.
   a. abrasive
   b. dental floss
   c. rubber cup
   d. a and b

8. In preparation for a coronal polishing procedure, the patient should be covered with _____.
   a. a patient napkin
   b. a lead apron
   c. protective eyewear
   d. a and c

9. Which members of the dental team are permitted to provide an oral prophylaxis?
   a. Dentist
   b. Dental hygienist
   c. Dental assistant
   d. a and b

10. To prevent injury to the gingival tissue, the rubber-cup stroke should be directed _____.
    a. away from the gingival tissue
    b. parallel to the gingival tissue
    c. toward the gingival tissue

11. When moving the rubber polishing cup from one area to another, what type of motion should be used?
    a. Patting
    b. Wiping
    c. Rubbing
    d. a and b

12. The use of a _____ is used on occlusal surfaces of teeth during coronal polishing.
    a. bristle brush
    b. rubber cup
    c. either of the above

13. When polishing the lingual aspect of the maxillary anterior sextant, the operator is seated at the _____ o'clock position.
    a. 6
    b. 8 to 9
    c. 10

14. The most common extrinsic stain found in children is _____.
    a. black line
    b. green
    c. orange

15. Saliva contamination of the tooth surface during sealant placement will interfere with the retention of the sealant on the tooth.
    a. True
    b. False

16. When placing dental sealants, protective eyewear should be worn by the _____.
    a. dental assistant
    b. patient
    c. a and b

17. Which of the following is a contraindication to the placement of a dental sealant?
    a. Deep pits and fissures
    b. Recently erupted tooth
    c. Decay on the proximal surface
    d. b and c

18. Which of the following types of sealant materials do NOT require mixing?
    a. Self-cured
    b. Light-cured

19. It is legal in every state for dental assistants to place dental sealants.
    a. True
    b. False

20. Another term for *conditioning* the tooth before the placement of sealants is _____.
    a. abrasion
    b. etching
    c. polishing
    d. drying

1. Before performing a coronal polish on 16-year-old Sydnie, the dental assistant noticed in the health history that Sydnie had been given the drug tetracycline as a young child. Sydnie stated that she repeatedly took the drug over a period of several months. What, if any, conditions might the dental assistant expect to see on Sydnie's teeth?

2. Mrs. Hansen telephones the dental office to notify the dentist that one of the dental sealants recently placed "just fell out of Pamela's tooth." The dental assistant recalls that Pamela was a very uncooperative child with a very plentiful flow of saliva, and moisture control during the procedure had been difficult. What could be the reason that the sealant did not stay in place?

3. Dr. Steiner advised Mr. Woolley that his 6-year-old daughter, Beth, should have dental sealants placed on her first permanent molars. Nevertheless, the insurance company does not provide coverage for dental sealants, and Mr. Woolley asks the dental assistant to explain again why the sealants are necessary. If you were that dental assistant, how would you respond?

4. Dr. Mackler asks the dental assistant to perform a coronal polish on a patient who is going to have some orthodontic brackets placed. The dental assistant notices some light calculus formation on the lingual surface of the mandibular anterior teeth. Because the calculus is light, the dental assistant thinks she can easily remove it before beginning the coronal polish. What would you do in this situation?

CHAPTER 22

Restorative Dentistry

http://evolve.elsevier.com/Robinson/essentials/

LEARNING OBJECTIVES	1. Pronounce, define, and spell the key terms.
	2. Define direct *restorative* and *esthetic dentistry* and discuss dental conditions requiring both types of treatment.
	3. Describe the process and principles of tooth preparation.
	4. Give the importance of the matrix system for:
	• Class II, III, and IV restorations.
	• Assembly and placement of a matrix system.
	5. Distinguish permanent and complex restorations and describe the procedures for the amalgam and composite restoration.
	6. Describe the use of direct veneers.
	7. Describe vital bleaching and its effects in esthetic dentistry.

KEY TERMS

cariology	operative dentistry	veneer
cavity	preparation	vital bleaching
esthetic dentistry	restorations	wedge
matrix	restorative dentistry	

Restorative dentistry, also described as operative dentistry, is an integral part of the general dental practice. The general dentist concentrates on evaluation, diagnosis, prevention, and treatment of the oral cavity, with an emphasis on cariology and biomaterials. This chapter introduces the background knowledge and describes the techniques necessary for the clinical dental assistant to be prepared when assisting with restorative procedures in a general dental practice.

Restorative dentistry is indicated when a tooth is to be restored back to its original structure with the use of either *direct* restorations or *indirect* restorations. Chapter 23 provides content involving indirect restoration.

Direct restorations are those that are completed within one visit. The most common direct restoration is the restoration of a tooth with the use of a composite resin material, dental amalgam, or a temporary material (Fig. 22.1).

Esthetic dentistry is allocated to improving the appearance of teeth by restoring imperfections with direct and indirect restorative materials or with the use of whitening techniques (Fig. 22.2). The common types of dental materials used are composite resin and tooth whitening.

Dental Conditions Requiring Restorative Dental Treatment

- Management and treatment of carious lesions by restoring the tooth with a permanent restoration
- Restoration of defects in tooth structure
- Replacement of failed restorations
- Abrasion or wearing away of tooth structure
- Erosion of tooth structure

Dental Conditions Requiring Esthetic Dental Treatment

- Discoloration attributable to extrinsic or intrinsic staining
- Anomalies caused by developmental disturbances
- Abnormal spacing between teeth
- Trauma

FIGURE 22.1 Removal of decay and replacement with a Class IV composite resin restoration.

Restoration Process

Regardless of the type of dental material selected, understanding the steps of a restorative procedure is important. The steps include examining the tooth in question, removing the decay or imperfection, **preparing** the tooth for placement of dental materials, and finishing the restoration.

To understand the different types of cavity classification, review the types of cavity classifications in Chapter 13. The most detailed part in restoring a tooth is the initial preparation. The purpose of cavity preparation is to remove the decay along with a small amount of healthy tooth structure, which, when completed, provides a solid foundation on which to place the restorative dental material as a final restoration (Fig. 22.3).

The dentist will use a high-speed handpiece with a variety of burs and hand instruments to accomplish this preparation step. Once the decay is removed, the dentist will use the high-speed handpiece with a differently shaped bur to place retentive grooves in the preparation. These small grooves in the tooth

allow the material to flow into the groove area, harden, and create the retentive result.

This decision on the type of restorative material to be used is based on the size, shape, and location of the preparation. With small preparations, a composite material can be directly placed over sound dentin. With deeper preparations, a cavity liner, base, and bonding material may be required before the final composite or amalgam material is placed.

Permanent Restoration

A permanent restoration can range from a small Class I restoration to an extensive Class II multisurface foundation. With the exception of steps added to the procedure by using supplementary accessories and dental materials, a restorative procedure will follow a standardized format.

- The assistant will communicate with the patient about the procedure and what to expect during treatment.
- The assistant will correctly position the patient for the dentist and specific area of the mouth.
- The dentist will evaluate the tooth to be restored.
- The dentist will administer local anesthesia (see Chapter 15).
- The assistant will prepare and apply the type of moisture control (cotton roll, dry angles, dental dam) to be used for the procedure (see Chapter 14).
- The dentist will prepare the tooth, which includes the high-speed dental handpiece with rotary instruments and examination and preparation hand instruments (see Chapter 12).
- The dentist will specify which dental materials are to be used (see Chapter 18).
- The assistant will prepare and assist in the placement of the dental materials.

FIGURE 22.3 Convenience form used for access to tooth decay.

FIGURE 22.2 Closure of a diastema using composite resin.

- The assistant will prepare and assist in checking the occlusion.
- The dentist will finish and polish the restoration.

Matrix Systems

When a tooth is prepared for a Class II, III, or IV restoration, at least one of the interproximal walls or surfaces of the tooth has been removed during the cavity preparation stage. With the addition of a matrix system, a temporary wall is created, against which the restorative material is placed until the material has set. A **matrix** is a metal or clear plastic strip used to replace the missing proximal wall of a tooth during placement of the restorative material. (*Matrix* is singular. The plural form is *matrices.*)

The universal retainer and matrix band is the system most commonly used when placing posterior restorations. The retainer firmly holds the matrix in place. Clear plastic matrices are used for anterior composite restorations.

Posterior Matrix Systems

The matrix systems have evolved for the class II restoration. There are two types of systems routinely used for the restorative procedure: the universal matrix system and the retainerless matrix system. The matrix band and universal retainer should be assembled before the procedure to save time during the procedure.

Universal Retainer

The universal retainer, also referred to as the Tofflemire retainer, is a device that holds the matrix band in position. The components of the universal retainer are described in the following box.

Retainerless Matrix System

A different type of matrix system other than the universal retainer is designed to secure a thick coated nonstick sectional matrix band with a tension ring. This system produces a tight anatomic contact for the placement of the composite resin and/or dental amalgam material (Fig. 22.4).

Matrix Bands

Matrix bands selected for Class II posterior restorations are made of a flexible stainless steel and are available in **universal** and **extension** sizes. The band wraps around the tooth, creating a temporary wall (Fig. 22.5).

Before the band and the retainer are assembled, the band should be **contoured** in the proximal area so the tooth can make proper contact with the adjacent tooth. To contour the band, place the band on a paper pad, using a burnisher or handle end of cotton pliers. Rub the inner surface of the band until the ends begin to curl. This thins the band and provides a normal curvature of the band to fit around the tooth.

See Procedure 22.1: Assembling a Matrix Band and Universal Retainer.

Components of a Universal Retainer

1. **Spindle:** This internal screw-like pin fits into the diagonal slot to hold the ends of the matrix band. When the retainer is assembled, the spindle point must be clear of the slot while the band is slid into the slot and then tightened.
2. **Outer guide slots:** Also known as guide channels, these slots are located at the end of the retainer and serve as channels to guide the loop of the matrix band. The channel selected is determined according to the quadrant that is being treated.
3. **Outer knob:** The outer knob is used to tighten or loosen the spindle within the diagonal slot and to hold the matrix band securely in the retainer. To tighten the spindle, turn the outer knob away from you. To loosen the spindle, turn the outer knob toward you. Be careful not to turn it

too far, or the diagonal slot vise will fall off the spindle. If this happens, then insert the end of the spindle into the diagonal slot vise and turn the outer knob away from you.
4. **Inner knob:** The inner knob is used to increase or decrease the size of the matrix band loop. The size of the loop formed by the band depends on the tooth to be restored. When the band is placed over the tooth, the size of the loop circumference should be larger than the tooth, and the band should be tightened after placement.
5. **Diagonal slot:** This slot is within the boxlike structure and is used to position the ends of the matrix band into the vise; the retainer is always positioned in the mouth with the diagonal slot facing toward the gingiva.

(From Bird DL, Robinson DS: *Modern dental assisting,* ed 11, St. Louis, 2015, Saunders.)

FIGURE 22.4 Sectional matrix system. A variety of sizes and shapes accommodate composite and amalgam restorative materials.

FIGURE 22.6 Assortment of wedges. (Courtesy Premier Dental Products Company, Plymouth Meeting, Pennsylvania.)

FIGURE 22.5 Three designs of the matrix band. (1) Universal bans. (2 and 3) Extension bands.

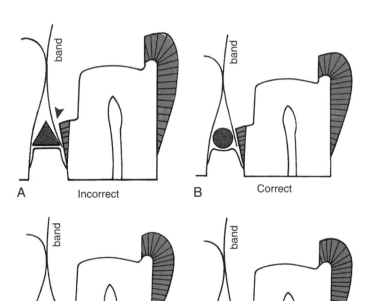

FIGURE 22.7 Proper placement of wedges. (From Heymann HO, Swift EJ, Ritter AV: *Sturdevant's art and science of operative dentistry,* ed 6, St. Louis, 2013, Mosby.)

Wedges

A wedge is triangular or round and supplied in wood or plastic (Fig. 22.6). The wedge is available in different sizes, depending on the location and space between the teeth.

Wedges are used for all Class II, III, and IV matrix systems. A wedge is placed into the lingual embrasure to hold the matrix band firmly against the gingival margin of the preparation. This placement allows the dentist to carve the restorative dental material back to the original normal contour with proximal contacts of the tooth. If the contact is not there, then the tooth could slightly drift, allowing food to impact the area, creating problems for the patient (Fig. 22.7).

Cotton pliers or Howe pliers are used to place the wedge firmly into the embrasure. If a universal retainer is used, then the retainer is situated from the buccal side of the tooth and the wedge is inserted from the lingual side.

See Procedure 22.2: Placing and Removing a Matrix Band and Wedge for a Class II Restoration (Expanded Function).

Anterior Matrix System

A clear plastic matrix strip is the matrix of choice for Class III and IV anterior restorations. Composite resins have inorganic filler particles that could be scratched or marked if a stainless-steel matrix system were used.

FIGURE 22.8 Placement of a retention pin for added internal strength.

The plastic matrix strip is supplied already contoured or as a clear flat strip that is contoured (rounded) to adapt to the shape of the tooth. To contour the strip, pull it lengthwise over the handle of a mouth mirror. The strip is placed interproximal (between the teeth) before etching the tooth and before the placement of the restorative material. The strip is then tightly pulled around the tooth to adapt the composite to the natural contour of the tooth. The matrix is held in place by hand or with a retainer clip until the composite is hardened from the light-cured process.

See Procedure 22.3: Placing a Plastic Matrix for a Class III or Class IV Restoration (Expanded Function).

See Procedure 22.4: Assisting in a Class II Amalgam Restoration, and Procedure 22.5: Assisting in a Class III or IV Composite Restoration.

Complex Restorations

If the loss of tooth structure is greater than the remaining natural tooth, then the dentist must decide whether to (1) move ahead and restore the tooth with an amalgam or a composite material or (2) change the treatment plan and replace the tooth structure with an indirect restoration. Bonding techniques and retention pins are best suited for use in teeth that require large restorations with little tooth structure remaining to provide strength and retention for the final restoration.

Retention pins provide internal strength to the placed material (Fig. 22.8). These pins are available in a variety of diameters (widths) and styles to fit all sizes of teeth. Because all retention pins are small (approximately one-half the size of a bur) and are easily dropped, the dental dam should be indicated for this procedure.

Veneers

The application of **veneers** is an esthetic procedure used to improve the appearance of teeth that are slightly abraded, eroded, or discolored from stains or from endodontic treatment. Veneers can also be used to improve the alignment of teeth or to close a diastema (Fig. 22.9).

A veneer is a thin layer of resin composite material that is directly bonded onto the tooth or is an indirect restoration that would be fabricated in the laboratory using a porcelain material and then cemented to the tooth surface.

Vital Bleaching

Vital bleaching, also referred to as tooth whitening, is a technique that involves the whitening of the external surfaces of the teeth. This desired whitening is completed for esthetic purposes, not for restorative purposes (Fig. 22.10).

Treatment Options

In-office treatment is a professionally applied tooth-whitening procedure that takes place in one appointment by using a

FIGURE 22.9 Veneers placed on teeth #8 and #9 to reduce discoloration and to cover stain. **A,** Before placement. **B,** After placement. (From Heymann HO, Swift EJ, Ritter AV: *Sturdevant's art and science of operative dentistry,* ed 6, St. Louis, 2013, Mosby.)

FIGURE 22.10 Tooth whitening used to treat extrinsic stains. **A**, Before placement. **B**, After placement.

whitening agent at a high concentration; a light or laser source is used to enhance the application.

With **at-home treatment**, the patient is under the care of a dentist and is provided a kit, which includes a custom tray and whitening material. The custom tray (see Chapter 19) is worn for a specific amount of time daily. The tray holds the gel-type material made of hydrogen peroxide, carbamide, and a thickening agent. The whitening process can take 2 to 6 weeks, depending on the strength of the gel and the length of time the tray is worn daily.

Over-the-counter whitening options include a variety of tooth-whitening products manufactured by oral health companies. These products are safe, reliable, and effective but will not achieve the dramatic changes that can be attained with the use of dentist-supervised products.

Ethical Implications

An important reason a patient is a part of your dental practice is because of the type of dental treatment they receive. The dental team's responsibility to the patient is to restore diseased teeth to a healthy normal state of function, which means providing the most up-to-date restorative care to your patients. The dental team's responsibility and obligation is to continually update their knowledge of procedures and materials.

When a specific intraoral task is delegated by a dentist to a clinical dental assistant, that task is considered an expanded function. To complete the task, two criteria must be met. (1) It must be legal in that specific state for the dental assistant to perform the function, and (2) the dental assistant must have received advanced training and proper credentials. You are placing your patient, yourself, and your dentist at risk by performing functions that you have not been trained to do.

Procedure 22.1

Assembling a Matrix Band and Universal Retainer

Equipment and Supplies

- Basic setup
- Universal retainer
- Matrix band
- Ball burnisher
- Paper pad

Procedural Steps

1. Rinse and dry the preparation.
2. Examine the outline of the cavity preparation using a mirror and explorer.
3. Determine the design of the matrix band to be used for the procedure.
Purpose: The band is selected according to the type of tooth and the depth of the cavity preparation.
4. Place the middle of the band on the paper pad and burnish this area with a burnisher.

Purpose: This creates a thin, slightly contoured area, where the contact will be located.
5. Hold the retainer with the diagonal slot facing you and turn the outer knob counterclockwise until the end of the spindle is visible and away from the diagonal slot in the vise.

6. Turn the inner knob until the vise moves next to the guide slots.

Purpose: The retainer is ready to receive the matrix band.

7. Bring together the ends of the band to identify the occlusal and gingival aspects of the matrix band. The occlusal edge has the larger circumference. The gingival edge has the smaller circumference.

8. With the diagonal slot of the retainer facing toward you, slide the joined ends of the band, *occlusal edge first (wider circumference),* into the diagonal slot on the vise.

9. Guide the band into the correct guide slots.

Purpose: The position of the band loop in the guide slots depends on whether the tooth being restored is maxillary, mandibular, right, or left.

10. Tighten the outer knob on the retainer to secure the band.

(Photos and content from Bird DL, Robinson DS: *Modern dental assisting,* ed 11, St. Louis, 2015, Saunders.)

Procedure 22.2

Placing and Removing a Matrix Band and Wedge for a Class II Restoration (Expanded Function)

Prerequisites for Performing This Procedure

- Mirror skills
- Operator positioning
- Dental anatomy
- Instrumentation

Equipment and Supplies

- Basic setup
- Prepared matrix band and retainer
- Wedge for each proximal space involved
- No. 110 pliers

Procedural Steps

Preparing the Band Size

1. If necessary, use the handle end of the mouth mirror to open the loop of the band.

Purpose: The band can become flattened or bent during placement in the retainer and may not easily slide onto the tooth preparation.

2. If necessary, adjust the size (diameter) of the loop to fit over the tooth by turning the inner knob.

Placing the Matrix Band and Universal Retainer

3. Position and seat the loop of the band over the occlusal surface, with the retainer parallel to the buccal surface of

Continued

the tooth. Ensure that the band remains beyond the occlusal edge by approximately 1.0 to 1.5 mm.

4. Securely hold the band in place by applying finger pressure over its occlusal surface. Slowly turn the inner knob clockwise to tighten the band around the tooth.
5. Use the explorer to examine the adaptation of the band.
Purpose: Gingival tissue or dental dam material can become trapped between the band and the proximal box of the cavity preparation.

6. Use a burnisher to contour the band at the contact area, creating a slightly concave area.

Placing the Wedge

7. Select the proper wedge size and shape.
Purpose: The size of the embrasure will determine the size and shape of the wedge for complete closure of the band and cavity preparation.

8. Place the wedge in the pliers so that the flat, wider side of the wedge is toward the gingiva.

9. Insert the wedge into the lingual embrasure next to the preparation and the band.
Note: If both proximal surfaces (mesial and distal) are being restored, then a wedge is inserted for each open contact.
10. Check the proximal contact to ensure that the seal at the gingival margin of the preparation is closed.

Removing the Universal Retainer, Matrix Band, and Wedge

11. After the dentist completes the initial carving of the restorative material, loosen the retainer from the band by placing a finger over the occlusal surface and slowly turning the outer knob of the retainer.
12. Carefully slide the retainer toward the occlusal surface, leaving the band around the tooth.
13. Gently lift the matrix band in an occlusal direction, using a seesaw motion.
Purpose: This step helps avoid fracturing the newly placed material.
14. Discard the matrix band into the sharp's container.
15. Using No. 110 pliers, grasp the base of the wedge to remove it from the lingual embrasure.
Purpose: The wedge remains in place to help prevent a fracture of the restoration when the matrix band is removed.
16. The restoration is now ready for the final carving steps.

(Photos from Bird DL, Robinson DS: *Modern dental assisting,* ed 11, St. Louis, 2015, Saunders.)

Placing a Plastic Matrix for a Class III or Class IV Restoration (Expanded Function)

Prerequisites for Performing This Procedure

- Mirror skills
- Operator positioning
- Dental anatomy
- Instrumentation

Equipment and Supplies

- Basic setup
- Clear matrix strip
- Wedges
- #110 pliers

Procedural Steps

1. Examine the contour of the tooth and preparation site, paying special attention to the outline of the preparation.

2. Contour the matrix strip.
3. Slide the matrix interproximal, ensuring that the gingival edge of the matrix extends beyond the preparation.

Purpose: If the matrix does not completely cover the preparation, the cavity preparation could be filled incorrectly.

Note: If a matrix is placed during the etching process, make sure a new matrix is used for placement of the composite resin material.

4. Using your thumb and forefinger, pull the band over the prepared tooth on the facial and lingual surfaces.
5. Using pliers, position the wedge within the gingival embrasure.

Note: The wedge can be positioned from the facial or the lingual side for anterior restorations.

6. After the preparation has been filled and light-cured, the matrix is removed.

(Photos and content from Bird DL, Robinson DS: *Modern dental assisting,* ed 11, St. Louis, 2015, Saunders.)

Assisting in a Class II Amalgam Restoration

Equipment and Supplies

- Restorative tray (basic setup, hand-cutting instruments, amalgam carrier, condensers, burnishers, carvers, articulating paper holder)
- Local anesthetic setup
- Dental dam setup
- High-volume oral evacuator (HVE) tip
- Saliva ejector
- High-speed and low-speed handpieces
- Assorted burs (dentist's choice)
- Matrix setup
- Dental liners, base, sealers, and bonding agents
- Premeasured amalgam capsules
- Dental floss
- Articulating paper
- Cotton pellets, cotton rolls, 2 × 2-inch gauze
- Dental floss

(From Boyd LRB: *Dental instruments: a pocket guide,* ed 5, St. Louis, 2015, Saunders.)

Continued

Procedural Steps

Preparing the Tooth

1. Transfer the mouth mirror and explorer to the dentist.
Purpose: The dentist examines the tooth to be prepared.
2. Assist in the administration of the local anesthetic agent.
3. Place and secure moisture control techniques (cotton roll, dental dam).

Preparing the Cavity

4. Transfer the mirror and the high-speed handpiece with cutting bur to the dentist.
5. During cavity preparation, use the HVE and air-water syringe, adjust the light, and retract the patient's cheek as necessary to maintain a clear field of vision for the dentist.
Purpose: With efficient placement and use of the HVE and air-water syringe, the dentist will maintain a clear operating field with comfort to the patient.
6. Transfer the explorer, excavators, and hand-cutting instruments as needed throughout the cavity preparation.

Placing the Base and Cavity Liner (Expanded Function)

1. After the examination, rinse and dry the preparation. Mix and place any necessary cavity liners and the base.

Placing the Matrix Band and Wedge (Expanded Function)

1. Assist in placing the preassembled universal (Tofflemire) retainer and matrix.
2. Assist in placing the wedge or wedges in the proximal box using cotton pliers or No. 110 pliers.

Placing the Bonding Agent (Expanded Function)

1. After the tooth is etched and primed, assist the dentist in preparing and placing the bonding material.

Mixing the Amalgam

1. Activate the capsule, place it in the amalgamator, close the cover, and set the timer for the time recommended by the manufacturer.
2. At the signal from the dentist, start the amalgamator.

3. Open the capsule and remove the pestle with cotton pliers. Drop the amalgam into the amalgam well.
4. Reassemble and discard the capsule.
Purpose: This step prevents mercury vapor from escaping into the air.

Placing and Condensing the Amalgam

1. Fill the smaller end of the amalgam carrier and transfer the carrier to the dentist.
2. Assist when necessary as the dentist exchanges the carrier for a condenser and begins to condense the first increments of amalgam with the smaller end of the condenser.

3. Assist as the process of placing and condensing the amalgam is repeated until the cavity is slightly overfilled.
4. When the cavity preparation is slightly overfilled, exchange the condenser for the burnisher so that the dentist can burnish the surface and margins of the restoration.
Purpose: This step strengthens the filled restoration by burnishing the excess mercury to the surface.

Initial Carving

1. Assist while the dentist uses an explorer and a discoid-cleoid carver to remove excess amalgam on the occlusal surface from between the matrix band and the marginal ridge of the tooth.
   Purpose: This step prevents the restoration from fracturing during the removal of the matrix band.

1. Assist in removing the universal retainer, matrix band, and wedge.

Final Carving

1. Transfer the amalgam carvers until the carving is complete.
2. Keep the tip of the HVE close to the restoration during the carving process.
   Purpose: All amalgam particles are removed as soon as possible.
   Note: This step is especially important when a dental dam is not used.

Occlusal Adjustment

1. Remove moisture control materials (cotton rolls, dental dam).
2. Place articulating paper on the teeth to be checked and instruct the patient to close the teeth together very gently.

Note: Heavy blue marks will appear on any high spots on the new restoration. If the patient bites too hard, then the restoration may fracture.

3. Assist with transfers as the dentist uses an amalgam carver to remove any remaining high spots.
Note: This step is repeated as often as necessary to bring the new restoration into proper occlusion.
4. Transfer a moist cotton pellet in cotton pliers to rub the surface of the amalgam gently.
   Purpose: Any remaining small surface irregularities are removed.

Postoperative Instructions

1. Caution the patient not to chew on the new restoration for a few hours.
   Purpose: Amalgam takes several hours to reach its maximum strength, and biting on it could cause the restoration to fracture.

DATE	TOOTH	SURFACE	CHARTING NOTES
	31	MO	1 carpule Xylocaine w/o epinephrine, dam isolation, liner/bonding/ Sybraloy. Pt tolerated procedure fine. T. Clark, CDA

Equipment and Supplies

- Restorative tray (basic setup, hand-cutting instruments, composite placement instrument, carvers, and articulating paper holder)
- Composite shade guide
- Local anesthetic setup
- Dental dam setup
- High-volume oral evacuator (HVE) tip
- Saliva ejector
- High-speed and low-speed handpieces
- Assorted burs (dentist's choice)
- Mylar matrix setup
- Dental liners, base, sealers, and bonding agents
- Composite material
- Curing light with protective shield
- Finishing burs and diamonds
- Dental floss
- Articulating paper
- Cotton pellets, cotton rolls, 2 × 2-inch gauze
- Dental floss
- Abrasive strips
- Articulating paper
- Polishing kit (disc and mandrel)
- Polishing paste

Procedural Steps

Preparing the Tooth

1. Transfer the mouth mirror and explorer to the dentist.
   Purpose: The dentist examines the tooth to be prepared.
2. Assist in the administration of the local anesthetic.
3. Assist in selecting the shade of the composite material.
4. Place and secure moisture control techniques (cotton roll, dental dam).

Preparing the Cavity

1. Transfer the high-speed handpiece and hand-cutting instruments so that the dentist can remove the decayed tooth structure. Use the HVE to maintain a clear operating field.
2. Rinse and dry the tooth throughout the procedure. If indicated, place a cavity liner.

Etching, Bonding, and Composite Placement

1. After the preparation is etched, rinse and dry according to the manufacturer's instructions.
2. Assist in placing the matrix strip. If indicated, then a wedge can also be placed.

B

3. Assist in the application of the primer and bonding resin, which are light-cured in accordance with the manufacturer's instructions.
4. Dispense the composite material on a paper pad or insert the capsule into a composite syringe, and transfer it along with the composite instrument to be placed into the preparation.

C

5. Assist as the matrix is pulled and tightly held around the tooth while the composite material is light-cured from the lingual and facial surfaces.

Assisting in a Class III or IV Composite Restoration—cont'd

5. Assist while the dentist uses polishing discs, points, and cups in the low-speed handpiece to polish the restoration.

Finishing the Restoration

1. Remove the matrix strip and wedge.
2. Assist with transfers as the dentist uses finishing burs or diamonds in the high-speed handpiece to contour the restoration.
3. If indicated, then transfer the finishing strips for smoothing the interproximal surface.
4. Remove the moisture control technique and use articulating paper to check the occlusion. Adjustments are made, as necessary.

DATE	TOOTH	SURFACE	CHARTING NOTES
	10	D	1 carpule Xylocaine w/o epinephrine, cotton roll isolation, etching/ bonding/ Silux shade YL. Pt tolerated procedure fine. T. Clark, CDA

(From Boyd LRB: *Dental instruments: a pocket guide,* ed 5, St. Louis, 2015, Saunders.)

Chapter Exercises

Multiple Choice

Circle the letter next to the correct answer.

1. The _____ circumference of the universal matrix band is placed toward the gingiva.
   a. wider
   b. narrow

2. For a complex restoration, the dentist may have to place a _____ in the cavity preparation of a tooth for internal strength.
   a. wedge
   b. liner
   c. veneer
   d. retentive pin

3. A _____ is a metal or plastic strip used to replace the missing interproximal wall of a tooth during the placement of the restorative dental material.
   a. wedge
   b. matrix
   c. retainer
   d. retentive pin

4. Which instrument would not be placed on the tray setup for a Class IV restorative procedure for tooth #6?
   a. Explorer
   b. Spoon excavator
   c. Articulating paper holder
   d. Amalgam carrier

5. In the placement of a matrix for a Class II amalgam restoration, the wedge would be positioned in the interproximal space from the _____ direction.
   a. buccal
   b. distal
   c. lingual
   d. mesial

6. Which restorative classification would require a clear plastic matrix system?
   a. Class I
   b. Class II
   c. Class III
   d. Class V

7. Tooth-whitening systems are esthetic procedures indicated for _____.
   a. endodontically treated teeth
   b. internal stains
   c. lightening the color of the external surfaces of teeth
   d. a and c

8. When placing the matrix band in a universal retainer, the diagonal slot should be facing _____.
   a. away from you
   b. toward you

9. To achieve the proper interproximal contour and contact of a restoration, a _____ must be inserted into the embrasure to restore proper contact.
   a. retentive pin
   b. wedge
   c. universal retainer
   d. matrix band

10. Which instrument would not be placed on the tray setup for an amalgam restorative procedure?
    a. Cotton pliers
    b. Wedge
    c. Shade guide
    d. Articulating paper holder

Apply Your Knowledge

1. You are assisting in a Class III restoration. (1) What tooth surfaces could be involved in a Class III restoration? (2) What type of moisture control isolation would best suit this procedure? (3) What type of matrix should be readied? (4) What restorative material should be set out?

2. While reviewing a new patient's health history, you notice that the patient does not like the color of her teeth. After talking with her more about this, you find that she drinks a lot of coffee, which seems to be staining her teeth. What technique could the dentist recommend to the patient to alter the color of her teeth? How would you explain this procedure to the patient?

3. You are assisting in the restoration of tooth #29. The tooth is charted to receive a mesio-occluso-distal (MOD) amalgam. (1) What type of matrix system will be used? (2) Describe the assembly of the matrix and any additional items needed to restore the proper contour of the tooth.

4. Dr. Smith is running behind and asks you to complete the etching, place the primer, and begin adding increments of the composite resin to the small Class I preparation. Are there any steps that you should not do?

CHAPTER 23

Prosthodontics and Digital Technology

http://evolve.elsevier.com/Robinson/essentials/

LEARNING OBJECTIVES	1. Pronounce, define, and spell the key terms.
	2. Describe indirect restorative dentistry and its role in prosthodontics.
	3. Discuss the impact of digital technology in prosthodontics.
	4. Discuss the following related to fixed prosthodontics:
	• Indications and contraindications to prescribing fixed prosthodontics.
	• Types of prosthetics, which include inlays, onlays, full crowns, veneers, and bridges.
	• Importance of provisional coverage.
	• Procedures associated with fixed prosthodontics.
	5. Discuss the following related to removable prosthodontics:
	• Function and components of a partial denture.
	• Functions and components of a full denture.
	• When an immediate denture is indicated.
	• How to reline a denture.
	6. Identify the types of dental implants and describe the surgical procedures for implantation.
	7. Describe home care instructions for fixed and removable prosthodontics and dental implants.

KEY TERMS

abutment	flange	post
articulator	framework	provisional coverage
bridge	gingival retraction	rests
core	implants	retainers
crown	inlay	saddle
edentulous	onlay	subperiosteal
endosteal	osseointegration	transosteal
fixed bridge	pontic	unit

Prosthodontics is a field of indirect restorative dentistry that provides treatment in a variety of fixed or removable prosthetic options. The term "indirect" is important to understand because it describes how the restoration is fabricated outside the mouth and then delivered to the patient.

Prosthodontics is divided into two specific categories: **fixed prosthodontics**, which involve the placement of a cast prosthesis that is cemented in place and cannot be removed by the patient, and **removable prosthodontics**, which involve the replacement of missing teeth with a prosthesis that the patient can freely take in and out of their mouth.

Dental implants provide a natural-looking and functional replacement for a single tooth or multiple teeth that incorporates the principles from fixed and removable prosthodontics with the use of a bone-anchored implant. Dental implants are now considered the standard of care in the replacement of a single tooth or multiple teeth.

Digital Technology in Prosthodontics

The introduction of digital technology has been a major advancement in the practice of fixed and removable prosthodontics and dental implants. It has allowed for an intraoral scan of a tooth preparation and the creation of a digital impression from a computer-assisted design, followed by the use of a computer-assisted manufacturing (CAD/CAM) system to create a virtual restoration and then the fabrication and delivery of a permanent restoration within a single dental appointment (Fig. 23.1A–C).

Major Benefits of Digital Technology
- Improved diagnostic data for treatment plan
- Less scheduled visits
- No use of conventional impression materials
- No need to place a provisional
- Greater comfort for the patient

Fixed Prosthodontics

The field of fixed prosthodontics is an area of prosthodontics focused on the restoration of teeth with a finished restoration either fabricated in the dental laboratory or through the use of digital technology. Table 23.1 illustrates the different types of indirect fixed prosthetics for a specific need.

Considerations for Prescribing Fixed Prosthodontics

Indications
- One or two adjacent teeth are missing in the same arch.
- Supportive tissues are healthy.
- Suitable abutment teeth are present.
- Patient is in good health and wants to have the prosthesis placed.
- Patient has the skills and motivation to maintain good oral hygiene.

Contraindications
- Supportive tissues are diseased or missing.
- Suitable abutment teeth are not present.
- Patient is in poor health or is not motivated to have the prosthesis placed.
- Patient has poor oral hygiene habits.
- Patient cannot afford the treatment.

Crown and Bridge Procedural Steps

Shade Selection

To ensure an exact match with a person's natural teeth, matching the shade is completed at the first appointment before the procedure begins. A **shade guide**, or electronic shade device, is used to match the natural tooth color (Fig. 23.2A–B). Natural light is best to capture the true color of a patient's teeth.

The shade selected is identified and noted on the patient's record and on the laboratory prescription. The shade guide is a semi-critical item that cannot withstand the heat of sterilization. After use, it must be disinfected.

Preparation

The fabrication of a single **unit** cast restoration (**inlay**, **onlay**, or crown) or a multiple unit (**bridge**) takes a minimum of two appointments if digital technology is not used. The *first appointment* involves taking preliminary impressions, preparing the tooth structure, taking final impressions, and placing a provisional restoration. The *second appointment* is for the *try-in* of the casting, adjustments, and final cementation of the completed restoration.

Tooth Preparation

During tooth preparation, the height and contour of the natural tooth or teeth are prepared to remove any diseased tooth structure and to prepare the tooth for the casting. The prepared tooth is shaped so that the cast restoration can fit into or over the preparation to resemble its natural tooth (Fig. 23.3).

If the coronal portion of the tooth is extensively decayed, fractured, or worn, then providing additional support for the crown may be necessary.

Core Buildups. A **core** buildup uses amalgam or core material to add onto the prepared natural tooth when there is not enough natural structure to hold a fixed restoration (Fig. 23.4). If an amalgam restoration is already in place, then this may be shaped and prepared for use as the core.

Pin Retention. Pin retention may be necessary to add strength to the core buildup for the crown. When pins are used, they are directly incorporated into the buildup material (Fig. 23.5).

Post and Core. If a tooth has been endodontically treated, then a **post** is placed into the pulp canal. The core is built up around the post to provide additional strength and stability for the crown (Fig. 23.6).

Gingival Retraction

For the laboratory technician to create an accurate fitting cast, a final impression is taken to prepare the working cast. As stated in Chapter 19, the final impression provides details of the preparation that extend below the finish line of the preparation. The best way to achieve this detail and not harm the tissue is with the use of the **gingival retraction cord**.

The gingival retraction cord temporarily pushes the gingival tissue away from the tooth and widens the sulcus, which allows the impression material to flow around all parts of the preparation.

Retraction cords are supplied as untwisted, twisted, or braided (Fig. 23.7). For easy application, the cord is moistened in water or in a **vasoconstrictor** solution and then twisted just before placement. Once placed, the cord will expand and open the sulcus, ready to receive the impression material.

To control hemorrhage from the preparation procedure, the retraction cord can be impregnated (saturated) with an astringent and a vasoconstrictor solution, which controls bleeding and short-term constriction of the tissue. Special caution must be taken if the patient is taking a blood thinner because of a cardiovascular condition; the patient should not receive a retraction cord prepared with a vasoconstrictor solution.

See Procedure 23.1: Placing and Removing the Gingival Retraction Cord (Expanded Function).

FIGURE 23.1 **A,** Intraoral scan of mandibular quadrant. **B,** Biogeneric proposal of the crown. **C,** Delivered ceramic crown. (From Heymann HO, Swift EJ Jr., Ritter AV: *Sturdevant's art and science of operative dentistry,* ed 7, St Louis, 2013, Mosby.)

TABLE 23.1

Types of Fixed Prosthodontics

Name	Description
Inlay (From Freedman G: *Contemporary esthetic dentistry*, St Louis, 2012, Mosby.)	An inlay cast restoration is made from either porcelain or gold, which is created to fit into a Class II preparation. The inlay restoration involves a portion of the occlusal surface and one or more proximal surfaces.
Onlay (Copyright iStock.com/Obencern.)	An onlay cast restoration is made from either porcelain or gold. The onlay restoration involves multiple surfaces, covering all of the occlusal and a portion of the proximal surfaces.
Crown 	A crown is a single cast restoration that completely covers the anatomic portion of a tooth. The materials used to make crowns are porcelain fused to metal (PFM), porcelain, or gold. PFM castings allow the esthetics of porcelain to be placed on the facial side of the crown or bridge and the strength of the metals on the occlusal, lingual, and proximal surfaces to provide strength for occlusion.

TABLE 23.1

Types of Fixed Prosthodontics—cont'd

Name	Description
Fixed Bridge (Courtesy Captek, The Argen Corporation, San Diego, California.)	The fixed bridge replaces one or more missing teeth adjacent to each other in the same arch. A bridge can be fabricated from PFM, porcelain, or gold. Because more than one tooth is involved, the parts of the bridge are as follows: • A unit indicates the number of teeth involved in the bridge (e.g., three teeth involved would be a three-unit bridge). • A *pontic* is the artificial tooth that it replaces in the bridge. • Abutments are the natural teeth involved in the bridge that support the pontics. At least one abutment is required.
Resin Bonded Bridge	Also referred to as a Maryland bridge. This type of bridge consists of a pontic that is made of porcelain with a winglike extension framework that is bonded into place on the lingual sides of the adjacent teeth.

FIGURE 23.2 A, Shade guide used to match the exact color of teeth. (Copyright iStock.com/Obencem) B, Placement of the VIA Easyshade V device (courtesy of VIA North America, Yhorba Linda CA)

FIGURE 23.3 A crown preparation reduces the height and contour of the teeth # 5 and #6.

FIGURE 23.4 Core build up on tooth #11.

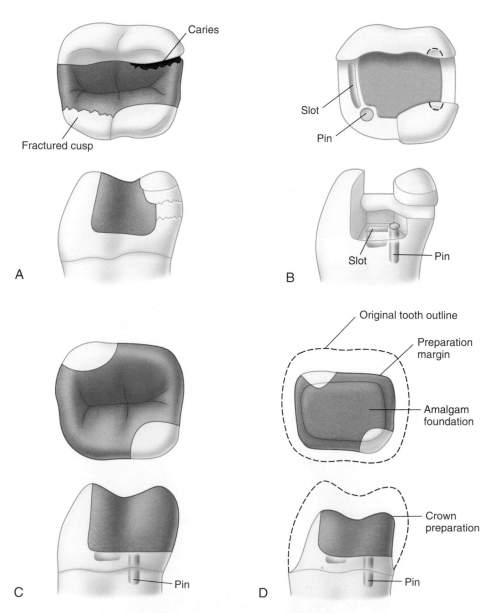

FIGURE 23.5 Pin retention placement. (From Heymann HO, Swift EJ Jr., Ritter AV: *Sturdevant's art and science of operative dentistry,* ed 6, St Louis, 2013, Mosby.)

FIGURE 23.6 Tooth #5 restored with a cast post and core.

FIGURE 23.7 Types of gingival retraction cords. (From Rosenstiel SF, Land MF, Fujimoto J: *Contemporary fixed prosthodontics,* ed 5, St Louis, 2016, Elsevier.)

Final Impression

After the prescribed time that the gingival retraction cord is within the sulcus, the retraction cord is removed, the sulcus is rinsed and dried, and the final impression is taken of the prepared tooth and surrounding tissue. (Refer to Chapter 19 for the procedure for taking final impressions.)

Provisional

A **provisional**, also known as a temporary, is a protective material that is temporarily placed for any type of indirect preparation from an inlay, onlay, or a single crown or for the abutment teeth for a bridge.

A provisional remains until the cast restoration or bridge is returned from the dental laboratory and readied for permanent cementation. This period may take from several days to a few weeks.

Specific Objectives for Provisional Coverage

- To reduce the sensitivity and discomfort of the prepared tooth
- To maintain function and esthetics of the tooth
- To protect the margins of the prepared tooth
- To prevent shifting of adjacent or opposing teeth

Types of Provisional Coverage. Several types of provisional coverage are available. The dentist will determine the type based on the needs of the patient. The construction and cementation of temporary coverage can be delegated to the expanded function dental assistant (EFDA) or to a registered dental assistant (RDA; Table 23.2).

See Procedure 23.2: Fabricating and Cementing a Custom Acrylic Provisional Crown.

Laboratory Prescription

After the first appointment, a laboratory prescription is completed by the dentist and sent to the laboratory along with the final impression and bite registration. The laboratory technician can fabricate a single crown or a bridge on the basis of a written prescription from the dentist. Also known as a work order or requisition, one copy of the prescription is included with the case, and another copy is retained with the patient record (Fig. 23.8).

Laboratory Working Days. The laboratory requires a specific number of working days to complete the cast restoration. This time must be a consideration when scheduling the patient's return visit.

See Procedure 23.3: Assisting in a Crown and Bridge Restoration.

Removable Prosthodontics

The field of removable prosthodontics is the area of prosthodontics involved in the replacement of missing teeth with a prosthesis that the patient is able to take in and out of the mouth. The two major types of removable prosthodontics are (1) removable partial dentures and (2) removable full dentures.

A **removable partial denture**, commonly referred to as a partial, replaces one or more teeth that are missing in a specific quadrant or arch (Fig. 23.9).

A **removable full denture**, commonly referred to as a denture, replaces all of the teeth that are missing in one arch (Fig. 23.10).

The laboratory technician plays an important role in the construction of these types of prostheses. The technician follows the

TABLE 23.2
Types of Provisional Materials

Types	Description
Preformed polymer crown	These shell-like crowns are available for posterior single crowns and for bridgework. The prostheses are supplied with a hybrid composite resin that bonds with the preformed crown.
Preformed polycarbonate crown	Made from a strong acrylic resin, the preformed polycarbonate crown is manufactured in a variety of sizes for anterior teeth where appearance is important. The crown is adapted to fit the prepared tooth using an acrylic laboratory bur and a Burlew wheel. It is then cemented.
Custom acrylic temporary (Copyright iSTock.com/Lighthaunter.)	Made from a tooth-colored acrylic resin, the material is loaded in a vacuum-formed custom tray or alginate impression, seated onto the prepared area, allowed to set, removed from the tray, and finished using acrylic burs and finishing stones. It is then cemented to provide temporary coverage of a single crown or bridge.

dentist's written prescription and works in close cooperation with the dentist in the fabrication of the prosthesis.

Partial Dentures

A removable partial denture receives its support and retention from the underlying tissue and from the remaining teeth that serve as abutments. The prosthesis is designed to distribute the forces of mastication between the abutments and the supporting tissue.

Considerations for Prescribing a Partial Denture

Indications

- Aids in eating and in maintaining good health.
- Improves appearance, confidence, and smile. This improvement is achieved by restoring the natural contours of the lips, cheeks, and face. The denture prevents the development of premature aging lines and wrinkles around the mouth.
- Corrects the effect of speech caused by the loss of teeth by closing the spaces left by the lost teeth.

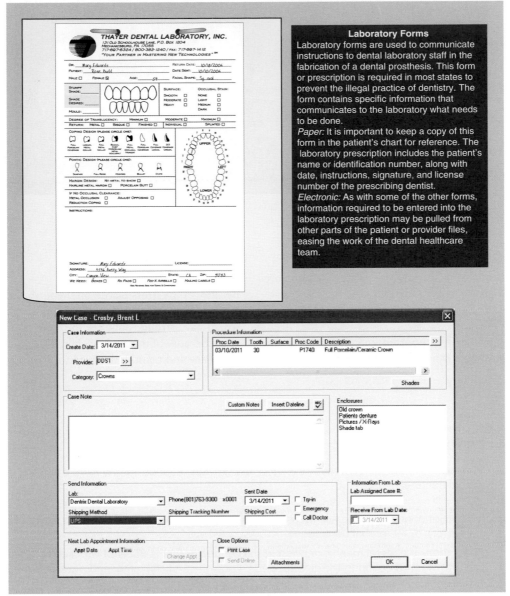

Laboratory Forms
Laboratory forms are used to communicate instructions to dental laboratory staff in the fabrication of a dental prosthesis. This form or prescription is required in most states to prevent the illegal practice of dentistry. The form contains specific information that communicates to the laboratory what needs to be done.
Paper: It is important to keep a copy of this form in the patient's chart for reference. The laboratory prescription includes the patient's name or identification number, along with date, instructions, signature, and license number of the prescribing dentist.
Electronic: As with some of the other forms, information required to be entered into the laboratory prescription may be pulled from other parts of the patient or provider files, easing the work of the dental healthcare team.

FIGURE 23.8 Laboratory prescription. (Form courtesy The Dental Record, Wisconsin Dental Associations, Milwaukee, Wisconsin. Dentrix screen shot courtesy Henry Schein Practice Solutions, American Fork, Utah. From Gaylor LJ: *The administrative dental assistant,* ed 3, St Louis, 2012, Saunders.)

- Corrects the positioning of the jaws necessary to prevent jaw joint problems.
- Protects the health of remaining oral tissues.
- Prevents other teeth from drifting into the gaps left by extractions.

Contraindications
- Lack of suitable teeth in the arch to support, stabilize, and retain the removable prosthesis
- Rampant caries and/or severe periodontal conditions that threaten the remaining teeth in the arch
- Lack of patient acceptance and/or chronic poor oral hygiene

FIGURE 23.9 Removable partial denture.

FIGURE 23.10 Full denture. (Courtesy Ivoclar Williams, Amherst, New York.)

Components of a Partial Denture

The basic components of a removable partial denture are described in Table 23.3.

Abutment Teeth

A partial denture is primarily supported and stabilized by the abutment teeth. Abutments can be remaining natural teeth or surgical implants.

Selection of Abutment Teeth

Because of the stress placed on them, abutment teeth must have strong roots and strong bone support. Canines and molars, which have strong roots, are the teeth best suited for this purpose. Because of their relatively weak root structure, individual maxillary and mandibular anterior incisors are least acceptable for use as abutments.

TABLE 23.3
Components of a Partial Denture

Framework	The framework is the cast metal skeleton that provides support for the saddle and the connectors of the partial denture.
Major connector	The major connector, also known as a bar, is the piece of rigid metal that joins the right and left quadrant framework of the partial denture.
Saddle	The saddle is a metal mesh extension of the connector that is covered with acrylic. The saddle rests on the oral mucosa covering the alveolar ridge, holds the artificial teeth, and provides some support for the prosthesis.
Retainers	A retainer, also known as a clasp, is the portion of the framework that directly supports and provides stability to the partial denture by partially circling an abutment tooth.
Rests	A rest is a metal projection on or near the clasp that is designed to control the extent of seating of the prosthesis.
Artificial teeth	Artificial teeth are constructed from acrylic or porcelain.

(Modified from Kratochvil FJ: *Partial removable prosthodontics,* Philadelphia, 1988, Saunders.)

Preparation of Abutment Teeth

Abutment teeth are prepared according to the type of rest selected. Preparation may involve one of the following options:

- Slight modification of the tooth itself
- Modification of an amalgam restoration if present
- Placement of a cast metal restoration with a recessed area to receive the rest or precision attachment

Final Impressions

A **final impression** is required for creating the **working casts** that are used by the laboratory technician for the construction of the partial denture.

Because this impression must be exact, a custom tray is made, and an elastomeric impression material is used. The dentist chooses the type of tray, the material, and the impression technique to be used (see Chapter 19).

In addition to the final impression, taking an impression of the opposing arch and obtaining an occlusal registration is necessary. Most commonly, this is an occlusal registration; the technique is described in Chapter 19.

Selecting the Artificial Teeth

The **shade** (color) and **mold** (shape) of the teeth are determined. The manufacturer of the artificial teeth provides a shade guide. To identify the teeth, the mold and shade numbers are imprinted by the manufacturer on the back of each tooth in the shade guide (Fig. 23.11).

When choosing the tooth shade and shape, the dentist considers the age and body size of the patient, the length of the lip, and the space to be occupied by the artificial tooth or teeth. The goal is to match the color, size, and shape of the patient's natural teeth as closely as possible.

The shade of the artificial teeth is examined using natural light for accuracy. When the selection has been made, the shape and shade of the artificial teeth are written in the patient's record.

This information, plus the name of the manufacturer and the material of the teeth, is also noted on the laboratory prescription to ensure that the technician will select the correct artificial teeth.

Laboratory Prescription

Before a case is sent to the laboratory, the dentist prepares a written prescription that includes all of the details concerning the construction of the prosthesis. The dentist must sign this prescription, and a copy is retained with the patient's records.

FIGURE 23.11 Artificial teeth. (Courtesy Ivoclar Vivadent, Amherst, New York.)

Try-In Appointment

An appointment is scheduled for the initial *try-in* of the prosthesis in the patient's mouth. At this point, the appliance consists of the cast **framework**, and the artificial teeth are set in wax.

At this visit, the dentist evaluates the fit, comfort, and function of the appliance. The shade, mold, and arrangement of the teeth are reviewed to ensure that their appearance is acceptable to the patient. If necessary, the dentist may alter the alignment of the teeth in the wax.

When the appliance is acceptable, another bite registration may be required to reflect any changes made during the try-in appointment. Any changes in the partial denture design are noted on the laboratory prescription. The wax-up and bite registration are disinfected and returned to the dental laboratory technician along with the prescription.

The laboratory technician finishes the partial denture as prescribed by the dentist. The completed prosthesis is delivered to the dental office in a sealed, moist container. (The acrylic **saddle** must be kept moist at all times to prevent warping.)

The appliance is disinfected and rinsed before the try-in of the appliance in the patient's mouth.

Delivery of the Partial Denture

A 20- to 30-minute appointment is usually adequate for the delivery of the partial denture. The day before the appointment, the assistant verifies that the case has been returned from the laboratory. See Procedure 23.4: Assisting in the Delivery of a Partial Denture.

Home Care Instructions to the Patient with a Partial Denture

- Maintain good oral hygiene.
- After meals, remove the partial and brush or rinse it to clean the **retainers**, **rests**, and saddles.
- Carefully brush and floss the abutment teeth and the remaining natural teeth to keep them free of food debris and plaque.
- When not wearing the partial, store the prosthesis in water or in a moist, airtight container. If the partial denture is allowed to get dry or too hot, the acrylic portion can warp.

Postdelivery Check

The patient is scheduled for a 10- to 20-minute postdelivery appointment within a few days after the delivery of the partial denture.

At this time, the dentist checks the mucosa for pressure areas and sore spots. If necessary, minor adjustments are made to the partial denture using a laboratory bur and a polishing lathe. When the dentist and patient are satisfied that the prosthesis is correctly functioning, the patient is given a recall appointment for several months later.

It is important that the patient regularly return for recall visits. The recall appointment should include dental prophylaxis and the evaluation of the function and fit of the prosthesis.

As time passes and individuals age, changes in the alveolar ridge and surrounding tissue may make it necessary to reline the partial denture.

Full Dentures

Full dentures, also known as complete dentures, are designed to restore the function and esthetics of the natural dentition when all of the natural teeth are missing. A complete denture receives all of its support and retention from the underlying tissue, the alveolar ridges, the hard and soft palates (maxillary), and the surrounding oral mucosa. Table 23.4 provides the components of the full denture and its description.

Considerations for Prescribing a Complete Denture

Indications

- The patient is edentulous in at least one arch.
- The remaining teeth cannot be saved.
- The remaining teeth cannot support a removable partial denture, and no available alternatives are acceptable.
- The patient refuses alternative treatment recommendations.

Contraindications

- When any other acceptable alternative is available, and teeth can be saved, or implants are completed
- Physical or mental illness affecting the patient's ability to cooperate during fabrication of the denture and to accept and/or wear the denture
- Hypersensitivity to denture materials (A hypoallergenic denture material may be indicated for these patients.)
- Patient not interested in replacing missing teeth

Denture Retention

Retention of a Maxillary Denture

Retention of a maxillary denture primarily depends on the suction seal known as the **post dam** or the posterior palatal seal, which is formed at the junction of the tissue and the posterior border of the denture.

Retention of a Mandibular Denture

Achieving good retention of a mandibular denture can be difficult. It lacks the broad suction area found in a maxillary denture, and the constant action of the tongue can dislodge it. Retention for a mandibular denture depends on the support of the remaining alveolar ridge and the suction that can be achieved between the prosthesis and the tissue covering the ridge.

The base and flange of a mandibular denture extend over the residual ridge and attached mucosa, down to the oblique ridge and mylohyoid ridges, and over the genial tubercles and retromolar pads.

Impressions for Diagnostic Casts of Edentulous Arches

Taking an alginate impression of an edentulous arch differs from taking other alginate impressions in three ways: (1) the height of the teeth is eliminated, (2) including more extensive tissue details is important, and (3) an edentulous tray is used to take this impression.

An edentulous tray is not as deep as other trays used for alginate impressions because the space required for the teeth is not needed. In addition, soft beading wax or rope wax should be attached to the edges of the tray to modify the borders for a custom fit.

This modification allows for **border molding**, also known as muscle trimming, to achieve closer adaptation of the edges of the impression of the tissue in the mucobuccal fold. Border molding is performed after the impression tray is in place. The dentist uses their fingers to gently massage the area of the face over these borders. Border molding shapes the wax-covered edges of the tray so these edges more closely approximate the tissue.

Final Impressions for Complete Dentures

Because accuracy is essential, an elastomeric impression material is selected for the final impressions for the making of working casts (Fig. 23.12). Because of the shape of the edentulous arch, custom trays are required for the final impression. The edges of the custom tray for an edentulous arch are modified with beading wax to allow for border molding. The edges of the completed tray should extend to 2 mm short of the mucobuccal fold.

Try-In of the Baseplate–Occlusal Rim Assembly

The **baseplate** is made of a semirigid material, such as self-curing or heat-cured resins. The **occlusal rims** are built of wax

---

TABLE 23.4
Components of a Full Denture

Name	Description
Base	The base covers the entire hard palate and fits over the residual alveolar ridge and surrounding gingival area.
	The base is usually constructed from denture acrylic; however, to provide additional strength, it may be reinforced with a metal mesh embedded in the acrylic.
Post dam	The post dam extends across the entire posterior of the denture from one buccal space across the back of the palate behind the maxillary tuberosity to the opposite buccal space.
Flange	The flange is an extension beyond the residual ridge and over the attached mucosa to the tuberosities and the junction of the hard and soft palates.
Artificial teeth	Denture teeth are made of acrylic or porcelain.
	Third molars are not included on dentures because of the need to provide space in the posterior region to allow the patient to close, chew, swallow, and speak normally.

FIGURE 23.12 Completed maxillary edentulous impressions. (Courtesy Ivoclar Vivadent, Amherst, New York.)

on the alveolar crest of the baseplate and are high and wide enough to occupy the space of the missing teeth.

The baseplate–occlusal rim assembly is used while (1) bite relationship records are made, (2) the casts are articulated, (3) the artificial teeth are arranged, and (4) the prosthesis is tried in the mouth.

The baseplate–occlusal rim assembly is returned to the dental office.

Before the try-in of the baseplate–occlusal rim assembly in the patient's mouth, it is removed from the articulator, disinfected, and rinsed. On the occlusal rims, the dentist records the:

- Vertical dimensions of the arches (i.e., the space occupied by the height of the teeth, which is considered normal occlusion)
- Occlusal relationships (e.g., centric, protrusive, retrusive, and lateral excursion movements) of the arches
- Smile line (i.e., number of teeth that normally show when the patient is smiling)
- Canine eminence (i.e., vertical line that indicates the location of the canines)

Selecting the Artificial Teeth

At this appointment, the dentist will select the shape, shade, and material of the artificial teeth to be placed in the denture. A full denture will have 14 teeth per arch. These factors are determined in the same way as the teeth of a partial denture.

When placing the teeth in the denture, the laboratory technician is able to modify the arrangement as requested to produce a more natural appearance for the patient, such as by slightly overlapping the mesial incisal margin of the maxillary lateral over the distal margin of the central incisor.

Occlusal Registration

During the construction of a complete denture, the laboratory technician must have an accurate and extensive record of the patient's occlusion. The technician uses this information to articulate the casts so that the completed prosthesis will replicate these normal motions.

The measurements most frequently used are the patient's bite registered in the following positions:

- **Centric relation** with the jaws closed, relaxed, and comfortably positioned
- **Protrusion** with the mandible placed as far forward as possible from the centric position
- **Retrusion** with the mandible placed as far posterior as possible from the centric position
- **Lateral excursion**, which is the sliding of the mandible to the left or right of the centric position

These exaggerated motions simulate the actual movements of the mandible as it functions in the acts of mastication, biting, yawning, and speaking. Various devices are used to obtain these measurements.

Wax Setup Try-In Appointment

The **wax setup** consists of the baseplate with the artificial teeth set in wax, which resembles gingival tissue. Shaping of the wax to simulate normal tissue contours, grooves, and eminence is known as **festooning**.

The complete denture try-in, which is fabricated in wax by the laboratory technician on an articulator, is returned to the dental office before the patient's appointment. An articulator, as shown in Fig. 23.13, is a laboratory device that simulates the movements of the mandible and the temporomandibular joint. The wax setup is removed from the articulator and disinfected before it is tried in the patient's mouth.

When the try-in has been approved and the denture is ready to process in the lab, the wax is replaced by acrylic and is ready for finishing, polishing and delivery.

See Procedure 23.5: Assisting in the Delivery of a Full Denture.

Home Care Instructions to the Patient with a Partial and Full Denture

The patient should be provided with written home care instructions to reinforce the following verbal instructions for daily care:

- With the denture removed, thoroughly rinse the oral tissues at least once daily.
- On removal, thoroughly clean all surfaces with a special denture brush and a nonabrasive denture cleanser. During cleaning, carefully hold the prosthesis over a sink with water to protect from accidental dropping.
- Do not soak in hot water or a strong solution.
- When not in the mouth, store dentures in a moist, airtight container to prevent drying and warping.
- Do not wear during sleep. It is important for the gingival tissues to be free from constant compression.

Relining of a Partial or Complete Denture

The purpose of relining a denture is to accommodate changes in the supporting tissue to ensure that the prosthesis properly fits. Relining is accomplished by placing a new layer of denture resin over the tissue surface of the appliance.

Impression for Laboratory Relining

- At the preliminary appointment, when it is agreed that relining is necessary, the patient is instructed that they will be without a denture for at least 8 to 24 hours while it is being processed in the laboratory.

FIGURE 23.13 Wax-up of a complete denture on an articulator.

- The impression is taken using the present (loose) denture as the impression tray. The dentist will use a zinc oxide–eugenol impression paste or elastomeric impression material. The material is allowed to flow into the tissue side of the denture.
- The denture is reseated in the mouth, and the patient is instructed to close in normal occlusion to hold the denture in place until the impression paste reaches a final set. The denture is removed and disinfected.
- The denture and written prescription are sent to the laboratory technician for relining.

Delivery of a Laboratory Relined Denture

- When the relined denture is returned from the laboratory, it is disinfected and rinsed before returning to the patient's mouth.
- If necessary, minor trimming may be accomplished with an acrylic bur in a straight handpiece. Minor polishing may be completed on the laboratory lathe with a sterile rag wheel with pumice paste. Note that the tissue-bearing surfaces are never polished; polishing will alter the fit of the appliance.
- The patient is dismissed and advised to return for a checkup of the tissue and adaptation of the prosthesis within a time specified by the dentist.

Immediate Dentures

An immediate denture is one that is immediately placed after extraction of the patient's teeth. During the healing process, the denture serves as a compress and bandage to protect the surgical area. The sterilized denture is rinsed with saline solution and positioned in the mouth. The patient returns in 24 hours for a postoperative checkup. During this time, the denture is to be continuously worn except when removed for cleaning. Daily visits continue until initial healing has started and the sutures are removed, which commonly occurs 48 to 72 hours after surgery. During each visit, the area is irrigated with a mild antiseptic solution, and the soft tissue is checked for pressure points. After the sutures have been removed and the dentist and patient are satisfied with the prosthesis, the patient is scheduled for another appointment within a few months.

Dental Implants

Dental implants are used to attach artificial teeth to anchors (similar to posts) that have been surgically embedded into a patient's mandible or maxilla. The implantation process involves several steps and can take from 3 to 9 months to complete. Depending on the type of implant, the steps will vary.

The placement of dental implants involves both surgery and the placement of the prosthesis. Several specialists, including an oral and maxillofacial surgeon, periodontist, prosthodontist, and or *implantologist* (general dentist with specialized training), can perform the procedure.

Considerations for Prescribing a Dental Implant

Indications

- To replace one or more teeth as single units without affecting adjoining teeth
- To support a bridge and to eliminate the need for a removable partial denture
- To provide support for a denture, making it more secure and comfortable
- To prevent bone loss and gum recession that often accompany bridgework and dentures
- To enhance the patient's confidence in smiling and speaking
- To improve the patient's overall psychological health
- To improve the esthetic appearance of the patient's teeth and mouth

Contraindications

- The financial investment is greater than that for a conventional bridge or denture.
- Treatment can take several months or longer to complete.
- As with any surgical procedure, implants convey a risk for infection and other complications.
- An implant may loosen, requiring replacement.
- Emotionally, the implant procedure may be challenging for some patients.
- *Bruxism* is a significant component of failed implants.

Types of Dental Implants

Endosteal Implant

Endosteal implants, also known as *osseointegrated* implants, are the most common type of dental implant. The implant is surgically placed into the maxilla or mandible. Each implant holds one or more prosthetic teeth. This type of implant is generally used as an alternative for patients that would be prescribed a crown, bridge, or partial denture.

Implants and abutment screws are commonly made from the metal **titanium** because of its compatibility with bone and oral tissues. Titanium implants can be coated with **hydroxyapatite**, a ceramic substance that rapidly osseointegrates the implant to the bone.

Components of Endosteal Implants

Endosteal implants have three components:

1. The *titanium implant* is surgically embedded into the bone during stage I surgery and is supplied as either a blade form, a cylinder form, or a screw form (Fig. 23.14).
2. The *titanium abutment screw* is screwed into the implant after osseointegration of the implant during stage II surgery.
3. The *abutment post* or *cylinder* attaches to the artificial tooth or denture.

Osseointegration (*osseo-* meaning bone) is the process by which the living cells of the bone naturally grow around the implanted dental supports. It refers to a bond that develops between living bone and the surface of an implant fixture. Osseointegrated implants are used to support, stabilize, and retain removable dentures, fixed bridges, and single-tooth implants.

For this type of implant, three appointments are required to complete the procedure. At the *first surgery,* implant fixtures are placed within receptor sites in the jawbone at predetermined

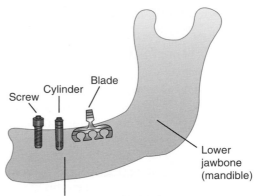

FIGURE 23.14 Diagram showing the types of endosteal implants. (From Darby ML, Walsh MM: *Dental hygiene, theory and practice,* ed 3, St Louis, 2010, Saunders.)

locations. The mucosa is sutured over the fixtures. After a 1- to 2-week healing period, the existing prosthesis (when applicable) may be removed and relined to adapt to the healed ridge.

A period of 3 to 6 months, the *osseointegration period,* is required to permit the fixture to osseointegrate or bond to the bone. Care must be taken during this healing period to avoid trauma to the mucosa overlying the implant sites.

At the *second surgery,* the endosteal implant fixture is exposed, and the abutment screw is connected to the anchor. This portion protrudes through the mucosa and connects the fixture to the prosthesis.

After both surgeries have been completed and tissues have healed, the patient begins the *restorative phase,* during which the final crown, bridge, partial denture, or full denture is fabricated. The entire implant process can require 3 to 9 months to reach completion (Fig. 23.15).

FIGURE 23.15 Stages of surgery Teeth # 20 and #21 with implants.

See Procedure 23.6: Assisting in an Endosteal Implant Surgery.

Subperiosteal Implant

A subperiosteal implant is a metal frame that is placed under the periosteum and *on top* of the bone. In contrast to an endosteal implant, a subperiosteal implant is *not* placed into the bone.

Subperiosteal implants are indicated for patients that do not have a sufficient alveolar ridge to support the endosteal-type implant. This type of implant is most frequently used to support a mandibular complete denture (Fig. 23.16).

Two surgical procedures are required for this type of implant. During the *first surgery,* the alveolar ridge is exposed, and impressions are taken of the alveolar ridge. After the impressions are taken, the tissue is repositioned over the ridge and is sutured back into place. The impression is sent to a dental laboratory, where a metal frame with posts is fabricated.

After the frame has been fabricated, the *second surgery* includes exposing the alveolar ridge and placing the metal frame over the ridge, and the tissues are repositioned and sutured into place.

FIGURE 23.16 Subperiosteal implant with full-arch denture prosthesis. (From Newman M, Takei T, Klokkevold P, Carranza F, editors: *Carranza's clinical periodontology,* ed 11, St Louis, 2012, Saunders.)

Transosteal Implant

The transosteal implant is inserted through the inferior border of the mandible and into the edentulous area. The most common type is the *transmandibular staple implant,* or fixed mandibular implant. These implants are primarily used in patients with severely resorbed ridges and only when no other options exist.

Maintenance of Dental Implants

Long-term maintenance is an integral part of treatment for patients with dental implants. Maintenance includes home care by the patient and periodic maintenance visits to the dental office.

The health of the peri-implant tissue is a critical factor in the success of dental implants. This tissue is similar to the gingival sulcus that surrounds a natural tooth. Peri-implant tissue responds to bacterial plaque with inflammation and bleeding, similarly to gingival tissues around a normal tooth.

Recall Visits

Recall visits are essential for the long-term success of implants. It is important that patients understand the need to maintain optimal plaque control with home care and frequent professional recalls. Patients should be scheduled at regular intervals for examination, radiography, prophylaxis, removal of fixed components, replacement of components, and relines and remakes as recommended.

Ethical Implications

Prosthodontics is an area of dentistry that relies on knowledge, technique, and communication with the patient and laboratory technician. Understanding the process of prosthodontics is important for the dental assistant.

The procedures of placing the retraction cord and the fabrication of a provisional may be legal for the CDA or RDA in the state in which you are practicing.

Placing and Removal of the Gingival Retraction Cord (Expanded Function)

Consider the following with this procedure: Confirm with state guidelines before performing this procedure. Personal protective equipment (PPE) is required for the health care team, the student is required to identify and prepare the instrument setup, moisture control is included to prevent contamination, and the procedure is to be documented in the patient record.

Prerequisites for Performing This Procedure

- Mirror skills
- Operator positioning
- Dental anatomy
- Instrumentation
- Fulcrum

Equipment and Supplies

- Basic setup
- Cotton rolls
- Cord-packing instrument
- Gingival retraction cord
- Dappen dish
- Scissors

Procedural Steps

Preparation

1. Rinse and gently dry the prepared tooth; isolate the quadrant with cotton rolls.
   Purpose: Dry tissue makes it easier to see the details of the gingival tissue and place the retraction cord.

2. Cut a piece of retraction cord 1 to 1 ½ inches in length, depending on the size and type of tooth under preparation. **Note:** The length is determined by the circumference of the prepared tooth and the placement technique to be used.

3. Use cotton pliers to form a loose loop of the cord.
   Purpose: This makes the cord easy to slip over the tooth, but the loop is not tied or knotted.

Placement

4. Make a loop in the retraction cord, slip it over the tooth, and position the loop in the sulcus around the prepared tooth.

5. Using the cord-packing instrument and working in a clockwise direction, pack the cord gently into the sulcus surrounding the prepared tooth, so that the ends are on the facial aspect.

Continued

Placing and Removal of the Gingival Retraction Cord (Expanded Function)—cont'd

Purpose: The ends in this position are easier to reach for removal of the cord.

6. Pack the cord into the sulcus by gently rocking the instrument slightly backward as the instrument is moved forward to the next loose section of retraction cord. Repeat this action until the length of cord is packed in place.

7. Overlap the cord where it meets the first end of the cord. The ends may be tucked into the sulcus on the facial aspect.
   Note: An alternative is to leave a short length of the cord sticking out of the sulcus. This makes it easier to grasp and quickly remove the cord.
   Optional: When a wider and deeper sulcus is required, two retraction cords may be placed with one on top of the other. Before the impression material is taken, remove the top cord. After the impression is completed, remove the second retraction cord.

8. The cord should be left in place for a maximum of 5 to 7 minutes. Instruct the patient to remain still to keep the area dry.

Purpose: This time allows the cord to push tissue away from the tooth and stay in this position.
Note: The exact time depends on the type of chemical retraction used.

Removal

9. Grasp the end of the retraction cord with cotton pliers and remove it in a counterclockwise direction (the reverse of the method used in packing).

10. Remove the retraction cord just before the impression material is placed.
    Note: Usually the operator removers the cord while the assistant prepares the syringe-type impression material.

11. Gently dry the area, and apply fresh cotton rolls.
    Note: The impression is taken immediately.

Documentation

12. Document the procedure.

Fabricating and Cementing a Custom Acrylic Provision Crown (Expanded Function)

Consider the following with this procedure: Confirm with state guidelines before performing this procedure. Personal protective equipment (PPE) is required for the health care team, the student is required to identify and prepare the instrument set-up, appropriate safety protocols are to be followed, and the procedure is to be documented in the patient record.

Prerequisites for Performing This Procedure

- Operator positioning
- Differentiation between cavity classifications and oral anatomy
- Knowledge of application technique
- Intraoral instrumentation
- Extraoral use of low-speed handpiece
- Mirror skills
- Fulcrum placement

Equipment and Supplies

- Basic setup
- Spoon excavator
- Alginate impression (obtained before preparation of the teeth)
- Separating medium
- Cotton rolls

Fabricating and Cementing a Custom Acrylic Provision Crown (Expanded Function)—cont'd

- Self-curing acrylic resin (liquid and powder)
- Spatula (small, cement type)
- Mixing container/dappen dish
- Scissors
- Surgical knife (optional)
- Burnisher ("beaver tail" or ball)
- Straight handpiece and mandrel
- Finishing diamond, discs, or burs
- Polishing discs or burs
- Articulating paper
- Pumice paste
- Lathe and sterile white rag wheel
- Provisional cementation setup

(From Rosenstiel SF, Land MF, Fujimoto J: *Contemporary fixed prosthodontics,* ed 5, St Louis, 2016, Elsevier.)

Procedural Steps

1. Obtain an alginate impression of the arch before the teeth are prepared.
   Purpose: You want the provisional coverage to be a replica of the tooth before the dentist prepares it.
2. Check the impression to be sure it is free of debris and tears in the area selected for construction of the provisional crown or bridge covering.
3. Disinfect the impression and keep it moist until needed.
   Purpose: If allowed to dry, the impression will be distorted and the provisional coverage will not fit.
4. Isolate the prepared tooth with cotton rolls to maintain moisture control.
5. Lightly apply petroleum jelly or a liquid medium to the prepared tooth to facilitate separation of the acrylic dough from the preparations.
6. If using the liquid/powder acrylic material, place the liquid monomer in the glass dappen dish; 10 drops of liquid

per unit is recommended. Quickly dispense the selected shade of self-curing powder (polymer) into the monomer until the powder is saturated.
   Important: Cover the monomer container immediately; this material is volatile.
   Note: If using the syringe-type acrylic material, skip to step 9.
7. Use a small spatula to blend the powder the liquid to a homogeneous mix.
8. Set the mixed material aside for 1 to 2 minutes until the resin reaches a doughy, less glossy stage.
   Important: Do not let the resin cure beyond this point.
9. Unwrap the alginate impression, and gently dry the area of the teeth to receive provisional coverage.
10. Remove the resin from the mixing container with a small spatula, and immediately place it within the area of the prepared teeth.
    Optional: Express the acrylic resin from a syringe directly into the impression.

11. Place the acrylic-loaded impression back into the patient's mouth on the prepared tooth or teeth.

12. Allow the material to reach an initial set, which takes approximately 3 minutes, and remove the tray from the patient's mouth.

Continued

Fabricating and Cementing a Custom Acrylic Provision Crown (Expanded Function)—cont'd

13. Carefully remove the provisional coverage from the alginate impression and place it onto the patient's teeth.
   Purpose: To avoid excess shrinkage during the final curing stage.
14. Mark the marginal border and contract points of the provisional coverage with a pencil to provide better visualization of the markings.

15. Trim the acrylic resin to within 1 mm of the gingival shoulder of the prepared tooth with an acrylic bur or stone.

Note: Any trimming completed by the EFDA/RDA must be completed outside the mouth with the low-speed handpiece and acrylic burs.

16. Check the occlusion, accuracy, and completeness of the provisional coverage and adjust as necessary. Remove the provisional coverage from the prepared tooth and complete the trimming with an acrylic bur.
17. Remove the provisional coverage and take it to the laboratory, where it is polished with a sterile white rag wheel and pumice on the laboratory lathe.
   Caution: Safety goggles must be worn throughout the trimming and polishing procedure. In addition, be aware that the rag wheel could remove a large bulk of acrylic or could overheat and cause distortion of the provisional coverage.
18. Temporarily cement the provisional coverage with provisional cement, such as zinc oxide-eugenol (TempBond [Kerr]) or intermediate restorative material.
19. Check the occlusion with articulating paper. If any reduction is required, the dentist will use an acrylic-trimming but.
20. Document the procedure.

Assisting in a Crown or Bridge Preparation

Consider the following with this procedure: Personal protective equipment (PPE) is required for the health care team, the student is required to identify and prepare the instrument setup, moisture control is included to prevent contamination, and the procedure is to be documented in the patient record.

Equipment and Supplies

- Local anesthetic agent setup
- Alginate impression setup
- Shade guide (for tooth-colored restoration)
- Large spoon excavator
- Additional hand instruments (dentist's choice)
- Gingival retraction setup
- Cotton rolls and gauze sponges
- High-volume oral evacuator (HVE) tip
- At this visit, setups are also required for the following:
  - Elastomeric impressions, which may include a custom tray
  - Occlusal (bite) registration
  - Provisional coverage fabrication, adjustment, and cementation supplies

(From Boyd LRB: *Dental instruments: a pocket guide,* ed 7, St Louis, 2021, Elsevier.)

Procedural Steps

Preliminary Steps

1. Assist in administration of the local anesthetic agent.
2. If an alginate impression is needed to fabricate the provisional coverage, the impression is obtained at this time. In addition, an alginate impression of the opposing arch is taken (see Chapter 46).

3. If a silicone two-step impression method is used, the first impression is obtained at this time.

4. If this procedure involves a tooth-colored restoration, the shade is selected at this time.

Tooth Preparation

5. Throughout the preparation, maintain a clear operating field by using the HVE to retract the lips and tongue and to remove water and debris.

6. The dentist uses diamond stones in the high-speed handpiece to remove all decay or fractured portions of the tooth.

   Purpose: Diamond stones are used during crown preparation because they can rapidly remove tooth structure.

(From Rosenstiel SF, Land MF, Fujimoto J: *Contemporary fixed prosthodontics,* ed 5, St Louis, 2016, Elsevier.)

Assistance

7. Assist in bur changes as necessary while the dentist reduces tooth bulk and completes the preparation using burs of different shapes.

8. Retraction cord is placed to reflect gingival tissue for the final preparation.

(From Rosenstiel SF, Land MF, Fujimoto J: *Contemporary fixed prosthodontics,* ed 5, St Louis, 2016, Elsevier.)

9. Assist in readying the final impression material.

10. Before transferring the light-bodied material, transfer cotton pliers for the dentist to remove the gingival retraction cord.

    Note: The dentist may want to rinse and dry the sulcus before applying the light-bodied material.

11. While the dentist is applying the light-bodied material, ready the try with heavy-bodied material.

12. Have the air-water syringe available for the dentist to "blow" air around the preparation.

    Purpose: This procedure thins out the material, allowing it to flow better within the sulcus and around the margins.

13. Retrieve the light-bodied material syringe from the dentist and transfer the tray, ensuring that the dentist can grasp the handle and insert the try property.

14. After the recommended time has passed for the material to set, the dentist will remove the tray.

15. The occlusal registration is obtained.

16. Provisional coverage is fabricated and is temporarily cemented to protect the prepared teeth (see Chapter 51).

17. The patient is scheduled for a cementation appointment and then dismissed.

    Note: Ensure that the laboratory has sufficient time to fabricate the crown before scheduling the patient for another appointment.

18. After the dentist writes the laboratory prescription, prepare the case and send it to the laboratory.

Documentation

19. Document the procedure.

Date	Tooth	Surface	Charting Notes
8/15	4	PFM	Crown prep, 2 cartridges Xylocaine w/epi, final impression, temporary made and cemented with tomp bond Shade C2 for porcelain. Pt tolerated procedure well. Reschedule in 2 weeks for cementation T. Clark, CD/M. Stewart, DDS

Assisting in the Delivery of a Partial Denture

Consider the following with this procedure: Personal protective equipment (PPE) is required for the health care team, and the procedure is to be documented in the patient record.

Equipment and Supplies

- Basic setup
- Articulating paper and holder
- Pressure indicator paste
- Low-speed and high-speed hand pieces
- Pressure-indicator paste
- Acrylic burs
- Finishing burs
- Three-pronged pliers

Procedural Steps

1. Remove partial from laboratory packaging: disinfect and rinse to prepare for try-in.
2. Seat the patient.
3. The dentist places the new partial denture in the patient's mouth.
4. The patient is instructed to close their teeth together.
5. To check the occlusion, assist in placing articulating paper on the *occlusion* surface or the mandibular teeth and ask the patient to simulate chewing motions. If the occlusion is too high, transfer hand piece with round carbide bur.
6. To detect *pressure points* (high spots) that could cause discomfort to the patient, apply pressure-indicator paste on the tissue surface of the prosthesis. The prosthesis in placed in the patient's month. These high spots on the prosthesis are adjusted as necessary.

7. Retainers are examined for tension on the natural abutment teeth. Transfer pliers to the dentist to adjust the tension on the retainers.
8. After adjustments have been made, the partial denture is polished on the laboratory lathe with the appropriate pastes and sterile buffing wheels.
9. Scrub the partial denture with soap, water, and a brush; disinfect and rinse; and return the partial denture to the treatment room for delivery to the patient.
10. Instruct the patient on placement, removal, and care of the partial denture.
11. Document the procedure.

Date	Tooth	Surface	Charting Notes
8/20	–	PFM	Delivered maxillary partial, minor adjustments made. Pt pleased with appearance and fit. Reschedule pt in 3 days for postdelivery check. T. Clark, CDA/L. Stewart, DDS T. Clark, CD/M. Stewart, DDS

Assisting in the Delivery of a Full Denture

Consider the following with this procedure: Personal protective equipment (PPE) is required for the health care team, and the procedure is to be documented in the patient record.

Equipment and Supplies

- Basic setup
- Dentures
- Hand mirror
- Articulating paper and holder
- High-speed and low-speed hand-pieces
- Pressure indicator paste
- Finishing burs
- Acrylic burs

Procedural Steps

1. Remove denture from laboratory packaging: disinfect and rinse to prepare for try-in.

2. Seat the patient.
3. Assist the patient in inserting the new denture into the patient's mouth.
4. Hand the patient a mirror and evaluate the shade and mold of the artificial teeth for natural appearance.
5. Ask the patient to perform facial expressions and the actions of swallowing, chewing, and speaking, using "a" and "the" sounds.
   Note: These sounds also are appropriate for exercises to help the patient learn to speak normally with the new denture.
6. Assist in checking the *occlusion* by placing articulating paper on the occlusal surface of the mandibular teeth and asking the patient to simulate chewing motions.
   Purpose: Cusps that are too high in contact will be marked with the color of the articulating paper.

Assisting in the Delivery of a Full Denture—cont'd

7. If the cusps are too high, the denture is removed from the mouth and is adjusted with a stone mounted on a straight hand-piece.

8. The denture is replaced in the mouth, and the procedure is repeated until the cusps appear to be in occlusion with the opposing arch.

   Note: If the denture must be taken into the laboratory for adjustment, it must be disinfected again before it is returned to the patient.

9. When the patient is pleased with the appearance, function, and comfort of the denture, another appointment is made for the postdelivery checkup.

10. After adjustments have been made, the partial denture is polished on the laboratory lathe with the appropriate pastes and sterile buffing wheels.

11. Scrub the denture with soap, water, and a brush; disinfect and rinse; return the denture to the treatment room for delivery to the patient.

12. Instruct the patient on placement, removal, and care of the denture.

13. Before dismissal, the patient is informed that learning to wear a new denture will take several days or weeks.

14. Document the procedure.

Date	Tooth	Surface	Charting Notes
8/28			Delivery of maxillary full denture. Pt pleased with change of canines. Teeth and shading good. Pt pleased with fit and appearance. Reschedule in 3 days for postdelivery check. T. Clark, CD/M. Stewart, DDS

Assisting in an Endosteal Implant Surgery

Equipment and Supplies

- Basic setup
- Local anesthetic
- Sterile surgical gloves
- Sterile surgical drilling unit
- Surgical irrigation tip
- Scalpel
- Periosteal elevator
- Implant instrument kit
- Implant kit
- Sterile saline solution
- Low-speed handpiece with contra-angle attachment
- Inserting mallet
- Suture setup
- Electrosurgical unit and tips (or tissue punch)
- 3% hydrogen peroxide with syringe
- Sterile cotton pellets
- Sterile 2 × 2–inch gauze sponges

(From Bird DL, Robinson DS: *Modern dental assisting,* ed 11, St Louis, 2015, Saunders.)

Continued

Procedural Steps

Stage I Surgery: Implant Placement

1. The surgical stent (template) is placed in position in the patient's mouth.
2. After achieving adequate anesthesia, the surgeon uses a *pilot drill* (similar to a Pesso bur) to drill through the stent and into the soft tissue on the ridge, creating a target point on the bone for the implant site.
   Note: All drilling of the bone is accomplished with generous amounts of sterile saline irrigation.
3. The surgeon removes the surgical stent and makes the incision at the implant site.

(From Newman M, Takei T, Klokkevold P, Carranza F, editors: *Carranza's clinical periodontology,* ed. 12, St Louis, 2015, Saunders.)

4. The mucoperiosteal tissues are reflected.

(From Newman M, Takei T, Klokkevold P, Carranza F, editors: *Carranza's clinical periodontology,* ed. 12, St Louis, 2015, Saunders.)

5. The surgeon smooths any sharp edges on the crest of the ridge. The crest should be at least 2 mm wider than the implant that is being used.
6. A variety of drill tips (similar to burs) are used to prepare the osseous receptor site.
7. The implant cylinder (with a plastic cap over the top of it) is partially inserted into the osseous receptor site.
8. The plastic cap is removed, and the implant is tapped into its final position with the inserting mallet.

9. The sterile sealing screw (also called a *healing collar*) is placed into the implant cylinder with the contra-angle screwdriver. Final tightening of the sealing screw is accomplished with the handheld screwdriver.

(From Newman M, Takei T, Klokkevold P, Carranza F, editors: *Carranza's clinical periodontology,* ed. 12, St Louis, 2015, Saunders.)

10. The retraction suture is removed, and the mucoperiosteal flaps are repositioned and sutured in place. The implant receptor is now covered by the tissue and is not visible in the mouth.

(From Newman M, Takei T, Klokkevold P, Carranza F, editors: *Carranza's clinical periodontology,* ed. 12, St Louis, 2015, Saunders.)

Osseointegration Period

1. A period of 3 to 6 months is required to permit the fixture or fixtures to osseointegrate or bond to the bone. During this period, the existing denture or provisional coverage can be adapted to the healed alveolar ridge for temporary use—a procedure usually performed by the *restorative dentist.* The goal of the restorative dentist is to provide patients with beautiful teeth and a beautiful smile, so they can continue their normal activities without delay.

Stage II Surgery: Implant Exposure

1. After local anesthesia is administered, the surgical stent (template) is repositioned.

2. A sharp instrument such as a periodontal probe is lowered through the opening in the stent to make bleeding points.

(From Bird DL, Robinson DS: *Modern dental assisting,* ed. 11, St Louis, 2015, Saunders.)

(From Bird DL, Robinson DS: *Modern dental assisting,* ed. 11, St Louis, 2015, Saunders.)

3. The stent is removed, and the mark on the soft tissue shows the position of the previously placed implant.

4. An electrosurgical loop is used to remove the soft tissue over the implant site by peeling it back one layer at a time until the titanium sealing screw is located. A special tissue punch can be used to remove the tissue from over the implant.

5. The implant is uncovered, and the sealing screw is removed.

(From Bird DL, Robinson DS: *Modern dental assisting,* ed. 11, St Louis, 2015, Saunders.)

(From Bird DL, Robinson DS: *Modern dental assisting,* ed. 11, St Louis, 2015, Saunders.)

6. The inside of the implant cylinder is cleaned with sterile cotton soaked in hydrogen peroxide.

7. A healing collar is screwed into the implant. This attachment will now extend above the mucosa.

(From Bird DL, Robinson DS: *Modern dental assisting,* ed. 11, St Louis, 2015, Saunders.)

8. The soft tissues are allowed to heal for 10 to 14 days before a permanent crown is fabricated.

Multiple Choice

Circle the letter next to the correct answer.

1. The portion of a fixed bridge that replaces the natural tooth is termed the _____.
   a. abutment
   b. clasp
   c. pontic
   d. retainer

2. A cast restoration that covers the proximal surfaces and most of the occlusal surface is called a(n) _____.
   a. inlay
   b. bridge
   c. onlay
   d. partial denture

3. The screw portion of the dental implant is commonly fabricated from what material?
   a. Bone graft
   b. Porcelain
   c. Titanium
   d. Enamel

4. A post and core is used to strengthen a restoration and improve retention in a(n) _____.
   a. badly decayed tooth
   b. fractured anterior tooth
   c. endodontically treated tooth
   d. implant

5. When a fixed bridge is created, there must be at least _____ of the bridge.
   a. one abutment
   b. one pontic
   c. two or more pontics
   d. two or more retainers

6. The use of a gingival retraction cord with epinephrine _____ recommended for a patient with cardiovascular disease.
   a. is
   b. is not

7. Provisional coverage can remain on a prepared tooth or teeth for a few days to _____.
   a. a few hours
   b. a few weeks
   c. a few months
   d. indefinitely

8. The saddle of a removable partial denture _____.
   a. holds the artificial teeth
   b. provides some support for the prosthesis
   c. rests on the oral mucosa covering the alveolar ridge
   d. attaches to the abutment teeth

9. Retention of the maxillary denture primarily depends on the _____.
   a. support of the alveolar ridge
   b. abutment teeth
   c. occlusion
   d. suction seal of the post dam

10. Osseo means the _____.
    a. occlusal portion of an implant
    b. gingival tissues surrounding the implant
    c. stent used in implant placement
    d. bone in which the implant is imbedded

Apply Your Knowledge

1. A patient calls the office and is having discomfort in her jaw on the same side that her crown was placed last week. You remember assisting in the cementation of this crown and that the crown fit great. What could be wrong?

2. Mr. Smith is scheduled for a lower partial denture. The partial will replace his molars on both sides. How many teeth will make up the partial denture? What teeth will become the abutment teeth for this prothesis?

3. Why is infection control so important during the preparation and procedure steps of a dental implant?

CHAPTER 24

Periodontics

http://evolve.elsevier.com/Robinson/essentials/

LEARNING OBJECTIVES

1. Pronounce, define, and spell the key terms.
2. Describe the characteristics of periodontal disease and include risk factors, signs, and symptoms.
3. Complete the following related to the periodontal examination:
   - Know which procedures are necessary for a comprehensive periodontal examination.
   - Understand why vertical bitewing radiographs are useful in periodontics.
   - Describe the mobility of teeth.
   - Know the instruments used in the periodontal examination and be able to explain the indications for use.
4. Explain the purpose of scaling, root planing, and gingival curettage.
5. Describe the indications and contraindications for the ultrasonic scaler.
6. Name and describe the types of periodontal surgeries.
7. Discuss instruments used in periodontal surgery.
8. Complete the following related to periodontal treatment and surgeries:
   - Know the purpose of antimicrobial and antibiotic agents in periodontal treatment.
   - Describe the five main reasons for periodontal surgery.
   - Describe periodontal surgery postop instructions.
   - Explain the purpose of periodontal surgical dressings and demonstrate the technique for proper placement.

KEY TERMS

gingival graft	periodontal dressing	scaling
gingivectomy	periodontal flap surgery	sulcus
gingivitis	periodontal pocket	supragingival/subgingival
gingivoplasty	periodontist	calculus
mobility	periodontitis	supragingival calculus
ostectomy	periodontium	ultrasonic scaler
osteoplasty	root planing	vertical bite-wing radiographs

Periodontal disease is the leading cause of tooth loss in adults. Fortunately, with early detection and treatment, it is possible for most people to keep their teeth for a lifetime. The **periodontist** (a dentist with advanced training in the specialty of periodontics) deals with the causes, prevention, and treatment of diseases of the tissue of the periodontium. The **periodontium** consists of the tissue that surrounds and supports the teeth (Fig. 24.1 and Table 24.1).

Periodontal Diseases

Most periodontal diseases begin as gingival inflammation caused by an accumulation of bacterial biofilm (see Chapter 20 for a discussion of biofilm plaque and calculus formation) adhering to the teeth, to calculus, and to fixed and removable restorations. Periodontal diseases and dental caries are caused by pathogenic (disease-causing) microorganisms found in microbial biofilm. Calculus is mineralized microbial biofilm.

FIGURE 24.1 Structures of the periodontium, junctional epithelium, gingival sulcus, periodontal ligaments, and cementum.

TABLE 24.1
Structures of the Periodontium

Name	Description
Gingivae	Commonly referred to as *gums,* this mucosa covers the alveolar process of the jaws and surrounds the necks of the teeth.
Epithelial attachment	This tissue is at the base of the sulcus where the gingiva attaches to the tooth.
Gingival sulcus	The sulcus is the space between the tooth and the free gingiva.
Periodontal ligaments	These tense connective fibers connect the cementum covering the root of the tooth with the alveolar bone of the socket wall.
Cementum	The cementum covers the root of the tooth; its primary function is to anchor the tooth to the bony socket with the attachments of the periodontal ligaments.
Alveolar bone	Alveolar bone supports the tooth in its position within the jaw. The alveolar socket is the cavity in the bone that surrounds the tooth.

General oral health depends on the daily removal of bacterial biofilm deposits.

Additional oral conditions and risk factors can also contribute to periodontal diseases (Table 24.2).

Signs and Symptoms

The following signs and symptoms are detected in patients with periodontal disease:
- Red, swollen, or tender gingiva
- Bleeding gingiva while brushing or flossing
- Loose teeth or movement of teeth
- Pain or pressure when chewing
- Pus around the teeth or gingival tissue

Gingivitis

Gingivitis is inflammation of the *gingival tissue* (Fig. 24.2). The gingivae appear red and swollen and tend to bleed easily. Gingivitis is *directly related* to the presence of bacterial biofilm on the

tooth surface and the amount of time that the biofilm is allowed to remain undisturbed (Biofilm plaque is discussed in Chapter 20).

Periodontitis

Periodontitis occurs as the infection from the gingivae progresses into the *alveolar bone*. Periodontitis is classified into *stages* according to the severity of the disease, which incorporates tooth loss, and management of the patient's periodontal therapy needs. Studies show that 47% of adults 30 years and older have some form of periodontal disease, with that percentage increasing to 70% of adults 65 years and older. Nevertheless, periodontitis can also be detected in children.

Stages of Periodontitis
Stage I—Mild periodontitis with probing depths less than 4 mm. Requires nonsurgical treatment, and no post-treatment tooth loss is expected. Has a good prognosis.

TABLE 24.2
Common Risk Factors for Periodontal Disease

Risk Factor	Rationale
Smoking	Smokers have a greater loss of attachment, bone loss, periodontal pocket depths, calculus formation, and tooth loss. Periodontal treatments are less effective in smokers than in nonsmokers.
Diabetes mellitus	Diabetes is a strong risk factor for periodontal disease. Individuals with diabetes are three times more likely to have attachment and bone loss. Persons who have diabetes under control have less attachment and bone loss than those with poor control.
Poor oral hygiene	Lack of good oral hygiene increases the risk for periodontal disease in all age groups. Excellent oral hygiene greatly reduces the risk for severe periodontal disease.
Osteoporosis	An association between alveolar bone loss and osteoporosis has been noted. Women with osteoporosis have increased alveolar bone resorption, attachment loss, and tooth loss compared with women without osteoporosis. Estrogen deficiency has been linked to decreases in alveolar bone.
HIV or AIDS	Gingival inflammation is increased around the margins of all teeth. Often patients with HIV or AIDS will develop necrotizing ulcerative periodontitis (NUP).
Stress	Psychologic stress is associated with depression of the immune system, and studies show a link between stress and periodontal attachment loss. Research is ongoing to determine the link between psychological stress and periodontal disease.
Medications	Some medications, such as tetracycline and nonsteroidal antiinflammatory drugs (NSAIDs), have a beneficial effect on the periodontium, and others have a negative effect. More than 400 medications, including diuretic, antihistamine, antipsychotic, antihypertension, and analgesic agents, can cause a decrease in salivary flow (xerostomia). Antiseizure drugs and hormones such as estrogen and progesterone can cause gingival enlargement.
Local factors	Overhanging restorations, subgingival placement of crown margins, orthodontic appliances, and removable partial dentures also may contribute to the progression of periodontal disease.

HIV, Human immunodeficiency virus; *AIDS,* acquired immunodeficiency syndrome.

Stage II—Moderate periodontitis with probing depths less than 5 mm; 3 to 4 mm horizontal bone loss and will require nonsurgical and surgical treatment. No tooth loss is expected. Good prognosis.

Stage III—Severe periodontitis with probing depths greater than 6 mm, with possible vertical bone loss and furcation involvement. Patient will require surgical and regenerative treatment. Fair prognosis.

Stage IV—Very severe periodontitis with probing depths greater than 6 mm, with vertical bone loss and furcation involvement. Fewer than 20 teeth present. Advanced surgical treatment / regenerative therapy needed. Questionable prognosis.

FIGURE 24.2 Gingivitis *(arrow).* (From Newman M, Carranza FA: *Carranza's clinical periodontology.* ed 12, Saunders, Saunders; 2015.)

Periodontal Examination

In addition to a thorough dental examination as described in Chapter 13, specialized procedures are necessary to diagnose and plan appropriate treatment for periodontal disease. A periodontal examination includes medical and dental histories, radiographic evaluations, examination of the teeth, examination of the gingivae and supporting structures, and periodontal charting, which consists of pocket readings and taking note of furcations, tooth mobility, exudate (pus), and gingival recession (Fig. 24.3).

Radiographs

Radiographs are a valuable aid for evaluating periodontal disease. The accuracy of a radiograph is critical in the diagnosis of periodontal disease because a distortion can result in a diagnostic error. **Vertical bite-wing radiographs** (Fig. 24.4) are exposed for a periodontal examination because they show generalized horizontal bone loss on both arches better than the traditional horizontal bite-wing radiographs.

FIGURE 24.3 Computer generated periodontal chart. (Courtesy Florida Probe Corporation. Gainesville, Florida.)

Examination of the Teeth

The examination of the teeth focuses on indications of periodontal disease or factors that can contribute to periodontal disease.

Dental Conditions that Can Contribute to Periodontal Disease

Pathologic migration—A shift in the position of the tooth or teeth caused by loss of periodontal support.

Clenching or bruxism—Bruxism places excessive biting forces on the teeth and may accelerate bone loss.

Defective restorations bridgework—Dental prostheses may retain plaque and increase the risk for periodontal disease.

Mobility—All teeth have some mobility. Mobility is recorded with the following scale: 0—normal, 1—slight mobility, 2—moderate mobility, 3—extreme mobility (Fig. 24.5).

FIGURE 24.4 Vertical bite-wing films can be used to cover a larger area of the alveolar bone.

FIGURE 24.5 Mobility is detected with the blunt ends of two instruments. (From Daniel SA, Harfst SA: *Mosby's dental hygiene concepts, cases, and competencies,* ed 2, Mosby, 2008.)

Examination of the Gingivae and Supporting Structures

The periodontal exam includes an assessment of the amounts of biofilm and calculus and of changes in gingival health, as well as an assessment of bleeding at the bone level and detection of periodontal pockets. A **periodontal pocket** occurs when disease causes the normal gingival **sulcus** to become deeper than normal (a normal sulcus measures 3 mm or less; Fig. 24.6).

The depth of the periodontal pocket is measured by using a periodontal probe. The dentist or dental hygienist will record six measurements for each tooth, (mesio-facial, facial, disto-facial, mesio-lingual, lingual, and disto-lingual; Fig. 24.7).

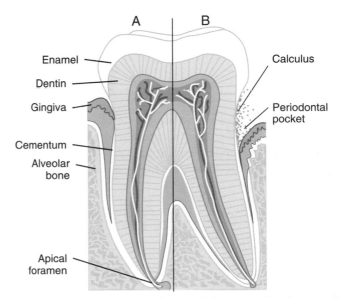

FIGURE 24.6 Cross-section of a tooth and associated anatomic structures. **A,** Illustrates the depth of a normal gingival sulcus. **B,** Illustrates a periodontal pocket.

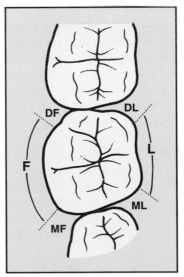

FIGURE 24.7 Six probing depths are taken for each tooth. *DF,* Distofacial; *DL,* distolingual; *F,* facial; *L,* lingual; *MF,* mesiofacial; *ML,* mesiolingual. (Modified from Perry DA, Beemsterboer P, Carranza FA: *Techniques and theory of periodontal instrumentation,* Saunders, 1990.)

FIGURE 24.8 Diagram showing probing of the periodontal pocket depth.

The **bleeding index** provides the severity of gingival inflammation and is measured by the amount of bleeding observed during probing. Several different indices can be used to measure bleeding. Each system is based on the principle that healthy gingivae do not bleed.

Instruments Used in the Periodontal Exam and Prophylaxis

Periodontal Probes

Periodontal probes, which are calibrated in millimeters, are used to locate and measure the depth of periodontal pockets (Fig. 24.8). On some periodontal probes, the tip is color-coded to make the measurements easier to read.

The manual probe is tapered to fit into the gingival sulcus and has a blunt or rounded tip. This probe is available in many designs, and selection depends on the personal preferences of the operator.

Automated computerized probes are accurate electronic devices used to measure the depth of periodontal pockets. With the probe, a thin, wire-like device is inserted into the sulcus, and data are recorded by a microcomputer. Voice-activated recording systems are becoming popular in periodontal assessment. The operator will speak the measurement, and the computer will automatically enter the information.

Explorers

Explorers are used to locate calculus deposits and provide tactile information to the operator about the roughness or smoothness of the root surfaces. Many styles of explorers are used in periodontal treatment, and they are longer and more curved than explorers used for caries detection. (Explorers are discussed in Chapter 12.)

The working ends of periodontal explorers are thin and fine, enabling them to be easily adapted around tooth surfaces. They are also long enough to reach the base of deep pockets and furcations. A furcation is the point at which the roots of a multi-rooted tooth diverge (Fig. 24.9).

FIGURE 24.9 Various styles of periodontal explorers. (Courtesy Hu-Friedy Manufacturing, Chicago, Illinois.)

Scalers

Sickle scalers are primarily used to remove large deposits of **supragingival calculus** (calculus above the gumline). A sickle scaler with a long straight shank is used to remove calculus from the anterior areas of the oral cavity (Fig. 24.10). A contra-angle sickle scaler, which is angled at the shank, is designed to remove calculus from the posterior teeth.

Chisel scalers are used to remove supragingival calculus in the contact area of the anterior teeth. The blade on the chisel scaler is slightly curved to adapt to the tooth surfaces (Fig. 24.11).

Hoe scalers are used to remove heavy supragingival calculus. Hoes are most effective when used on buccal and lingual surfaces of the posterior teeth (Fig. 24.12).

Curettes

Curettes are used to remove **supragingival** (above the gumline) and **subgingival** (below the gumline) **calculus**, to smooth rough root surfaces (root planing), and to remove the diseased soft tissue lining of the periodontal pocket (soft tissue curettage). Curettes have a rounded end, unlike a scaler, which has a pointed end (Fig. 24.13). Two basic designs of curettes are available: the universal curette and the Gracey curette.

Universal curettes are designed so that one instrument is able to adapt to all tooth surfaces (hence the name *universal*). Two cutting edges are found on each side of the blade. Universal curettes resemble the spoon excavators used in restorative dentistry (Fig. 24.14).

Gracey curettes have one cutting edge and are specific to an area, which means that they are designed to adapt to specific

FIGURE 24.10 Curved sickle scaler. (From Boyd LRB: *Dental instruments: a pocket guide,.* ed 5, Saunders, 2015.)

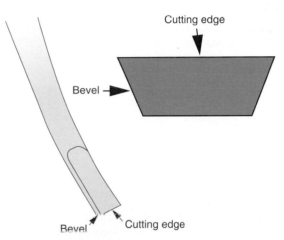

FIGURE 24.11 The chisel has a single blade with a firm shank. The cutting edge is at the end of the instrument so that when it is pushed against a deposit, the leading edge engages the calculus. (From Daniel SA, Harfst SA: *Mosby's dental hygiene concepts, cases, and competencies,* ed 2, Mosby, 2008.)

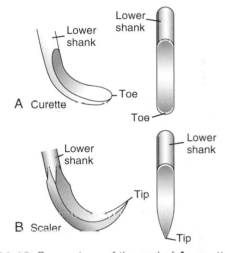

FIGURE 24.13 Comparison of the end of **A**, curette (rounded), and **B**, scaler (pointed).

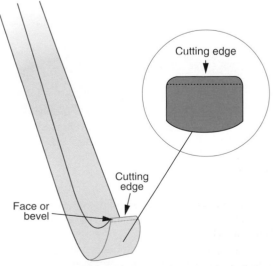

FIGURE 24.12 The hoe has one blade with a firm shank.

tooth surfaces (mesial or distal). Treatment of the full dentition requires the use of several Gracey curettes (Fig. 24.15).

Ultrasonic Scaler

The **ultrasonic scaler** rapidly removes calculus and significantly reduces hand fatigue for the operator. Newer styles and slimmer instrument tips have been designed to allow for better access to subgingival pockets.

The ultrasonic scaler converts very-high-frequency sound waves into mechanical energy in the form of very rapid vibrations (20,000 to 40,000 cycles per second) at the tip of the instrument. A spray of water at the tip prevents the buildup of heat and provides a continuous flush of debris and bacteria from the base of the pocket (Fig. 24.16). Contraindications and precautions must be considered for pediatric patients and for people with certain medical and oral conditions.

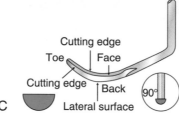

FIGURE 24.14 The universal curettes. **A,** Barnhart ½. **B,** Ratcliff ¾. **C,** The arrows indicate the cutting edges on a universal curette. (From Boyd LRB: *Dental instruments: a pocket guide,* ed 5, Saunders, 2015.)

FIGURE 24.15 Assorted Gracey curettes. (Courtesy Hu-Friedy Manufacturing, Chicago, Illinois.)

Indications for Using the Ultrasonic Scaler

- Removal of supragingival calculus and difficult stains
- Subgingival periodontal removal of calculus, attached biofilm, and endotoxins from the root surface
- Cleaning of furcation areas
- Removal of deposits before surgery
- Removal of orthodontic cement (debonding)
- Removal of overhanging margins of restorations

Contraindications and Precautions for Using the Ultrasonic Scaler

- Tissue in young patients is sensitive to ultrasonic vibrations.
- Vibrations and heat may damage the pulp tissue of primary and newly erupted permanent teeth.
- A patient can transmit an infectious disease by aerosols.

FIGURE 24.16 **A,** Positioning of the ultrasonic scaler. **B,** Ultrasonic scaler with water source turned on. (Courtesy Hu-Friedy Manufacturing, Chicago, Illinois.)

- A compromised patient is open to infection.
- Materials can be aspirated into the lungs of patients with respiratory problems.
- An ultrasonic scaler can stimulate the gag reflex in the patient who has a swallowing problem.

FIGURE 24.17 Kirkland and Orban interdental knives.

FIGURE 24.18 Scaling, root planing, and curettage. (From Newman M, Carranza FA: *Carranza's clinical periodontology,* ed 12, Saunders, 2015.)

- Consultation with the patient's cardiologist may be necessary because, theoretically, an ultrasonic scaler can possibly disrupt a pacemaker (although no cases have been reported). The newer models of scalers have protective coatings.
- The vibrations of the ultrasonic scaler tip can remove the areas of remineralization that begin to cover the demineralization.
- Exposed dentin structures can cause tooth sensitivity.
- Some restorative materials, such as porcelain, amalgam, composite resins, and laminate veneers, can be damaged by an ultrasonic scaler.
- The ultrasonic scaler will damage titanium surfaces.

Periodontal Surgical Instruments

Periodontal Knives

Kirkland knives are one of the most common type of knives used in periodontal surgery. These instruments are usually double-ended with kidney shaped blades.

Orban knives are used to remove tissue from the interdental areas. They are shaped similar to spears and have cutting edges on both sides of the blades (Fig. 24.17).

Pocket Markers

Pocket markers are similar in appearance to cotton pliers; however, one tip is smooth and straight, and the other tip is sharp and bent at a right angle. The smooth tip of the pocket marker is inserted into the base of the pocket. When the instrument is pressed together, the sharp tip makes small perforations in the gingivae, which are referred to as *bleeding points* and are used to outline the area for a gingivectomy.

Periodontal Treatment Procedures

The realm of periodontal treatment ranges from the basic dental prophylaxis to the most sophisticated periodontal surgeries involving tissue grafts and implants of bone.

The method of treatment depends on the severity of the disease and the amount of tissue destruction that has occurred.

Many general dentists provide basic periodontal services, such as scaling and root planing, and refer more complex cases involving surgery to the periodontist. Regardless of the treatment plan, ongoing good daily oral hygiene is essential for the success of any type of periodontal therapy.

Dental Prophylaxis

- A dental prophylaxis, commonly referred to as a *prophy,* involves the complete removal of calculus, soft deposits, biofilm, and stains from all supragingival and unattached subgingival tooth surfaces. The dentist and the dental hygienist are licensed to perform this procedure.
- See Procedure 24.1: Assisting with a Dental Prophylaxis.
- A dental prophylaxis is indicated for patients with healthy gingivae as a preventive measure and is most commonly performed during recall appointments. A dental prophylaxis is also the primary treatment for gingivitis.

Scaling, Root Planing, and Gingival Curettage

Scaling and root planing are indicated as the initial treatment before periodontal surgery. In some cases, gingival curettage is also indicated (Fig. 24.18).

Scaling

During scaling, scalers are used to remove supragingival calculus from the tooth surface, and curettes are used to remove subgingival calculus. Some areas on the root surface may remain rough after calculus removal. This roughness occurs because the cementum has become necrotic (dead) or because the scaling has produced grooves and scratches.

Root Planing

Root planing follows scaling procedures to remove any remaining particles of calculus and necrotic cementum embedded in the root. After root planing, the surfaces of the root are smooth and glasslike. Smooth root surfaces resist new calculus formation and are easier for the patient to keep clean.

Gingival Curettage

In addition to scaling and root planing, some areas in the mouth may require a procedure called *gingival curettage*. (*Curettage* means scraping or cleaning with a curette.) Gingival curettage, also referred to as *subgingival curettage*, consists of scraping the gingival wall of a periodontal pocket to remove necrotic tissue from the pocket wall.

Postoperative Instruction After Scaling and Curettage

Most patients appreciate the dental assistant explaining postoperative instructions to them so that they have the opportunity to ask questions. Postoperative instructions are an important legal consideration; therefore providing written postoperative instructions for the patient to take home is wise.

Discomfort. Mild discomfort may be noted for a few hours after the local anesthetic agent has worn off. Usually a mild analgesic drug, such as acetaminophen (Tylenol) or ibuprofen (Advil), is adequate for relieving this discomfort.

Diet. A normal diet is recommended; however, avoiding very spicy foods, citrus fruits, and alcoholic beverages is recommended.

The patient is also advised not to smoke. Smoking irritates the tissue and delays healing.

Home Care. Good home care is essential for the success of scaling and curettage. Normal home care should be resumed the following day.

Antimicrobial and Antibiotic Agents

The dentist may prescribe antimicrobial and/or antibiotic agents for use in conjunction with periodontal treatment.

Tetracycline is an antibiotic used for the treatment of periodontitis, juvenile periodontitis, and rapidly destructive periodontitis.

Chlorhexidine rinse twice daily is the most effective agent available to reduce biofilm and gingivitis, but chlorhexidine can cause some temporary brown staining of the teeth, tongue, and resin restorations.

Metronidazole is used in treating rapidly progressing periodontitis. It is not prescribed to treat juvenile periodontitis because metronidazole is not effective against the type of bacteria found in this disease.

Fluoride mouth rinses have been shown to reduce bleeding by delaying bacterial growth in the periodontal pockets.

Periodontal Surgery

Periodontal surgery may be recommended for the following reasons:
- To reduce or eliminate periodontal pockets
- To create or improve access to the root surface
- To treat osseous (bone) defects
- To correct mucogingival defects
- To create new tissue attachment

Gingivectomy

A **gingivectomy** is the surgical removal of diseased gingival tissue or the removal of gingival tissue for cosmetic reasons.

This surgical procedure is performed to reduce the depth of the periodontal pocket and remove fibrous gingival tissue. It involves making bleeding points with pocket markers and removing the gingival tissue with periodontal knives and surgical scissors. After healing, cleaning the area when the pockets have been reduced is easier for the patient.

It can also be performed with the use of lasers, which offer a faster healing process with reduced discomfort postoperatively.

Gingivoplasty

A **gingivoplasty** involves surgical reshaping and contouring of the gingival tissue. The presence of deep periodontal pockets with fibrous tissue is the primary indication for both the gingivectomy and the gingivoplasty. Often, the two procedures are simultaneously performed. During the gingivoplasty procedure, the gingivae is recontoured using periodontal knives, rotary diamond burs, curettes, and surgical scissors. Gingival margins are thinned and given a scalloped edge.

See Procedure 24.2: Assisting with Gingivectomy and Gingivoplasty.

Periodontal Flap Surgery

Periodontal flap surgery involves separating the gingivae from the underlying tooth roots and alveolar bone, similar to the flap of an envelope. When the flap is elevated (lifted up), the dentist has excellent visibility and may perform one or more of the following procedures:
- Thorough scaling and root planing of exposed root surfaces
- Moving the flap laterally (to the side) to cover the root surfaces of an adjacent tooth that does not have adequate tissue coverage (this procedure is called a *laterally sliding flap*.)
- Recontouring (reshaping) the underlying bone
- Closing the flap and suturing it into place after the surgery is completed (Fig. 24.19; a periodontal pack is usually placed after flap surgery.)

Gingival Grafting

Some patients may benefit from a **gingival graft**, a procedure during which tissue is taken from one site in the patient's mouth and placed on another. The palate is frequently used as the donor site. A section of tissue is removed and then carefully positioned and sutured into the recipient area. The donor site on the palate is usually covered with a periodontal dressing until it has healed (Fig. 24.20).

Osseous Surgery

Osseous (bone) surgery is performed to remove defects and to restore normal contours in the bone. There are two types of bone surgeries: *osteoplasty* and *ostectomy*. Each one requires surgically exposing the bone and recontouring it with a rotary diamond stone or bone chisel.

Osteoplasty

In **osteoplasty**, or additive surgery, the bone is contoured and reshaped. In addition, bone may be *added* through *bone grafting* that replaces missing bone with material from the patient's

FIG. 24.19 Periodontal flap procedure. (Courtesy Dr. Joseph Schwartz, Portland Oregon.)

FIGURE 24.20 **A** and **B,** Presurgical recession of gingival tissues. **C** and **D,** Healed tissues after gingival graft surgery. (Courtesy Dr. Christine Ford, Santa Rosa, California.)

own body (an artificial, synthetic, or natural substitute). This procedure is useful for patients with bone defects caused by periodontal disease.

Ostectomy

In an **ostectomy**, or subtractive surgery, bone is removed. This type of procedure is necessary when the patient has large exostoses (bony growths). For example, an ostectomy is performed if a patient needs a denture and the bony growth would interfere with the comfort and fit of the denture.

Periodontal Dressing

A periodontal dressing is similar to a bandage over a surgical site. Periodontal dressings (periopacks) are used to:

- Hold the flaps in place
- Protect the newly forming tissue
- Minimize postoperative pain, infection, and hemorrhage
- Protect the surgical site from trauma during eating and drinking
- Support mobile teeth during the healing process

Types of Periodontal Dressings

For most surgical procedures, a periodontal dressing is placed to protect the area from postoperative irritation, trauma, saliva contamination, and gingival detachment. A variety of materials are used for periodontal dressings. The most common materials are zinc oxide–eugenol and noneugenol dressings.

Zinc Oxide–Eugenol Dressing. Zinc oxide–eugenol dressings are supplied as a powder and liquid that are mixed before using. The material may be mixed ahead of time, wrapped in wax paper, and frozen for future use. This type of dressing has a slow set, which allows for longer working time. It sets to a firm and heavy consistency and provides good support and protection for tissues and flaps.

Some patients are allergic to the eugenol and experience redness and burning pain in the area of the dressing.

Noneugenol Dressing. Noneugenol dressing is the most widely used type of periodontal dressing. The material is supplied in two tubes—one contains the base material and the other contains the accelerator.

The material is easy to mix and to place; it has a smooth surface for patient comfort. Noneugenol dressing has a rapid setting time if exposed to warm temperatures and cannot be mixed in advance and stored.

See Procedure 24.3: Preparing and Placing Noneugenol Periodontal Dressing, and Procedure 24.4: Removing a Periodontal Dressing.

Postperiodontal Surgery

Instructions

Postoperative instructions are provided to the patient in both verbal and written form. These instructions should include information about discomfort, periodontal dressing, rinsing the mouth, diet, activity, home care, and postoperative visits.

Discomfort

Mild-to-moderate discomfort can be expected, especially during the first 24 hours. If indicated, pain medication is prescribed.

Periodontal Dressing

If bleeding is present under the dressing, then the patient is instructed to call the dental office immediately. Small pieces of the periodontal dressing may break off. If no pain or bleeding occurs, then the dressing does not usually have to be replaced.

Rinsing

The patient should not rinse their mouth for the first 24 hours. After 24 hours, a warm salt-water rinse (1 tsp of salt in 8 oz of warm water) is indicated.

Diet

A normal diet is recommended. Avoiding hard foods, alcoholic beverages, citrus fruit, and spicy foods is recommended.

Activity

Avoid excessive exercise for the first few days, which allows a firm clot to form in the surgical area.

Home Care

The areas of the mouth that were not involved in the surgery should be brushed and flossed normally. The areas of the periodontal dressing should be gently cleaned using a soft toothbrush.

Postoperative Visit

Approximately 1 week after surgery, the dressing will be removed for a postoperative check. Usually after the dressing is removed, it is not necessary to replace it.

Ethical Implications

Failure to diagnose periodontal disease at an early stage is a leading complaint in malpractice lawsuits. Ethically, it is incumbent on the dental professional to educate and instruct patients about periodontal care. Careful documentation related to issues of patient education, compliance with home care advice, and referrals to periodontists must be prepared.

From an ethical and legal standpoint, including a periodontal evaluation as part of every dental examination is essential.

Procedure 24.1

Assisting with a Dental Prophylaxis

Goal

To assist competently with a dental prophylaxis procedure.

Equipment and Supplies

- High-volume evacuator (HVE) tip or saliva ejector
- Basic instrument setup
- Scalers, universal curette
- Prophy angle
- Rubber polishing cup and brushes
- Polishing agent
- Dental floss and/or tape
- Preprocedural mouth rinse

Procedure 24.1

Assisting with a Dental Prophylaxis—cont'd

(From Bird DL, Robinson DS: *Modern dental assisting*. ed 11, Saunders, 2015.)

Procedural Steps

1. Assist with the transfers as the operator uses an explorer to locate interproximal and subgingival calculus.
   Note: The operator must have good access and visibility during this procedure.
2. Use the HVE as necessary, and retract the lips, tongue, and cheeks to improve visibility and access as the operator uses scalers and curettes to remove all calculus and biofilm.
3. The operator checks for and removes any remaining calculus.
4. The operator polishes the teeth using polishing paste, a rubber cup, and bristle brushes.
5. The operator removes any remaining interproximal debris with dental floss or tape.
6. Provide oral hygiene instructions appropriate to the individual needs of the patient.

Procedure 24.2

Assisting with Gingivectomy and Gingivoplasty

Goal

To assist the dentist competently in performing gingivectomy and gingivoplasty periodontal procedures

Equipment and Supplies

- High-volume evacuator (HVE) tip and surgical aspirating tip
- Local anesthetic setup
- Scalpel and blades
- Surgical periodontal knives
- Surgical tissue retraction forceps
- Periodontal pocket marker
- Tissue tweezers
- Scalers and curettes
- Diamond burs and sterile stones
- Suture needle and sutures
- Hemostat and surgical scissors
- Periodontal surgical dressing materials
- Sterile gauze sponges
- Sterile irrigation solution (water or saline)

Typical series of periodontal surgical instruments, divided into two cassettes. **A,** *From left,* Mirrors, explorer, probe, series of curettes, needle holder, rongeur instrument, and scissors. **B,** *From left,* Series of chisels, Kirkland knife, Orban knife, scalpel handles with surgical blades (#15C, #15, #12D), periosteal elevators, spatula, tissue forceps, cheek retractors, mallet, and sharpening stone. (Courtesy Hu-Friedy Mfg. Co., LLC, Chicago, Illinois.)

Continued

Assisting with Gingivectomy and Gingivoplasty—cont'd

Procedural Steps

Role of the Dental Assistant

1. Set out the patient's health history, radiographs, and periodontal chart.

   Purpose: The dentist needs to review the case before surgery.

2. Assist in the administration of the local anesthetic agent.

3. Anticipate the dentist's needs and be prepared to transfer and retrieve surgical instruments when needed.

   Purpose: This step saves time and makes the procedure less stressful.

4. Have gauze ready to remove tissue from the instruments, as necessary.

   Purpose: Periodontal surgery can generate heavy bleeding.

5. Provide oral evacuation and retraction.

   Purpose: Good access and visibility are critical for the dentist, and the patient will be more comfortable.

6. Irrigate with sterile saline.

   Purpose: Irrigation keeps the surgical site clean and free of debris.

7. If sutures are used, then prepare the suture needle and suture material and position them in a hemostat or needle holder. Transfer them to the dentist when requested.

   Purpose: This step simplifies the procedure for the dentist and increases patient comfort.

8. Place, or assist with the placement of, the periodontal dressing.

   Purpose: The dressing acts as a bandage to protect the surgical site.

   Note: Check your state's Dental Practice Act before placing a periodontal dressing without assistance.

9. Wipe any blood or debris from the patient's face. Provide postoperative instructions to the patient.

   Purpose: This step ensures that the patient clearly understands the postoperative instructions as necessary for personal well-being and to address legal considerations.

Role of the Dentist

1. The dentist administers the local anesthetic agent.

   Purpose: In addition to pain control, local anesthesia aids visibility by constricting blood vessels and reducing the amount of blood at the surgical site.

2. The dentist marks the pockets on the facial and lingual gingivae by using the periodontal pocket marker.

   Purpose: The bleeding points indicate the pocket depth and thus the point for the initial incision.

3. The dentist uses a scalpel or a periodontal knife to incise the gingiva at a 45-degree angle, following along the bleeding points. The incision is beveled to create a normally contoured, free gingival margin.

4. The dentist removes the gingival tissue along the incision line using surgical knives.

5. The dentist tapers the gingival margins and creates a scalloped marginal outline.

   Purpose: This marginal outline creates an attractive and healthy appearance.

6. The dentist shapes the interdental papillae using interdental knives.

   Purpose: This step contours the interdental grooves.

7. The dentist performs scaling and root planing of the root surfaces.

   Purpose: This step removes any residual calculus that was inaccessible before surgery.

8. The dentist places sutures if needed.

9. The dentist irrigates the surgical site and then covers it with a periodontal dressing.

   Purpose: Periodontal dressing protects the surgical site.

   Note: In some states, the placement and removal of the periodontal dressing are delegated to the dental assistant (expanded function).

Preparing and Placing Noneugenol Periodontal Dressing

Goal

To prepare and assist the dentist in placing a noneugenol periodontal dressing.

Equipment and Supplies

- Paper mixing pad (supplied by the manufacturer)
- Wooden tongue depressor
- Noneugenol dressing (base and accelerator)
- Paper cup filled with room-temperature water
- Saline solution
- Plastic type of filling instrument

Procedural Steps

Mixing the Material

1. Extrude equal lengths of the two pastes on the paper pad.
2. Mix the pastes with a wooden tongue depressor until a uniform color has been obtained (2 to 3 minutes).
3. When the paste loses its tackiness, place it in the paper cup filled with room-temperature water.
4. Lubricate gloved fingers with saline solution.

Purpose: This step prevents the material from sticking to the gloves.

5. Roll the paste into strips approximately the length of the surgical site.

Placing the Dressing

1. Press small triangle-shaped pieces of dressing into the interproximal spaces.

2. Adapt one end of the strip around the distal surface of the last tooth in the surgical site.
3. Bring the remainder of the strip forward along the facial surface, and gently press the strip along the incised gingival margin.
4. Gently press the strip into the interproximal areas.

5. Apply the second strip in the same manner from the lingual side.
6. Join the facial and lingual strips at the distal surface of the last tooth at both ends of the surgical site.
7. Apply gentle pressure on the facial and lingual surfaces.
8. Check the dressing for overextension and interference with occlusion.

Purpose: Excess packing irritates the mucobuccal fold and floor of the mouth.

9. Remove any excess dressing and adjust the new margins to remove any roughness.

Purpose: If the pack is not properly adapted, it can break off.

Goal

To remove a periodontal dressing.

Equipment and Supplies

- Spoon excavator
- Suture scissors (if sutures are present)
- Dental floss
- Warm saline solution
- Irrigating solution
- High-volume evacuator (HVE) tip or saliva ejector

Procedural Steps

1. Gently insert the spoon excavator under the margin.
2. Use lateral pressure to pry the dressing gently away from the tissue.

Purpose: The area may still be sensitive, and the newly healed tissue is delicate and easily injured.

3. If sutures are embedded in the dressing material, cut the suture material free. Gently remove the sutures from the tissue.

Purpose: Accidentally pulling the sutures could be painful for the patient and might open the wound.

4. Gently use dental floss to remove all fragments of dressing material from the interproximal surfaces.

Purpose: Remaining fragments could cause discomfort for the patient and result in tissue irritation.

5. Gently irrigate the entire area with warm saline solution to remove superficial debris.

6. Use the HVE tip or saliva ejector to remove fluid from the patient's mouth.

Chapter Exercises

Multiple Choice

Circle the letter next to the correct answer.

1. The leading cause of tooth loss in adults is _____.
   a. periodontal disease
   b. root caries
   c. occlusal trauma
   d. root abscess
2. The most common periodontal disease and the easiest one to treat is _____.
   a. gingivitis
   b. early periodontitis
   c. advanced periodontitis
   d. refractory periodontitis
3. How many periodontal probing measurements are taken for each tooth?
   a. 4
   b. 6
   c. 8
4. Curettes that are designed with two cutting edges are called _____.
   a. universal curettes
   b. Gracey curettes
5. The procedure in which the gingival wall of the pocket is scraped is called a _____.
   a. gingival curettage
   b. gingivectomy
   c. gingivoplasty
6. A periodontal examination and diagnosis include _____.
   a. evaluation of radiographs
   b. medical and dental histories
   c. periodontal probing
   d. all of the above
7. The primary cause of gingivitis and most forms of periodontal disease is _____.
   a. calculus
   b. defective restorations
   c. food debris
   d. dental biofilm
8. The depth of a periodontal pocket is measured with a(n) _____.
   a. curette
   b. explorer
   c. periodontal probe
   d. pocket marker
9. Which dental professional(s) is (are) licensed to perform a dental prophylaxis?
   a. Dental assistant
   b. Dentist
   c. Dental hygienist
   d. b and c
10. What surgical procedure is required to reshape the bone to remove defects and to restore normal contour?
    a. Gingivectomy
    b. Gingivoplasty
    c. Osteoplasty
    d. Root planing
11. The procedure that removes calculus, soft deposits, and stains from all unattached tooth surfaces is known as _____.
    a. dental prophylaxis
    b. curettage
    c. root planing
    d. scaling
12. To locate calculus deposits, a(n) _____ is used.
    a. explorer
    b. curette
    c. periodontal probe
13. In charting mobility, moderate mobility is recorded as _____.
    a. 0
    b. 1
    c. 2
    d. 3
14. Which of the following instruments is used to outline the area for a gingivectomy?
    a. Periodontal knife
    b. Periodontal probe
    c. Pocket marker
15. During the first 24 hours after a gingivectomy, the patient can expect _____.
    a. bleeding from under the dressing
    b. mild-to-moderate pain
    c. severe pain
    d. a and c

Apply Your Knowledge

1. Jimmie, a 9-year-old, is brought into your dental office for a checkup. The dentist notes that Jimmie has gingivitis around the lingual surfaces of his mandibular molars. What do you think is the likely cause of this localized gingivitis?
2. Mrs. Georgette Pearson is a very pleasant woman in her mid-60s. Her periodontal charting shows generalized pocketing between 6 and 8 mm. In addition, the mobility for most teeth is recorded as 2. Based on her records, Mrs. Pearson is in what stage of periodontitis?
3. The dentist has asked you to give Mr. Matthews postoperative instructions after a gingivectomy. What would you include in your instructions to Mr. Matthews?
4. You are responsible for setting up a periodontal instrument cassette. At first glance, what is the distinguishing characteristic between a scaler and a curette? Then, how will you distinguish between a universal curette and a Gracey curette?

CHAPTER 25

Endodontics

http://evolve.elsevier.com/Robinson/essentials/

LEARNING OBJECTIVES

1. Pronounce, define, and spell the key terms.
2. Describe the subjective and objective components of an endodontic diagnosis.
3. Describe the role and use of radiographic images in endodontics.
4. Describe how an endodontic diagnosis is presented to the patient.
5. Explain the assistant's role in the use of an electric pulp vitality test.
6. Identify the specialized instruments used in endodontic treatment, including the use of the operating microscope.
7. Explain the assistant's role in preparing and assisting in the placement of disinfectants, medicaments, and dental materials in endodontics.
8. Discuss the dental assistant's role in an endodontic procedure.
9. Discuss surgical endodontic techniques.

KEY TERMS

apicoectomy
control tooth
debridement
direct pulp cap
endodontist
gutta-percha

hemisection
indirect pulp cap
irreversible pulpitis
necrotic
nonvital
obturation

pulpectomy
pulpotomy
retrograde restoration
reversible pulpitis
root amputation
sealer

Endodontics is the specialty in dentistry involved in the prevention, diagnosis, and treatment of diseases of the dental pulp. Endodontic treatment, which is often referred to as *root canal therapy,* provides an effective means of saving a tooth that might otherwise require extraction because of extensive decay or fracture in the tooth.

The general dentist is licensed to care for simple endodontic cases; however, most dentists will refer a patient in need of pulp therapy to an endodontist, who specializes in this area of dentistry. Endodontic treatment does not include the placement of a final restoration after root canal therapy. Once endodontic treatment has been completed, the patient returns to their general dentist or specialist for the placement of a permanent fixed restoration.

Endodontic Diagnosis

The endodontic diagnosis is made through an examination that has both subjective and objective components.

The **subjective** portion of the **examination** includes the assessment of symptoms or problems described by the patient. These include the patient's description of the *location, intensity,* and *duration* of the pain. Specific questions to ask a patient include:

- Is there oral pain when you bite down or chew?
- Do you experience any sensitivity to hot or cold?
- Have you noticed any swelling in the gingiva surrounding the tooth?

The **objective examination** includes the patient's medical and dental histories, radiographic images, clinical examination, and pulp vitality tests. Table 25.1 describes the types of tests completed to determine a tooth's vitality.

The **medical history** may provide information about conditions that could contribute to the pain the patient is experiencing. One example is that a patient with severe allergies may be experiencing unexplained dental pain in the maxillary anterior region.

The **dental history** may provide information concerning injury to a tooth or recent dental treatment that might help explain the pain the patient is experiencing.

A control tooth is used during each type of pulp testing procedure, providing the dentist with a comparison of a healthy tooth with an infected tooth in terms of level of sensitivity. A healthy tooth (of the same type) in the opposite quadrant is

TABLE 25.1
Diagnostic Testing of Vital Teeth

Diagnostic Test	Description
Percussion test	Tapping on the incisal or occlusal surface with a mouth mirror handle provides the dentist with the ability to determine whether the inflammation process has extended into the periapical tissue.
Palpation test	Firm pressure is applied to the mucosa above the apex of the root. This pressure helps the dentist determine whether the inflammation process has extended into the periapical tissue.
Cold test	Ice, dry ice, or ethyl chloride is used to determine the pulp response to a cold temperature.
Heat test	A small piece of heated gutta-percha or the end of an instrument is heated and placed on the occlusal or incisal surface of the tooth to determine the pulp response.
Electric pulp test	A small electrical stimulus is delivered to the pulp. A small quantity of toothpaste is used to establish an adequate contact to conduct the current from the pulp tester to the tooth.

FIGURE 25.1 Radiograph showing extensive decay into the pulp. (From Johnson W: *Color atlas of endodontics,* Philadelphia, 2002, Saunders.)

FIGURE 25.2 Abscess *(arrow)* associated with mandibular first molar, resulting from extensive decay into the pulp. (Courtesy Margaret Fehrenbach, RDH, MS)

selected as a control tooth. For example, if the maxillary right first premolar (tooth #5) is the suspected tooth, then the control tooth will be the maxillary left first premolar (tooth #12).

See Procedure 25.1: Assisting in Electric Pulp Vitality Testing.

Diagnostic Conclusions

Once the subjective and objective tests have been completed, a diagnosis is presented to the patient.

Normal pulp indicates no subjective symptoms or objective signs. The tooth responded normally to sensory stimuli, and a healthy layer of dentin surrounds the pulp. **Necrosis,** also referred to as **necrotic** or **nonvital,** is when the tooth does not respond to sensory stimulus.

Pulpitis indicates that pulpal tissues have become inflamed. Pulpitis can be clinically described as follows: **reversible pulpitis** occurs when the pulp is irritated from decay or moisture, and the patient is experiencing pain to thermal stimuli. By eliminating the irritant and placing a sedative material, the pulp may be saved. **Irreversible pulpitis** shows symptoms of lingering pain. Clinical diagnostic findings show that the pulp is incapable of healing, which would indicate the need for root canal therapy or extraction (Fig. 25.1).

Periradicular abscess is an inflammatory reaction to pulpal infection (Fig. 25.2). The lesion can be chronic, which would be asymptomatic with little or no discomfort, or acute, which would be associated with pain, tenderness, pus formation, and swelling.

Periodontal abscess is an inflammatory reaction caused by bacteria entrapped in the periodontal sulcus. Most often, a patient will experience rapid onset, pain, tenderness to pressure, pus formation, and swelling.

A **periradicular cyst** develops at or near the root of a necrotic tooth. This type of cyst occurs as an inflammatory response to pulpal infection and necrosis of the pulp.

Use of Radiographic Imaging in Endodontics

Digital radiography is a necessity in endodontics. The endodontist will request a **periapical image** to expose the full length of the tooth and the periapical tissue immediately surrounding the tooth in question.

FIGURE 25.3 Initial radiograph showing the second molar in question. (From Johnson W: *Color atlas of endodontics*, Philadelphia, 2002, Saunders.)

FIGURE 25.4 Final instrumentation radiograph. (From Johnson W: *Color atlas of endodontics*, Philadelphia, 2002, Saunders.)

A minimum of four images are exposed throughout an endodontic procedure. The following list describes when a radiograph is required and at what stage of treatment:

1. **Initial radiographic image:** A periapical image of the tooth in question is exposed and completed at the diagnostic stage (Fig. 25.3).
2. **Working length radiograph:** A periapical image is exposed to determine the length of the canal. Detecting the canal length is easier with the file remaining in the tooth.
3. **Final instrumentation radiograph:** A periapical image of the tooth is taken with the final size of the file in all canals involved (Fig. 25.4).
4. **Root canal completion radiograph:** A final periapical image is exposed of the completed canal that has been filled and temporized with an intermediate restorative material (Fig. 25.5).

FIGURE 25.5 Completion radiograph. (From Johnson W: *Color atlas of endodontics*, Philadelphia, 2002, Saunders.)

Instruments in Endodontics

Endodontic instruments and accessories are designed to be flexible and to fit into the pulpal canal. To provide uniformity between manufacturers, the American Dental Association (ADA) has standardized the numbering and color-coded system used for files.

Files are supplied in different diameters, ranging from size 08 (the smallest) to size 140 (the largest). Files are available in various diameters and designs, based on their specific function. See Table 25.2 for images and descriptions of the hand and rotary instruments most commonly used in the practice of endodontics.

Microscopic Endodontics

The development of the operating microscope in the field of endodontics has essentially changed the practice of endodontics, resulting in a more efficient, effective, and patient-friendly endodontic procedure. Endodontic procedures can be completed in less time because of the greater visibility of the root canal anatomy, with the final product reducing procedural errors (Fig. 25.6).

Benefits of Using the Operating Microscope
- Locates cracks and fractures that are not clinically visible or palpable with an explorer
- Locates canals obstructed by mineralization that are reduced in size
- Access to the canal without causing damage to dentin
- Removing materials, posts, or separated files
- Removing canal obstructions
- Repairing perforations
- Facilitating in surgery such as root-end resection and retro filling materials

Disinfection and Filling Materials in Endodontics

In treating an endodontically affected tooth, the dental assistant will prepare and assist in the disinfection and placement of medications and dental materials for the pulpal canal (Fig. 25.7).

TABLE 25.2
Instruments and Armamentarium Used for Endodontic Procedures

Name	Description
Endodontic explorer	The endodontic explorer is a double-ended instrument with the working ends at an angle. The working end is long enough to enter and locate canal openings.
Endodontic spoon excavator	The endodontic spoon excavator is a double-ended instrument similar to other spoon excavators except that the shank is long, allowing the instrument to reach into the tooth and canal.
Endodontic K-type file	The endodontic K-type file has a twisted design and is used in the initial debridement (cleaning) of the canal and during the later stages of shaping and contouring the canal.
Hedström file	The Hedström file provides cutting efficiency because of the design and is used for final enlargement of the canal.
Reamer file	The reamer file is similar in design to the K-type file but with cutting edges farther apart. Its functions are to remove dentin structure and to smooth and increase the size of the canal.
Broaches	Broaches, which have tiny fishhook-like barbs along the shaft, are used to remove the bulk of the pulp tissue. They are also useful for removing fragments of paper points that become lodged in the canal. They are not used to shape or enlarge the canal.

Continued

TABLE 25.2

Instruments and Armamentarium Used for Endodontic Procedures—cont'd

Name	Description
Gates Glidden bur	The Gates Glidden bur is a football-shaped bur that is used on a low-speed handpiece. The bur has a very long shank with a latch-type attachment that is operated in a clockwise direction. These burs are not end-cutting, which means that the cutting edge is only on the sides of the bur.
Pesso file	A Pesso file is primarily used when the tooth requires a parallel post-preparation for the placement of the final restoration. This file is adapted to the low-speed handpiece.
Lentulo spiral	The Lentulo spiral is a twisted wire instrument used in the low-speed handpiece to spin sealer, cements, or calcium hydroxide pastes into the canal.
Double-ended Glick no. 1 instrument	The paddle-shaped end of the double-ended Glick no. 1 instrument is designed for the placement of temporary restorations, and the rod-shaped plugger at the opposite end is ideal for the removal of excess gutta-percha. The plugger end is graduated at 5-mm increments and can be heated for the placement or removal of gutta-percha.
Endodontic spreader	The endodontic spreader is a long, pointed working tip instrument. The dentist uses this instrument to obturate (fill) the canal by spreading the gutta-percha points in a lateral direction.

TABLE 25.2

Name	Description
Endodontic plugger 	The endodontic plugger is a long, flat-ended working tip instrument. The dentist uses this instrument to condense and adapt the gutta-percha points to the canal in a lateral direction.
Millimeter ruler 	A millimeter ruler is a small ruler that accurately measures files and instruments used in the pulpal canal.
Rubber stop(s) 	Rubber stops are small, round pieces of rubber or plastic that prevent the files from perforating the apex of the tooth during instrumentation. The dentist uses a precise radiograph and a millimeter ruler to measure the length of the canal. The rubber stop is precisely placed at the predetermined working length of the canal on the file.
Paper points 	Paper points are made of absorbent paper rolled into long, narrow points. A paper point is held with locking pliers and inserted into the canal to absorb the irrigating solution and to dry the canal.

Figures of the endodontic explorer, endodontic spoon excavator, endodontic spreader, and endodontic plugger courtesy Hu-Friedy Manufacturing Company, Chicago, Illinois. Figures of the K-type file, Hedström file, and reamer file courtesy Premier Dental, Plymouth Meeting, Pennsylvania. Figures of the broach, Pesso file, double-ended Glick no. 1 instrument, millimeter ruler, rubber stops, and paper points from Boyd LRB: *Dental instruments: a pocket guide,* ed 5, St. Louis, 2015, Saunders. Figure of the Gates Glidden bur from Johnson W: *Color atlas of endodontics,* Philadelphia, 2002, Saunders. Figure of the Lentulo spiral instrument from Walton RE, Torabinejad M: *Principles and practice of endodontics*, Philadelphia, 1989, Saunders.

FIGURE 25.6 Operating endodontic microscopic. (From Hargreaves KM, Berman LH, Rotstein I: *Cohen's pathways of the pulp,* ed 11, St Louis, 2016, Elsevier.)

FIGURE 25.7 Materials needed for the preparation and obturation of the pulpal canal. *Top,* Sterile irrigating solution. *Bottom,* Sterile paper points and syringe used with irrigating solution. *Left and center,* Files. *Right,* Gutta-percha points.

FIGURE 25.8 **A,** Gutta-percha is the most widely used obturation material. It has benefits of being biocompatible, radiopaque, and easy to manipulate. Various obturation techniques with gutta-percha are currently practiced, including warm vertical compaction and lateral compaction. Because many root canal systems are quite complex, use of a cold filling system minimizes the risk for voids caused by shrinkage. **B,** The Obtura Max is a heated gutta-percha delivery system used to deliver warm gutta-percha to the root canal system for obturation. (**A,** Courtesy Coltene/Whaledent, Cuyahoga Falls, Ohio. **B,** Courtesy Obtura Spartan Endodontics, Algonquin, Illinois.)

Disinfection

In endodontics, disinfection is a key element of the overall treatment. Antimicrobial irrigants are used during root canal treatment as a standard of practices during root canal therapy to remove all bioburden. The following solutions are used in the cleaning and shaping:

- *Sodium hypochlorite* (NaOCl), commonly known as *household bleach,* has the ability to dissolve organic tissue. It is diluted with equal parts of sterile water for use as an irrigation solution. A 5- to 6-mL disposable plastic syringe with a special 27-gauge needle. This solution is used during the instrumentation phase to increase time within the canal.
- Ethylenediaminetetraacetic acid (EDTA) is used at the end of the preparation phase to remove inorganic debris and the smear layer from the canal walls.

- *Chlorhexidine* (CHX) is used as a final flush. It is a clear, colorless liquid with disinfectant and bleaching properties for endodontics.
- *Parachlorophenol (PCP)* is a colorless, crystalline toxic phenol compound that is used as an antimicrobial agent for disinfecting the pulp canal.

Root Canal–Filling Materials

Gutta-percha points is a natural rubber material made from the Palaquium gutta tree. It is heated and compressed to fill or **obturate** the pulpal canal after treatment has been completed. Gutta-percha is an organic substance that is solid at room temperature and becomes soft and pliable when heated. This radiopaque material is supplied in various sizes and is followed by a sealer (Fig. 25.8).

Root Canal Sealers

A root canal sealer is a cement type of material that seals out unfilled voids during the obturation process. Several cements, including calcium hydroxide, zinc oxide–eugenol, and glass ionomer, can be used as a sealer for root canal therapy. These materials are designed to have little shrinkage and are easy to place, radiopaque for detection in a radiograph, nonstaining to the teeth, bacteriostatic, gentle on the periapical tissue that surrounds them, and able to resist moisture.

Formocresol is a mixture of formaldehyde and cresol in a water-glycerin base. This type of solution is used as a sealer for pulpotomy of deciduous teeth and as an intracanal medicament for permanent teeth during root canal therapy.

Pulp Therapy

The choice of endodontic treatment depends on the diagnosis. The first line of treatment in pulpal therapy is an attempt to stimulate pulpal regeneration and save the pulp. When pulpal therapy is not effective, the endodontist will move to a more extreme measure, including root canal therapy or surgery.

Pulp Capping

In an attempt to save the pulp, a covering of calcium hydroxide is placed over an exposed or nearly exposed pulp to encourage the formation of secondary dentin at the site of injury.

An indirect pulp cap is indicated when a thin partition of dentin is still intact. The pulp has not yet been exposed, but the pulp may become exposed when decay that is near the pulp is removed. The goals are (1) to promote pulpal healing by removing most of the decay and (2) to stimulate the production of reparative dentin through the placement of calcium hydroxide.

A direct pulp cap is indicated when the pulp has been slightly exposed. With a direct pulp cap, the tooth is still vital; however, it may become infected, requiring additional treatment, or it may become necrotic and require root canal therapy. When a direct pulp cap is performed, it is necessary to inform the patient that problems may develop later and that periodic monitoring is essential.

Pulpotomy

A pulpotomy involves the removal of the coronal portion of an exposed vital pulp. This procedure is completed to preserve the vitality of the remaining portion of the pulp within the root of the tooth. Pulpotomy is often indicated for vital primary teeth, teeth with deep carious lesions, and emergency situations.

Pulpectomy

A pulpectomy, also referred to as *root canal therapy*, involves the complete removal of the dental pulp.

Overview of Root Canal Therapy

Root canal therapy consist of five steps of treatment: (1) anesthesia and pain control, (2) isolation of the operating field, (3) access preparation, (4) debridement and shaping of the canal, and (5) obturation.

Anesthesia and Pain Control

The anesthetic techniques of choice for endodontic treatment are infiltration (supraperiosteal injection) for maxillary teeth and nerve blocks for mandibular teeth (see Chapter 15). A local anesthetic agent is administered any time vitality (life) remains in the tooth to be treated. If the tooth is nonvital, then the endodontist may advise the patient that a local anesthetic agent is not necessary.

After the pulp has been removed, a local anesthetic agent may or may not be administered during subsequent visits, depending on the patient's preference. Inflamed and infected tissues are difficult to anesthetize. Because endodontic procedures generally involve inflamed pulp or periapical tissues or both, obtaining an adequate level of anesthesia can be a problem. Injecting an additional local anesthetic solution directly into the pulp may be necessary. In addition, sedatives (oral or inhalation) may be used for patients who are apprehensive about the procedure.

Isolation of the Operating Field

The standard of care established by the ADA for endodontic treatment requires the use of a dental dam. Once the dam is placed, disinfecting the tooth, the dental dam clamp, and the surrounding dental dam material with an iodine solution or a sodium hypochlorite solution is necessary.

Access Preparation

During access preparation, the dentist uses a high-speed handpiece and a round bur to create an opening in the coronal portion of the tooth for the instrumentation to reach the root canals. Access is gained through the occlusal surfaces of the posterior teeth and the lingual surfaces of the anterior teeth.

Estimated Working Length

The dentist must know the length of the completed canal preparation and root canal filling. Problems that result from inaccurate measurement of length include (1) perforation of the apex, (2) over instrumentation or under instrumentation of the canal length, (3) overfilling or underfilling of the canal, and (4) postoperative pain.

Because exact apex locations vary and are not always visible on radiographs, the working length is estimated and is termed the *estimated working length*. The estimated working length is determined by selecting a reference point on the tooth, usually the highest point on the incisal or occlusal surface. On a periapical radiograph, a millimeter endodontic ruler is used to measure the distance from the reference point to the apex of the tooth. From this measurement, all files are measured to the exact length, and rubber stops are used for placement. It is extremely important that the tooth length as represented on the radiograph be accurate and not distorted.

An electronic apex locator is a supplemental technique that can be used to facilitate the identification in the apex of the root canal (Fig. 25.9). The use of an electronic apex locator as an aid to endodontic therapy can reduce the number of diagnostic radiographs required for determining the estimated working length.

FIGURE 25.9 Electronic apex locator. (Courtesy Kerr Corporation, Orange, California.)

FIGURE 25.10 Rotary handpiece used for endodontics. (From Johnson W: *Color atlas of endodontics,* Philadelphia, 2002, Saunders.)

Debridement, Disinfection, and Shaping of the Canal

The purposes of debridement, disinfection, and shaping of the canal are the use of specific shaped files and canal disinfection to (1) remove bacteria, necrotic tissue, and organic debris from the root canal and (2) smooth and shape the canal so that the filling material can be completely adapted to the walls of the canal.

Rotary files are similar to hand files but are latch-type files placed in a high-torque, low-rpm handpiece designed for nickel-titanium (NiTi) rotary instruments (Fig. 25.10). These groups of instruments are becoming more popular than traditional hand instruments because of their makeup, ease in use, and efficiency.

Obturation

After the canal has been debrided to the desired size and shape, it is dried; the canal is now ready to be obturated or filled by the

FIGURE 25.11 The apex of the mesiofacial root has been surgically removed. (From Johnson W: *Color atlas of endodontics*, Philadelphia, 2002, Saunders.)

endodontist using gutta-percha and then sealed. If the tooth has more than one canal, then each canal is individually filled, and each canal requires a properly fitted and sealed gutta-percha point.

See Procedure 25.2: Assisting in Root Canal Therapy.

Surgical Endodontics

Root canal therapy is successful approximately 90% to 95% of the time. In exceptional situations, however, surgical endodontic techniques must be used to save a tooth from extraction.

Apicoectomy involves the surgical removal of the apical portion of the root with the use of a tapered fissure bur in a high-speed handpiece (Fig. 25.11).

Retrograde restoration, also referred to as root end filling, is completed when the apical seal is not adequate.

Root amputation is a surgical procedure that is used to remove one or more roots of a multirooted tooth without removing the crown.

Hemisection is a procedure during which the root and the crown are cut lengthwise and removed.

▢ Ethical Implications

Endodontic therapy is an area of dentistry in which the dental team is almost always working with a patient who is in pain. It is important that the patient understand the steps involved in determining the origin of the pain. Communicating to the patient about what to expect throughout the procedure is the dental team's responsibility.

For a root canal to be effectively completed, remembering that accuracy is the number-one criterion when exposing diagnostic and working radiographic images and measuring and preparing endodontic files.

Assisting in Electric Pulp Vitality Testing

Equipment and Supplies

- Electric pulp tester
- Toothpaste
- Electric pulp testing kit(Courtesy SybronEndo, Orange,

California.)

Procedural Steps

1. Describe the procedure to the patient and explain that the patient may feel a tingling or warm sensation.
2. Identify the teeth to be tested (the suspect tooth and the control tooth), and then isolate these teeth and thoroughly dry them.

Set the dial (current level) at zero.

1. Place a thin layer of toothpaste on the tip of the pulp tester electrode.
   Purpose: The toothpaste provides adequate contact to conduct a current from the pulp tester to the tooth.
2. Test the control tooth first.

3. Place the tip of the electrode on the facial surface of the tooth at the cervical third.
4. Gradually increase the level of the current until the patient feels a sensation. Document the level at which the response occurred in the patient's record.
5. Repeat the procedure on the suspect tooth.

DATE	TOOTH	SURFACE	CHARTING NOTES
	7	—	Pt complained of pain. Tooth #10 used as control tooth. Vitality test showed tooth still responding to sensation.
			T. Clark, CDA/L. Stewart, DDS

Equipment and Supplies

- Basic setup
- Local anesthetic agent setup (optional)
- Dental dam setup
- High-speed handpiece with burs (dentist's choice)
- Low-speed handpiece with latch attachment
- 5- to 6-mL syringe with 27-gauge needle
- Broaches and Hedström and K-type files (assorted sizes and lengths)
- Rubber instrument stops
- Paper points
- Gutta-percha points
- Endodontic sealer supplies
- Endodontic spoon excavator
- Endodontic explorer
- Double-ended Glick no. 1 instrument
- Lentulo spiral instrument
- Millimeter ruler
- Locking cotton pliers
- Sodium hypochlorite solution
- Hemostat
- High-volume evacuator (HVE) tip

(From Boyd LRB: *Dental instruments: a pocket guide,* ed 5, St. Louis, 2015, Saunders.)

Procedural Steps

Preparing the Field of Operation

1. Assist in the administration of the local anesthetic agent (if applicable).
2. Assist with the preparation and placement of the dental dam.
   Note: Expose only the tooth being treated.
3. Swab the antiseptic solution over the exposed tooth, the clamp, and the surrounding dental dam.

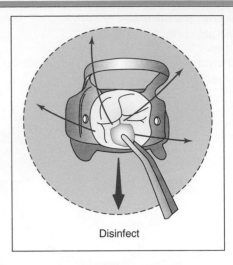

Disinfect

Removing the Pulp

1. The dentist enters the coronal portion of the tooth with a carbide bur and removes the decay and infected tooth structure.

Once the canals are located with the endodontic explorer, the pulp tissue is removed with intracanal instruments.

Assisting in Root Canal Therapy—cont'd

2. The canals are gently disinfected with the sodium hypochlorite solution. Excess solution is removed with the HVE tip.
3. The dentist uses a small endodontic file to rub the irrigation solution against the walls of the canal and pulp chamber.
   Purpose: The solution acts as a disinfectant to destroy bacteria in the canal and to wash away debris. This step is called *biochemical cleaning.*

Cleaning and Shaping the Canal

1. The dentist inserts files into the canal and moves them up and down with short strokes.
   Purpose: During this motion, the cutting edges of the files will remove dentin and debris from the walls of the canal.

2. Transfer larger files to the dentist to clean and shape the canals.
   Purpose: The increase in the size of the files is used to enlarge the diameter of the canal.
3. The rubber stop must be placed on the file at the desired working length for each canal.
4. Thoroughly irrigate the canals at frequent intervals during this shaping and cleaning process.
   Purpose: Irrigation prevents the dentin shavings from clogging the cutting edges of the instruments.
5. Transfer paper points for insertion into the canals until the points come out dry.

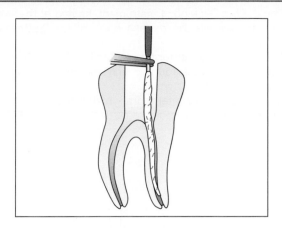

Preparing to Fill the Canal

1. Select an appropriately sized gutta-percha point and cut it to the predetermined length. This length is called the *trial point.*
2. Take a periapical radiograph of the tooth with the trial point in the canal; this is the working length radiograph.
3. If the radiograph does not show the tip of the trial point within 1 mm of the apex of the root, then the point is repositioned, and another radiographic image is taken.
4. At the signal from the dentist, prepare a thin mix of sealer on a sterile glass slab.
   Purpose: The sealer is used to ensure a perfect seal at the apical foramen.

Filling the Canal

1. The master cone is removed from the canal, coated with sealer, and reinserted by the dentist.
2. The dentist inserts the finger spreader into the canal within 1 mm of the working length. The spreader is rotated counterclockwise to spread the sealer around the canal and to create space for the other cones.
3. Continue transferring gutta-percha points to fill the canal.

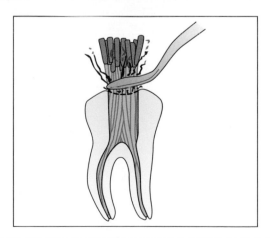

Continued

4. Transfer the Glick no. 1 instrument, heated at the working end, to remove the excess ends of the gutta-percha points.
5. Transfer the plugger for the dentist to compact vertically.
6. Continue steps 2 through 5 until the canal is completely filled and sealed.
7. The dentist places a temporary restoration.

8. Expose a posttreatment radiograph.
9. The dentist checks the occlusion and adjusts as needed.

Posttreatment Instructions and Follow-up

1. Instruct the patient to call the practice immediately if indications of a problem arise, such as swelling or pain.

2. Remind the patient that a return to their regular dentist is necessary to have a final restoration placed.
3. Request that the patient return to the endodontist for follow-up examinations at intervals ranging from 3 to 6 months.

Purpose: Follow-up appointments enable the endodontist to ensure that the treatment is successful and that no complications have developed.

DATE	TOOTH	SURFACE	CHARTING NOTES
	30	—	Root canal therapy, 2 carp. Xylocaine w/ epinephrine, dam isolation, tooth opened, maximum file used #70, working length 24 mm, canal disinfected with NaOCl, gutta-percha working/posttreatment radiographs. Pt tolerated procedure well. Return for postoperative check in 1 week. T. Clark, CDA/L. Stewart, DDS

Multiple Choice

Circle the letter next to the correct answer.

1. Before treatment, the patient seeking endodontic treatment should be informed that _____.
   a. all root canal treatments are successful, and no further treatment will be required
   b. they will need to complete the restorative phase of the procedure with their general dentist
   c. patients never experience postoperative pain
   d. the chance exists that the tooth may still need to be extracted

2. Root canal therapy is not recommended when the _____.
   a. diagnosis is reversible pulpitis
   b. patient has a medical condition that precludes any dental treatment
   c. tooth has severe periodontal involvement
   d. all of the above

3. After the irrigation of a pulpal canal, the canals are dried with _____.
   a. cotton pellets
   b. paper points
   c. quick blasts of air
   d. gutta-percha

4. To place the sealer and cement into the pulpal canal, a _____ is inserted into a low-speed handpiece.
   a. flexible K-type file
   b. Gates Glidden bur
   c. Lentulo spiral
   d. Pesso file

5. After the placement of the dental dam, the tooth should be _____.
   a. wiped with an alcohol wipe
   b. wiped with an antiseptic
   c. wiped with hydrogen peroxide
   d. wiped with sodium hypochlorite

6. _____ have tiny fishhook-like barbs along the shaft and are used to remove the bulk of the pulpal tissue.
   a. Broaches
   b. Endodontic explorers
   c. Hedström files
   d. Pesso files

7. The pulpal canal is filled with which final dental material?
   a. Amalgam
   b. Calcium hydroxide
   c. Composite resin
   d. Gutta-percha

8. During endodontic treatment, the canals would be disinfected with _____.
   a. 2% glutaraldehyde
   b. alcohol
   c. iodine
   d. diluted sodium hypochlorite

9. During pulp testing, if the suspected tooth is #4, then the control tooth should be tooth #_____.
   a. 5
   b. 13
   c. 20
   d. 29

10. A _____ is a football-shaped, rotary instrument with its cutting edge on the sides rather than at the end.
    a. K-type file
    b. broach
    c. Pesso file
    d. Gates Glidden bur

Apply Your Knowledge

1. You are assisting the endodontist with root canal therapy on tooth #3. The dentist indicates that all roots are to be treated today. How many roots are in the maxillary right first molar? How would these roots appear on a radiographic image?

2. A patient calls the office in reference to experiencing severe pain in the lower right jaw. What specific questions could be asked of the patient to help identify what kind of pain the patient is having, and which teeth could possibly be involved?

3. You are a clinical dental assistant in a pediatric dental office, and the child has extensive decay in a primary molar. The decay has not affected the pulp at this point. What would you suspect the diagnostic conclusion to be? What procedure will the dentist complete at this stage in the child's treatment?

CHAPTER 26

Oral and Maxillofacial Surgery

http://evolve.elsevier.com/Robinson/essentials/

LEARNING OBJECTIVES

1. Pronounce, define, and spell the key terms.
2. Define the specialty of oral and maxillofacial surgery.
3. Discuss the surgical environment for surgical procedures.
4. Identify and describe the function of instruments used for surgical procedures.
5. Describe the importance of the chain of asepsis throughout a surgical procedure.
6. Describe the surgical assistant's role in oral surgery.
7. Discuss the types of procedures practiced in this specialty.
8. Describe the types of postoperative care provided after a surgical procedure.

KEY TERMS

alveolitis
alveoloplasty
asepsis

extraction
impaction
luxate

oral and maxillofacial surgery (OMFS)
sutures

Oral and maxillofacial surgery (OMFS) is the specialty of dentistry that involves the diagnosis, surgery, and treatment of diseases, injuries, and defects of the oral and maxillofacial region.

The general dentist is qualified to perform basic surgical procedures, such as single tooth extractions, in their practice. For more complicated procedures, however, dentists will refer their patient to an oral and maxillofacial surgeon.

Description of Oral and Maxillofacial Procedures

- Extraction of decayed teeth that cannot be restored
- Surgical removal of impacted teeth
- Extraction of nonvital teeth
- Preprosthesis surgery to smooth and contour the alveolar ridge
- Removal of teeth for orthodontic treatment
- Removal of root fragments
- Reconstructive surgery
- Removal of cysts and tumors
- Biopsy of a questionable area
- Treatment of fractures of the bones of the face and jaws
- Surgery to alter the size or shape of a facial bone
- Surgery of the temporomandibular joint
- Surgical implants
- Reconstructive surgery
- Surgical repair of cleft lip and cleft palate
- Salivary gland surgery

Surgical Environment

Oral surgery, even when performed in the general dental office, is just as much a surgical procedure as one performed in a hospital surgical unit. It is essential for the dental team to have the patient's clinical record, emergency equipment, anesthetic supplies, and surgical instruments readied before seeing a patient for a surgical procedure.

Patient Record

The dentist must have a complete patient record, which includes a current medical history, radiographic images showing the area to be treated, recorded vital signs, appropriate charting of treatment, and the type of pain control methods that are prescribed before, during, and after surgery.

Signed Consent

Once the procedure has been reviewed with the patient or legal guardian, it is important that the responsible party sign a release form indicating that they understand the procedure to be performed and any possible complications that may occur.

Oral Surgery Instruments

Oral surgery instruments have specific uses and are designed to separate the tooth from the socket, to retract surrounding tissue, to loosen and elevate the tooth within the socket, and to remove the tooth from the socket. The oral surgery instruments most commonly used in surgical procedures are provided in Table 26.1. Because all surgical instruments are classified as critical instruments, they must be sterilized and remain in their packaging until ready for use.

Extraction Forceps

Extraction forceps are available in many different shapes and designs to accommodate the dentist's needs in grasping teeth with different crown shapes, root configurations, and locations within the mouth. The goal is to remove the tooth in one piece with the crown and root intact.

Forceps are used to remove teeth from the alveolar bone after they have been slightly loosened in the socket by the application of elevators. The handles, which are held firmly in a palm grasp, provide the surgeon with the necessary leverage to luxate and remove the tooth (**luxate** means to rock back and forth). See Table 26.2 for the commonly used surgical forceps.

Surgical Asepsis

Establishing and maintaining the chain of asepsis in a surgical procedure means that the instruments, surgical drapes, and gloves worn by the dental team must be sterile from setup to completion of the procedure. (**Asepsis** means the absence of pathogenic microorganisms.) Contact with anything that is not sterile will break the chain of asepsis and contaminate the surgical area.

See Procedure 26.1: Performing a Surgical Scrub and Procedure 26.2: Performing Sterile Gloving.

Surgical Procedures

When preparing for a surgical procedure, specific criteria must be met for a smooth, efficient performance of the procedural steps. Every surgical procedure requires preparation and advance planning by the dental team.

TABLE 26.1
Oral Surgery Instruments

Name of Instrument	Description of Use
Periosteal elevator	A periosteal elevator separates and retracts the periosteum from the bone that is holding the tooth in its socket.
Straight elevator	A straight elevator is used to apply leverage against the tooth to loosen it from the periodontal ligament and to ease the extraction.
Root tip picks	Root tip picks are used to remove root tips, tooth fragments, or debris that may have broken away from the tooth during the extraction.
Surgical curette	A surgical curette resembles a large spoon excavator and is used after an extraction to clean the interior of the socket or to remove diseased tissue.
Rongeur	A rongeur is a scissors-shaped instrument with short blades used to trim alveolar bone. The rongeur instrument is commonly used after multiple extractions to remove sharp projections and to shape the edentulous ridge.
Bone file	The bone file is a flat working instrument with large cutting grooves. The bone file is used with a push-pull motion to smooth the surface of the bone after using the rongeur instrument or to smooth the rough margins of the alveolus.

Continued

TABLE 26.1
Oral Surgery Instruments—cont'd

Name of Instrument	Description of Use
Scalpel	A scalpel is a surgical knife used to make a precise incision into soft tissue. Scalpel blades are available in many sizes and styles. 1. A one-piece disposable instrument consisting of a scalpel blade and handle. 2. Reusable Bard-Parker handle. 3. #12 single use blade to attach to the Bard-Parker. 4. #15 single use blade to attach to the Bard-Parker.
Hemostat	A hemostat has beaks with serrations or grooves and a locking mechanism on the handle, which makes it useful for grasping and holding an object or tissue.
Needle holder	The needle holder resembles the hemostat, but the beaks are straight with fine serrations to grasp a suture needle firmly.
Surgical scissors	Surgical scissors are available in fine straight or curved blades and are used to trim soft tissue.
Tissue retractors	Tissue retractors are used to grasp and hold soft tissue during surgical procedures. Extreme care must be taken when retracting tissue to prevent trauma or damage to the tissue.
Surgical chisel and mallet	A surgical chisel and mallet are used to split a tooth for easy removal by tapping the mallet on the chisel, which helps in the removal of a tooth or to reshape bone.
Surgical aspirating tip	A surgical aspirating tip is used in a surgical procedure. The smaller tip easily fits into the socket or surgical site.

(All images courtesy Hu-Friedy, Chicago, Illnois.)

TABLE 26.2
Dental Forceps

Name/Number of Forceps	Description of Use
Maxillary universal forceps/# 150	For the extraction of maxillary centrals, laterals, canine, premolars, and roots.
Universal maxillary forceps/#10S	For the extraction of maxillary molars.
Maxillary forceps **# 88R** **#88L**	For the extraction of maxillary and right and left first and second molars. Notice the design of the beak to fit into the trifurcation of the molars.
Maxillary root tip forceps	For the extraction of maxillary roots remaining in the socket.

Continued

TABLE 26.2

Dental Forceps—cont'd

Name/Number of Forceps	Description of Use
Mandibular universal forceps/#151	For the extraction of mandibular centrals, laterals, canine, premolars, and roots.
Universal mandibular forceps/# 16	Commonly referred to as "cowhorn" because of the shape of the beaks. For the extraction of mandibular first and second molars.
Mandibular forceps/# 17	For the extraction of mandibular first and second premolars. Notice the design of the beak to effectively fit into the bifurcation of the tooth.
Mandibular anterior forceps	For the extraction of mandibular anterior teeth. Beaks of forceps are serrated for a better grasp.
Mandibular root tip forceps	For the extraction of mandibular roots remaining in the socket

(Images from Boyd LRB: *Dental instruments: a pocket guide,* ed 7, Elsevier, 2021.)

Surgical Assistant's Role in Oral Surgery

Advance Preparation

- Review the patient record and prepare radiographic images.
- Confirm that the consent forms are signed and available for review.
- Verify that any information requested from the patient's physician has been received.
- If a prosthesis will be delivered to the patient, then determine whether the dental laboratory has returned it.
- Verify that the appropriate surgical setup has been prepared and sterilized.
- Contact the patient and provide preoperative instructions for taking any premedication and instructions for eating or drinking after midnight.
- Instruct the patient to have someone drive them and stay during the procedure.

Treatment Room Preparation

- Prepare the treatment room by placing protective barriers on anything that may be touched during the procedure.
- Keep surgical instruments in their sterile wraps until ready for use. If a surgical tray has been set out, then open it and place a sterile towel over the instruments.
- Have the appropriate pain control medications (e.g., local anesthesia, nitrous oxide–oxygen inhalation, intravenous [IV] sedation) ready for administration.
- Have the necessary postoperative instructions ready to provide to the patient.

Patient Preparation

- Update the patient's medical history and all laboratory reports.
- Check that the patient has taken their prescribed premedication. If not, the surgeon should be immediately alerted.
- Illuminate radiographic images.
- Take the patient's vital signs to determine a baseline and record the signs in the patient's record.

- Prepare any additional monitoring equipment to be applied.
- Seat and drape the patient. (To protect the patient's clothing, a large drape is often used, in addition to a patient towel.)
- Adjust the chair into a comfortable reclining position. If general anesthesia is to be administered, then place the patient in a supine position.

During Surgery

- Maintain the chain of asepsis.
- Assist in the administration of local anesthetic medications.
- Monitor the administration of nitrous oxide and IV sedation (refer to Chapter 14 for a description of these procedures).
- Transfer and receive instruments.
- Aspirate and retract as needed.
- Maintain a clear surgical field with adequate light.
- Monitor the patient's vital signs, oximetry, and electrocardiogram (ECG; refer to Chapter 11 for a description of these procedures).
- Steady the patient's head and mandible, if necessary, during the use of a mallet and chisel.
- Observe the patient's condition and anticipate the surgeon's needs.

After Surgery

- Stay with the patient until they have sufficiently recovered to leave the office.
- Give verbal and written postoperative instructions to the patient and to the responsible person who has accompanied the patient.
- Confirm a postoperative visit as directed by the dentist.
- Update the patient's treatment records, including a copy of any new prescriptions given to the patient.
- Return the patient's records to the business assistant.
- Break down and disinfect the treatment area.
- Transport all contaminated items to the sterilization center.

Types of Surgical Procedures

Forceps Extraction

Forceps extraction is often described as a *routine* or *simple* **extraction**. These terms are misleading because all extractions are considered surgical procedures. Using these terms implies that the extraction can be completed without extensive instrumentation.

A forceps extraction is performed on a tooth that is fully erupted, has a solid intact crown, and can be firmly grasped with the forceps. Most routine forceps extractions will not require the placement of **sutures**.

See Procedure 26.3: Assisting in a Forceps Extraction.

Multiple Extractions

When several teeth are to be extracted at the same time, the forceps extraction procedure is essentially the same. If the teeth being extracted are proximal to one another, however, then the alveolar socket will have bony projections where the teeth have been removed. The dentist must then complete an alveoloplasty. Alveoloplasty involves surgically contouring and smoothing

the remaining bone to provide a properly contoured ridge for proper healing and also for a bridge, partial, or denture, if one is to be placed. It is common for sutures to be placed so the gingival area will heal uniformly.

See Procedure 26.4: Assisting in Multiple Extraction and Alveoloplasty.

Removal of Impacted Teeth

The term complex extraction is used when conditions exist that require additional skill, effort, and instrumentation to remove a tooth. The extraction of an impacted mandibular third molar is an example of a complex extraction. (An impacted tooth is one that has not erupted. It may be partially or totally covered by tissue and/or bone.)

In the case of a tissue impaction, a scalpel would be used to expose the unerupted tooth. For a bony impaction, the dentist would first use the scalpel. Then, with the use of a surgical bur, the dentist would go through bone to gain access to the tooth for removal. As a rule, if a scalpel has been used to expose tissue, then sutures are placed for proper healing.

Steps in Assembling a Scalpel

See Fig. 26.1.
1. Hold handle of scalpel with nondominant hand.
2. With dominant hand, grip blade with forceps, avoiding contact with cutting edge.
3. Place blade partway over handle fitting and engage slots.
4. Slide blade until it clicks into position.

See Procedure 26.5: Assisting in the Removal of an Impacted Tooth.

Suture Placement

Sutures provide several functions for the healing process of a surgical site. They (1) help control bleeding, (2) promote healing, and (3) assist in creating an even attachment of tissue. Therefore, when a scalpel is added to the tray setup, suture equipment is also added.

The suture needle is circular in shape and held in a hemostat or a needle holder. Suture needles are supplied already threaded and in a sterile pack (Fig. 26.2). The surgeon uses a technique that will use the least amount of suture material but will still promote the healing process.

Sutures are available in both **absorbable** and **nonabsorbable** varieties. Absorbable suture materials include plain catgut, chromic catgut, and polydioxanone. These sutures are readily absorbed by the body and do not have to be removed.

Nonabsorbable suture materials include silk, polyester fiber, and nylon. Black silk suture material is popular because it is strong, durable, and easy to manipulate. Nonabsorbable sutures, as a rule, are removed 5 to 7 days after surgery.

See Procedure 26.6: Assisting in Suture Placement, and Procedure 26.7: Performing Suture Removal (Expanded Function).

Immediate Postoperative Care

In addition to directions from the dentist, the assistant will provide postoperative instructions to the patient and to the individual accompanying the patient. Instructions for home care should be provided in both written and verbal forms.

Control of Bleeding

The patient is given the following instructions regarding the control of bleeding:
1. Avoid rinsing or spitting during the first 12 hours.
2. A pressure pack made of folded sterile gauze has been placed over the socket to control bleeding and to encourage clot formation.
3. Keep the pack in place for a minimum of 30 minutes. If the pack is removed too soon, then clot formation may be disturbed, and increased bleeding may occur.
4. If bleeding increases or does not stop, then call the dental office.
5. Do not disturb the clot with your tongue or by vigorously rinsing your mouth.
6. Strenuous work or physical activity should be restricted for a few days.

Control of Swelling

The patient is given the following instructions regarding the control of swelling:
1. The dentist may recommend the use of a nonsteroidal anti-inflammatory drug (NSAID) such as ibuprofen before and after surgery. (An NSAID is helpful in preventing and controlling swelling and also relieves pain.)
2. During the first 24 hours, a cold pack is placed in a cycle of 20 minutes on and 20 minutes off.
3. After the first 24 hours, external heat may be applied to the area of the face to enhance circulation and to promote healing.
4. After the first 24 hours, the patient can gently rinse the oral cavity with warm saline solution (1 tsp of salt to 8 oz of warm water) every 2 hours to promote healing.

Alveolitis (Dry Socket)

After a tooth is extracted, healing immediately begins with blood filling the socket and forming a clot. An open wound such as this will heal itself from the inside first. The clot is important in this process because it protects the wound and is later replaced by granulation tissue and, ultimately, by bone.

Failure of the process can result in **alveolitis**, also known as *dry socket*. This very painful condition commonly occurs 2 to 4 days after the extraction of a tooth.

Treatment for alveolitis is to have the patient immediately come in, irrigate the socket with warm saline solution, and pack the socket with medicated gauze (**iodoform**), which contains a topical antiseptic medication that soothes the nerves and covers the exposed bone to allow the healing process to begin.

FIGURE 26.1 Steps in placement of scalpel blade.

FIGURE 26.2 An example of suture material. (From Boyd LRB: *Dental instruments: a pocket guide,* ed 7, Elsevier, 2021.)

The specialty area of oral and maxillofacial surgery is one that requires the dental team to be prepared at all times for the care of a patient. Developing a surgical conscience is especially important for the surgical assistant. Most surgical procedures are invasive, and the assistant must always preserve the integrity of the sterile field, monitor the patient's vital signs throughout the procedure, be ready to assist, and be alert to the needs of the surgeon and the patient. Oral surgery can be a traumatic experience for a patient, and it takes the entire dental team to be empathetic, supportive, and, most of all, in control of the procedure and the patient.

Procedure 26.1

Performing a Surgical Scrub

Equipment and Supplies
- Orange stick
- Antimicrobial soap, such as chlorhexidine gluconate
- Sterile surgical scrub brush
- Sterile disposable towels

Procedural Steps

1. Remove all jewelry.
2. Cover your hair and place protective eyewear and mask before performing a surgical scrub.
   Purpose: Once your hands are scrubbed, they should not touch anything.
3. With water running, use the orange stick to clean under your nails. Discard the stick and rinse your hands without touching the faucet or the inside of the sink.

4. Wet hands and forearms up to the elbows with warm water and then dispense approximately 5 mL of antimicrobial soap into cupped hands.

5. Use the surgical scrub brush to scrub the hands and forearms for 7 minutes.

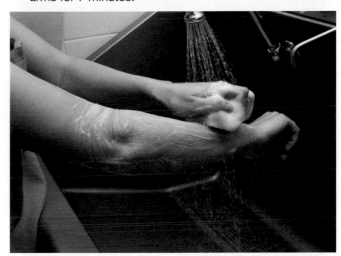

6. Thoroughly rinse the hands and forearms with warm water. Keep your hands up and above waist level.
   Purpose: Keeping your hands above the waist allows the water to run toward the elbows, keeping the hands clean.
7. Dispense another 5 mL of antimicrobial soap and repeat the scrub.
8. Wash for an additional 7 minutes without using a brush. Rinse so the contaminated water runs down the arms and off the elbows.
9. Dry hands and arms with a sterile towel. Use a patting motion, and continue up the forearms.
10. Keep your hands above your waist before donning your sterile gown.

(Photos from Hupp JR, Ellis E III, Tucker M: *Contemporary oral and maxillofacial surgery*, ed 6. Mosby, 2014.)

Procedural Steps

1. The glove package should already be opened before the surgical scrub. Be sure to touch only the inside of the package at this point.
   Note: The open glove pack is a sterile field.

2. Glove your dominant hand first.
   Purpose: Applying the second glove is more difficult, and you will have greater dexterity with your dominant hand.

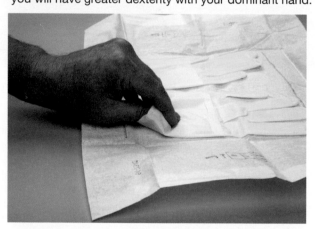

3. Pull the glove over the hand, touching only the folded cuff.
   Purpose: Remember to touch only the inside of the glove.

4. With your dominant hand gloved, slide your forefingers under the cuff of the other glove.
   Purpose: You can touch the sterile portion of the glove only with your dominant hand.

5. Pull the glove up over your other hand.

6. Unroll the cuff from your gloves.

(Photos from Hupp JR, Ellis E III, Tucker M: *Contemporary oral and maxillofacial surgery,* ed 6. Mosby, 2014.)

Equipment and Supplies

- Local anesthetic agent setup
- Basic setup
- Periosteal elevator
- Elevator (dentist's choice)
- Forceps (dentist's choice)
- Surgical curette
- Sterile gauze sponge
- Surgical aspirator tip

Procedural Steps

1. Assist in the administration of a local anesthetic agent.
2. Transfer the explorer for the dentist to probe the area to determine the level of anesthesia.
3. Transfer the periosteal elevator for the dentist to loosen the gingival tissue gently and to compress the alveolar bone surrounding the neck of the tooth.

(Courtesy Dr. Edward Ellis III.)

4. Transfer an elevator (most often straight) as requested by the dentist to loosen the tooth.
5. The dentist places the beaks of the forceps on the tooth and firmly grasps the tooth around and below the cementoenamel junction.

(Courtesy Dr. Edward Ellis III.)

6. The tooth is luxated in the socket to compress the bone and enlarge the socket. When luxation is complete, the tooth can be freely lifted from the socket.
7. The dentist examines the tooth to ensure that the root is intact.
8. When the tooth is removed, use the aspirating tip to debride the surgical site.
9. Fold several sterile gauze sponges into a tight pad to form a pressure pack. Retract the cheek and place the folded gauze over the extraction site.
10. Instruct the patient to bite firmly on the pack for at least 30 minutes.
    Purpose: This pressure aids in controlling bleeding and in blood clotting.
11. Slowly move the dental chair to an upright position.
12. Provide the patient with postoperative instructions.

DATE	TOOTH	SURFACE	CHARTING NOTES
	4	—	Extraction, Vital signs within normal range, 2 carpules Xylocaine 1/50,000. Pt tolerated procedure well. Postoperative instructions given. T. Clark, CDA/L. Stewart, DDS

Equipment and Supplies

- Forceps extraction setup
- Additional elevators and forceps (dentist's choice)
- Rongeur
- Curettes
- Bone file
- Scalpel
- Suture material and needle
- Needle holder or hemostat
- Suture scissors
- Sterile saline solution

(From Boyd LRB: *Dental instruments: a pocket guide,* ed 5, Saunders, 2015.)

Procedural Steps

1. Follow steps 1 through 9 in Assisting in Forceps Extraction (see Procedure 26.3) until all the teeth have been extracted.
2. After the teeth have been extracted, the dentist uses the rongeur to trim the alveolus. After each cut with the rongeur, have a sterile gauze available to remove debris from the cutting ends carefully.

(From Boyd LRB: *Dental instruments: a pocket guide,* ed 5, Saunders, 2015.)

3. After the rongeur is used, transfer the bone file to the dentist to finish smoothing any rough margins. After each stroke with the file, use a clean sterile gauze square to remove debris from the grooves.

(From Boyd LRB: *Dental instruments: a pocket guide,* ed 5, Saunders, 2015.)

(From Boyd LRB: *Dental instruments: a pocket guide,* ed 5, Saunders, 2015.)

4. Irrigate and aspirate the surgical site with sterile saline solution to remove bone fragments. The dentist repositions the mucosa over the ridge and sutures it into place.

(From Hupp JR, Tucker MR, Ellis E: *Contemporary oral and maxillofacial surgery,* ed 6, Mosby, 2014.)

5. Place pressure packs made of sterile gauze sponges as needed. Provide the patient with postoperative instructions, both verbal and written, and complete the patient's dismissal.

DATE	TOOTH	SURFACE	CHARTING NOTES
	22–27	—	Vitals: P 90 bpm, BP 140/90 mm Hg. Extractions, 3 carpules Xylocaine 1:20,000, alveoloplasty, 8 nylon sutures placed. Pt tolerated procedure well. Postoperative instructions provided. Prescription for Tylenol w/ Codeine, and Penicillin 500 VK. Pt to return in 1 wk for suture removal and check. T. Clark, CDA/L. Stewart, DDS

Equipment and Supplies

- Forceps extraction setup
- Scalpel, #15 blade and handle
- Additional elevators and forceps (surgeon's choice)
- Rongeur
- Bone file
- Curettes
- Root tip picks
- Surgical scissors
- Conventional high-speed handpiece with surgical bur or mallet and chisel
- Irrigating syringe
- Sterile saline solution
- Sterile suture material and needle
- Needle holder or hemostat
- Suture scissors
- Sterile gauze sponges

(From Boyd LRB: *Dental instruments: a pocket guide,* ed 5, Saunders, 2015.)

Procedural Steps

Surgical Preparation

1. The surgeon determines that adequate anesthesia has been achieved.
2. Transfer the scalpel for the surgeon to make the initial incision along the ridge through both the gingival mucosa and the periosteum.

(From Boyd LRB: *Dental instruments: a pocket guide,* ed 5, Saunders, 2015.)

3. The periosteal elevator is used to retract the tissue from the bone.
4. Once the incision is made, continuously evacuate blood, debris, and saliva from the surgical site.
5. A surgical mallet and chisel or a surgical handpiece with surgical burs will be used to remove the bony covering from the impacted tooth.

Removing the Impacted Tooth

1. When the surgeon has uncovered the impacted tooth, it can be luxated and lifted from the alveolus with an elevator or extraction forceps.

2. In some cases, the tooth is lodged between bone and another tooth. This position may necessitate sectioning the crown of the impacted tooth with the mallet and chisel or a surgical bur.
3. After the tooth has been removed, the surgical site is curetted, irrigated, and evacuated to remove all debris and infectious material.
4. After a thorough debridement, the surgeon returns the mucoperiosteal flap to its normal position over the wound and sutures it into place.
5. Slowly return the patient to an upright position.
6. Provide the patient with postoperative instructions.

DATE	TOOTH	SURFACE	CHARTING NOTES
	18	—	Vitals: P 80 beats/min, BP 130/82 mm Hg. Extraction, N$_2$O sedation, 2 carpules Xylocaine 1:20,000; incision using #12 blade, tooth removed in sections; 2 gut sutures placed. Pt tolerated procedure well. Prescription for Tylenol w/ Codeine, and Penicillin 500 VK Postoperative instructions Provided. Pt to return in 1 wk. T. Clark, CDA/ L. Stewart, DDS

Equipment and Supplies

- Suture material
- Hemostat
- Needle holder
- Suture scissors
- Sterile gauze sponges

Procedural Steps

1. Remove the suture material from its sterile package.
2. Using the needle holder, clamp the suture needle at the upper third.

   Purpose: If you clamp too close to the thread, then you may cause the suture to detach from the needle; if you clamp too close to the needle end, then you may damage the needle point.

(Copyright iStock.com/propeller.)

3. Transfer the needle holder to the surgeon while grasping the hinge, which allows the surgeon to grasp the handle of the instrument.

(Copyright iStock.com/megaflop.)

4. Retract the tongue or cheek to provide a clear line of vision for the surgeon as the sutures are placed.
5. After tying each suture and if directed by the surgeon, use the suture scissors to cut the sutures, leaving approximately 2 to 3 mm of suture material beyond the knot.

(Copyright IStock.com/Lighthaunter.)

6. Retrieve the suturing supplies from the surgeon and replace them on the surgical tray.
7. Record the numbers and types of sutures placed in the patient's record.

Performing Suture Removal (Expanded Function)

Equipment and Supplies

- Basic setup
- Suture scissors
- Sterile cotton gauze
- Cotton-tip applicator

Procedural Steps

1. The surgeon examines the surgical site to evaluate healing. If healing is satisfactory, then the sutures may be removed.
2. Swab the site with an antiseptic agent to remove any debris.
3. Use cotton pliers to hold the suture gently away from the tissue to expose the attachment of the knot. Gently slip one blade of the suture scissors under the suture. Cut near the tissue.

4. Use the cotton pliers to grasp the knot, and gently tug it so that the suture slides through the tissue.
   Note: Never pull ("yank") the knot through the tissue.

5. If bleeding occurs, then irrigate the surgical site with an antiseptic solution or warm saline solution. Briefly apply a compress to the surgical site to promote clotting.
6. Count the sutures that have been removed and compare this number with the number indicated in the patient's record.

DATE	TOOTH	SURFACE	CHARTING NOTES
	—	—	Suture removal, 3 nylon sutures removed. Pt. healing well, with no complications. T. Clark, CDA/L. Stewart, DDS

Chapter Exercises

Multiple Choice

Circle the letter next to the correct answer.

1. A bone file is used to _____.
   a. debride the socket
   b. loosen gingival tissue
   c. smooth the rough margins of the alveolus
   d. remove bone over an impacted tooth

2. The term *universal* means that a forceps may be used _____.
   a. anywhere in the mouth
   b. on the left side of the dental arch
   c. on the right side of the dental arch
   d. b and c

3. Nylon and silk sutures _____ absorbed by the body.
   a. are
   b. are not

4. A rongeur is used to _____.
   a. loosen gingival tissue
   b. remove infected tissue
   c. trim alveolar bone
   d. retrieve root fragments

5. The common term for alveolitis is _____.
   a. dry socket
   b. impaction
   c. excessive bleeding
   d. extraction

6. During a surgical procedure, _____ are to be worn.
   a. examination gloves
   b. over gloves
   c. sterile gloves
   d. utility gloves

7. A(n) _____ is used to control immediate postoperative bleeding.
   a. gauze pressure pack
   b. heating pad
   c. ice pack
   d. moistened tea bag

8. Periosteal elevators are used to _____.
   a. remove clots and debris from the socket after the extraction
   b. remove the tooth from the socket
   c. separate the periosteum from the surface of the bone
   d. remove gauze from the surgical site

9. The surgical reshaping of the alveolar ridge is known as a(n) _____.
   a. alveolitis
   b. alveoloplasty
   c. gingivectomy
   d. impaction

10. Sutures that are not resorbed by the body are commonly removed in _____ days.
   a. 1 to 2
   b. 3 to 4
   c. 5 to 7
   d. 10 to 14

Apply Your Knowledge

1. You are assisting in a forceps extraction on tooth #4. List the surgical instruments that would be set up for this procedure.

2. A patient calls the office after hours describing extreme pain 2 days after having her wisdom teeth extracted. You remember the patient because the procedure took longer than expected because the teeth were impacted. What might this patient be experiencing?

3. You have identified the problem in the previous question. How do you instruct this patient to relieve her pain and discomfort?

CHAPTER 27

Pediatric Dentistry

http://evolve.elsevier.com/Robinson/essentials/

LEARNING OBJECTIVES	1. Pronounce, define, and spell the key terms.
	2. Describe the appearance and setting of a pediatric dental office.
	3. Discuss the behavioral management techniques used for pediatric patients.
	4. Explain the stages of child behavior and how they affect your approach when providing care.
	5. Describe techniques for caring for a challenging patient.
	6. Discuss patients with special needs.
	7. Describe the types of procedures commonly provided in a pediatric dental practice.
	8. Describe the types of traumatic injuries that can be commonly seen in a pediatric practice.

KEY TERMS

autonomy
avulsed
cross-bite

rapport
space maintainer
stainless steel crowns

Pediatric dentistry is a specialized area of dentistry that is focused on providing oral health care to infants, children, adolescents, and individuals of any age with special needs. The emphasis of the pediatric dental practice is on developmental guidance, early detection, prevention, and treatment of dental diseases. It is common for a child to continue seeing their pediatric dentist until the age of 18 to 21 years old.

> **Clinical Procedures Provided for a Pediatric Patient**
> - Preventive care
> - Restorative procedures
> - Pulp therapy
> - Surgical procedures
> - Space maintenance
> - Preventive and interceptive orthodontics

Pediatric Dental Office

The design of a pediatric dental office should portray a cheerful, pleasant, and nonthreatening atmosphere to a child. Many pediatric dental offices are designed with several dental chairs arranged in one large treatment area or bay (Fig. 27.1). This design provides reassurance from one child to another when they can see other children being treated. An open-bay design can be psychologically effective because children are often hesitant to express fear or to misbehave in the presence of other children.

The pediatric office will also have a "quiet room." This treatment area is separate from the open area and is used for children whose behavior may upset other children.

Behavioral Management Techniques

Children are treated differently from adult patients, and the techniques used to manage a child's behavior depend on the age of the child (see Table 27.1 for the stages of behavior). Members of the dental team in a pediatric office will make modifications in the way they practice dentistry for several reasons: age, size, and how the child is behaving (Fig. 27.2).

Guidelines for Child Behavior

The development of trust between the parent and child and the dentist serves as the basis for a productive, effective means of providing dental health care. Dental procedures can be accomplished for patients of all ages if the dental team practices the following procedural guidelines:
- Be honest with the child.
- Consider the child's point of view.
- Always "tell, show, and do."
- Give positive reinforcement.

FIGURE 27.1 Example of a pediatric dental office. (Courtesy Patterson Dental, St. Paul, Minnesota.)

TABLE 27.1
Stages of Behavior

Age Range	Behavioral Characteristics
Birth to 2 years of age	Children may act friendly toward strangers but then become afraid of them. They may experience fear of separation from a parent. Toddlers are too young to be expected to cooperate with dental treatment. If the parent is with the child, then the initial examination is easier.
3–5 years of age	Children are learning to follow simple instructions at this age. They want *autonomy*. Allow children at this age to make choices (e.g., ask them to choose the flavor of fluoride).
6–11 years of age	Children in this age group are in the period of socialization. They want to learn the rules. They have overcome most of their fears.
12–20 years of age	In this age group, young people have acquired self-certainty and a sexual identity. They will seek leadership and develop their own ideals.

FIGURE 27.2 Patient at a pediatric dental office.

Challenging Patient

Treating an anxious, fearful, or uncooperative child can be challenging for the dentist, assistant, parents, and especially the child (Fig. 27.3). In some situations, a child will remain uncooperative, despite the fact that the dental team has used every possible approach to provide a positive dental experience. Occasionally, a child's behavior during treatment requires a more assertive management style to be used to protect them from possible injury. Voice control (speaking calmly but firmly) will usually prevent the need for additional steps.

In certain cases, some form of restraint may be required for the patient's protection. A **restraint** can be pharmacologic or physical. If the dentist knows that restraint will be needed, then a premedication can be prescribed to calm and ease the patient before treatment. Mild sedation, such as nitrous oxide–oxygen or a sedative, may benefit an anxious child. A

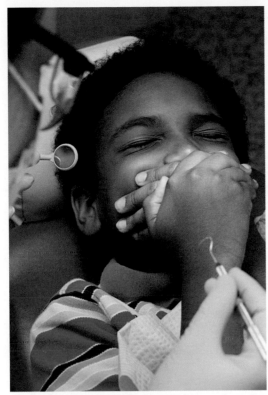

FIGURE 27.3 Anxious patient. (©iStock/XiXinXing)

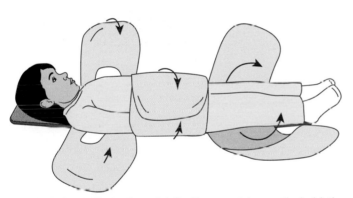

FIGURE 27.4 Protective stabilization used to gently hold the patient still during treatment.

protective stabilization wrap, which is a temporary stabilization for a child, can also be used (Fig. 27.4). This device gently *hugs* or wraps around the child's arms, legs, and middle section during a procedure to help keep a patient's movement or activity to a minimum for their protection.

Patients with Special Needs

Physical and mental challenges can slow or challenge a child's physiologic and social growth. An intellectual disability is a state of functioning that begins in childhood and is characterized by limitations in intelligence and adaptive skills. Examples include down syndrome, autism, and cerebral palsy. Each diagnosis can influence how individuals are able to care for themselves and what role the parents and caregivers may be required to take on for maintaining daily physical and oral health needs.

The pediatric dentist receives extensive education and training to care for patients with special needs. The severity of each individual patient's disorder dictates whether treatment is provided in the pediatric dental office or in the hospital setting. An evaluation of a patient's medical and social history will help determine necessary modifications to the treatment plan.

Examination of the Pediatric Patient

According to the American Academy of Pediatric Dentistry, the first dental appointment for a child should take place around their first birthday. This initial examination is often the first dental experience for a child. The rapport that is developed with the child during this initial examination can establish a positive attitude toward dental health that will last for the child's lifetime. (**Rapport** means a feeling of ease or comfort.)

The child's parent or legal guardian must provide consent (permission) before any dental treatment is provided for a child younger than 18 years of age.

Medical and Dental Histories

The parent or guardian completes the **medical history form** for the child under the age of 18 years, which includes information about the child's general health background (Fig. 27.5). If medical problems are noted, then the dentist may choose to contact the child's pediatrician to obtain a more complete medical background.

The **dental history** includes information about the eruption pattern of the teeth, past dental problems and care, fluoride intake, and current oral hygiene habits.

General Appraisal and Behavioral Assessment

A general appraisal addresses physical conditions and developmental levels. It also includes vital signs and baseline health data for emergency situations.

A behavioral assessment is used to evaluate the communication skills of the patient and to determine whether behavioral management techniques are necessary.

Intraoral Examination

The intraoral examination requires the use of a mouth mirror, an explorer, and air from an air/water syringe. Young children may be hesitant and only allow fingers and the mouth mirror in their mouths.

Ideally, each of the 20 primary teeth should be examined. In addition to charting the erupted teeth, the occlusion is analyzed to determine spacing and crowding and the presence or absence of teeth.

Radiographic Examination

A radiographic examination is necessary for the dentist to make a complete diagnosis, but young children often have difficulty with the radiographic procedure, and the radiographic examination may have to be deferred until the child can comprehend the need to remain still and follow directions. When radiographs are possible, techniques are available that can be helpful for introducing the procedure to the child.

Child Health/Dental History Form

ADA American Dental Association®
America's leading advocate for oral health

Patient's Name				Nickname	Date of Birth
LAST	FIRST	INITIAL			

Parent's/Guardian's Name	Relationship to Patient

Address				
PO OR MAILING ADDRESS		CITY	STATE	ZIP CODE

Phone			Sex M ☐ F ☐
Home	Work		

Have you (the parent/guardian) or the patient had any of the following diseases or problems? .... ☐ Yes ☐ No
1. Active Tuberculosis, 2. Persistent cough greater than a three-week duration, 3. Cough that produces blood?
If you answer yes to any of the three items above, please stop and return this form to the receptionist.

Has the child had any history of, or conditions related to, any of the following:

☐ Anemia	☐ Cancer	☐ Epilepsy	☐ HIV +/AIDS	☐ Mononucleosis	☐ Thyroid
☐ Arthritis	☐ Cerebral Palsy	☐ Fainting	☐ Immunizations	☐ Mumps	☐ Tobacco/Drug Use
☐ Asthma	☐ Chicken Pox	☐ Growth Problems	☐ Kidney	☐ Pregnancy (teens)	☐ Tuberculosis
☐ Bladder	☐ Chronic Sinusitis	☐ Hearing	☐ Latex allergy	☐ Rheumatic fever	☐ Venereal Disease
☐ Bleeding disorders	☐ Diabetes	☐ Heart	☐ Liver	☐ Seizures	☐ Other_____
☐ Bones/Joints	☐ Ear Aches	☐ Hepatitis	☐ Measles	☐ Sickle cell	

Please list the name and phone number of the child's physician:

Name of Physician _____Phone _____

Child's History

	Yes	No
1. Is the child taking any prescription and/or over the counter medications or vitamin supplements at this time? .... 1. ☐ ☐		

If yes, please list: _____

2. Is the child allergic to any medications, i.e. penicillin, antibiotics, or other drugs? If yes, please explain: _____ 2. ☐ ☐
3. Is the child allergic to anything else, such as certain foods? If yes, please explain: _____ 3. ☐ ☐
4. How would you describe the child's eating habits?_____
5. Has the child ever had a serious illness? If yes, when: _____ Please describe: _____ 5. ☐ ☐
6. Has the child ever been hospitalized?.. 6. ☐ ☐
7. Does the child have a history of any other illnesses? If yes, please list: _____ 7. ☐ ☐
8. Has the child ever received a general anesthetic? .... 8. ☐ ☐
9. Does the child have any inherited problems?.. 9. ☐ ☐
10. Does the child have any speech difficulties?.. 10. ☐ ☐
11. Has the child ever had a blood transfusion?.. 11. ☐ ☐
12. Is the child physically, mentally, or emotionally impaired?............................ 12. ☐ ☐
13. Does the child experience excessive bleeding when cut? .... 13. ☐ ☐
14. Is the child currently being treated for any illnesses? .... 14. ☐ ☐
15. Is this the child's first visit to a dentist? If not the first visit, what was the date of the last dentist visit? Date: _____ 15. ☐ ☐
16. Has the child had any problem with dental treatment in the past? .... 16. ☐ ☐
17. Has the child ever had dental radiographs (x-rays) exposed? .... 17. ☐ ☐
18. Has the child ever suffered any injuries to the mouth, head or teeth? .... 18. ☐ ☐
19. Has the child had any problems with the eruption or shedding of teeth? .... 19. ☐ ☐
20. Has the child had any orthodontic treatment? .... 20. ☐ ☐
21. **What type of water does your child drink?** ☐ City water ☐ Well water ☐ Bottled water ☐ Filtered water
22. **Does the child take fluoride supplements?** .... 22. ☐ ☐
23. **Is fluoride toothpaste used?** .... 23. ☐ ☐
24. How many times are the child's teeth brushed per day? _____ When are the teeth brushed?_____ 24. ☐ ☐
25. Does the child suck his/her thumb, fingers or pacifier?................................ 25. ☐ ☐
26. At what age did the child stop bottle feeding? Age _____ Breast feeding? Age _____
27. Does child participate in active recreational activities? .... 27. ☐ ☐

NOTE: Both doctor and patient are encouraged to discuss any and all relevant patient health issues prior to treatment.
I certify that I have read and understand the above. I acknowledge that my questions, if any, about inquiries set forth above have been answered to my satisfaction. I will not hold my dentist, or any other member of his/her staff, responsible for any action they take or do not take because of errors or omissions that I may have made in the completion of this form.

Parent's/Guardian's Signature _____Date _____

For completion by dentist
Comments _____
_____
_____
_____

For Office Use Only: ☐ Medical Alert ☐ Premedication ☐ Allergies ☐ Anesthesia Reviewed by_____
Date _____

© American Dental Association, 2006
Form S707

To Reorder call 1-800-947-4746
or go online at www.adacatalog.org

FIGURE 27.5 Example of child's health and dental history form.

FIGURE 27.6 A space maintainer is used to reserve the space until the permanent tooth erupts.

Pediatric Procedures

The procedures described in this chapter are introduced to help maintain the health of the primary, mixed, and permanent dentition through early adult years.

Preventive Dentistry

Prevention is one of the most encompassing areas of a pediatric dental practice. It not only involves the complete dental team in educating the patient and parents, but it also reaches to the community and local school systems. The role of the pediatric dentist is to communicate preventive dental health in such areas as oral hygiene, fluoride use, nutrition, and preventive and protective procedures.

Oral Hygiene

Oral hygiene instructions are geared toward improving a child's brushing and flossing techniques. Eventually, this learning process is intended to lead to cleaner teeth and healthier gums. When children are encouraged to develop the habit of effectively brushing twice a day with fluoride toothpaste and flossing once a day, they will maintain proper oral habits throughout their lives (see Chapter 20).

Nutrition

The best diet is one that is healthy, balanced, and naturally supplies all the nutrients a child needs to grow. Chapter 20 describes the types of foods that children should eat for normal growth and identifies foods that can increase decay.

Topical Fluorides

Fluorides have played a primary role in bringing about the decline in dental caries; however, for many children, decay is still a major dental problem. Often, these children are those who have not had the benefits of fluoride from birth. Professional topical application of fluoride is especially important in controlling caries in children. (Fluorides are discussed in Chapter 20.)

Sealants

Sealants are a routinely preventive procedure provided in a pediatric office. Sealants protect the grooves and pitted surfaces of teeth, especially the chewing surfaces of molars and premolars, where most decay is detected. Sealants are made of a clear or tooth-colored composite resin and are applied to the pits and fissures to help keep them free from cavities. (See Chapter 21 for further discussion.)

Preventive and Interceptive Orthodontics

It is never too early to start evaluating a child's oral and facial (orofacial) development. The pediatric dentist is the first to identify malocclusion, crowded or crooked teeth, and habits that can affect the dentition. The pediatric dentist can actively intervene or can refer the patient to an orthodontist to guide the teeth as they emerge in the mouth. Early preventive and interceptive orthodontic treatment can prevent more extensive treatment later.

Preventive orthodontics can prevent or eliminate irregularities and malpositions in the developing dentofacial region. Preventive orthodontics can include:

- Control of decay to prevent the premature loss of primary teeth, which may result in loss of space for the eruption of permanent teeth
- Use of a space maintainer to save space for the eruption of permanent teeth (Fig. 27.6) (Space maintainers most often are cemented in place and retained until the permanent tooth erupts.)
- Use of appliances cemented in place to correct oral habits, such as thumb sucking, which can affect the permanent dentition (Fig. 27.7)
- Early detection of genetic and congenital anomalies that may influence dental development
- Supervision of the natural exfoliation (shedding) of the primary teeth (If retained for too long, the primary teeth may cause the permanent teeth to erupt out of alignment or to be impacted.)

Interceptive orthodontics allows the dentist to intercede or correct problems as they develop. For example, a **cross-bite**

FIGURE 27.7 Example of a fixed appliance to discourage thumb sucking. (Courtesy Dr. Frank Hodges.)

FIGURE 27.8 Example of a fixed appliance to correct cross-bite. (Courtesy Dr. Frank Hodges.)

FIGURE 27.9 Palatal expansion appliance used to widen the maxillary arch. (Courtesy Dr. Frank Hodges.)

occurs when one or both sides of the maxillary teeth are positioned lingual to the mandibular teeth. Interceptive orthodontics includes the following:
- Extraction of primary teeth that can contribute to malalignment of the permanent dentition
- Correction of a cross-bite through the use of a removable or fixed appliance (Fig. 27.8)
- Correction of a jaw size discrepancy through the use of a removable or fixed appliance (Fig. 27.9)

FIGURE 27.10 Copper T-band used for primary molars. **A,** In preparation for closing the band. **B,** End of band held in place by closing tabs.

- Extraction of primary or permanent teeth to correct overcrowding

Sports Safety

The fields of sports medicine and dentistry have documented the benefits of wearing protective face equipment during recreational sports that might injure the mouth area. Many states have regulations that require athletes in school contact sports to wear protective mouth guards to help prevent traumatic injuries to the teeth.

Commercial or custom mouth guards may be used. Commercial mouth guards are supplied as kits. The material is heated in warm water, placed in the individual's mouth, and molded to fit the arch.

Custom mouth guards are created in the dental office. An alginate impression is obtained of the player's maxillary arch, and a diagnostic cast is created. The mouth guard is vacuum formed from the cast.

Restorative Procedures

Restorative procedures, described in Chapter 22, are also performed on primary teeth. The dentist follows many of the same restorative principles as with permanent teeth in the placement of amalgam, composite, glass-ionomer cement, and preformed metal crowns. The major difference is the size and shape of the teeth.

Moisture Control

Because of the size of the mouth and less area to control moisture during a procedure, the use of cotton rolls or the dental dam may need to be adapted for the area. When preparing the dental dam, isolating the tooth receiving the restoration and the tooth behind or distal for the dental clamp works best.

Matrix Systems for Primary Teeth

The matrix systems most commonly used on primary teeth are the (1) T-band, which is a small, copper T-shaped band that, when the top portion of the T is bent, provides an adjustable band to fit around the circumference of a primary molar (Fig. 27.10), and the (2) spot-welded band, which is form-fitted around the tooth using No. 110 pliers. The band is then removed and placed in a smaller form of a welder that fuses the metal together to make a custom band.

For anterior teeth, the use of a plastic matrix, also referred to as celluloid strips, or mylar strip is placed interproximal for the placement of the composite resin and the final stages of polymerization.

Pulp Therapy

The primary objective of pulp therapy in a pediatric setting is to stimulate and preserve pulpal regeneration of a primary tooth. The two most common factors that affect the pulpal health of primary teeth are deep decay and traumatic injury. Decay is more likely to affect the posterior teeth, and trauma is more likely to affect the anterior teeth.

Indirect and direct pulp capping is indicated for a young permanent tooth to promote pulpal healing and to stimulate the production of reparative dentin.

Pulpotomy

Pulpotomy is the complete removal of the coronal portion of the dental pulp in a primary tooth. The goal of this procedure is to remove the portion of the pulp that is inflamed but maintain the healthy vital pulp tissue in the canals of the primary tooth.

See Procedure 27.1: Assisting in Pulpotomy of a Primary Tooth.

Stainless Steel Crowns

Stainless steel crowns are used in the treatment of posterior primary molars. This type of crown is considered the treatment of choice over large multisurface amalgam restorations for primary molars (Fig. 27.11). Stainless steel crowns are available in a variety of sizes.

FIGURE 27.11 Stainless steel crowns are trimmed and contoured to fit properly.

Indications for Use of Stainless Steel Crowns

- Restoration of primary or permanent teeth with extensive decay
- Restoration of primary teeth after pulpotomy or pulpectomy procedures
- Permanent restoration after accidental fracture of a tooth
- Temporary restoration of a fractured tooth
- Restorations for patients who have difficulty maintaining good oral hygiene, such as disabled children

---

Types of Stainless Steel Crowns

Two types of stainless steel crowns are commonly used in pediatric dentistry.

Pretrimmed crowns have straight sides but are festooned to follow a line parallel to the gingival crest. They must be trimmed and contoured to fit the tooth. (*Festooned* means trimmed. *Contoured* means shaped to fit.)

Precontoured crowns are already festooned and contoured. Some additional trimming and contouring may be necessary but usually only minimally.

See Procedure 27.2: Assisting in the Placement of a Stainless Steel Crown.

Traumatic Injury

An injury to the tooth of a young child can have serious and long-term consequences, including discoloration and possible loss of the tooth. Many injuries to primary teeth commonly

FIGURE 27.12 Traumatized maxillary incisor. (Courtesy Dr. Frank Hodges.)

occur at 1½ to 2½ years of age (the toddler stage). The teeth most frequently injured in the primary dentition are the maxillary central incisors (Fig. 27.12). These types of injuries can have damaging effects on permanent teeth forming directly below the roots of the primary teeth.

Common causes of dental injury to children include falling, bicycle accidents, sports injuries, and possible child abuse. For more information, see Table 27.2.

Fractured Anterior Teeth

Fractures of anterior teeth are common emergencies in a pediatric dental practice.

The business assistant should instruct the parents of a child with a fractured tooth to come to the office immediately. Complete documentation of the accident, clinical examination,

TABLE 27.2
First Aid for Dental Emergencies

Dental Emergency	Instructions for Parents
Toothache	• Rinse out mouth with warm water. • If there is swelling, place cold compress on cheek. • Do NOT place aspirin on the gum or on the aching tooth. • Take the child to the dentist.
Broken Tooth	• Rinse mouth from injured area with warm water. • Place cold compress in the area of the injury. • Immediate dental attention is necessary.
Knocked-Out Tooth	• Handle the tooth by the crown, not the root portion. • Rinse tooth gently under running water but do NOT scrub. • Inspect the tooth for fractures. • Do NOT pack a baby tooth back in the socket. • A permanent tooth can be placed back in socket if possible. • If you cannot reinsert the tooth, transport the tooth in a cup of milk or cool water. • Prompt care by the dentist is recommended.
Bitten Lip, Tongue, or Cheek	• Apply ice to bruised area. • If there is bleeding, apply firm by gentle pressure with a gauze or cloth. • If bleeding does not stop after 15 minutes or cannot be controlled by simple pressure, take the child to the emergency center.

Adapted from flyer (Courtesy Dr. John Christensen.)

vitality testing, and radiographs are almost always part of the emergency visit (Fig. 27.13).

The plan of treatment is to delay restorative treatment for 3 to 6 weeks to prevent further trauma to the pulp of an injured tooth. This delay gives the pulp a greater opportunity to recover without additional injury.

In the meantime, the dentist provides temporary relief by covering all exposed dentin with calcium hydroxide to prevent thermal sensitivity and places an interim covering of resin material. Radiographs and vitality tests are taken at subsequent appointments to determine the status of the injured tooth.

If the pulp shows vitality, then a definitive restorative procedure can be performed on the injured tooth.

Avulsed Teeth

Permanent teeth that have been avulsed, which means that the tooth has come completely out of the tooth socket, can be replanted with varying degrees of success (Fig. 27.14). Primary teeth are not usually replanted. (**Avulsed** means torn away or removed by force.)

The more quickly a tooth can be repositioned, the greater the chance for success. The highest success rate occurs when the permanent tooth is replanted within 30 minutes of the accident.

FIGURE 27.13 Fracture of an anterior tooth. (Courtesy Dr. Frank Hodges.)

FIGURE 27.14 Avulsion of maxillary central incisors. (Courtesy Dr. Frank Hodges.)

Reporting Abuse and Neglect

Dentists, dental hygienists, and dental assistants may be the first to recognize signs of abuse and may be instrumental in enhancing the victim's chances of obtaining assistance. Abuse can occur inside or outside of the homes. Because many injuries occur around the mouth, neck, face, and head, members of the dental health team are in an excellent position to recognize the signs of abuse and to report cases of suspected abuse to authorities. Many states identify dental professionals as mandated reporters. In these states, dental professionals must report suspected abuse if they observe signs of abuse or if they have reasonable suspicion of abuse. The report may be made to a social work agency, a county welfare or probation department, or a police or sheriff's department.

Indicators of Child Abuse and Neglect

Behavioral Indicators
- Child is wary of adult contacts.
- Child is apprehensive when other children cry.
- Child is afraid to go home.
- Child is frightened of parents.
- Child exhibits overly compliant, passive, and undemanding behaviors to avoid confrontation with abuser.
- Child lags in development of motor skills, toilet training, socialization, or language.

Dental Neglect or Abuse
- Child has untreated rampant caries that is easily detectable by a layperson.
- Child has untreated pain, infection, bleeding, or trauma affecting the orofacial region.
- Child has injuries or tears to the labial frenum, indicating forced feedings.

Other Indicators
- Child displays cigarette burns or bite marks.
- Child displays cuts, bleeding, or finger marks on ears or "cauliflower ear."
- Child displays bald or sparse spots on scalp, indicating malnutrition or hair pulling.
- Child is dirty, is unkempt, or has poor oral hygiene.
- Child is dressed inappropriately for weather to conceal bruises or injuries (e.g., long sleeves on a hot day).
- Child shows evidence of poor supervision, such as repeated falls downstairs, repeated ingestion of harmful substances, or being left alone in a car or on the street.
- Mentally or physically disabled children are especially vulnerable and are often targets for abuse because of the difficulties caregivers face in meeting the needs of these children.

Ethical Implications

The provision of dental care to children is a responsibility of the dental team. The image and memories that a child has of their dental experiences will be carried with them throughout life. Use words and terminology that are age appropriate and creates a nonthreatening experience when you explain a procedure as you speak to a child. Allow children to ask questions but be ready to answer questions in a nonthreatening manner. Many expanded functions can be completed by the certified dental assistant in the pediatric office. Make certain that you have the current knowledge and skill required for these procedures.

Procedure 27.1

Assisting in Pulpotomy of a Primary Tooth

Equipment and Supplies

- Local anesthetic agent setup
- Basic setup
- Dental dam setup
- Low-speed handpiece
- Round burs
- Spoon excavators (various sizes)
- Sterile cotton pellets
- Formocresol
- Zinc oxide–eugenol (ZOE) base
- Final restorative material and instruments for placement

Procedural Steps

1. The local anesthetic agent is administered.
2. The dental dam is placed.
3. The dentist will use a round bur in the low-speed handpiece to remove the caries and expose the pulp chamber.
4. Transfer a spoon excavator for the dentist to remove all pulp tissue inside the coronal chamber.
5. Transfer a sterile cotton pellet moistened with formocresol for the dentist to place in the pulp chamber for approximately 5 minutes to control hemorrhaging.
6. Once bleeding is controlled, the pulp chamber is filled with ZOE paste, to which a drop of formocresol has been added.
7. The ZOE base and the final restoration are placed.

DATE	TOOTH	SURFACE	CHARTING NOTES
	C	—	Pulpotomy, 1 carpule Xylocaine, 1:100,000 w/o epinephrine. Dam isolation, tooth opened, formocresol placed. ZOE base, amalgam. Pt tolerated procedure well. T. Clark, CDA/L. Stewart, DDS

Procedure 27.2

Assisting in the Placement of a Stainless Steel Crown

Equipment and Supplies

- Basic setup
- Local anesthetic agent setup
- Dental dam setup
- Low-speed and high-speed handpieces
- High-volume evacuator (HVE) tip
- Friction grip burs (dentist's choice of diamond or carbide)
- Spoon excavator
- Selection of stainless steel crowns
- Crown and bridge scissors
- Contouring and crimping pliers
- Mandrel
- Finishing and polishing discs
- Mounted green stones
- Cotton rolls
- Cementation setup
- Dental floss
- Articulating paper and holder

Procedural Steps

Preparing the Tooth

1. After the local anesthetic agent has been administered and has taken effect, the dental dam is applied.
2. The dentist will use the high-speed handpiece and a tapered diamond or carbide bur to prepare the tooth by a method similar to that used for a cast crown (see Chapter 23).

Assisting in the Placement of a Stainless Steel Crown—cont'd

3. The dentist reduces the entire circumference of the tooth and the height of the tooth.
4. Dental caries are removed with hand instruments and burs.

Selecting and Sizing the Stainless Steel Crown

1. The crown is selected and tried on the prepared tooth for fit.
2. The stainless steel crown is properly sized when it fits snugly on the prepared tooth and has both mesial and distal contact.
3. Clean and sterilize any crowns that were tried in the mouth but not used, then return them to storage.

Trimming and Contouring the Crown

1. The dentist will use a crown and bridge scissors to reduce the height of the crown until it is approximately the same height as the adjacent teeth.

1. The dentist may use a green stone to smooth the rough edges of the crown along the cervical margin.
2. The cervical margin of the crown may be polished with a rubber abrasive wheel.
3. The occlusion is checked and adjusted as needed.
4. The dentist uses contouring pliers to crimp the cervical margins of the crown toward the tooth to obtain a tight fit and a proper cervical contour.

Cementation

1. Thoroughly rinse and dry the tooth. Place cotton rolls to maintain dry conditions.

2. Mix the permanent cement (polycarboxylate is often selected).
3. Line the crown with the cement and transfer the patient to the dentist for placement.

4. Transfer an explorer to the dentist to remove the excess cement from around the tooth.
5. Use dental floss to remove any remaining cement from the interproximal areas.

6. Use the air-water syringe and HVE tip to rinse the patient's mouth before dismissal.

(From Duggal MS, Curzon MEJ, Fayle SA, et al: *Restorative techniques in pediatric dentistry. Saunders, 1995;* and Hatrick CD, Eakle WS: *Dental materials: clinical applications for dental assistants and dental hygienists, ed 3. Saunders, 2016.*)

DATE	TOOTH	SURFACE	CHARTING NOTES
	L	—	Placement of stainless steel crown, 1 carpule Xylocaine1:100,000 w/o epinephrine. Dental dam isolation, crown cemented w/ Duralon. Pt tolerated procedure well. T. Clark, CDA/L. Stewart, DDS

Multiple Choice

Circle the letter next to the correct answer.

1. The types of procedures provided in a pediatric dental office include _____.
   a. pulp therapy
   b. restorative procedures
   c. preventive procedures
   d. all of the above

2. The age groups served by a pediatric dental practice include _____.
   a. infants through 2 years of age
   b. 3 to 5 years of age
   c. 13 to 18 years of age
   d. all of the above

3. What is unique about the treatment areas of a pediatric practice?
   a. Dental chairs are isolated from each other.
   b. More than one dentist will use a dental chair.
   c. An open-bay concept is present.
   d. Chairs are situated for the parents to sit in the dental treatment area.

4. At what stage of life does a child first want control and structure of their environment?
   a. Birth to 2 years of age
   b. 3 to 5 years of age
   c. 6 to 11 years of age
   d. 12 to 20 years of age

5. At what phase of orthodontics would a pediatric dentist intercede in getting a patient to stop sucking their thumb?
   a. Interceptive
   b. Preventive
   c. Corrective
   d. a and b

6. Stainless steel crowns are _____.
   a. considered to be permanent restoration for a primary tooth
   b. indicated when rampant decay is present
   c. used for primary molars
   d. all of the above

7. What endodontic procedure is commonly performed on primary teeth?
   a. Apicoectomy
   b. Pulpectomy
   c. Pulpotomy
   d. Retrograde

8. What type of matrix system is recommended for primary molars?
   a. Universal metal band
   b. T-band
   c. Mylar matrix
   d. Palodent

9. The teeth most frequently injured by toddlers are the _____.
   a. mandibular incisors
   b. mandibular molars
   c. maxillary incisors
   d. maxillary molars

10. A tooth that was knocked completely out of its socket is said to be _____.
    a. avulsed
    b. extruded
    c. exfoliated
    d. luxated

Apply Your Knowledge

1. Your next patient is 3 years old, and you are in the reception area ready to escort him to the treatment area, but the patient begins to cling to his mother. What do you do?

2. You will be applying sealants to the primary molars of a 5-year-old. Your plan is to use cotton rolls as your moisture control method. You notice that this child has a hard time keeping the cotton roll on the lingual side by the tongue. The cotton roll will not stay in place. Any suggestions on how you can maintain a dry field and still complete the procedure?

3. Dr. Stewart has asked you to take a preliminary impression for a space maintainer. As soon as you try to put in the impression tray, the child gags. How do you think the child is going to handle the impression material, and how will you get the impression?

4. An emergency patient has just arrived. A 2-year-old patient has fallen and hit her front tooth. You have been asked to take a periapical radiograph of the area. Describe the best technique for obtaining a radiograph on a young child.

CHAPTER 28

Orthodontics

http://evolve.elsevier.com/Robinson/essentials/

LEARNING OBJECTIVES	1. Pronounce, define, and spell the key terms.
	2. Identify the classifications of malocclusion and indications for orthodontic treatment.
	3. Describe the types of skills used by the orthodontist to make a diagnosis and treatment plan.
	4. List and describe the four categories of orthodontic treatment.
	5. Identify and describe the use of orthodontic instruments.
	6. Describe the components of fixed appliances, attachments, auxiliaries, and arch wires, and demonstrate the following procedures:
	• Place and remove elastomeric ring separators.
	• Assist in the fitting and cementation of orthodontic bands.
	• Assist in the direct bonding of orthodontic brackets.
	• Place arch wires.
	• Place and remove ligature ties.
	7. Discuss oral hygiene and dietary instructions, as well as adjustment visits and completed treatments for the orthodontic patient.

KEY TERMS	arch wires	fixed appliances	retainer
	auxiliaries	headgear	separator
	bands	malocclusion	tipping
	cephalometric	removable appliances	

Orthodontics is the specialty of dentistry that includes the diagnosis, prevention, interception, and treatment of all forms of malocclusion of the teeth and surrounding structures. (**Malocclusion** is an abnormal or a malpositioned relationship of the maxillary teeth to the mandibular teeth when occluded.) Refer to Chapter 4 for normal occlusion.

Types of treatment include straightening teeth that are rotated, tilted, improperly aligned, crowded, or unevenly spaced; correcting bite problems; and surgically aligning the upper and lower jaws.

Angle Classifications of Malocclusion

The system developed by Dr. Edward H. Angle is used to describe and classify occlusion and malocclusion. In this system, the key to understanding a person's *bite* is identifying the relationship of the permanent first molars when the patient is in centric occlusion. Refer to Chapter 4 for normal occlusion. See Fig. 28.1 for further clarification of malocclusion.

Indications for Orthodontic Treatment

Orthodontic treatment may be necessary as a result of any combination of the following conditions:

• Psychosocial influences on patients, such as self-esteem, and negative feelings about their appearance attributable to malocclusion and dental facial deformities
• Oral function, such as chewing problems from malocclusion, jaw discrepancies, speech sounds, and temporomandibular joint pain
• Dental disease, such as dental decay, and periodontal disease affected by malocclusion

Class	Model	Arch Relationships	Descriptions
Class I		*Molar:* MB cusp of the maxillary first molar occludes with the MB groove of the mandibular first molar. *Canines:* Maxillary occludes with the distal half of the mandibular canine and the mesial half of the mandibular first premolar.	Dental malalignment(s), such as crowding or spacing, present (see text). Mesognathic profile.
Class II	Division 1	*Molar:* MB cusp of the maxillary first molar occludes (by more than the width of a premolar) mesial to the MB groove of the mandibular first molar. *Canines:* Distal surface of the mandibular canine is distal to the mesial surface of the maxillary canine by at least the width of a premolar.	*Division 1:* Maxillary anteriors protrude facially from the mandibular anteriors, with deep overbite. Retrognathic Profile.
	Division 2		*Division 2:* Maxillary central incisors are upright or retruded, and lateral incisors are tipped labially or overlap the central incisors with deep overbite. Mesognathic profile.
Class III		*Molar:* MB cusp of the maxillary first molar occludes (by more than the width of a premolar) distal to the MB groove of the mandibular first molar. *Canines:* Distal surface of the mandibular mesial to the mesial surface of the maxillary by at least the width of a premolar.	Mandibular incisors in complete cross-bite. Prognathic profile.

Note: This system deals with the classification of the permanent dention.
MB, Meslobuccal.
Data from Fehrentach MJ, Popowics T: *Illustrated dental embryology, histology, and anatomy,* ed 4, St Louis, 2016, Saunders.
Images copyright Elsevier Collection.

FIGURE 28.1 Angle classification of malocclusion.

Records Visit and Treatment Planning

The first orthodontic appointment is scheduled to obtain records required by the orthodontist to make a diagnosis and create a treatment plan. The patient's diagnosis is based on information from three major sources:
1. Interview with the patient and/or the parent or guardian
2. Clinical examination of the patient
3. Assessment of diagnostic records

Interview Information

Through an interview with the patient and/or the parent or guardian, the orthodontist gathers important information about their desire to improve the appearance and function of their teeth.

Medical and Dental History

A thorough medical and dental history is necessary to provide a comprehensive understanding of the physical status of the patient and to evaluate specific orthodontic-related concerns.

FIGURE 28.2 Facial analysis from frontal and profile views. (From Proffit WR, Fields HW, Sarver DM: *Contemporary orthodontics,* ed 5, St Louis, 2013, Mosby.)

Physical Growth Evaluation

Because orthodontic treatment in children is closely related to growth stages, evaluating the patient's physical growth status is necessary. Questions will include how rapidly they have recently grown, such as a growth spurt, and what signs of sexual maturing are evident.

Social and Behavioral Evaluation

Motivation for seeking treatment is important. What outcome can the patient and parent or guardian expect as a result of treatment? How cooperative or uncooperative is the patient likely to be? The major motivation for orthodontic treatment for children can be the parent or guardian's desire for treatment; however, the child's willingness and cooperation are essential.

Adults seek orthodontic treatment for themselves for many reasons, including improving personal appearance, correcting the function of their teeth, and also having the ability to seek out orthodontic treatment because of insurance through an employer or self-insurance. Exploring the reasons that the patient is seeking treatment at this time is important.

Clinical Examination

The purpose of the orthodontic clinical examination is to document and evaluate the facial aspects, occlusal relationship, and functional characteristics of the jaws. At the records visit, the orthodontist decides which diagnostic records are required for the patient.

Evaluation of Facial Form

Facial form analysis is the visual examination of the face. It provides information that cannot be gathered from dental radiographs and diagnostic casts (Fig. 28.2).

Frontal evaluation (from the front)—the orthodontist examines the face to determine:
- Bilateral symmetry
- Size proportions of midline-to-lateral structures
- Vertical proportions

Profile evaluation (from the side)—the orthodontist examines the face in profile to:
- Determine whether the jaws are proportionately positioned
- Evaluate lip protrusion
- Evaluate the vertical facial proportions

Evaluation of Oral Health

A thorough hard and soft tissue examination and an oral hygiene assessment must be completed before orthodontic treatment begins. If problems are detected, the patient is referred for preventive and restorative treatment before orthodontic treatment is started.

Diagnostic Records

Diagnostic records include photographs, radiographic images, and diagnostic casts that provide data related to tooth angulation, dental crowding, and the presence of unerupted teeth. When possible, having these records available at the time of the clinical examination is best.

Photographs

Photography is useful as an aid in patient identification, treatment planning, case presentation, case documentation, and patient education and instruction. See Chapter 13 for techniques used in a dental office.

Extraoral Photographs. Two standard extraoral photographs are taken: (1) the frontal view, with lips in a relaxed position; and (2) a profile view of the patient's right side, with lips in a relaxed position (Fig. 28.3).

FIGURE 28.3 Extraoral photographs. **A,** Frontal view. **B,** Profile view from the right side.

Intraoral Photographs. Three standard intraoral photographs are also required: (1) the full direct view, which includes all teeth in occlusion; (2) the maxillary occlusal view, which includes the palate and all maxillary occlusal surfaces; and (3) the right buccal view, which includes the distal of the canine to the distal of the last molar (Fig. 28.4).

Cephalometric Radiographs

A **cephalometric** radiograph is an extraoral radiograph that is exposed from a side view, showing how the major functional skeletal structures of the face are related to each other (Fig. 28.5). This type of radiographic image makes it possible for the orthodontist to measure and evaluate dentofacial proportions and to clarify the anatomic basis for a malocclusion.

Diagnostic Casts

Evaluation of the occlusion requires impressions for diagnostic casts and a record of the patient's occlusion, enabling the casts to be articulated. Alginate impressions and diagnostic casts are discussed in further detail in Chapter 19.

For orthodontic purposes, the bases of the diagnostic casts are trimmed to a symmetric shape that is oriented to the midline of the palate, which makes detecting asymmetry within the dental arches easier. The casts are polished to provide a more acceptable case presentation for the patient (Fig. 28.6).

Case Presentation

The orthodontist studies the information gathered and develops a treatment plan and a cost estimate for the patient in preparation for the case presentation.

Approximately an hour is reserved for the case presentation visit, and the patient—and parent or responsible adult if the patient is a child—should be present. This presentation includes the approximate length of treatment, the fees involved, and a clear statement of the responsibility of the patient in helping ensure the successful completion of the treatment.

Orthodontic Treatment

Orthodontic treatment can be divided into four broad categories: (1) preventive, (2) limited, (3) interceptive, and (4) comprehensive.

Preventive Orthodontic Treatment

Preventive orthodontic procedures are designed to prevent or minimize the degree of severity of future orthodontic problems. The pediatric or general dentist commonly provides and oversees most of this type of treatment.

Preventive orthodontic treatment includes:
- Care to prevent premature loss of primary teeth
- If a tooth is lost, a space maintainer to save the space for the permanent tooth
- Correction of oral habits, such as thumb sucking, which may affect the development and alignment of the permanent dentition (Thumb sucking is not considered a problem until the permanent teeth are in position.)
- Early detection of developmental factors that may cause malocclusion
- Supervision of the natural exfoliation of the primary teeth (Primary teeth retained too long may cause the permanent teeth to erupt out of alignment or to be impacted.)

Limited Orthodontic Treatment

This category of orthodontic treatment involves an isolated area that would not involve the entire dentition. Examples of this category would be to correct crowding teeth in only one arch, to open a space or to upright a tooth to allow an adjacent tooth to move into the space, and to treat for the closure of one or more spaces.

FIGURE 28.4 Intraoral photographs showing a patient's front view in occlusion **(A)**, maxillary occlusal view **(B)**, and right buccal view **(C)**.

Interceptive Orthodontic Treatment

Interceptive treatment is an extension of preventive and/or limited orthodontic treatments but can also include localized tooth movement in an otherwise normal dentition.

Interceptive orthodontic treatment usually occurs in the transitional dentition and may include such procedures as the redirection of a tooth that has erupted out of position, correction of an isolated cross-bite, or recovery of lost space where overall space is not adequate.

Another interceptive step is the serial extraction of primary or permanent teeth to correct critical overcrowding in the arch, which is performed only when more conservative methods of treatment will not be effective. When extractions are required, the orthodontist refers the patient to a general dentist or to an oral and maxillofacial surgeon.

Comprehensive Orthodontic Treatment

Comprehensive orthodontic treatment involves coordinated diagnosis and treatment, leading to an improvement of the patient's craniofacial dysfunction and/or dentofacial deformity, including anatomic, functional, and esthetic relationships. This type of treatment can use fixed or removable orthodontic appliances.

Fixed appliances, commonly known as braces, are attached to the teeth and assist in tooth movement (Fig. 28.7). The application is discussed later in this chapter.

Removable appliances, which can be placed and removed by the patient, provide a wide range of treatment options.

The other type of removable appliance is the retainer, which is versatile in its use. A retainer is primarily used after comprehensive treatment or in tipping teeth. (**Tipping** is the movement

FIGURE 28.5 **A,** Cephalometric radiograph. **B,** Cephalometric landmark and points. **C,** Cephalometric analysis. *ANS,* Anterior nasal spine; *Gn,* gnathion; *Go,* gonion; *Me,* menton; *Na,* nasion; *Or,* orgitale; *Pog,* pogonion; *Point A,* innermost point on the contour of the premaxilla between the ANS and the incisor; *Point B,* innermost point on the contour of the mandible between the incisor and the bony chin; *PNS,* posterior nasal spine. (From Proffit WR, Fields HW, Sarver DM: *Contemporary orthodontics,* ed 5, St Louis, 2013, Mosby.)

FIGURE 28.6 Diagnostic model that is digitally produced from a laser scan of the cast and displayed for space analysis. (From Proffit WR, Fields HW, Sarver DM: *Contemporary orthodontics,* ed 5, St Louis, 2013, Mosby.)

of a tooth into a more upright position.) Additional information on retainers is provided later in this chapter.

Orthodontic **alignment technique** is an orthodontic approach used today for the positioning of the teeth. **Invisalign** is one brand of this technology. The vacuum-formed clear aligner (similar in design and fit to the thermoplastic vacuum–formed tray) is a series of clear *aligners* designed by the computer. The customized aligners are fabricated and worn at 2-week intervals (Fig. 28.8). Although not suitable to treat all cases of malocclusion, this alignment system is increasingly the system of choice because of its ease of use.

Instruments for Orthodontics

Orthodontics requires the use of highly specialized instruments. See Table 28.1 for the names of the most common types of orthodontic instruments and their descriptions of use.

FIGURE 28.7 Full braces. (From Boyd LRB: *Dental instruments: a pocket guide,* ed 5, St Louis, 2015, Saunders.)

FIGURE 28.8 Invisalign is an alignment system used to correct malocclusion.

Fixed Orthodontic Appliances

Through the use of fixed appliances, a tooth can be moved in six directions: (1) mesially, (2) distally, (3) lingually, (4) facially, (5) apically, and (6) occlusally. Fixed appliances are also used when rotating (turning) or moving a tooth to the left or right within its socket.

The principle components of fixed appliances are bands, brackets, arch wires, and auxiliaries.

Orthodontic Bands

Bands are preformed stainless steel rings fitted around the teeth and cemented in place. Buttons, tubes, and cleats may also be attached to a band to hold the arch wire and power products. (A **power product** is anything that is elastic and is used to create tooth movement; Fig. 28.9).

TABLE 28.1
Orthodontic Instruments and Their Uses

Instrument	Description of Use
Orthodontic scaler	Aids in bracket placement, removal of elastomeric rings, and removal of excess cement or bonding material.

Continued

TABLE 28.1

Orthodontic Instruments and Their Uses—cont'd

Instrument	Description of Use
Ligature director	Guides the elastic or wire ligature tie around the bracket. In addition, the operator can guide the cut tie under the arch wire.
Band plugger or pusher	Has a serrated end to help seat maxillary molar bands.
Bite stick	
Bracket placement tweezers	Is a long-tip reverse action tweezers that is used to carry and place the brackets directly on the facial surface of the tooth.
Bird-beak pliers	Is useful in forming or bending wires for fixed or removable appliances.
Three-prong pliers	Is used to contour or bend the arch wire for tooth movement.

TABLE 28.1
Orthodontic Instruments and Their Uses—cont'd

Instrument	Description of Use
Distal end cutter 	Is used to cut the end of the arch wire once it has been placed in the buccal tube.
Pin and ligature cutter 	Is used to cut the ligature wire after its placement around the bracket and in the removal of the arch wire.
Weingart utility pliers 	Helps guide the arch wire into the brackets.
Band remover 	Removes bands without placing stress on the tooth, which would result in discomfort to the patient.
Orthodontic hemostat 	Helps twist the ligature tie around the bracket.

(Photographs from Boyd LRB: *Dental instruments: a pocket guide,* ed 5, St Louis, 2015, Saunders.)

FIGURE 28.9 Molar band showing the attachments of tubes and cleats to hold the arch wire, headgear, and elastics. (From Boyd LRB: *Dental instruments: a pocket guide,* ed 4, St Louis, 2012, Saunders.)

Use of Separators Before Banding

Tight interproximal contacts can make it impossible to seat a band properly; therefore the teeth must be separated before fitting and placing the bands. A separator is used for this purpose.

The two items commonly used for separation are steel separating springs and elastomeric separators. Both work on the same principle. A week before the banding appointment, a separator is placed to force the mesial and distal spaces of the tooth slightly apart. By the time of the banding appointment, the required space is present.

See Procedure 28.1: Placing and Removing Elastomeric Ring Separators (Expanded Function).

Selecting Bands

The manufacturer supplies preformed bands of different sizes in a tray. These bands are set up to fit specific teeth (e.g., UL = upper left).

At chairside, bands can be selected by visually inspecting them and by estimating the size of the tooth. The band is removed from the tray with sterile cotton pliers and fitted around the tooth. If a band is tried in the mouth but is not selected, then it must be sterilized before returning it to the tray.

An alternative approach is to select, adapt, and fit the bands on the patient's diagnostic cast. This method eliminates the lengthy process at chairside, and minor alterations can be accomplished at chairside, as necessary.

Fitting Maxillary Bands

Initially, a maxillary band is positioned over the tooth using finger pressure on the mesial and distal surfaces. This pressure brings the band down close to the height of the marginal ridges. Then a **band pusher** is used on the mesiobuccal and distolingual edges to push the band into place.

Fitting Mandibular Bands

Initially, a mandibular band is positioned with finger pressure on the proximal surfaces. A **band seater** is placed along the buccal margins, and the patient's biting force is used to seat the band into place.

FIGURE 28.10 Example of an edgewise bracket bonded to a central incisor. (From Proffit WR, Fields HW, Sarver DM: *Contemporary orthodontics,* ed 5, St Louis, 2013, Mosby.)

Cementing Bands

Cementing orthodontic bands is similar to cementing cast restorations; the difference is that the cementation is exclusively to enamel. Glass ionomer or polycarboxylate cement is regularly selected for orthodontic purposes. The consistency of the cement should be slightly thicker than the consistency of the cement for an inlay or a crown because the escape of excess from the margins of a band is not the same problem as it is from beneath a cast restoration.

See Procedure 28.2: Assisting in the Fitting and Cementation of Orthodontic Bands.

Bonded Brackets

The edgewise bracket is the most universal type of bracket and is attached to a stainless-steel backing pad that is bonded to the enamel surface of the tooth. (The term **edgewise** describes a type of bracket.) These brackets are designed with four tie wings; the arch wire is placed in the bracket and is either ligated (attached) to it or is self-ligating (Fig. 28.10).

See Procedure 28.3: Assisting in the Direct Bonding of Orthodontic Brackets.

Arch Wires

The arch wire serves as a pattern for correcting the dental arch (Fig. 28.11). When the arch wire is attached (ligated), a force is transmitted through the brackets to the teeth. Arch wires are designed to be round, square, or twisted and are available in different gauge sizes. The orthodontist will make the decision regarding which wire to use, based on the stage of treatment and the type of movement required. Bending the arch wire causes the tooth or teeth to move in the desired direction.

See Procedure 28.4: Placing Arch Wires (Expanded Function).

FIGURE 28.11 Examples of arch wires. (From Boyd LRB: *Dental instruments: a pocket guide,* ed 5, St Louis, 2015, Saunders.)

FIGURE 28.13 Elastomeric ties. (Courtesy DynaFlex, St. Louis, Missouri.)

FIGURE 28.12 Ligature wires. (Courtesy DynaFlex, St. Louis, Missouri.)

FIGURE 28.14 Elastic chain ties. (From Graber LW: *Orthodontics: current principles and techniques,* ed 5, St Louis, 2012, Mosby.)

Ligating the Arch Wire

Once the arch wire has been positioned, it must be ligated (tied) to be held in place. The four types of ligature ties are:

1. **Wire ligatures:** Thin wires are twisted around the bracket to hold the arch wire in place (Fig. 28.12).
2. **Elastomeric ties:** These ligature ties are made of a plastic or rubberlike material and are available in many colors (Fig. 28.13).
3. **Elastic chain ties:** These are continuous, round rings that form a chain. Commonly referred to as Os, elastic chain ties are used to close the space between the teeth or to correct rotated teeth (Fig. 28.14).
4. **Continuous wire ties:** Although similar to wire ligatures, continuous wire ties are primarily used to close spaces where two or more teeth are to be ligated (tied) together.

See Procedure 28.5: Placing and Removing Ligature Ties (Expanded Function).

Elastics

Elastics, commonly referred to as rubber bands, are placed between the maxillary and mandibular arches to bring about tooth movement. On the basis of the movement required, the orthodontist determines where and when the elastics are to be placed (Fig. 28.15).

The patient is instructed on how to place and remove these elastics and is encouraged to wear them regularly as directed.

FIGURE 28.15 Elastics. (From Proffit WR, Fields HW, Sarver DM: *Contemporary orthodontics,* ed 5, St Louis, 2013, Mosby.)

Auxiliaries

Auxiliaries are added to the brackets and bands, making it possible to attach the arch wire to the tooth. The combination of these auxiliaries with the arch wire creates the forces required to move the teeth.

FIGURE 28.16 Headgear. (From Graber LW: *Orthodontics: current principles and techniques,* ed 5, St Louis, 2012, Mosby. Adapted from McNamara, JA Jr., Brudon, WL: *Orthodontics and dentofacial orthopedics.* 2001, Needham Press, Ann Arbor, MI.)

Headgear tubes are round tubes commonly placed on maxillary first molar bands. They are used for the insertion of the inner bow of a face-bow appliance.

Edgewise tubes are rectangular tubes gingivally placed to the plane of the main arch wire. These tubes should be present on the facial surfaces of the upper and lower first molars to receive the arch wire.

Labial hooks are hooks located on the facial surfaces of the first and second molar bands for both arches. These hooks hold the interarch elastics.

Lingual arch attachments are cleats or brackets located on the lingual portion of the bands for stabilization of the arch to reinforce anchorage and tooth movement.

Headgear

Another aspect of the treatment phase in fixed appliances is the use of headgear to control growth and tooth movement. Headgear is made up of two parts: (1) face bow and (2) traction device (Fig. 28.16).

Face Bow

The face bow is used to stabilize or to move the maxillary first molar distally, creating more room in the arch. The intraoral part of the face bow fits into the buccal tubes of the maxillary first molars. The outer part of the bow attaches to the traction device.

Traction Devices

The traction device applies the extraoral force used to achieve the desired treatment results. Four types of traction devices are available: high-pull, cervical, combination, and chin cap.

Oral Hygiene and Dietary Instructions

Oral Hygiene

Orthodontic appliances will harbor areas of food and plaque that can be trapped and hidden, making brushing more difficult. Good oral hygiene during orthodontic treatment is imperative.

If the patient does not properly take care of their mouth, then the results can include rampant caries and periodontal disease.

Dietary Instructions

Poor eating habits are an additional concern with patients in orthodontic treatment. The patient should be reminded to use good sense when selecting foods and to avoid those that can weaken or break bands and bonds or bend arch wires.

Examples of foods to be avoided are ice, hard foods such as popcorn and nuts, and sticky foods such as caramel candy and chewing gum.

Adjustment Visits

Throughout active orthodontic treatment, the patient must regularly return for adjustments. At these appointments, the orthodontist reviews the patient's progress and makes adjustments, as necessary.

Although these visits are brief, each is extremely important, and the necessity of keeping each appointment should be stressed to the patient.

Checking the Appliance

At each adjustment appointment, the chairside assistant is responsible for examining the patient's appliance and looking for:
- Loose, broken, or missing arch wires or ligature ties
- Loose brackets and bands
- Loose, broken, or missing rubber bands

Bands

Loose bands can result from a break in the cement seal, from poor eating habits, or from the use of elastics, headgear, or other types of power products.

A loose band can be spotted by its appearance. Bands are checked with an explorer or a scaler, and loose bands slide up and down on the tooth. Unless the band has been distorted, it can be cleaned and recemented.

Bonded Brackets

Two primary problems are associated with bonded attachments: (1) An attachment can become loose or come off the surface of the tooth; and (2) on rare occasions, the bracket may break loose from the pad of the bond.

Most bonds are replaced unless the orthodontist elects to leave the attachment off because it is not necessary for the current phase of treatment.

Arch Wires

Poor eating habits and the patient picking or playing with the appliance can bend the arch wire. Bent or broken wires must be reshaped or replaced.

The patient should be advised to call the office if a problem develops between appointments. The orthodontist should promptly make repairs without waiting for the regular adjustment appointment.

When checking for bends in the arch wire, the assistant also looks for broken wires. Some breaks are hard to see. A tooth that moves out of alignment or a complaint of a sore tooth can be an indication of a problem; it should be investigated.

Completed Treatment

Once the patient has completed the treatment phase of orthodontics, the bands and bonded attachments are removed.

Bands are removed with band-removing pliers. The cushioned tip of the pliers is placed on the distobuccal cusp, and the blade edge of the pliers is used against the buccogingival margin of the band. Then the band is gently lifted upward. If necessary, this process is repeated on the mesial and lingual aspects. Any cement left on the teeth after debanding can be easily removed by scaling with a hand instrument or with an ultrasonic scaler.

Bonded brackets must be removed without causing damage to the enamel surface. Removal can be completed by creating a fracture within the resin bonding material or between the bracket and the resin and then removing the residual resin from the enamel surface.

Retention

Although a patient may believe that their treatment is complete when the fixed appliances are removed, an important stage in orthodontic treatment lies ahead. If excellent long-term results are to be achieved, then orthodontic control of tooth position and occlusal relationships must be gradually, not abruptly, withdrawn. Retention is necessary to:

- Allow gingival and periodontal tissues the required time to heal from changes that occurred during treatment.
- Support the teeth that are in an unstable position to ensure that pressure from the cheeks and tongue does not cause a relapse.
- Control changes caused by growth.

The **positioner** is a custom appliance made of rubber or pliable acrylic that fits over the patient's dentition after orthodontic treatment. The positioner is designed to retain the teeth in their desired position and to permit the alveolus to rebuild support around the teeth before the patient wears a retainer.

The **retainer** is the most commonly placed appliance after fixed orthodontics. It is worn to passively retain the teeth in their new position after removal of the orthodontic bands. The retainer also encourages some tooth movement to close band spaces and provides control of the incisors.

▮ Ethical Implications

As a chairside assistant in an orthodontic practice, you must realize the importance of your role in the care of a patient's treatment. You may see one patient on a regular basis for 2 years. The accomplishments of the dental team in the orthodontic office for a patient can change a person's perception of their own dental function and dental appearance.

The assistant's role in this specialty is to prepare all of the diagnostic records for the orthodontist, to assist in the placement of fixed orthodontics, and to assist in adjustments during the many visits thereafter. Always be certain that the functions you are performing in the orthodontic office are legal functions for you to complete in the state in which you are practicing.

Equipment and Supplies

- Elastomeric separators
- Separating pliers
- Floss
- Orthodontic scaler

(From Boyd LRB: *Dental instruments: a pocket guide,* ed 5, St Louis, 2015, Saunders.)

Procedural Steps

Placing Elastomeric Ring Separators

1. Place the separator over the beaks of separating pliers.
2. Stretch the ring, and then use a see-saw motion to push it gently through the contact.

(From Proffit WR, Fields HW, Sarver DM: *Contemporary orthodontics,* ed 5, St Louis, 2013, Mosby.)

3. An alternative method is to use two loops of dental floss to stretch the ring and to guide it into place.

(From Proffit WR, Fields HW, Sarver DM: *Contemporary orthodontics,* ed 5, St Louis, 2013, Mosby.)

4. This type of separator can be left in place for up to 2 weeks.

Removing Elastomeric Ring Separators

1. Slide an orthodontic scaler into the doughnut-shaped separator.
2. Use slight pressure to remove the ring from under the contact.

Assisting in the Fitting and Cementation of Orthodontic Bands

Equipment and Supplies

- Basic setup
- Preselected orthodontic bands
- Chilled glass slab
- Spatula (stainless steel)
- Gauze sponges
- Band pusher
- Band seater
- Scaler
- Band remover
- Contouring pliers
- Isopropyl alcohol
- Masking tape
- ChapStick or utility wax
- Selected cement

(From Boyd LRB: *Dental instruments: a pocket guide,* ed 5, St Louis, 2015, Saunders.)

Procedural Steps

Preparation

1. Place each preselected orthodontic band on a small square of masking tape with the occlusal surface on the tape and the gingival margin of the band upright.
   Purpose: This step keeps the bands in order and prevents the cement from flowing out of the other side.
2. Wipe any buccal tubes or attachments with ChapStick or utility wax.
   Purpose: This step prevents the cement from getting into or around these areas.

Mixing and Placing the Cement

1. The teeth are isolated and dried.
2. At a signal from the orthodontist, dispense the cement according to the manufacturer's directions, then quickly mix the cement until it is homogeneous.

3. Hold the band by the margin of the masking tape. The gingival surface is upright, and the cement spatula is placed on the margin of the band.
4. Wipe the spatula over the margin, allowing the cement to flow into the circumference of the band.

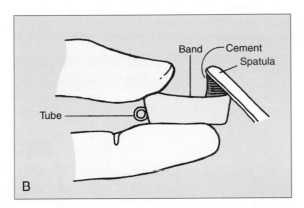

5. Transfer the cement-filled band to the orthodontist, who inverts the band over the tooth.
6. Transfer the band seater. The orthodontist places it on the buccal margin of the band.
7. The patient is instructed to bite gently on the band. This action forces the band down onto approximately the middle third of the tooth crown.
8. Excess cement is forced out from under the gingival and occlusal margins of the bands and is allowed to harden.
9. This process is repeated until all of the bands have been seated.

Removing Excess Cement

1. After the cement has reached its final stage of setting, a scaler or an explorer is used to remove excess cement from the enamel surfaces.
2. The patient's mouth is rinsed, flossed, and checked to ensure that all of the excess cement has been removed.

DATE	TOOTH	SURFACE	CHARTING NOTES
	—	—	Upper and lower bands cemented w/glass ionomer on first molars, UR-22, UL-24, LL-21, LR-22. Schedule for bonding. T. Clark, CDA/L. Stewart, DDS

Equipment and Supplies

- Brackets (type specified by the orthodontist)
- Cotton rolls or lip retractors
- Prophy cup
- Pumice
- Bonding setup
- Bracket placement tweezers
- Orthodontic scaler

(From Boyd LRB: *Dental instruments: a pocket guide,* ed 5, St Louis, 2015, Saunders.)

Procedural Steps

Preparing the Teeth

1. The tooth surface must be cleaned with a prophy cup and pumice slurry and then rinsed and dried.
2. Use cotton rolls or retractors to isolate the teeth.
3. An etchant gel is placed on the facial area of the tooth that is to receive the bonding agent. This gel remains on the tooth for the manufacturer's specified time and then is rinsed and thoroughly dried.

(From Proffit WR, Fields HW, Sarver DM: *Contemporary orthodontics,* ed 5, St Louis, 2013, Mosby.)

Bonding the Brackets

1. The orthodontist applies a liquid sealant, usually the monomer of the bonding agent, to the prepared tooth surface.
2. Mix a small quantity of bonding material and places it on the back of the bracket. Bracket placement tweezers are used to transfer the bracket to the orthodontist.

3. Transfer the orthodontic scaler. The orthodontist will place the bracket and move it into its final position with a scaler.
4. The orthodontist uses the scaler to remove the excess bonding material immediately before light-curing the material.

(From Proffit WR, Fields HW, Sarver DM: *Contemporary orthodontics,* ed 5, St Louis, 2013, Mosby.)

DATE	TOOTH	SURFACE	CHARTING NOTES
	—	—	Edgewise brackets bonded on maxillary 5-1/1-5 and mandibular 4-1/1-4. Light arch wire placed. T. Clark, CDA/L. Stewart, DDS

Placing Arch Wires (Expanded Function)

Prerequisites for Performing This Procedure

- Mirror skills
- Operator positioning
- Dental anatomy
- Instrumentation
- Fulcrum

Equipment and Supplies

- Preformed arch wires
- Patient's diagnostic casts (or previously used arch wire)
- Weingart pliers
- Bird-beak pliers
- Torquing pliers
- Distal end cutter

(From Boyd LRB: *Dental instruments: a pocket guide,* ed 5, St Louis, 2015, Saunders.)

Procedural Steps

Measuring the Arch Wire

1. Preformed wires are measured before they are placed in the mouth. The wire should be long enough to extend past the end of the buccal tube on the molar band but not so long that it injures the patient's tissues.

2. Measure the wire by trying it on the patient's diagnostic model or by holding it against the arch wire that is being replaced.

3. If the orthodontist has to place any bends in the wire, then additional wire must be allowed for the length.

Positioning the Arch Wire

1. Locate the mark at the center of the arch wire.
   Purpose: This location indicates the midline or the center of the arch form.

2. Position the wire in the mouth with the mark between the central incisors.

(From Proffit WR, Fields HW, Sarver DM: *Contemporary orthodontics,* ed 5, St Louis, 2013, Mosby.)

3. Place the arch wire in the main arch wire slot of the buccal tube.

4. Use the Weingart pliers to slide the wire in on either side of the arch and to position the wire within the bracket slots.

5. Check the distal ends to determine whether they are securely positioned or are too long or too short.

Equipment and Supplies

- Ligature ties
- Ligature director
- Hemostat
- Ligature cutter

(From Boyd LRB: *Dental instruments: a pocket guide,* ed 5, St Louis, 2015, Saunders.)

Placing Wire Ligatures

1. Holding the ligature between the thumb and the index finger, slide the wire between these fingers so that only the section that wraps around the bracket is exposed. Make sure to work toward the midline.
2. Slide the ligature around the bracket, using the ligature director to push the wire against the tie wing.
3. Twist together the ends of the ligature. Place the hemostat approximately 3 to 5 mm from the bracket, and snugly twist the wire against the bracket.

(From Boyd LRB: *Dental instruments: a pocket guide,* ed 5, St Louis, 2015, Saunders.)

4. After all teeth have been ligated, use a ligature cutter to remove the excess wire, leaving a 4- to 5-mm pigtail.

(From Boyd LRB: *Dental instruments: a pocket guide,* ed 5, St Louis, 2015, Saunders.)

5. Use the ligature director to tuck the pigtails under the arch wire toward the gingiva at the interproximal space.

(From Boyd LRB: *Dental instruments: a pocket guide,* ed 5, St Louis, 2015, Saunders.)

6. Repeat this procedure until all ligatures have been cut and tucked away.
7. Run a finger along the arch to ensure that there are no protruding wires that could injure the patient.

Removing Ligature Ties

1. Using the ligature cutter, place the beaks of the pliers at the end of the twisted wire and snip it off; make sure to hold on to the cut portion.
2. Carefully remove a portion of the wire.
3. Do not twist or pull as you cut and remove the ligatures.

Multiple Choice

Circle the letter next to the correct answer.

1. In the definition of Angle classification, a prognathic profile would be viewed in a Class _____ malocclusion.
   a. I
   b. II
   c. III

2. Indications for orthodontic treatment include _____.
   a. psychosocial influences
   b. oral function
   c. dental disease
   d. all of the above

3. The arch wire serves as a(n) _____.
   a. pattern that gives the dental arch its shape
   b. attachment for labial hooks
   c. item directly bonded to the teeth
   d. a and b

4. Ligature wire ties are twisted and tightened around a bracket with the use of a(n) _____.
   a. bird-beak pliers
   b. explorer
   c. hemostat
   d. scaler

5. Dentofacial proportions are most effectively evaluated on a _____ radiographic image.
   a. cephalometric
   b. panoramic
   c. periapical

6. Using orthodontic separators is necessary for the placement of _____.
   a. arch wires
   b. bands
   c. bonded brackets
   d. ligatures

7. The patient should be educated on _____ when wearing braces.
   a. oral hygiene procedures
   b. speech patterns
   c. dietary instructions
   d. a and c

8. To determine the correct length of an arch wire, it can be measured _____.
   a. on the radiograph
   b. in the patient's mouth
   c. on the patient's diagnostic casts
   d. b or c

9. When preparing the facial surface of the teeth for bonding brackets, _____.
   a. a preliminary impression is taken
   b. the teeth are isolated using cotton rolls or retractors
   c. the teeth are cleaned with a prophy cup and pumice
   d. b and c

10. Buccal tubes on molar bands are designed to hold the _____ securely.
    a. main arch wire
    b. brass separators
    c. elastomeric ligatures
    d. headgear

Apply Your Knowledge

1. You are assisting in a records appointment. As an expanded function dental assistant (EFDA) or a registered dental assistant (RDA) in the practice, what responsibilities could be assigned to you, and what will the orthodontist complete?

2. A patient is coming to the orthodontic office to have separators placed. The patient record indicates that you will be banding the maxillary and mandibular first molars. Where are the separators placed for this patient?

3. A patient is scheduled for an appliance check, and you notice the patient's buccal mucosa is inflamed and irritated. What could have caused this? How could this irritation be alleviated for the patient?

4. You are assisting in a bonding procedure. Describe the steps involved in the application of brackets.

CHAPTER 29

The Job Search

http://evolve.elsevier.com/Robinson/essentials/

LEARNING OBJECTIVES

1. Pronounce, define, and spell the key terms.
2. Define your personal career goals.
3. Identify the types of employment opportunities for the dental assistant.
4. Complete the following related to the job search:
   - List different types of sources for employment leads.
   - Name three social media sites for job prospects.
5. Prepare a resume, cover letter, and job application form.
6. Describe techniques for a successful job interview and prepare a follow-up letter.
7. Describe methods of negotiating salaries and benefits.
8. Discuss the steps for terminating employment.

KEY TERMS

career	follow-up letter	resume
cover letter	interview	social media
Facebook	LinkedIn	Twitter

A **career** in dental assisting offers many exciting employment opportunities in a variety of settings. Your knowledge, skills, and credentials enable you to select a position in which you will be recognized as a valuable member of the dental health care team.

Personal and Professional Goals

Before beginning your search for employment, it is important to determine your own realistic personal desires and professional goals, which should include: *happiness* in your daily life, *income* that meets your living expenses and lifestyle, *freedom* to establish your own path in life and work, *peace* about who you are and your purpose, *joy* in finding the right role or position for you at this time, *balance* in your work and life, *fulfillment* by living up to your highest and best potential, and *confidence* of your ability

Ask yourself, "What is important to me in a job?" and "What type of career do I want?" Then you can establish concrete career goals that focus on your talents and accomplishments.

"Your Dream Job"

Rank the following job characteristics in order of importance to you, and use them as a guide when seeking employment:
- Set working hours
- Flexible working hours
- No need to relocate
- Pleasant coworkers
- Responsibilities
- Attractive office
- Informal work environment
- More formal work environment

- Job security
- Type of practice
- Vacation time
- Sick leave
- Profit sharing
- Childcare allowance
- Good salary
- Distance from home
- Medical and dental insurance
- Retirement plan
- Vision plan
- Excellent infection control
- Written job description
- Involvement in planning
- Recognition for your work
- Understanding of personal problems
- Paid continuing education
- Holidays
- Dues to professional organization

Career Opportunities

Private Practice

Private practice in a general practice or in a specialty practice can provide an opportunity for you to gain experience at chairside, in the business office, and in the dental laboratory. Many dental assistants find great personal pride and fulfillment in joining a private practice. In addition, they enjoy developing a close rapport with the patients and with other members of the dental team.

Corporate Dentistry

Corporate dentistry, also referred to as the Dental Support Organization or "DSO," is the corporation version of a dental office setting. This type of environment is increasing because of the cost of operating a private practice. The organization controls all business and management of the practice, which includes hiring and training all employees and associates, obtaining equipment, marketing and promotion, and setting fees for service.

Insurance Company

If you think you might enjoy a challenging career in business and administration, then consider working for a dental insurance company. Dental insurance companies are continually looking for talented dental assistants with knowledge of the processing of insurance claims and customer service. These companies will train you in the specifics of their own operation.

Sales Representative

If you enjoy sales and traveling, then you might find a rewarding career as a representative for a dental manufacturing or supply company. These positions often include travel opportunities, entertaining, commissions, and bonuses. Other opportunities with dental manufacturers involve the areas of research and development.

Public Health and Government Programs

Public health and other government-supported dental facilities function at the federal, state, and local levels. Dental public health programs promote dental health through organized community efforts. Dental assistants may be employed in programs in which dental services are provided at no cost or at a minimal cost to patients who are eligible to receive care. Public health practices almost always involve a team effort with other professionals such as physicians, nurses, social workers, and nutritionists.

Dental School

Dental assistants with a business or clinical background can be employed at a dental school. An assistant would be an asset to the faculty and to the dental students in many areas in a school. Employment in a dental school provides the assistant with the stimulation of working in an educational setting with faculty, students, and patients. In addition, opportunities for staff members to attend continuing education courses are offered.

Hospital

Many university-based hospitals have a fully staffed dental clinic. Patients seen in this clinic are generally those who have been diagnosed with an acute or infectious disease and must receive their dental care while either as an in-patient or as an out-patient in a hospital setting.

Teaching

A career in teaching dental assisting might be another consideration. Teaching in a dental assisting program is a challenging and rewarding career. The American Dental Assistants Association (ADAA) accreditation states that a dental assisting instructor must hold certification by the Dental Assisting National Board (DANB) or registration as a dental assistant and should be working toward a bachelor's degree.

If you think you would enjoy teaching, then consider taking college courses on a part-time basis while gaining valuable work experience in the dental office.

Marketing Your Skills

Once you have narrowed your potential areas of interest for employment, knowing where to begin your search for employment is important. Table 29.1 lists several traditional sources for employment leads.

Job Search on the Internet

Social media is an extremely powerful tool when looking for employment opportunities. Many job opportunities can now be found on the Internet through a search result like "dental assisting jobs near me." The three major social media sites associated with job searches are LinkedIn, Facebook, and Twitter.

LinkedIn

LinkedIn is the largest professional network site in the world. Members connect with each other and directly with employers. Most employers prefer LinkedIn because it is widely viewed as the most businesslike and professional of the social networks (https://www.linkedin.com).

TABLE 29.1
Employment Search

Type of Traditional Advertisement	Description
Classified advertisements	The newspaper classified section and online advertisements such as Craigslist (www.craigslist.org) post jobs daily. You type in "dental assisting" and a list is displayed with the city location. After clicking on the posting, the advertisement describes the position and include a telephone number to call or a request to submit a resume.
Employment agencies	The purpose of an agency is to connect a person with a vacancy. Some agencies charge the employee a fee to find them a position. Other agencies charge the employer the fee.
Professional organizations	Local dental societies and dental-assisting organizations frequently serve as informal employment information centers. Professional journals also have a classified section of possible job opportunities.
Campus placement	Most formal dental assisting programs offer a placement service with practicing dentists in the area. Dentists frequently contact local schools for new employees.
Dental sale's representatives	When seeking employment, connect with a local dental sale's representative. They frequently know when a dentist is looking for a qualified dental assistant.

Facebook

Facebook is the largest social networking website. Most dentists will have a Facebook page for their dental practice. They may also have a Facebook page for marketing and recruiting.

It is necessary that you keep your Facebook wall suitable for viewing by potential employers or sufficiently protected by your privacy settings. Remove any photos or items that are politically divisive or could be considered offensive

Twitter

Twitter is a free social networking service that enables its users to send and read messages known as *tweets*. Entering the phrase "dentalassistingjobs" in quotations in the search window means you want that exact phrase to be searched. By placing spaces between each word, it will pull up twitter posts for each of the words mentioned

Seeking Employment

Whether you choose to pursue your job search through the use of social media or with a traditional method, you will need to follow specific steps that are important in securing your new position.

Telephone Contact

If your first contact with a prospective employer is made by telephone, then identify yourself and explain your reason for calling. This first impression over the telephone is extremely important; if you do not make a good first impression, then you may not get a second chance to prove yourself in an interview. You may be asked to submit a completed application or a resume before being granted an interview.

Cover Letter

A well-written cover letter serves to introduce you to a prospective employer and markets your skills and qualifications at the same time. It also serves to create interest on the part of the reader to look at your resume. A variety of approaches and styles are available, but general guidelines should be followed (Fig. 29.1).

> ### Guidelines for a Cover Letter
> - Prepare a one-page typed letter (never handwritten).
> - Be brief, professional, and neat.
> - Address the cover letter to a specific person.
> - Identify the position for which you are applying.
> - Request an interview.
> - Give contact numbers where you can be reached.
> - Thank the recipient for their consideration.

Resume

A resume is a concise written statement that highlights your individual qualities and skills that would be valuable to a prospective employer. A resume communicates a maximum amount of information through a minimum number of words (Fig. 29.2). The primary purpose of a resume is to convince a prospective employer that you are an outstanding candidate for employment and that it would be worth their time to interview you in person.

The time and effort you devote to developing your own resume is a worthwhile investment in your future. Your resume should highlight your educational and professional accomplishments. There is no single correct way to write a resume; however, certain guidelines will assist you in preparing a good resume.

> ### Guidelines for Writing a Resume
> - Be 100% honest.
> - Be easy to read and understand.
> - Reflect your uniqueness.
> - Stress your assets (avoid information that could screen you out).
> - Focus on important information.
> - Avoid containing personal pronouns (e.g., I, my, me).
> - Stimulate the interest of the reader.
> - Use language appropriate to the profession.

Heading

The heading includes four items: full name (with credentials [CDA, RDA], if appropriate), complete address, cellular telephone number, and e-mail address. These items can be centered at the top of the page.

Professional Objective

A professional objective is a clear statement of the type of position you are seeking. It should not be too narrowly stated, however, because that might limit your job opportunities.

Education

List your most recent to least recent education. If you have a college degree, then do not list your high school graduation. If you have taken special courses or have received honors that may be of interest to your potential employer, then you may want to make note of them in the education section.

Professional Experience

List your most recent to least recent work experiences. Provide the date (month and year only) of your employment, your

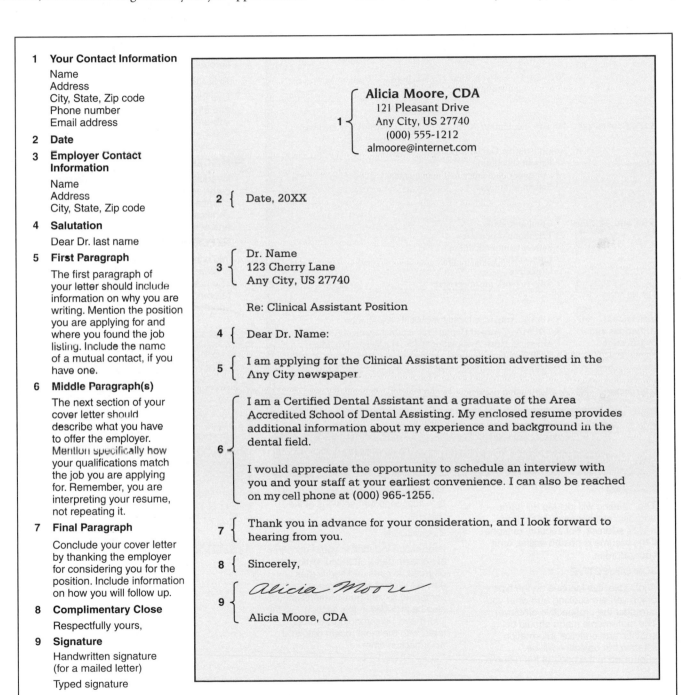

1 **Your Contact Information**
Name
Address
City, State, Zip code
Phone number
Email address

2 **Date**

3 **Employer Contact Information**
Name
Address
City, State, Zip code

4 **Salutation**
Dear Dr. last name

5 **First Paragraph**
The first paragraph of your letter should include information on why you are writing. Mention the position you are applying for and where you found the job listing. Include the name of a mutual contact, if you have one.

6 **Middle Paragraph(s)**
The next section of your cover letter should describe what you have to offer the employer. Mention specifically how your qualifications match the job you are applying for. Remember, you are interpreting your resume, not repeating it.

7 **Final Paragraph**
Conclude your cover letter by thanking the employer for considering you for the position. Include information on how you will follow up.

8 **Complimentary Close**
Respectfully yours,

9 **Signature**
Handwritten signature (for a mailed letter)
Typed signature

---

1 {
Alicia Moore, CDA
121 Pleasant Drive
Any City, US 27740
(000) 555-1212
almoore@internet.com

2 { Date, 20XX

3 {
Dr. Name
123 Cherry Lane
Any City, US 27740

Re: Clinical Assistant Position

4 { Dear Dr. Name:

5 { I am applying for the Clinical Assistant position advertised in the Any City newspaper.

6 {
I am a Certified Dental Assistant and a graduate of the Area Accredited School of Dental Assisting. My enclosed resume provides additional information about my experience and background in the dental field.

I would appreciate the opportunity to schedule an interview with you and your staff at your earliest convenience. I can also be reached on my cell phone at (000) 965-1255.

7 { Thank you in advance for your consideration, and I look forward to hearing from you.

8 { Sincerely,

9 {
Alicia Moore

Alicia Moore, CDA

FIGURE 29.1 Sample cover letter. (From Bird DL, Robinson DS: *Modern dental assisting,* ed 11, St. Louis, 2015, Saunders.)

Ima Graduate

1234 Valley Boulevard
Canyon View, CA 12345
Cell phone (123) 555-7890
imagraduate@comcast.com

Objective Interested in obtaining a position as an administrative dental assistant. Offering excellent skills in patient communication, appointment scheduling, and computer applications. Enjoy working as a member of a professional healthcare team.

Education

2014–2015	Canyon View Junior College	Canyon View, CA
	Administrative Dental Assistant	
	Certification of Completion	

| 2010-2014 | Canyon View High School | Canyon View, CA |
| | Diploma | |

Work Experience January–September 2015 Canyon View Dentistry
 Canyon View, CA
Administrative Dental Assistant
- Patient scheduling
- Computer data entry and management
- Patient relations

Skills and Abilities

- Computer skills
- Telephone procedures
- Patient communications
- Enthusiastic team member
- Organized
- Able to work unsupervised

Professional
Affiliations and
Certification
- ADAA, American Dental Assistants Association
- CDPMA, Certified Dental Practice Management Assistant
- American Heart Association, CPR–Healthcare Provider
- Radiology Certification

References 7 Available upon request

4 WORK HISTORY

This section can also come under the heading **Work Experience, Employment History, Professional Experience,** or **Experience.** In this section you will list the name and location of each company or organization, starting and ending dates, and a brief description of your duties. You can also list volunteer work experience, especially if it demonstrates skills and abilities that will enhance your job qualifications (non-paid training can also be listed). List the experience in chronological order.

5 SKILLS AND ABILITIES

Use this section to highlight skills, abilities, and strengths that are pertinent to the job you are applying for. Statements should be action-oriented, begin with verbs, and be concise.

6 MISCELLANEOUS

Headings and information include such items as extracurricular activities, clubs, memberships in professional organizations, certification, volunteer activities, awards, and achievements.

7 REFERENCES

You can include two professional references or state: References furnished upon request. The use of references is optional. When listing references state the name, title or occupation, address, and telephone number.

ORDER OF INFORMATION
Prime space is the top one-third of the page, so list the most important sections first.

MECHANICS
Typed on one page, easy to read, with correct spelling, grammar, and punctuation. Eliminate unessential words or phrases.

MARGINS
The finished resume should appear balanced, centered from top to bottom and left to right.

PAPER
Use heavy stock standard size (8.5" x 11") resume paper of good quality (white, cream, or light gray). Print on high-quality setting or have professionally printed. Pages should be free of streaks, fading, or correction fluid.

A resume is a summary of your skills, abilities, education, and work experience. The completed resume serves as an introduction; depending on your resume, you may or may not obtain an interview.

1 HEADING

The heading will include full name, address, cell phone number, and e-mail address. For security reasons if the resume is posted online, omit your address.

2 JOB OBJECTIVE

A job objective focuses on the type of job you are seeking and what you can offer the prospective employer. The statements made should be specific and concise. Information listed in the objective will be supported in the body of the resume.

The objective is considered one of the most important sections of the resume.

3 EDUCATION

Information included in your education statement: dates attended, diplomas, degrees, awards and certificates earned. Workshops and seminars that contribute to your qualifications should also be included in this section. List the information in chronological order (start with the most recent date and work back in time).

FIGURE 29.2 Sample resume.

position or title, the employer's name and location, and your responsibilities and accomplishments.

Note: If you are a recent graduate with minimal or no work experience, then you might wish to list your education first. If your strength is your experience, then list it first. Remember, the purpose of your resume is to make you shine!

Certifications

List your certification or registration, such as cardiopulmonary resuscitation (CPR) certification, and any other appropriate certification information. Emphasize any career-related affiliations, such as membership in the ADAA.

It is not recommended that personal data be included in your resume. Under the federal regulations governed by the Equal Employment Opportunity Commission, employers should not ask questions regarding race, color, religion, gender, national origin, marital status, and childcare arrangements unless they relate to bona fide occupational qualifications. Nevertheless, you may be required to submit verification of citizenship or appropriate alien status.

References

Although references are not required, if you choose to provided references, then be certain to contact those you list to get their permission before you provide their names. Your references should be individuals who can address your character as a person and your job-related skills.

Volunteer Experience

If you have done any volunteer work, then list it. Even if it does not pertain to dentistry, it will exhibit a quality in you that can be admired by the employer. Do not list this category if it does not apply to you.

Awards and Scholarships

List any scholarships or awards you have received. Do not list this category if it does not apply to you.

See Procedure 29.1: Preparing a Professional Resume.

Job Application

Before the interview, you may be asked to complete an application form, which can serve as the initial basis of your conversation with the dentist or office manager. When completing this form, follow the directions exactly and make certain that the information you provide is accurate, neat, and complete. Read the entire application before you begin filling in the answers. By doing this, you are less likely to make errors or give information on the wrong line. Bringing a copy of your resume for reference as you fill out the application is also a good idea.

Interview

An interview can be an excellent experience, one in which you discuss your assets and accomplishments; or it can be an unpleasant experience, during which questions are asked of you, and the wrong answer could mean losing the job.

Controlling your nerves, projecting a positive image, and participating in the interview are your responsibility. Remember, not only will the dentist and staff members decide whether you are the assistant they are looking for, but you will also determine whether this job is right for you and whether you would be happy working in this office. Table 29.2 lists some tips that will help you do your best during your next interview.

Federal and state equal employment opportunity laws have a significant impact on the way employers may recruit and select employees. Employers may not discriminate on any legally recognized basis, including but not limited to race, age, color, sex,

TABLE 29.2
Tips for a Good Interview

Be prepared	Make a list of all the pertinent questions you would like to ask and points you would like to make.
Be honest	Do not be afraid to say, "I don't know." Then follow up by saying that you will find out.
Be prompt	Arrive approximately 15 minutes early. Never be late or too early. If for any reason you are delayed, then telephone and reschedule the interview.
Be aware	Do not divulge too much personal information. Questions about age, spouses, and children, among other personal information, are optional for you to answer. Keep the conversation about business.
Make eye contact	When you maintain eye contact, even during difficult questions, you display self-confidence.
Show enthusiasm	Be enthusiastic about your career potential, your interests, and your abilities. Remember, you must "sell" yourself. Be honest about your abilities.
Discuss salary if asked	Know the salary ranges in the area in which you are looking. Do not introduce salary negotiations; however, if asked what salary you are seeking, then answer without fear of rejection. Know your worth.
Be aware of body language	Pay attention to the way you nonverbally communicate. Sit upright, do not slouch or fidget, and avoid gestures and postures that show boredom or hostility.
Avoid multiple interviews	Do not arrange for more than one interview in the morning or afternoon.
Say "thank you"	Thank the interviewer at the end of the interview and follow up with a thank-you note to help remind the interviewer about you and to indicate your continued interest.

religion, creed, national origin, physical or mental disability, marital status, or veteran status. Box 29.1 lists the guidelines from the Equal Employment Opportunity Commission regarding questions that may and may not be legally asked during interviews.

Preparation

Rereading your resume before each interview will ensure that you present yourself as a well-organized person with a calm and positive manner. It is also a means of helping you recall facts, through association, that are not on the resume but will probably come up in the interview.

Appearance

Your appearance is especially important. In selecting your clothing, you want your appearance to reflect the fact that you are a neat, well-organized, and a competent professional.

Do not wear a uniform or scrubs to an interview. Wearing conservative business attire is best. Keep only enough jewelry and makeup to enhance your attire, not overwhelm it.

Arrival

Plan to arrive 15 minutes before the scheduled time of the interview. If the interview is scheduled in a geographic area with which you are unfamiliar, it is advisable to make a "dry run" to find the office before the interview. In addition, make sure you arrive alone. Although you may think you need moral support, having a person accompany you would appear unprofessional.

Interviewing Professionally

The first 10 minutes of your interview are the most critical; during this time, both you and the interviewer will have formed a first impression. You may be nervous but try to relax and be natural.

A smile; direct eye contact; the words, "Hello, I'm (first name and last name). It's a pleasure to meet you"; and a firm but gentle handshake are essential for creating a positive and professional first impression (Fig. 29.3).

Many questions will be asked and answered on both sides. Try to answer all questions courteously, completely, and honestly. Be prepared for a variety of questions, and feel free to ask questions if it seems to be an appropriate time. Remember that your attitude and motivation during the interview are important determining factors. You want to convey a positive attitude without overselling yourself.

Concluding the Interview

Let the prospective employer (or office manager) conclude the interview. If you think the interview has concluded, then you could say, "I would like to thank you for your time." Make the interviewer aware of your interest in the position and that you would like to be seriously considered for the role.

Make sure to extend your hand for a final handshake, and again, use direct eye contact before you say, "I look forward to hearing from you." Within the first week after the interview, you will have developed some intuition of how the interview went and whether the office is the one in which you would like to pursue employment.

Box 29.1 What You May and May Not Be Asked During an Interview*

What Applicants MAY NOT Be Asked

- Age or date of birth
- Previous address
- Religion or race
- Mother's surname
- Marital status or maiden name
- Number or ages of children
- Who will care for your children
- Spouse or parent's place of employment
- Parents' residence
- Whether you own or rent your residence
- Questions about your ability to speak a foreign language (unless job relevant)
- Questions about arrests
- Membership in social organizations
- Visible physical characteristics (e.g., scars, burns, missing limbs)
- Health status
- Psychologic well-being
- Past injuries or diseases
- Loans, financial obligations, wage attachments, or personal bankruptcies

What Applicants MAY Be Asked

- Reasons for termination of previous employment
- References
- Work schedules
- Previous work experience
- Job-related attitudes about previous assignments or present position
- Career interests
- Job duties
- Job training
- Education
- Qualifications for duties related to the position
- Verification of citizenship or appropriate alien status

*Guidelines from the Equal Employment Opportunity Commission, U.S. Department of Labor.

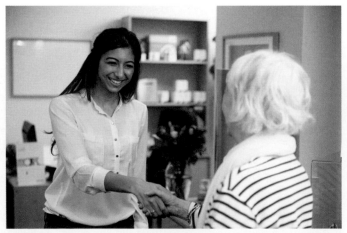

FIGURE 29.3 Your first impression is extremely important. (Copyright © iStock.com/monkeybusinessimages.)

Follow-up Letter

A thank-you letter is an excellent way to follow up with an employer after an interview. It serves to remind the employer of your interview, to accentuate your qualifications, to reaffirm your interest in the position, and to help you stand out in the interviewer's mind. The follow-up letter should be sent within 48 hours, should be addressed to the person with whom you interviewed, and should reaffirm your interest in the position in the practice. Make sure the letter is thoughtful and sincere (Fig. 29.4).

Once you have landed the right position, it is also courteous to call or send a note to those offices with whom you have interviewed to let them know that you have found a position.

Salary Negotiations

Although salary and benefits are not the only factors to be considered when you are accepting a job, they are important issues that need to be clarified.

The interviewer may ask, "What do you expect in terms of salary?" If you have a definite and realistic idea, then by all means state it. Keep in mind that education, experience, and skills are important factors that should be considered in a fair and equitable salary and benefits package.

As you negotiate a compensation package with the dentist, you should realize the importance of the total dollar value when benefits are added to salary, the number of hours you will be working, and the working conditions.

Alicia Moore, CDA
121 Pleasant Drive
Any City, US 27740
(000) 555-1212
almoore@internet.com

Date, 20XX

Dr. Name and Staff
123 Cherry Lane
Any City, US 27740

Dear Dr. Name and Staff:

Thank you for taking time out of your busy schedule to interview me last Tuesday, October 25th. I enjoyed our conversation and am very enthusiastic about the possibility of working with you and your staff.

I know that my clinical and communication skills would be an asset to your practice. Please do not hesitate to call me should you have any other questions.

Again, thank you for your consideration. I look forward to hearing from you in hopes that you have reached a decision favorable to both of us.

Sincerely,

Alicia Moore

Alicia Moore, CDA

FIGURE 29.4 Sample follow-up letter. (From Bird DL, Robinson DS: *Modern dental assisting,* ed 11, St. Louis, 2015, Saunders.)

The negotiating discussion offers an excellent opportunity to ask about the frequency of reviews, salary increases, and opportunities to advance in the practice.

Job Termination

There may come a time when you will have to terminate employment. It should be ended in a professional manner. If your practice has an employee handbook, follow the procedures for resigning your position. The employer should always learn—directly from you—of your intention to resign, not from another employee in the office.

The most common time frame for notifying your employer is 2 weeks. If asked, then help select and train your replacement. The time between giving notice and departing is an important period of employment. Those employees who slack off in the final weeks should expect a less-than-positive recommendation. Commit yourself to leaving your job with honor and dignity. Remember, the last impression is the one that will always be remembered.

If your employment is terminated by your employer, then your departure should be handled in accordance with the terms of your employment agreement. Severance pay, which is the equivalent of salary for the notice period, is paid if your employer terminates your employment and is typically paid with the final paycheck.

Exit Professionally: Tips for Terminating Employment

- Give adequate notice to your employer.
- Leave on a positive note. Do not vent anger and/or frustrations.
- Do not burn your bridges with angry remarks about others.
- Avoid new job-hunting activities during office hours.
- Do not slack off your duties during your last 2 weeks.
- When possible, find and train your replacement.

Ethical Implications

The dental profession is a small community. Dentists socially and professionally interact with each other. They have formed connections through schools, dental societies, community and service organizations, and social activities.

Keeping good ties between you and former employers and coworkers is always a good idea. At some time in the future, these individuals can be valuable assets and can provide crucial help for future employment. During your career in the dental profession, you will find people who will enter and exit and enter your life again. Never allow angry words or unprofessional behavior to burn the bridges behind you.

Your professional reputation can spread; therefore always demonstrate ethical behavior at every job, from the first day to the last day.

Procedure 29.1

Preparing a Professional Resume

Goal

To prepare a resume to be used for seeking employment.

Procedural Steps

1. Keep the resume to one page (see Fig. 29.2).
2. Use standard letter size (8½ × 11) white or ivory rag paper.
3. Use common typefaces.
4. Use 1-inch margins on all sides.
5. Use a 12-point font size.
6. Ensure that the resume is neat and error free.
7. Keep the content concise and easy to read.

Chapter Exercises

Multiple Choice

Circle the letter next to the correct answer.

1. Dental assistants may be employed in which of the following areas?
   a. Private practice
   b. Education
   c. Dental sales
   d. All of the above

2. The purpose of a cover letter is to _____.
   a. introduce yourself to the prospective employer
   b. market your skills and qualifications
   c. create interest for reading your resume
   d. all of the above

3. Which information should NOT be included in a resume?
   a. Certifications
   b. Family
   c. Professional objective
   d. Professional experience

4. On a resume, your education should be listed _____.
   a. most recent to least recent
   b. top of the page
   c. least recent to most recent
   d. last item on the page

5. It is recommended that you arrive how early for an interview?
   a. 30 minutes early
   b. 15 minutes early
   c. Exactly on time
   d. Within the hour of the appointment

6. Which of the following is (are) NOT appropriate for a job interview?
   a. Casual wear
   b. Heavy makeup
   c. Scrubs
   d. All of the above

7. After an interview, you should _____.
   a. telephone the office and thank them once again
   b. send a thank-you letter
   c. fax an additional copy of your resume
   d. all of the above

8. When leaving a job, what is the usual minimum amount of notice that should be given to the employer?
   a. 24 hours
   b. 1 week
   c. 2 weeks
   d. 1 month

9. Which of the following social media sites is the largest for professional networking?
   a. Twitter
   b. Facebook
   c. LinkedIn

10. A resume communicates a minimum amount of information in a maximum amount of space.
    a. True
    b. False

Apply Your Knowledge

1. During a clinical internship in an orthodontic office, you decide that you would like to work in an orthodontic office after graduating from the dental-assisting program. You have an interview scheduled with Dr. Marcus, an orthodontist, and she is concerned about your lack of experience. What might you say to convince Dr. Marcus that you will make an excellent orthodontic assistant, despite your lack of experience?

2. Linda, an outgoing and experienced dental assistant, has finally had it with the inner-office politics and quarreling among the staff members. She decides it's time to look for another job, but before leaving she plans on sharing with her coworkers what she thinks of them, and then discussing with the doctor what she thinks of his management policies. What risk do you see in this plan?

3. Trang Li has just graduated from a dental-assisting program and is nervous about going for her first job interview. As a friend and classmate, how could you help her prepare?

4. An education in dental assisting can lead to a variety of career opportunities. Identify those areas in which a dental assistant can be employed and think about which ones might interest you.

GLOSSARY

A

absorbed dose Amount of energy imparted by ionizing particles to unit mass of irradiated material at a place of interest (16)

abutment Tooth, root, or implant used for support and retention of a fixed or removable prosthesis (23)

act of commission Performance of an act that a "reasonable and prudent professional" would not perform (2)

act of omission Failure to perform an act that a "reasonable and prudent professional" would perform (2)

active learning An approach to instruction, where the learner participates in the learning activities (20)

acute infection Infections of short duration but possibly of severe course of disease (5)

acute myocardial infarction Medical term for heart attack, which is a life-threatening condition. Typically a result of a blockage of one or more coronary arteries (10)

acute radiation exposure Large dose of radiation that is absorbed in a short period as in a nuclear accident (16)

aerosol 1. Suspension of fine solid particles or liquid droplets in air or another gas 2. Substance dispensed as a component of a gas or vapor suspension (5)

air-powder polishing A specially designed handpiece with a nozzle that delivers a high-pressure stream of warm water and sodium bicarbonate to rapidly and efficiently remove stains (21)

ala of the nose Wing-like tip on the outer side of each nostril (3)

ALARA principle Acronym for "As Low As Reasonably Achievable" (The ALARA principle pertains to radiation exposure encountered when taking x-ray images; it requires that every possible precaution be taken to limit radiation levels when exposing the patient or technician to radiation.) (16)

alcohol Transparent colorless liquid that is mobile and volatile (Alcohols are organic compounds formed from hydrocarbons by the substitution of hydroxyl radicals for the same number of hydrogen atoms.) (7)

alcohol-based hand rubs Waterless antiseptic agents that are alcohol-based products available in gels, foams, or rinses (6)

alginate Salt of alginic acid (e.g., sodium alginate), which, when mixed with water in accurate proportions, forms an irreversible hydrocolloid gel used for making impressions (19)

allergen Substance capable of producing an allergic response (Common allergens are pollens, dust, drugs, and food.) (10)

alloy Metallic substance composed by combining two or more metallic elements (18)

alveolar socket Cavity or space within the alveolar process that surrounds the root of a tooth (3)

alveolitis Inflammation of a socket after a tooth is extracted and a blood clot fails to form (also described as a *dry socket*) (26)

alveoloplasty Surgical shaping and smoothing of the margins of the tooth socket after the extraction of the tooth, generally in preparation for the placement of a prosthesis (26)

amalgam Alloy used for restoring teeth (Mercury is one of the constituents in amalgam.) (18)

amalgamator Mechanical device used to triturate the ingredients of dental amalgam into a mass (11)

analgesia Insensibility to pain without loss of consciousness; a state during which a painful stimulus is not perceived or interpreted as pain (Analgesia is usually induced by a drug.) (15)

anaphylaxis A severe life-threatening allergic reaction from the exposure of an allergen (10)

anatomic crown All of the tooth covered by enamel (4)

anatomy Science of the form, structure, and parts of organisms (3)

anesthetics Drugs that generally or locally produces a loss of feeling or sensation (15)

angina pectoris A medical term for chest pain due to coronary heart disease (A severe pain behind the sternum that sometimes radiates to the arms, neck, or mandible is characteristic of angina pectoris.) (10)

angle of the mandible Lower posterior of the ramus (3)

anode The positive charged electrodes in the x-ray tube (16)

anterior Toward the front surface of the mouth or tooth (3)

anterior naris Nostril; plural, nares (3)

antianxiety Technique or drug used to prevent or relieve anxiety (15)

antigen Substance that causes your immune system to stimulate the production of an antibody (10)

antiseptic Substance for preventing growth of a disease-causing microorganism (7)

apex Tapered end of each root tip (4)

apical Pertaining to the end portion of the root (4)

apicoectomy Surgical procedure to remove the tip of a tooth root in endodontic therapy (25)

arch wires Contoured metal wires that provide force when guiding the teeth in movement for orthodontics (28)

articulator Dental laboratory device that simulates mandibular and temporomandibular joint movement when models of the dental arches are attached to it (23)

asepsis The absence of bacteria, viruses, and other microorganisms (26)

asthma Respiratory disease often associated with allergies and characterized by sudden recurring attacks of labored breathing, chest constriction, and coughing (10)

attached gingivae Fibrous attachments of the gingival tissues to the teeth (3)

autoclave Instrument used for sterilization by means of moist heat under pressure (8)

automatic processing techniques
Efficient methods of processing dental film from the developer to the fixer, rinsing, and drying (17)

automix Mixing technique available for use with dental materials (The unique automix system device provides a homogeneous mix with the appropriate amount of material without waste.) (19)

autonomy Childhood process of becoming independent (27)

auxiliaries Attachments located on the brackets and bands that hold arch wires and elastics (28)

avulsed Torn away or dislodged by force (27)

B

background radiation Level of ionizing radiation present in the environment in a particular location, such as a dental setting (16)

bacteria Small, unicellular microorganisms that morphologically vary in shape and size; spherical (cocci), rod-shaped (bacilli), spiral (spirochetes), or comma-shaped (vibrios) (5)

bacterial endocarditis Inflammation of the heart valves and lining of the heart as the result of a bacterial infection (5)

bands Stainless steel rings cemented to molars that hold the arch wire and auxiliaries for orthodontics (28)

bifurcation Division into two parts or branches, such as any two roots of a tooth (4)

bioburden Blood, saliva, and other bodily fluids (7)

biofilm A collection of one or more types of microorganisms that can grow on surfaces (Dental plaque is a biofilm; hence, the term *oral biofilm*.) (7, 20, 21)

biologic monitor Instrument that verifies sterilization by confirming that all spore-forming microorganisms have been destroyed (8)

bisecting angle technique Angle at which a periapical x-ray image is taken; this is accomplished by placing the film/receptor as close to the tooth as possible, with the central x-ray beam directed perpendicular to an imaginary line that bisects the angle formed by long axis of tooth. (17)

bite registration Taking an impression of a patient's upper and lower teeth in the bite position to assist in the making and fitting of a fixed or removable prosthesis (19)

bite-wing image Radiographic image that shows the maxillary and mandibular crowns of the teeth, providing a clear image of interproximal surfaces (17)

blood pressure Pressure of circulating blood against the walls of blood vessels within the arteries (9)

bloodborne diseases A disease that can be transmitted via contaminated blood and/or other bodily fluids (5)

Bloodborne Pathogens (BBP) Standard Standard from the Occupational Safety and Health Administration (OSHA) designed to protect employees against occupational exposure to bloodborne and disease-causing organisms (6)

bonding Technique used to adhere restorative materials and orthodontic attachments to the teeth (18, 28)

brachial Related to the arm (brachium), as in brachial artery (9)

breach of contract Failure, without legal excuse, to perform an obligation or duty specified in a contract (2)

bridge Fixed prosthesis to replace missing teeth (23)

buccal Referring to structures closest to the cheek (3)

burs Rotary cutting instruments of steel or tungsten carbide that are designed with various cutting shapes (12)

C

calculus Calcium and phosphate salts in saliva that become mineralized and adhere to tooth surfaces (20, 21)

canthus Fold of tissue at the corner of the eyelids (3)

career 1. Chosen pursuit; profession or occupation 2. General course or progression of one's working life or one's professional achievements (29)

carotid Related to either one of the two major arteries on each side of the neck that carries blood to the head (3, 9)

carpal tunnel syndrome (CTS) Pain associated with continued flexion and extension of the wrist (11)

cassette Holder for extraoral films for radiographic imaging (17)

cathode Negative electrode in the x-ray tube (16)

cavity A damaged area within a tooth caused by decay (also referred to as *caries*) (22)

cavity classifications Standard classifications that describe the types and locations of decay or restorations (Carious lesions are classified according to the surfaces of the tooth on which they occur [e.g., lingual, buccal, occlusal], the type of surface [e.g., pit, fissure, smooth], and numeric grouping.) (13)

cells Basic building blocks of all living things (3)

cements Type of dental materials that provide a bond of a direct restoration and the tooth (18)

cementoenamel junction Point at which the enamel of the crown and the cementum of the root of a tooth meet (4)

cementum Specialized, calcified connective tissue that covers the anatomic root of a tooth (4)

Centers for Disease Control and Prevention (CDC) Nonregulatory federal agency that issues recommendations on health and safety (6)

centric Having an object centered, such as maxillary teeth centered over mandibular teeth in correct relation (19)

cephalometric Extraoral radiograph image that shows the bones and soft tissue areas of the facial profile (28)

cerebrovascular accident (CVA) Also referred to as a *stroke*; a sudden loss of brain function caused by blockage or rupture of a blood vessel in the brain (10)

certified dental assistant (CDA) Person who successfully passes the Dental Assisting National Board Examination or State Board and remains current with continuing education requirements (2)

certified dental technician (CDT) Dental laboratory technician who passes the proper written examination (1)

cervical collar Leaded device that is positioned around the throat during radiographic procedures to protect the thyroid gland from exposure to radiation (17)

charge-coupled device (CCD) Solid-state image sensor used in intraoral digital imaging (17)

chemical label Identifies all hazardous ingredients and safety precautions for a product (A chemical label is required by the Hazard Communication Standard.) (6)

chemical vapor sterilization Process during which chemical vapors are created under heat and pressure for the sterilizing procedure (8)

chlorine dioxide Effective, rapid-acting environmental surface disinfectant or chemical sterilant (7)

chronic infection Pathogens with slow growth promoting an infection of long duration (5)

chronic radiation exposure Exposure to small amounts of radiation that are repeatedly absorbed over a long period, the effects of which may not be observed until years after the original exposure (16)

civil law Category of law that is about conflict resolution between individuals (2)

clean areas Places where sterilized instruments, fresh disposable supplies, and prepared trays are stored (8)

clinical crown Portion of the tooth that is visible in the oral cavity (4, 21)

collimation Restricting and confining the x-ray beam to a given area to reduce the overall dose to the patient and scattered radiation (16)

collimator Lead disc within the x-ray tube (rectangular or circular) designed to limit the dimension of a beam of radiation (16)

Commission on Dental Accreditation of the American Dental Association (CODA) Commission that accredits dental and dental assisting, dental hygiene, and dental laboratory educational programs (1)

composite resin Restorative material used for its esthetic purposes (The chemical makeup of composite resin includes an organic resin matrix, inorganic fillers, and a coupling agent.) (18)

contact point Area of the mesial or distal surface of a tooth that touches the adjacent tooth in the same arch (4)

contaminated area Place in the sterilization center where contaminated items are taken for precleaning (8)

contract law A legally binding agreement between two or more parties that is enforceable by law (2)

contrast Radiation quality or kVp; shows the differences in degrees of blackness on a radiograph (16)

control panel Master switch, indicator light, selector buttons, and exposure button on the x-ray machine (16)

control tooth Healthy tooth used as a standard to compare questionable teeth of similar size and structure during pulp vitality testing (25)

core Central part of or support for an indirect restoration (The core can be prepared from an existing amalgam restoration, a composite material, or reinforced glass ionomer cement.) (23)

cover letter Letter of introduction sent with other documents (e.g., resume) that provides more information (29)

critical instruments Items used to penetrate soft tissue or bone (7)

cross-bite Tooth that is not properly aligned with its opposing tooth (27)

cross-contamination Direct transfer of an infection from one person to another or indirectly from one person to a second person via an object or exposure (5)

crown Portion of the tooth covered by enamel (23)

cumulative radiation Exposure to radiation, resulting in a cumulative effect over a lifetime (16)

cumulative trauma disorder Condition caused by repetitive motion and overflexion and overextension of the wrist (11)

curing Act of polymerization of preventive and restorative dental materials (18, 21)

cusp Major elevation on the masticatory surfaces of the canines and posterior teeth (4)

D

debridement Process of removing or cleaning out the pulpal canal (25)

demineralization Loss of minerals from the tooth; initial stage of tooth decay (20)

demographics Personal information about patients, such as address, employer, as well as statistical characteristics of populations (9)

density Overall darkness or blackness of a radiographic image (16)

dental assistant Oral health care professional qualified to provide supportive procedures for the dentist and patients (1)

dental auxiliary Dental assistant, dental hygienist, and dental laboratory technician qualified to perform specific dental work under the direction and supervision of a dentist (2)

dental dam Thin, stretchable material that becomes a barrier when applied to select teeth during preventive and restorative dental care (14)

dental decay Destruction of tooth structure by certain types of bacteria, beginning on the external surface by demineralization of enamel or exposed cementum (20)

dental health care team Dentist, dental assistant, dental hygienist, and dental laboratory technician (The purpose of the dental health care team is to provide quality oral health care for the patients of the practice.) (1)

dental laboratory technician Professional who performs dental laboratory services, such as fabricating crowns, bridges, and dentures, as

specified by the dentist's written prescription (1)

dental operatory Dental treatment room and control center of the clinical area (11)

dental public health Specialty that promotes oral health through organized community efforts (1)

dental sealant Resin dental material that is placed in the occlusal pits and fissures of teeth to prevent dental caries (21)

dental specialties Eleven fields recognized by the American Dental Association (ADA): dental anesthesiology, dental public health, endodontics, oral and maxillofacial pathology, oral and maxillofacial radiology, oral and maxillofacial surgery, oral medicine, orthodontics, pediatric dentistry, periodontics, and prosthodontics (1)

dentin Portion of the tooth that lies between the enamel or cementum and the pulp (4)

dentinal fiber Fibers found in dental pulp that project into dentinal tubules (4)

dentinal tubules Microscopic canals found in dentin (4)

dentist Individual educated and licensed to diagnosis, prevent, and treat diseases and conditions of the mouth (1)

diabetes Metabolic disorder characterized by high blood glucose levels and insufficient insulin (10)

diagnosis The act of identifying a disease from its signs and symptoms (13)

diagnostic cast Stone or plaster model fabricated from dental structures for the purpose of study and treatment planning (19)

diagnostic quality image Radiographic image that has been properly placed, exposed, and processed (17)

diastolic Blood pressure reading from the rhythmic relaxation and dilation of the heart chambers (9)

digital image Electronic representation of a radiographic, a film, or an x-ray image (17)

digital imaging Filmless method of capturing and displaying an intraoral image by using an image sensor, an electronic signal, and a computer to process and store the image (16)

digitize Process of scanning a traditional film-based radiograph into a digital image (17)

direct pulp cap Application of a material to the exposed pulp to stimulate repair of the injured pulpal tissue (25)

direct supervision Level of supervision during which the dentist is physically present when the dental auxiliary performs a delegated function (2)

direct transmission Pathogens transferred directly into the body by direct contact or droplet spread (5)

disclosing agents Coloring agents that make plaque visible when applied to teeth (20)

disinfection Process of cleaning with a chemical to destroy bacteria or render them inactive (7)

distal Farther away from the trunk of the body; opposite of proximal (3)

Doctor of Dental Surgery (DDS) Type of degree that some dental schools award to dentists upon graduation (1)

Doctor of Medical Dentistry (DMD) Type of degree that some dental schools award to dentists upon graduation (1)

dose equivalence A measure of the biological damage to living tissue as a result of radiation exposure (16)

dry heat sterilizer Type of sterilization method for instruments that uses dry heated air (8)

duration Time from induction to complete reversal of anesthesia (15)

E

edentulous Without teeth (23)

embrasure Triangular space in a gingival direction between the proximal surfaces of two adjoining teeth in contact (4)

emergency Unforeseen occurrence or a combination of circumstances that calls for immediate action or remedy; pressing necessity; exigency (10)

enamel 1. Hard tissue covering the anatomic crown of the tooth 2. Outermost layer or covering of the coronal portion of the tooth that overlies and protects the dentin (4)

enamel prisms Another term for the enamel rods that make up the enamel structure (4)

endodontics Dental specialty that diagnoses and treats diseases of the pulp (1)

endodontist Dentist who practices endodontics, which focuses on the causes, diagnosis, prevention, and treatment of diseases of the dental pulp and their sequelae (25)

endogenous An intrinsic stain acquired from within the structure of the tooth, such as in tooth development (21)

endosteal Type of dental implant to replace a missing tooth (23)

epilepsy Neurologic disorder that exhibits sudden, recurring seizures of motor, sensory, or psychic malfunctioning (10)

ergonomics The study of a person's working environment and how to fit a workplace to the user's needs (11)

esthetic dentistry Type of dentistry that improves the appearance of teeth by disguising defects and whitening teeth (22)

etching Process of preparing the tooth surface with the use of an acid product (21, 22)

ethics Moral standards of conduct; rules or principles that govern proper conduct (2)

evacuator Instrument used to remove saliva, blood, water, and debris during a dental procedure (14)

exfoliation Normal process of shedding the primary teeth (4)

exogenous Growing or originating from an agent, organism, or external sources (21)

exothermic Characterized by the release of heat from a chemical reaction (18)

expanded function Specific intraoral function delegated to an auxiliary with the required advanced skill and training (11)

expanded function dental assistant (EFDA) Assistant who has received additional training and is legally permitted to provide certain intraoral patient care procedures beyond the duties traditionally performed by a dental assistant (1)

extraction Removal of a tooth from the oral cavity by means of elevators and/or forceps (26)

extrinsic stain Stain that appears within the structure of the tooth caused by external sources (21)

extrude To push or force out (19)

F

Facebook Popular free social networking website that allows registered users to create profiles, upload photos and videos, send messages, and keep in touch with other users (29)

Federation Dentaire Internationale (FDI) System Recognized method of dental charting used to identify and designate permanent and primary and deciduous teeth within the oral cavity (4)

film duplicating Process of copying a radiographic image (17)

filter Aluminum disc placed in the x-ray unit at the position indicator device (PID) to absorb less penetrating x-ray beams (16)

filtration Use of aluminum filters to remove long (less penetrating) wavelengths from a primary x-radiation beam (16)

fixed appliance Intraoral appliance that is cemented in place or attached by a bonding material (28)

fixed bridge Dental prosthesis with artificial teeth cemented in place and supported by attachment to natural teeth (23)

flange Part of a full or partial denture that extends from the teeth to the border of the denture (23)

fluoride Mineral that naturally occurs in food and water and is used for the prevention of tooth decay (Fluoride can be delivered through systemic and topical methods.) (20, 27)

fluoride varnish Concentrated topical fluoride that is applied to the teeth to prevent tooth decay (20)

fluorosis An overexposure to fluoride during a child's early years of life (the appearance is faint white lines or streaks on the teeth) (20)

focusing cup A shallow depression on the surface of the cathode of an x-ray tube, which keeps the electrons beam towards the focal spot of the anode (16)

follow-up letter Letter used to follow up with a potential employer after an interview (29)

force To cause a physical change through energy and strength, such as push and pull (18)

forced air sterilizer Also referred to as a *rapid heat transfer sterilizer*; a type of sterilization that circulates hot air throughout the chamber at high velocity, which permits the rapid transfer of heat energy from the air to the instruments, reducing the time needed for sterilization (8)

fossae Pits, indentations, grooves, or depressions (4)

framework Metal skeleton of a removable partial denture (23)

friction-grip Type of bur that has a short and smooth shank that has no retention grooves (12)

frontal plane Vertical plane that divides the body into anterior (front) and posterior (back) portions (3)

F-speed film A conventional intraoral dental x-ray film that provides good image quality with 60% less radiation per exposure (16)

fulcrum Finger rest within the mouth that is used when holding an instrument or handpiece for a specified time (21)

fungi Group of spore-producing organisms, which include mushrooms, yeasts, and molds (5)

G

galvanic An electrochemical reaction between two dental restorations come together (18)

general supervision Level of supervision given by a licensed dentist who has examined the patient and is available for consultation, diagnosis, and evaluation (2)

genetic changes Mutations that affect future generations (17)

gingival graft Surgical procedure where gingival tissue is removed from a donor site and attached (grafted) to another site (24)

gingival retraction Displacement of gingival tissue by the use of a retraction cord for tooth preparation and impressions (23)

gingivectomy Surgical removal of diseased gingival tissue (24)

gingivitis Inflammation of gingival tissue (24)

gingivoplasty Surgical reshaping and contouring of gingival tissue (24)

glabella Smooth surface of the frontal bone and also the anatomic part directly above the root of the nose (3)

Globally Harmonized System (GHS) of Classification and Labeling of Chemicals International system of labeling and classifying chemicals that will be the same regardless of where in the global market the chemical is manufactured or used (6)

glutaraldehyde Environmental Protection Agency (EPA)–registered high-level hospital disinfectant (7)

grasp Manner in which a dental instrument is held during use (11)

gutta-percha Permanent filling material for root canal therapy (25)

H

handpiece Essential electrical instrument to hold rotary instruments used by every dental personnel for routine procedures in general and specialty procedures (12)

hazard classes Classification system used to categorize hazardous materials that have similar properties (6)

Hazard Communication Standard (HCS) Occupational Safety & Health Administration (OSHA) standard regarding employees' "right to know"

about hazardous chemicals in the workplace (6)

hazard statement Statement on a chemical label that indicates the specific hazard of a chemical (6)

hazardous waste Waste that poses a danger to humans or to the environment (6)

headgear External orthodontic appliance used to control growth and tooth movement (28)

hemisection Procedure in which a tooth with two roots is cut lengthwise and removed (25)

hepatitis A virus (HAV) Type of hepatitis that is very contagious and is spread from person to person via the oral-fecal route and blood of people who are infected (5)

hepatitis B virus (HBV) A serious viral disease transmitted by bodily fluids, which include saliva, that may result in acute and chronic illness, affecting the liver (5)

hepatitis C virus (HCV) Type of hepatitis that is largely transmitted by blood transfusion or percutaneous inoculation, such as when intravenous drug users share needles (5)

hepatitis D virus (HDV) A liver infection caused by HDV virus that occurs in people who are infected with HBV (5)

Health Insurance Portability and Accountability Act (HIPAA) Federal regulations that ensure privacy regarding a patient's health care information (9)

HIV Human immunodeficiency virus; a bloodborne viral disease that attacks and weakens or destroys the immune system (5)

holding solution Used for instruments that cannot be immediately cleaned after a dental procedure (8)

horizontal angulation Position of the x-ray tube head in a horizontal plane to produce open contacts (17)

host Living cells that may be human, animal, plant, or bacteria in which viruses live and replicate (5)

host susceptibility Ability of a host cell to resist the invasion of a virus (5)

hyperglycemia High level of blood glucose when the body does not produce or use enough insulin (10)

hyperventilation Abnormally fast or deep breathing (10)

hypoglycemia Condition when blood glucose level is too low (10)

I

impaction Tooth that has not erupted (26)

implant An artificial tooth that is surgically placed into the mandible or maxilla (23)

implied consent Patient's permission, which indicates consent for treatment (2)

impression Negative reproduction of teeth and soft tissues in the mouth (19)

indirect pulp cap Placement of dental material to prevent necrosis when decay is in close proximity to the pulp (25)

indirect supervision Level of supervision for credentialed dental auxiliary when performing delegated functions according to the instructions of the dentist, who is not necessarily physically present; also known as general supervision (2)

indirect transmission Indirect transfer of organisms to a susceptible person, which can occur by handling contaminated instruments or by touching contaminated surfaces and then touching the face, eyes, or mouth (5)

induction Time from injection to effective anesthesia (15)

infectious disease Diseases by many pathogens, which include bacteria, viruses, fungi, and parasites (5)

infectious waste Term used to identify waste to be disposed of according to applicable federal, state, and local regulations (6)

inferior Lower in position; closer to the feet (3)

informed consent Permission granted by a patient after being informed of the advantages, disadvantages, and alternatives of a procedure (2)

inlay Cast restoration designed for Class II cavity preparation (23)

innervation Distribution of an anesthetic agent to the surrounding nerves (3)

intrinsic stain Stain developed from within the structure of the tooth (21)

instrument Tool or appliance specifically designed for a technique or application in a dental procedure (12)

instrument processing Procedure to prepare contaminated instruments for sterilization and reuse on the next patient (8)

interdental aids Special devices recommended as aids for cleaning between teeth with large or open interdental spaces and under fixed bridges (20)

International Standards Organization (ISO) System Numbering system that assigns a two-digit number to each tooth (The first number is the quadrant; the second number is the tooth.) (4)

interview Formal meeting between an employer and applicant for the assessment of qualifications (29)

iodophors Environmental Protection Agency (EPA)–registered intermediate-level hospital disinfectant with tuberculocidal action (7)

ionization Process during which electrons are removed from atoms, causing the harmful effects of radiation in humans (16)

irreversible hydrocolloid Dental material of choice when taking preliminary impressions (*hydro* means water, and colloid means a *gelatinous* substance) (19)

irreversible pulpitis Condition in which the pulp is incapable of healing, requiring root canal therapy (25)

isolation Technique that isolates and protects a tooth from oral fluids and debris during a surgical or restorative procedure, usually through the application of a dental dam or the use of cotton rolls (14)

K

Kells, C. Edmund (1856–1928) New Orleans dentist credited with employing the first dental assistant (1)

L

label elements Labeling system used for chemical elements (6)

latch-type Shank of dental bur with a small groove at the end to mechanically lock into a contra-angle attachment, which fits on the low-speed handpiece (12)

latent image Invisible image on the x-ray film after exposure but before processing (17)

latent infection Persistent infection with recurrent symptoms that "come and go" (5)

latent period Interval between exposure to ionizing radiation and the appearance of symptoms (16)

lateral Relating to the side or away from the midline (3)

lateral surface of the tongue Sides of the tongue (3)

leakage radiation Escape of radiation from within the source, except for the useful beam (16)

legal Permitted by law (2)

licensure Granting of a license to practice a profession (2)

light-cured Technique to polymerize a dental material with a curing light (21)

lingual Surface of teeth closest to the tongue (3)

LinkedIn Business-oriented social networking service primarily used for professional networking (29)

luxate To dislocate, as a tooth from its socket (26)

M

malaligned Displaced out of line, such as teeth that are displaced from a normal relation to the line of the dental arch (28)

malocclusion A misalignment from maxillary and mandibular arches (deviated from a Class I normal occlusion) (28)

mandibular Lower jaw (3)

manipulate Process of adapting an instrument to a procedure (12)

manual processing Procedure to process an exposed x-ray film in processing chemicals, which causes the image to become visible on the film (17)

masticatory mucosa Oral mucosa that covers the hard palate, dorsum of the tongue, and gingiva (3)

matrix Band that provides a temporary wall for the restoration of a tooth (22)

maxillary Upper jaw (3)

maximum permissible dose (MPD) Amount of radiation a person may be exposed to without being harmed (16)

medial Toward or nearer to the midline of the body (3)

medically compromised Individual who may be ill, in pain, or physically challenged (9)

mental protuberance Part of the mandible that forms the chin (3)

midsagittal plane Imaginary line that divides the patient's face into right and left sides (3)

mists Droplets of particles larger than those generated by the aerosol spray (Mists, such as those that result from coughing, can transmit a respiratory infection.) (5)

mixed dentition Stage at which both deciduous and secondary teeth have erupted (4)

mobility Loosening of a tooth in the alveolar socket because of the destruction of periodontal fibers (24)

model trimmer Dental lab machine used to trim stone or plaster models (19)

mucogingival junction Distinct junction in the gingival tissue where the alveolar membrane meets with the attached gingivae (3)

mucous membrane Smooth tissue that lines the oral cavity and other canals and cavities of the body (3)

MyPlate Online graphic guide designed to help consumers think about building a healthy plate and to offer more information to build a healthier plate at mealtimes (20)

N

nasion Midpoint between the eyes just below the eyebrows (3)

necrotic Term used to describe a tooth that does not respond to sensory stimulus (25)

nitrous oxide–oxygen Combination of gas and oxygen used as an analgesic and sedative agent to ease a patient's anxiety (15)

noncritical instruments Items that come into contact with only intact skin (7)

nonvital Not containing a living nerve (25)

numbering systems Simplified means of identifying the teeth for charting and descriptive purposes (4)

O

object-film distance (OFD) Distance between the object being radiographed and the film or cassette (16)

obturation Process of filling a root canal (25)

occlusal image Image exposed or photographed used to examine larger area of the upper or lower jaw (13, 16)

occupational exposure A skin, eye, mucous membrane contact, or percutaneous injury with blood or any other potentially infectious materials (6)

Occupational Safety & Health Administration (OSHA) Federal agency charged with establishing guidelines and regulations regarding worker safety (6)

onlay Cast restoration designed to cover the occlusal and proximal surfaces of posterior teeth (23)

operating zones Working positions of the dental team members during a procedure; based on a "clock concept" (11)

operative dentistry Term used to describe restorative and esthetic dentistry (22)

opportunistic infection Infection caused by nonpathogenic organisms, which occurs in individuals whose resistance is decreased or compromised (5)

oral and maxillofacial radiology Dental specialty involved in the diagnosis of disease through various forms of imaging, including x-ray films (radiographs) (1)

oral and maxillofacial surgery (OMFS) Dental surgical specialty that diagnoses and treats conditions of the mouth, face, upper jaw (maxilla), and associated areas (1, 26)

oral biofilm A variety of microorganisms that adheres to all tissues and surfaces in the oral cavity, which can cause periodontal disease and dental caries (20)

oral pathology Dental specialty that diagnoses and treats diseases of the oral structures (1)

oral prophylaxis Complete removal of calculus, debris, stain, and plaque from the teeth (21)

organs Several types of tissues grouped together to perform a single function (e.g., heart, lungs, kidneys) (3)

orthodontics Specialty of dentistry designed to prevent, intercept, and correct skeletal and dental problems (1, 28)

ortho-phthalaldehyde (OPA) Chemical used in high-level disinfection (7)

osseointegration A direct connection between living bone and an endosseous implant (23)

ostectomy Surgery involving the removal of bone (24)

osteoplasty Surgical procedure involved with bone alteration, reshaping, or bone grafting (24)

P

Palate Described as the roof of the mouth, where bone and soft tissue divide the nasal cavity and oral cavity (3)

Palmer Notation System Method of charting that uses symbols, numbers, and letters to indicate a tooth in each of the four quadrants (4)

panoramic radiography A two-dimensional image that captures the entire mouth with a view of the upper and lower jaws and surrounding structures and tissues (17)

paralleling technique Intraoral technique where the periapical film is placed parallel to the long axis of a tooth (17)

parenteral transmission Act of transmitting bloodborne pathogens through needlestick injuries, human bites, cuts, abrasions, or any break in the skin (5)

pathogen Disease-producing microorganism (5)

patient of record Individual who has been examined and diagnosed by the dentist and has had treatment planned (2)

patient record Document that is managed by the dentist for each patient in a dental practice (9)

pediatric dentistry Dental specialty involved with neonatal through adolescent patients and patients with special needs in these age groups (1, 27)

percutaneous Through the skin, such as a needlestick, cut, or human bite (6)

periapical Apex and the surrounding area of a tooth (4)

periapical views Images that show the whole tooth from the crown to the root tip and its surrounding structures (17)

periodontal dressing Surgical dressing applied over a surgical site for protection, similar to a bandage (24)

periodontal flap surgery Also referred to as *flap surgery*, where tissue is pulled back from the underlying tooth roots and alveolar bone, similar to the flap of an envelope (24)

periodontal ligament System of collagenous connective tissue fibers that connect the root of a tooth to its alveolus (4)

periodontal pocket Deepening of the gingival sulcus beyond normal, resulting from periodontal disease (24)

periodontics Dental specialty involved with the diagnosis and treatment of diseases of the supporting tissue (1, 24)

periodontist Dentist with advanced education in the art and science of examination, diagnosis, and treatment of diseases affecting the periodontium (1, 24)

periodontitis Inflammatory disease of the supporting tissue of the teeth (24)

periodontium Structure that surrounds, supports, and is attached to a tooth (4, 24)

permanent dentition The 32 teeth of adulthood that replace or are added to the complement of deciduous teeth (4)

permucosal Through mucous membranes, such as in exposure to the eyes or mouth (6)

personal protective equipment (PPE) Items such as clothing, masks, gloves, and eyewear to minimize exposure to illnesses and injury (6)

pestle Object that pounds or pulverizes a material (18)

philtrum Rectangular area from under the nose to the midline of the upper lip (3)

phosphor storage plates (PSPs) Thin flexible plates the size of conventional x-ray film that have been coated with phosphor crystals (16)

photon Smallest amount of electromagnetic radiation, which has no weight or mass (16)

physiology Study of the functions of the human body (3)

pictogram Graphic elements used on a hazard label to identify the specific hazard class and category (6)

pits and fissures Small pinpoint depressions located at the junction of developmental grooves on the primary parts of the occlusal surfaces of posterior teeth and the lingual surfaces of the maxillary incisors (21)

plaque Soft deposit on teeth that consists of bacteria and bacterial byproducts (20)

plaque control Preventive methods to remove plaque, such as brushing, flossing, interdental cleaning aids, and antimicrobial solutions (20)

plaster A quick setting gypsum material used for pouring preliminary impressions to make diagnostic models (19)

point of entry Position on the patient's face where the central beam is directed (17)

polyether Elastic-type impression material that provides a good accuracy and surface detail of the dentition (19)

polymerization Chemical reaction or light activation of two or more monomers that reach a final setting (18)

polysulfide One of the first elastomeric final impression materials, also referred to as a *rubber base* (It is supplied as a two-paste system—the base and the catalyst.) (19)

pontic Artificial tooth that replaces a missing natural tooth within a bridge (23)

portal of entry Manner in which a pathogen enters a susceptible host necessary to cause an infection (5)

position indicator device (PID) The LED-lined cone that directs the x-ray beam and is round or rectangular in shape and available in two lengths (short, 8 inch, and long, 16 inch) (16)

post Prefabricated pin that accurately fits within the pulpal canal of an endodontically treated tooth to provide added strength and stability to the final restoration (23)

posterior Toward the back (3)

postural hypotension Form of low blood pressure that occurs when standing and may result in dizziness and fainting (10)

precleaning Removal of bioburden and other materials before disinfection or sterilization (7)

preventive dentistry Program of patient education, with the use of fluorides, application of dental sealants, proper nutrition, and plaque control to prevent dental disease. (18)

primary dentition Also referred to as deciduous or "baby teeth"; comprised of 20 teeth, which exfoliate as they are replaced by the permanent teeth (4)

primary radiation Primary beam emitted from the target in an x-ray tube (16)

process indicators Tapes, strips, or tabs with heat-sensitive chemicals that change color when exposed to a certain temperature (8)

process integrators Strips placed into packages that change colors when exposed to a combination of heat, temperature, and time (8)

professionalism Demonstration of specialized skills and knowledge in a manner that meets the standards of a profession (2)

prosthodontics Dental specialty that provides fixed and removable restoration and replacement of natural teeth (1, 23)

provisional coverage Temporary protective crown or bridge that is temporarily cemented to a prepared tooth for a single crown or to abutment teeth for a bridge (23)

proximal Close to the trunk of the body (3)

pulp Chamber of a tooth that is made up of the nerve, blood vessels, and connective tissue (4)

pulpectomy Procedure to remove the infected or diseased pulp from a tooth (25)

pulpotomy Procedure that involves the removal of the coronal portion of a vital pulp from a tooth (25)

R

radiation monitoring Used to protect the operator by measuring the radiation within the vicinity of a radiation source; occupational exposure to radiation (16)

radiograph Image produced on a sensitive plate or conventional dental film (1, 17)

radiolucent Image on a radiograph that appears in ranges from shades of gray to black (16)

radiopaque Image on a radiograph that appears in ranges from shades of light gray to total white or clear (16)

rapport A relationship in which people or a group of people understand each other's feelings or ideas and communicate well (29)

reciprocity System that allows a credentialed professional from one state to obtain a license in another state without retesting (2)

refractory periodontitis Progressive inflammatory destruction of the periodontal attachment in spite of adequate treatment and proper oral hygiene (24)

registered dental assistant (RDA) Dental assistant who has met the qualifications required by the state that issues the registration (1)

registered dental hygienist (RDH) Dental hygienist who has passed credentials set up by the state they are practicing in (1)

regulated waste Infectious waste that requires special handling, neutralization, and disposal (6)

remineralization Reparative process that occurs naturally and daily inside the mouth (20)

removable appliance Appliance designed so that it can be removed and replaced by the patient, such as a retainer (28)

res gestae (Latin, *things done*) Statements made by any person present at the time of an alleged negligent act that are admissible as evidence in a court of law (2)

respiration Act or process of inhaling and exhaling; breathing (9)

rests Metal projections on a removable or fixed prosthesis designed to control the seating as it is positioned in the mouth (23)

restorations Use of dental materials to restore teeth to a functional permanent unit (22)

restorative dentistry Type of dentistry that restores teeth to their original structure by removing decay and restoring defects (22)

resume Brief account of one's professional or work experience and qualifications, often submitted with an employment application (29)

retainer 1. Device used to hold attachments and abutments of a removable prosthesis in place 2. Appliance used for maintaining the positions of the teeth and jaws after orthodontic treatment (23, 28)

retention Result of adhesion, mechanical locking, or both in keeping restorative material in place (18)

retrograde restoration Root end filling, which is completed when the apical seal is not adequate (25)

reversible pulpitis Form of pulpal inflammation in which the pulp remains healthy enough to save (25)

risk management Variety of ways to identify, evaluate, reduce, or eliminate potential harm to patients, staff, and visitors within an organization (2)

Roentgen, William Conrad Bavarian physicist (1845–1923) who discovered x-ray images, or radiographs, in 1895 (1)

root amputation Dental procedure during which one root is removed from a multiroot tooth (25)

root planing Procedure that smooths the surface of a tooth by removing subgingival bacteria (plaque and calculus) (24)

rotary Part or device that rotates around an axis (12)

rubber-cup polishing Technique used to remove plaque and stains from the coronal surfaces of the teeth (21)

S

saddle 1. Part of a denture that fits the oral mucosa of the basal seat, restores the normal contours of the soft tissue of the edentulous mouth, and supports the artificial teeth 2. Portion of a denture that overlies the soft tissue, usually fabricated of resin or combinations of resins and metal (23)

safety data sheet (SDS) Standardized forms completed by the manufacturer providing occupational safety and health data for the components and use of a product (6)

sagittal plane Any anteroposterior plane of the body parallel to the median sagittal plane (3)

scaling Removal of plaque and calculus from the teeth with the use of hand and ultrasonic instruments (24)

scanning A diagnostic imaging technique the produces images on a PC (17)

scatter radiation Form of secondary radiation that occurs when an x-ray beam has been deflected from its path by interaction with matter (16)

sealer Dental material used to fill the space around silver or gutta-percha points in a pulp canal (25)

secondary radiation X-radiation that is created when the primary beam interacts with matter (16)

sedation The administering of a sedative drug to produce a state of calm or sleep (15)

semicritical instruments Items that come into contact with oral tissues but do not penetrate soft tissue or bone (7)

sensor-holding device Instrument that holds the image receptor in the patient's mouth during radiography exposure (17)

separator Elastomeric ring or steel separating spring placed interproximal to force the mesial and distal spaces of the tooth slightly apart (28)

septum 1. Tissue that divides the nasal cavity into two nasal fossae 2. Dental dam material located between the holes of the punched dam (3, 14)

sharps Pointed or cutting instruments, including needles, scalpel blades, orthodontic wires, and endodontic instruments, which can be potentially infectious (6)

sign Indication of the existence of something; an objective evidence of a disease (10)

signal word Two words that are used on the safety data sheet: "Warning" for less severe hazard categories and "Danger" for more severe hazard categories (6)

silicone A siloxane material widely used in dentistry as an impression material (19)

sodium fluoride (NaF) An organic compound used as a caries-preventing agent, in the fluoridation of drinking water, toothpaste, and as a topical fluoride (20)

sodium hypochlorite Surface disinfectant commonly known as household bleach (7)

social media Internet-based applications dedicated to community-based input, interaction, content sharing, and collaboration (29)

somatic changes Effects of radiation that can cause illness and are responsible for poor health (e.g., cancer, leukemia, cataracts) but are not passed on to offspring (16)

source-film distance Distance from the focal spot of an x-ray tube to the radiographic film; also known as *target-object distance* (16)

space maintainer Fixed or removable appliance designed to preserve the space created by the premature loss of a tooth (27)

sphygmomanometer Instrument used for measuring blood pressure in the arteries (9)

spore 1. A unit of sexual or asexual reproduction for survival. 2. Biological indicators or spore tests are used to monitor sterilization (5, 8)

stainless steel crown Preformed steel crown used for the restoration of badly decayed primary teeth (27)

Standard Precautions Standard of care designed to protect health care providers from pathogens that can be spread by blood or any other bodily fluid, excretion, or secretion (6)

stannous fluoride Type of antibacterial agent used in oral health care products such as toothpaste (It has been shown to be useful in treating dental hypersensitivity.) (20)

static air sterilizer Sterilizing method that circulates heat, similar to an oven (Heat is transferred from the static [nonmoving] air to the instruments in approximately 1–2 hours.) (8)

sterilization Process that kills all microorganisms (8)

stethoscope Instrument used for listening to sounds produced within the body; commonly used to detect a heartbeat (13)

stone Abrading instrument or tool (19)

strain Distortion or change produced as a result of stress (18)

stress Internal reaction or resistance to an externally applied force (18)

subgingival Area below the gingivae (24)

subperiosteal Situated or occurring under the periosteum and on top of the bone (23)

subsupine Lying-down position in which the patient's head is lower than the feet (below the heart); used in emergency situations (11)

sulcus Groove or depression on the surface of a tooth and surrounding the tooth (24)

superior Above another portion or closer to the head (3)

supine Lying-down position in which the patient's head, chest, and knees are at the same level (11)

supragingival Area above the gingivae (24)

surface barriers Fluid-resistant materials used to cover surfaces likely to become contaminated (7)

suture 1. An immovable junction between two bones, such as in the skull 2. Surgical stitch or seam to hold edges of a wound or incision (3, 26)

symptom A subjective evidence of a disease; something that is apparent to the patient (10)

syncope Loss of consciousness caused by insufficient blood to the brain; also referred to as *fainting* (10)

synthetic phenol An Environmental Protection Agency (EPA)–registered intermediate-level hospital disinfectant with broad-spectrum disinfecting action (7)

syringe Instrument consisting of a needle, barrel, and plunger used to inject liquid into a cavity or under the skin (15)

systemic fluoride A primary method of fluoride delivery that is ingested from water and supplements and then circulated throughout the body (20)

systolic Rhythmic contraction (first sound recorded on blood pressure reading) when blood forces against the artery wall (9)

T

tele dentistry Type of technology used to deliver virtual dental care, guidance, treatment, and education (10)

temperature Degree of heat or cold of a body or an environment (9)

thermometer Instrument for measuring temperature (9)

tipping Type of tooth movement in which the root of the tooth is facially or lingually tipped to correct the angle of the crown of the tooth (28)

tissue A distinct type of specialized cells united in the performance of a particular function (3)

tooth preparation Involves the use of rotary and hand instruments to prepare the tooth structure to receive a restorative material or fixed or removal prosthesis (22)

tooth whitening Noninvasive method of lightening the color of dark or discolored teeth; commonly known as *vital bleaching* (18)

topical fluorides Fluorides that are directly applied to teeth through toothpaste, mouth rinses, and fluoride treatments (20)

torque Twisting or turning force (12)

tort law Involvement in an act that brings harm to a person or damage to property (2)

toxic waste Waste that can have a poisonous effect (6)

trabeculae A porous lattice design of supportive and connective tissue that provides structural support to spongy bone (3)

tragus Cartilaginous projection anterior to the external opening of the ear (3)

transosteal Type of implant that is inserted through the inferior border of the mandible and into the edentulous area (23)

transverse plane Imaginary plane that divides the body into superior (upper) and inferior (lower) portions; also known as the *horizontal plane* (3)

tray Device made from plastic or metal that can hold or carry impression material to the oral cavity (19)

treatment plan In dentistry, a schedule of procedures and appointments designed to restore, step by step, the oral health of a patient (13)

trifurcation Area of the tooth in which three roots divide (4)

trigeminal nerve Fifth cranial nerve that provides motor innervation to the muscles of mastication and sensory innervation to the face, jaws, and teeth (3)

trituration Process of mechanically mixing a material, such as by using an amalgamator to mix an alloy and mercury to create a dental amalgam (18)

tubehead Tightly sealed, heavy metal housing that contains the x-ray tube that produces dental x-rays (16)

tuberculosis Infectious disease caused by *Mycobacterium tuberculosis* and characterized by the formation of tubercles in the tissue (5)

Twitter Online social networking service that enables users to send and read short messages called "tweets" (29)

U

ultrasonic cleaner Device used in the sterilization center that loosens and removes debris by sound waves traveling through a liquid (8)

ultrasonic scaler Handheld device used for rapid calculus removal that operates on high-frequency sound waves (24)

unit Each component of the fixed bridge (23)

Universal National System Numbering system (1–32 for the permanent teeth and 1–20 for the primary teeth) that begins with the maxillary right and concludes at the mandibular right (4)

Universal Precautions Based on the concept that all human blood and certain bodily fluids (including saliva) are to be treated as if known to be infected with the bloodborne diseases (6)

V

vasoconstrictor Type of drug that constricts (narrows) blood vessels and is used to prolong anesthetic action (15)

veneer Thin layer of composite resin or porcelain bonded or cemented to a prepared facial surface (22)

vertical angulation Angle measured within the vertical plane at which the central ray of the x-ray beam is projected, relative to a reference in the horizontal or occlusal plane (17)

vertical bite-wing radiograph Bite-wing film or receptor placed in the mouth with the long portion of the film or receptor in a vertical direction (24)

virulence Strength of a pathogen's ability to cause disease; also known as *pathogenicity* (5)

viruses A submicroscopic infectious agents that replicates only inside the living cells of an organism (Most viruses have either RNA or DNA in the genetic material.) (5)

viscosity Physical property of fluids for resistance to flow (19)

vital bleaching Procedure in which a chemical oxidizing agent (sometimes in combination with light) is used to lighten tooth discolorations (22)

vital signs Clinical measurements used to evaluate a person's general physical condition (9)

W

wedge Wooden or plastic triangular device placed in the embrasure to provide the contour needed when restoring a Class II lesion (22)

white spot Earliest sign of demineralization (20)

Z

zygomatic arch Arch formed by articulation of the temporal process of the zygomatic bone with the zygomatic process of the temporal bone (3)

Page numbers followed by "*f*" indicate figures, "*t*" indicate tables, and "*b*" indicate boxes.

Orthodontics (Continued)
   diagnostic records, 461
     interview information, 460
   retention after, 471
   scaler, 465t–467t
   separators used in, 468, 472b
   serial extraction for, 463
   treatment, 462
     comprehensive orthodontic treatment, 463
     interceptive orthodontic treatment, 463
     limited orthodontic treatment, 462
     preventive orthodontic treatment, 462
Ortho-phthalaldehyde, 89
Orthostatic hypotension, 134
OSHA. see Occupational Safety & Health Administration (OSHA)
Osseointegrated implants, 389
Osseointegration, definition of, 389
Osseous surgery, 410
Ostectomy, 410–411
Osteoplasty, 410
Osteoporosis, as periodontal risk factor, 403t
Outer guide slots, 363b
Outer knob, 363b
Ovaries, 21, 22f, 23
Over-the-counter, 366
Ownership, of dental records and radiographs, 256
Oxygen, 132

P
Packaging, for sterilization, 100
Pain control, 213, 425. see also Anesthesia
   analgesic agents for, 221
   documentation of, 222
   local anesthesia for, 214
   methods for, 218
   topical anesthesia for, 213, 214f
Pain medication, allergies to, 116f
Palatal anesthesia, 215, 215f
Palatal expansion appliance, 452f
Palatal innervation, 31f
Palatal surfaces, 44
Palate, soft, 28
Palmer Notation System, 45, 49b
Palpation, 181t–182t
Palpation test, 419t
Pancreas, 21
Panoramic imaging, 256, 258f
Panoramic radiographs
   advantages and disadvantages of, 259t
   equipment for, 256, 259t
     preparing, 283b
   guidelines for exposing, 259
   patient for, 284b
   positioning, 285b
Panoramic radiography, 256
Panoramic unit, 259f
Pantothenic acid, 334t–335t
Paper points, for endodontics, 421t–423t
Papillae, 32
Parachlorophenol (PCP), 424
Paralleling technique, for radiography, 246, 246f, 266b–274b
Paranasal sinuses, 24, 28f
   types of, 24b
Parathyroid gland, 35f
Parenteral transmission, of disease, 55

Paste system, impression materials and, 312, 312f
Pathogens, 51, 55f
Pathologic migration, in periodontal disease, 404b–405b
Patient protection, 236
Patient records. see Records, patient
Patients
   admitting and seating, 155b–156b
   assessment and monitoring of, in nitrous oxide analgesia, 219
   autonomy, 13
   dental. see also Examination, dental
     challenging, 448
     clinical examination of, 120f
     dental history of, 116f
     medical history of, 116f
     record of, 113b, 432
     registration of, 113b
     responsibilities to, 113b
     with special needs, 449
   dental decay in, high risk for, 333b
   education, in preventive dental care, 338
   health status of, 215
   and informed consent, 16
   positioning in coronal polishing technique, 349
   precautions for, in sealants, 353
   questions commonly asked by, in sealants, 351b
   record, 13
Pediatric dental office, 447, 448f
Pediatric dentistry, 4, 447
   appraisal and behavioral assessment in, 449
   clinical procedures provided for, 447b
   defined, 447
   dental office in, 447, 448f
     behavioral management techniques, 447, 448f
     challenging patient, 448
     guidelines for child behavior, 447
     patients with special needs, 449
   examination of pediatric patient, 449
     general appraisal and behavioral assessment, 449
     intraoral examination, 449
     medical and dental histories, 449
     radiographic examination, 449
   intraoral examination in, 449
   medical and dental histories of, 449
   orthodontics in, 451
   patient in, 448f
   and prevention, 451
   procedures for, 451
     oral hygiene, 451
     preventive and interceptive orthodontics, 451
     preventive dentistry, 451
     pulp therapy, 453
     restorative procedures, 452
     sports safety, 452
     stainless steel crowns, 453, 453f
     traumatic injury, 453
   radiographic examination in, 449, 451b
   restorative procedures for, 452
   special needs patients in, 449
   and sports safety, 452
   traumatic injury in, 453, 453f

Pediatric patients, 237
   examination of, 449
Pediatric procedures, 451
Pellicle formation, 327b
Percussion test, 419t
Percutaneous, defined, 57
Percutaneous exposure, 64
Perforated tray, 309t
Periapical, 41
Periapical abscess, charting symbols for, 186t–191t
Periapical image, 419
Periapical radiographs, 245t
Periapical view, 249
Periodontal abscess, 419
Periodontal chart, 404f
Periodontal diseases, 327–328, 401
   antimicrobial and antibiotic agents, 410
   examination for, 403
     gingivae and supporting structures in, 405, 405f
     radiographs of, 403, 405f
     teeth, 404
   instruments for
     curettes, 406, 407f–408f
     explorers, 406, 406f
     probes, 406, 406f
     scalers, 406, 407f
   postperiodontal surgery, 412
   risk factors for, 403t
   scaling, root planing, and gingival curettage for, 409, 409f
   signs and symptoms of, 402
   stages of, 402b–403b
   surgery, 410
   surgical instruments for
     knives, 409
     pocket markers, 409
   treatment procedures for, 409
     antimicrobials for, 410
     prophylaxis for, 409
   ultrasonic scaler, 407, 408b–409b, 408f
   voice-activated recording systems for, 406
Periodontal dressing, 412, 416b
   types of, 412
Periodontal exam, 406
Periodontal flap procedure, 411f
Periodontal flap surgery, 410
Periodontal knives, 409, 409f
Periodontal ligament injection, 216, 216f
Periodontal pockets, in periodontal disease, 404b–405b, 405f, 405, 406f
Periodontal probes, 161t–162t, 406, 406f
Periodontal tissue, examination of, 183
Periodontics, 4, 401
Periodontist, 401
Periodontitis, 328, 402
Periodontium, 401, 402f, 402t
Periodontium, of tooth, 43f
Periosteal elevator, 433t–434t
Periosteum, 24
Peripheral nervous system, 21
Periradicular abscess, 419f, 419
Periradicular cyst, 419
Permanent dentition, 38–39
   facial and buccal view of, 39f
   in quadrants, 40, 40f
   in sextants, 41, 41f
   teeth, types of, 42f